Studies in Systems, Decision and Control

Volume 358

The series "Studies in Systems, Decision and Control" (SSDC) covers both new developments and advances, as well as the state of the art, in the various areas of broadly perceived systems, decision making and control–quickly, up to date and with a high quality. The intent is to cover the theory, applications, and perspectives on the state of the art and future developments relevant to systems, decision making, control, complex processes and related areas, as embedded in the fields of engineering, computer science, physics, economics, social and life sciences, as well as the paradigms and methodologies behind them. The series contains monographs, textbooks, lecture notes and edited volumes in systems, decision making and control spanning the areas of Cyber-Physical Systems, Autonomous Systems, Sensor Networks, Control Systems, Energy Systems, Automotive Systems, Biological Systems, Vehicular Networking and Connected Vehicles, Aerospace Systems, Automation, Manufacturing, Smart Grids, Nonlinear Systems, Power Systems, Robotics, Social Systems, Economic Systems and other. Of particular value to both the contributors and the readership are the short publication timeframe and the world-wide distribution and exposure which enable both a wide and rapid dissemination of research output.

Indexed by SCOPUS, DBLP, WTI Frankfurt eG, zbMATH, SCImago.

All books published in the series are submitted for consideration in Web of Science.

More information about this series at http://www.springer.com/series/13304

Diego Oliva · Said Ali Hassan · Ali Mohamed
Editors

Artificial Intelligence for COVID-19

Springer

Editors
Diego Oliva
Department of Computer Sciences
University of Guadalajara
Guadalajara, Jalisco, Mexico

Said Ali Hassan
Operations Research and Decision Support
Department, Faculty of Computers
and Artificial Intelligence
Cairo University
Giza, Egypt

Ali Mohamed
Operations Research Department, Faculty
of Graduate Studies for Statistical Research
Cairo University
Giza, Egypt

ISSN 2198-4182 ISSN 2198-4190 (electronic)
Studies in Systems, Decision and Control
ISBN 978-3-030-69743-3 ISBN 978-3-030-69744-0 (eBook)
https://doi.org/10.1007/978-3-030-69744-0

This Springer imprint is published by the registered company Springer Nature Switzerland AG
The registered company address is: Gewerbestrasse 11, 6330 Cham, Switzerland

Preface

Artificial Intelligence (AI) is an area of science that emphasizes intelligent machines that work and behave like humans. Machines can often act and react like humans only if they have much information relating to the world. AI has become an essential part of technology and represents incredibly exciting and powerful techniques. It is used to solve many real-world problems of growing interdisciplinary interest and practical importance.

This book contains several different types of articles that provide access to the state of AI art. It covers all major areas of the concepts, methods, tools and leading AI results in the domain of recent developments. The information contained in the book explores different areas of AI; machine and deep learning; advanced image processing; computational intelligence; IoT; robotics and automation; optimization; mathematical modelling; neural networks; information technology; big data, data processing; data mining and likewise. We intend to cover the breadth and depth of AI, presenting general overviews of the scientific issues and detailed discussions of techniques and essential system material in AI for real-world applications. The book's overarching purpose is to provide a collected and connected set of reflections about AI and its influences as the field advance. The participants represent diverse specialties, geographic regions and career stages. The included chapters develop theory, algorithms, programs, policies and systems design to ensure that these systems can inspire innovations and provide intelligent advice to government agencies and non-government organizations to combat against COVID-19. The book is a long-term investigation of AI's field and its influences on defending against the COVID-19 pandemic and broadly benefit individuals and society.

The book features a wealth of real applications, case studies and illustrations for COVID-19 emerging pandemic along with the theoretical concepts, algorithms and procedures. With this diversity and interdisciplinary subject matter, we are trying to build bridges that scientists can cross in other fields. These applications cover a wide variety of different specialties that include many diverse directions in the field of combating against COVID-19 like: relation between numbers of handwashing facilities and COVID-19 deaths; big data analysis for COVID-19; data interpretation of COVID-19 cases using R programming; AI applications to COVID-19; ANN and fuzzy classifier to diagnose COVID-19; QoL barometer for well-being during pandemics; deep and machine learning models for COVID-19; using X-ray images; information and communication technology application in COVID-19 pandemic; robotics and automation for COVID era; COVID-19 machine learning forecasting models; optimization of the international trade activities in COVID-19 period; IoT applications for COVID-19; scheduling disinfection process for COVID-19; forecasting of COVID-19 using SIR; modified SEIR; logistic growth and Holt's models; text mining for COVID-19 analysis; mathematical modelling the spread of COVID-19; information technology in health emergency control; big data in COVID-19 assistance; proactive detection of people infected by COVID-19; online learning problems during COVID-19 period; modelling of population density effect on the infectiousness and mortality rates of COVID-19; AI; chat-bots; solitude; people and a therapeutical blending; prevention guidelines based on cognitively inspired AI and data mining for COVID-19; AI for diagnosis and treatments for COVID-19; factors affecting medical mask purchase decision and Harris hawks optimization for classification of COVID-19 gene.

The book is useful as a valuable reference for AI theoretical and practical professionals because of its comprehensive coverage and a large number of detailed algorithms. It is intended primarily for researchers, decision-makers and practitioners in AI and many application disciplines. It will also be of interest to graduate level for rich case studies and projects.

The editors hope that this book will help the readers share their fascination with Artificial Intelligence and applications. They expect that the proactive guidance stemming from the chapters will have broad global relevance and are making plans for future contributions to expand the scope of the studies.

Finally, we wish to acknowledge the book authors who have made distinguished and fruitful efforts to complete the various chapters of the book. The book contents will enrich the world library in the vital field of Artificial Intelligence with all its multiple specializations and applications.

Guadalajara, Mexico — Diego Oliva
Giza, Egypt — Said Ali Hassan
Giza, Egypt — Ali Wagdy Mohamed
2021

Contents

Simulation of the Relation Between the Number of COVID-19 Death Cases as a Result of the Number of Handwashing Facilities by Using Artificial Intelligence

Sajedeh Norozpour

Abstract Artificial intelligence has recently been one of the most commonly discussed topics of discussion in the world. The need for efficient and reliable energy has been a growing fact in many sectors of the sciences. More importantly, the need for predictive analysis has become essential for most of the forecasting variables. On the other hand, there has been a notable relationship and overlaps between artificial intelligence and simulation due to the decrease in the use of hardware, while the sophistication of the software application increases. Algorithms used in simulation also allow expert systems to think in the direction and line of complex models and systems, which may always change dynamically or that may have an inclusion of the stochastic processes. The following paper begins with an introduction of artificial intelligence and its relationship to modeling and simulation. The study has involved a critical review of different pieces of literature on the value of artificial intelligence in modeling and simulation and also finds out the model of the relationship between the COVID-19 death rate and the number of handwashing materials.

Keywords Artificial intelligence · Simulation and modeling · COVID-19 · Death rate · Handwashing materials

1 Literature Review

The general meaning of AI is the ability of a computing machine to perform activities that would otherwise require human reasoning and decision-making, such as speech recognition, visual distinction, and performing decision-making processes and analytics [1]. However, this definition is inherently misrepresented as to what is logical, and the discussion has always been open to debate. By that definition, an internal controller of the house, such as a thermostat, can be considered intelligent because it can sense and change the temperature [2]. It is not the same as artificial intelligence, with which a drone selects and designs approaches without

S. Norozpour (✉)
Department of Civil Engineering, Istanbul Gelisim University, Istanbul, Turkey
e-mail: snorozpour@gelisim.edu.tr

D. Oliva et al. (eds.), *Artificial Intelligence for COVID-19*, Studies in Systems, Decision and Control 358, https://doi.org/10.1007/978-3-030-69744-0_1

significant intervention from humans, which is usually perceived when it comes to autonomous ordnances system. Additionally, another key factor to consider when talking about autonomous ordinances is the growing inability to liberate independence from the commercial autonomy of military drones. With the growth of the business sector to develop autonomous land and air systems, there is no doubt that there is evidence of a shift in the military's AI capability to the business. Therefore, restricting autonomous innovation for military purposes may not be realistic, as it can also be commercially available in the lower end of the market for consumers. Also, the divergent improvement in the market of the autonomous corporate structure would result in governments and armies that would no longer dominate, resulting in unsafe and dangerous AI systems, both semi-autonomous and autonomous.

One concept that has usually been interlinked with AI is drone swarming, a form of modeling and simulation. The technology behind drone swarming allows drones to make decisions autonomously based on shared decisions from other drones [3]. This has proven to be promising as it can revolutionize drone applications in military warfare. Countries such as China have succeeded in developing drone swarm technology. On the other hand, the US has been testing a ' Low-Cost Unmanned aerial vehicle Swarming Technology (LOCUST), a drone swarming program that employs AI on several drones to help in data gathering in the battlefield [3]. Swarms can revolutionize e military as they are applicable in every area of national and homeland security. For example, the marine forces can use swarms of drones to search the ocean for enemy submarines. Drones can also be deployed in large areas to help identify enemy hideouts and help eliminate their air defense systems. Furthermore, drone swarms can act as a shield by helping intercept incoming hypersonic missiles. Furthermore, the drones can be equipped with chemical, biological, radiological, and nuclear (CBRN) sensors, which can help identify and devise solutions to such threats.

The fate of artificial intelligence in combat scenarios is primarily linked to specialists' capacity to develop systems that have an autonomous capability of using knowledge and logical reasoning based on the data being fed [4]. Currently, there are no such systems in operation. Most drones on-site are controlled remotely, which means that a human continues to legitimately control a drone after a certain distance, for example, via an additional virtual link such as a satellite feed. Most unscrewed military aircraft develop just a little, and gradually they gain semi-autonomy, which means that they can navigate and land by themselves without any human input [5]. However, almost all of them require some degree of human input to complete their combat operations. Even drones that take off and fly to a specific target to take pictures and then go back to base still operate on an automated system but cannot be compared to some of the operations of an autonomous let alone a semi-autonomous drone.

Although the current systems are more programmed to be automatic rather than autonomous, more research continues to be carried out within the scope of autonomy. In many countries, airplanes, land, water, and underwater vehicles have gradually improved their military capabilities, with varying results [5]. In the United States, certain types of independent helicopters are under development. A sales representative can operate the aircraft with a cell phone and are currently under development by countries such as the USA, Europe, and China. Autonomous drones are under rapid research and development across the world. However, the offices that make these systems still find it difficult to make a qualitative leap in operational execution [6]. There are many reasons for the failure to develop these innovations, including unexpected costs and unforeseen technical problems. However, authoritarian and social boundaries are also barriers to the implementation of autonomous UAS. The United States, for example, has struggled to launch autonomous drones into operation mainly because of the hierarchical struggle and the prioritization of crewed aircraft [7].

For some soldiers, the drone systems are only suitable for rescue operations, but they put the rule at risk as long as they are qualified to perform the most recognized and advanced tasks. However, other hierarchical problems restrict the operational use of autonomous aircraft, and an increasingly dangerous problem is the commercialization of AI drone technology for businesses. However, cargo delivery services like UPS, FedEx, and DHL are looking into military drone technology in the delivery of cargo [8]. An allegorical arms competition takes place in the company's group to improve autonomous systems. The improvement in autonomous military systems was, at best, moderate and constant and did not reflect the progress made in independent commercial contexts, such as driverless vehicles and, in particular, drones.

Several roboticists and military experts have argued that autonomous drones should not be regarded as a threat on ethical grounds but should be a more preferred option than human fighters. According to roboticist Ronald C. Arkin, future autonomous drones will have the ability to make a better judgment on the battlefield based on the fact that they do not need to be fed with a self-preservation program, which is more common in humans. In this case, the drones will have the ability to make ethical decisions avoiding the need to "shoot first and ask questions later" scenarios [9]. Furthermore, autonomous drones will not be plagued by human emotions, such as fear in a combat scenario. The systems will be able to handle a lot of information being fed compared to humans and thus improve some of the battlefield outcomes.

There are many positive aspects of expanding AI's combat work. Focusing on AI skills increases AI's ability to verify authentic or wrong approaches decisively [5]. Intelligent drones can be designed to reduce the number of acts of war against individuals, e.g., For example, the massacre of civilians or prisoners of war, the destruction of civilian property by non-military personnel, the torture of prisoners, and devastation while limiting collateral damage due to instances of helplessness and confrontation [4]. Artificial intelligence will be more competent than humans and modern combat strategies and methods. Errors are also greatly reduced in the war zone. It is currently possible to accurately calculate and see the degree of destruction of an attack, which will now result in minor injuries due to an unpredictable attack [10]. The additional violation of human rights in the types of aggression, agony, etc. is eliminated with the method at the right time because AI is the predominant method or strategy of combat.

Drone swarms offer customization and flexibility to military commanders allowing them to add or remove drones in the formation when necessary. However, this requires a new form of inter-drone communication protocol that allows for drones to be easily added or removed from a swarm. As such, the drones should easily accommodate drones added or removed from the swarm either from the command or from hostile action [11]. The adaptability of intelligent drone swarms means that the drones can easily adapt to the needs of the situation and alleviate the commanders from small tasks such as managing the drones. The customization of drone swarms means that the size of the swarm can be adjusted depending on the mission.

Furthermore, military commanders can easily customize the drones with sensors, weapons, or other payloads depending on the needs of the mission. Drone swarms can also easily break into small groups or merge as a unit, which can easily change battlefield dynamics [11]. For example, a drone swarm can break into small groups to conduct reconnaissance in a particular area. If they spot an adversary, they can easily merge to eliminate the target.

2 Aim of the Research

Global concerns about the value of artificial intelligence have been raised about modeling and simulation. When simulation and modeling have been used, one of the critical areas is military and security areas. Moreover, previous studies have also added the value of National Language Processing (NLP) as a form of simulation. Modeling has been applied in artificial intelligence to provide a link between human language and computer language. Currently, there has been an increase in the use of Unmanned Aircraft Systems (UASs) in military and commercial environments has led to a heated discussion on the ban on "killer robots" [12]. These autonomous machines, which can operate on the ground or in the air, hypothetically when combined with "artificial intelligence" (AI), can autonomously execute missions. These give rise to the underlying idea of the use of artificial intelligence in simulation and modeling. The debate, which involves many stakeholders and scopes, raises a serious topic of whether AI systems should be allowed to carry out these combat operations, especially when there is a likelihood that there will be human casualties. Considering the complex issue at hand, the functional importance of AI is necessary. However, how artificial intelligence relates to simulation must be discussed deeply.

The value of artificial intelligence ranges from a variety of departments: from security departments to defense departments. The research aims at knowing the importance of artificial intelligence in simulation and modeling. Besides, this article aims to include how artificial intelligence is used in simulation and other modeling programs such as drone swan. The paper also aims at identifying the benefits and applications of artificial intelligence in other governmental and economic departments. For instance, artificial intelligence may be used to model future armed conflicts and mitigations against such conflicts among nations.

2.1 Statement of the Problem

Many studies have been conducted on the future of Information and Technology and programming in the world. This has come up with many issues concerning the future growth of artificial intelligence. Currently, most of the economic sectors in many countries are being run by programs based on artificial intelligence. Moreover, many studies have also been carried out on the importance and negative effects of artificial intelligence. As the world grapples with COVID-19, every ounce of technological innovation and ingenuity harnessed to fight this pandemic brings us one step closer to overcoming it. Artificial intelligence (AI) and machine learning are playing a key role in better understanding and addressing the COVID-19 crisis. Machine learning technology enables computers to mimic human intelligence and ingest large volumes of data to quickly identify patterns and insights.

In the fight against COVID-19, organizations have been quick to apply their machine learning expertise in several areas: scaling customer communications, understanding how COVID-19 spreads, and speeding up research and treatment.

However, this study decided to explore the link between artificial intelligence and modeling and simulation. Previously, little studies had been conducted in that area, and this study finds it as an opportunity to explore such an area. The case example used for this study is the model illustration of the COVID-19 deaths due to the number of handwashing facilities.

2.2 Research Methodology

This part of the study includes a series of methodological approaches for the study. The study on artificial intelligence and its importance on simulation and modeling follows a secondary study model. The study relies on secondary sources of data and follows a qualitative model of analysis. The main source of data for this study is the previous scholarly articles on artificial intelligence. Besides, the study also follows a quantitative approach of study to model and simulate the relationship between the numbers of COVID-19 death cases as a result of the number of handwashing facilities.

2.3 Research Setting and Research Paradigm

The availability of scientific data has allowed many researchers to do further studies on the relationship that might exists between artificial intelligence and simulation and modeling. Both the quantitative and qualitative research paradigm has been implemented for the data collection.

2.4 Limitations of the Method

The method used for this study was based on a qualitative approach to study using secondary sources of data. The fundamental impediment to the use and reliance of secondary data is that the accuracy of the secondary data used may not be fully known because of no accuracy with the information provided. Besides, some of the secondary sources of data might be too old for use in data analysis, and at the same time, the secondary sources may fail to fit the research model and framework. This is because the area of artificial intelligence is dynamic. Besides, the study has also used a quantitative research approach.

3 Results and Discussion

In this study, we wish to know how artificial intelligence may be applied to determine the future number of COVID-19 death cases due to the number of handwashing facilities. In this way, the study wishes to apply simulation and modeling in finding the relationship. The dataset used for the study has been sourced from Coronavirus Pandemic (COVID-19) data. For the model, the dependent variable is the number of COVID-19 deaths, while the independent variable is the number of handwashing facilities. The sample data used is represented in Table 1. (Data retrieved from https://ourworldindata.org/coronavirus-data)

Using the data in Table 1, the study developed a model, which would also be essential for simulation purposes. The model is summarized as follows;

Table 1 Sample coronavirus pandemic (COVID-19) Data

Death rate	Handwashing facilities	Death rate	Handwashing facilities
597.029	37.746	344.094	47.964
278.364	83.741	137.973	83.841
276.045	26.664	303.74	19.351
341.01	94.043	190.968	85.198
559.812	83.241	318.949	4.472
298.003	34.808	266.653	55.182
170.05	88.469	140.448	80.635
176.957	90.083	525.432	89.827
235.848	11.035	167.295	90.65
217.066	79.807	202.812	24.64
204.299	25.383	182.634	7.96
329.635	97.164	331.43	7.876
269.048	11.877	298.245	41.047
293.068	6.144	155.898	76.665
270.892	66.229	336.717	17.45
244.661	2.735	382.474	6.403
435.727	16.603	373.159	77.159
280.995	5.818	430.548	22.863
124.24	65.386	240.208	84.169
261.516	15.574		

Summary output								
Regression statistics								
Multiple R	0.138792							
R Square	0.019263							
Adjusted R Square	−0.00724							
Standard error	112.2751							
Observations	39							
ANOVA								
	df	SS	MS	F	Significance F			
Regression	1	9161.054	9161.054	0.726739	0.399427			
Residual	37	466411	12605.7					
Total	38	475572.1						
	Coefficients	Standard Error	t Stat	P-value	Lower 95%	Upper 95%	Lower 95.0%	Upper 95.0%
Intercept	308.9056	31.33775	9.857299	6.78E-12	245.4093	372.4019	245.4093	372.4019
X Variable 1	-0.45735	0.536492	−0.85249	0.399427	−1.54439	0.629682	−1.54439	0.629682

The model can, therefore, be represented as:
$Y = 308.9056 - 0.45735X$

which implies that, the rate of COVID-19 fatalities = 308.9056 – 0.45735 (number of handwashing facilities).

The results show that there is a negative relationship between the two variables. I.e., the rate of COVID-19 fatalities will increase with a decrease in the number of handwashing facilities. Given the regression model above, then we can simulate it. The simulation results will show the minimum value of the dependent variable, the first quartile, the median value, mean, third quartile, and the maximum value of the dependent variable. Given the independent variable data, we have the following:

Mean = 47.84

Standard deviation = 33.95

Suppose we simulate from the model;

$Y = 308.9056 - 0.45735X + \varepsilon$; assume ε is approximately normally distributed with mean 0 and $X \sim N(47.84;33.95)$, $\beta_0 = 308.9056$ and $\beta_1 = -0.45735$.

We have the following R output:

```
> set.seed (39)
> x < −rnorm (39, 47.84, 33.95)
> e < −rnorm (39, 0, 2)
> y < −308.9056-0.45735*x + e
> Summary(y)
```

The summary would output the minimum value of the dependent variable, the first quartile, the median value, mean, third quartile, and maximum value. As such, it would be easy to model the rate of fatalities of COVID-19 due to the number of handwashing facilities using artificial intelligence techniques.

4 Conclusion

The idea of artificial intelligence is a critical technological tool in current society. The study has explored the relationship between artificial intelligence and modeling and simulation by exploring the COVID-19 data. Through the study, it is evident that artificial intelligence can be used to model and simulate the relationship between two or more variables. The study has employed both qualitative and quantitative approaches to find the results. More specifically, the study has used a quantitative approach to find out the relationship between the COVID-19 death rate and the number of handwashing materials in different countries. The relationship between the two variables has been represented in a model. Therefore, the data model is essential in simulating the future expectations of the dependent variable (COVID-19 death rates). Therefore, it is true that artificial intelligence has a great interdependence with simulation and modeling of future outcomes and data.

References

1. Stuart, R., Peter, N.: Artificial Intelligence—A Modern Approach 3rd edn. (2016)
2. Rodriguez, C., Robinson, R.: Enhancing Dengue Fever Modeling Through a Multi-scale Analysis Framework–A Case Study in the Central Valley of Costa Rica (2013)
3. Allison, J., Amako, K., Apostolakis, J., Arce, P., Asai, M., Aso, T., Bagli, E., et al.: Recent developments in Geant4. Nuclear Instruments and Methods in Physics Research Section A: Accelerators, Spectrometers, Detectors and Associated Equipment, vol. 835, pp. 186–225 (2016)
4. Kibble, R.: Can an unmanned drone be a moral agent? Ethics and accountability in military robotics. In: Gunkel, D.J., Bryson, J.J., Torrance, S. (eds.), The machine question: AI, ethics and moral responsibility (Proceedings of symposium "Machine Question: AI, Ethics, and Moral Responsibility"AISB/IACAP 2012), pp. 62–67 (2012)
5. Allen, G., Chan, T.: Artificial Intelligence and National Security. Belfer Center for Science and International Affairs, Cambridge, MA (2017)
6. Harwood, R.: The Challenges To Developing Fully Autonomous Drone Technology. Ansys, Com (2019)
7. Spinetta, L., Cummings, M.L.: Unloved Aerial Vehicles: Gutting its UAV Plan, the Air Force Sets a Course for Irrelevance (2012)
8. James, W.: Holding Aloft the Banner of Ethiopia: Caribbean Radicalism in Early-Twentieth Century America. Verso Books (2020)
9. Arkin, Ronald C.: The case for ethical autonomy in unmanned systems. J. Military Ethics **9**(4), 332–341 (2010)
10. Cass, Kelly: Autonomous weapons and accountability: seeking solutions in the law of war. Loy. LAL Rev. **48**, 1017 (2014)
11. Kallenborn, Z.: The Era Of The Drone Swarm Is Coming, And We Need To Be Ready For It - Modern War Institute." Modern War Institute, 2020. https://mwi.usma.edu/era-drone-swarm-coming-need-ready/
12. Human Rights Watch: Arms: New Campaign To Stop Killer Robots. Human Rights Watch. https://www.hrw.org/news/2013/04/23/arms-new-campaign-stop-killer-robots (2013)
13. Ackerman, S.: Pentagon: A Human Will Always Decide When A Robot Kills You. WIRED (2020)
14. Lin, L., Hou, Z.: Combat COVID-19 with artificial intelligence and big data. J Travel Med 27(5) (2020):taaa080
15. Kumar, A., Gupta, P.K., Srivastava, A.: A review of modern technologies for tackling COVID-19 pandemic. Diabetes & Metabolic Syndrome: Clinical Research & Reviews (2020)

Big Data and Data Analytics for an Enhanced COVID-19 Epidemic Management

Joseph Bamidele Awotunde, Rasheed Gbenga Jimoh, Idowu Dauda Oladipo, Muyideen Abdulraheem, Taibat Bolanle Jimoh, and Gbemisola Janet Ajamu

Abstract The transmission features of the COVID-19 epidemic have still not been properly recognized in the sense of global environmental changes. Likewise, the pace of global development, increased population size, nuanced encounters, and lack of medical security in developing countries all contribute to the complexities of COVID-19 prevention and regulation. The COVID-19 seems to have a greater impact on the global economy when compared to severe acute respiratory syndrome (SARS) that occurs in 2013. The bone of contention is how to fight the spread of these infectious diseases and how to contains it spread from human-to-human. Most countries depended on the observation of classic steps to monitor diseases and public health to contain the COVID-19 pandemic, similar to those used with SARS in 2003. Data in the healthcare sector are usually huge and not easy to handle, this results from the enormous way by which data grows in the healthcare sector, the rate at which data are been produced, and the variety of various data in the healthcare system contributed to this growth. Also, the rate at which these data are been captured, stored, analyzed, and retrieved in healthcare has swiftly from the aged paper-based storage technique to the use of digital techniques and methods. Hence, the application of advanced

J. B. Awotunde (✉) · M. Abdulraheem
Department of Computer Science, University of Ilorin, Ilorin, Nigeria
e-mail: awotunde.jb@unilorin.edu.ng

M. Abdulraheem
e-mail: muyideen@unilorin.edu.ng

R. G. Jimoh · I. D. Oladipo · T. B. Jimoh
National Examinations Council, Zonal Office, Ilorin, Nigeria
e-mail: jimoh_rasheed@unilorin.edu.ng

I. D. Oladipo
e-mail: odidowu@unilorin.edu.ng

T. B. Jimoh
e-mail: bolanlejimoh80@gmail.com

G. J. Ajamu
Department of Agricultural Extension and Rural Development, Landmark University, Omu Aran, Nigeria
e-mail: ajamu.gbemisola@lmu.edu.ng

D. Oliva et al. (eds.), *Artificial Intelligence for COVID-19*, Studies in Systems, Decision and Control 358, https://doi.org/10.1007/978-3-030-69744-0_2

technologies which includes virtualization and cloud computing allows for huge and effective data processing in the healthcare system. Thereby rapidly turning the healthcare system into a big data industry. Nevertheless, in these modern days, the improvement in the information and communication technologies (ICT) brings the advancement of varied data from new sources in the healthcare system. Therefore, this chapter discusses the possible application of big data and analytics to improve conventional public health approaches to tackle the COVID-19 pandemic to control, manage, identify and avoid COVID-19 and reduce the effect on health implicitly associated with COVID-19. The significant applications of big data and challenges are presented. Leveraging big data and intelligent analytics becomes expedient in other to enjoy their use for COVID-19 disease outbreak and public health.

Keywords Big data · Coronavirus · Big data analytics · COVID-19 pandemic · Healthcare · Diagnosis

1 Introduction

The scientific research centered on generating new data through the performing of basic experiments to answer specific questions related to any infectious diseases. The collection and storing of a huge amount of data digitally are growing exponentially. This may require patients to receive care at various hospitals within a region, thus underrepresent or over-represent key clinical feature studies single-site. The coronavirus disease 2019 (COVID-19) epidemic poses a growing threat to the world. We are more connected than ever before, our cities are increasingly densely populated and in recent years the world has witnessed successive waves of the new severe acute respiratory syndrome (SARS), Ebola virus, Zika virus and recently COVID-19 and influenza infectious diseases threats global pandemics.

The coronavirus (COVID-19) pandemic is playing thoughtful havoc in socio-communal systems, humanity, and creates economic crises worldwide [1]. Many strategies have been used to managed and curtailed the COVID-19 outbreak, but many countries are still helpless in fighting and containing the outbreak. The epidemiology complexity and the rapidly evolving disease patterns of the COVID-19 demand a couturier approach by government, researchers, and medical experts in dealing with this overwhelming pandemic. Similarly, other methods such as social distancing, the use of facemask, isolated of confirmed patients among others have developed in crucial and manage the COVID-19 pandemic.

The pandemic originated from China in a town called Wuhan, but it has spread to 213 other countries globally. As of August 28, 2020, the World Health Organization (WHO) has reported a total of 24,926,312 COVID-19 cases with 840,662 deaths, and 17,799,210 patients recovered successfully from this deadly disease. This has been confirmed by WHO that COVID-19 spread and transmitted from wild animals illegally sold in the Huanan Seafood Wholesale Market in Wuhan [2]. According to the recent report, ages between 30 and 79 years, approximately 86.60% are susceptible to COVID-19 pandemic of all patients infected so far, thus have a median age of 47 years [3].

The men are noted to exhibit a higher propensity for this outbreak, though researches have not reported significant gender preponderance [4]. Human-to-human has been identified as the major mode of transmission of COVID-19 pandemic, and the National Health Commission ofChina, has identified droplets, direct exposure, feces, respiratory aspirates, and aerosols transmission has a carrier of COVID-19 pandemic [5]. Although research has not provided concrete evidence about sporadic reports about the vertical transmission of SARS-CoV-2 it has been shown that these also can be a possible way of spread COVID-19 [6, 7].

The data science analysis is newly evolving, intending to empower health care systems and organizations to connect to harness information and convert it to usable knowledge and preferably personalized clinical decision making. The application of big data in the area of infectious diseases has introduced several changes in the information accumulation models using analytics. The processing, accumulation, and accrual of big data in healthcare are possible through the rapidly evolving field of Big Data Analytics (BDA), thus offers the capacity to understand, rationalize and use big data to serve different purposes.

Improvement in information technology and data computing has greatly changed researches on population-based by encouraging easy access to a huge amount of data. Sometimes, such database links are referred to as "big data" [8, 9]. In other to make efficient use of these data for researches in clinical health or public health, the researchers need to widen researches further than the traditional surveillance model, as operating with big data differs from focusing on performing narrow analysis, treatment-oriented clinical data. Therefore, leveraging on Big data to reflect accurately on the heterogeneous population it represents becomes expedient [10, 11]. This endeavor needs a swift research environment that can adopt a quick advancement in computing technology to at all-time combine data while making use of new methods to reduce their complexity [9, 10]. Also, trends and patterns which make it easy to diagnose and treat patients are been revealed by big data.

The Mutual collaboration that exists in the healthcare sector results in the generation of a huge amount of data from various sources [10, 12, 13]. This has a result of huge figures of varied sections and departments including physicians of different disciplines, ranging from the nurses, the pathologists, radiologists, and laboratory technologists which collaborates efforts to achieve unified goals towards bringing medical costs and mistakes down to the barest minimum. And also to provide excellent and standardized healthcare services. Various stakeholders that work collaboratively in the health sector get data from different sources. This source includes data gotten from patient's observation, imaging reports from scans, interview and test results, insurance, and bills, summaries of patient discharges, reports from pharmacists, case notes from physicians, admission notes of the hospitals, feedback from social media and journals of medical articles.

Consequently, the application of advanced technologies which includes virtualization and cloud computing allows for huge and effective data processing in the healthcare system. Thereby rapidly turning the healthcare system into a big data industry. Nevertheless, in these modern days, the improvement in the information and communication technologies (ICT) brings the advancement of varied data from new sources in the healthcare system. The 21st century is an age of big data affecting every aspect of human life, including biology and medicine [14, 15]. The move from paper medical records to Electronic Health Record (EHR) systems has resulted in an unprecedented increase in data [16]. Big data thus offers a great opportunity for doctors, epidemiologists, and specialists in health policy to make evidence-driven decisions that will eventually enhance patient care [17, 18]. "Big data is not only a modern reality for the biomedical scientist but an imperative that needs to be fully grasped and used in the search for new knowledge" [19, 20].

Therefore, this chapter discusses the possible application of big data and BDA to improve conventional public health approaches to tackle the COVID-19 pandemic to control, manage, and identify infected patients, thus reduce the effect on health implicitly associated with the outbreak. The remaining part of this chapter is organized thus: Sector 2 discusses the growth of data in healthcare, the challenges, and the importance of big data in COVID-19. Section 3 presents the big data privacy and ethical challenges in COVID-19. Section 4 discusses BDA in the COVID-19 epidemic. Finally, Sect. 5 concludes the chapter.

2 Big Data and Big Data Analytics for COVID-19

The era of big data impacting all parts of people's lifespan, including genetics and medicine in this 21st century [14, 21]. The transition from paper patient reports to Electronic Health Record (EHR) systems resulted in exponential data development [22]. Big data thus creates a tremendous incentive for physicians, epidemiologists, and public policy experts to take evidence-driven action that will inevitably strengthen patient safety [23, 24]. There are various technologies like IoT devices and sensors in the modern age that contribute greatly to the massive growth of Big Data. Current advances in the fields of computation, storage, and connectivity have created vast data sets, extracting valuable information from this immense volume of data would bring value to science, government, industry, and society.

Through embracing biosensors, wearable devices, and mHealth, the volume of biological data collected has expanded [25]. According to a study by Cisco [26, 27], the total amount of data produced by IoT sensors and devices will hit 847 ZB (Zettabytes) by 2021. The vast volume of data cannot be processed, collected, and controlled with conventional methods. BDA is the method of analyzing broad data sets comprising a range of data types [28] to uncover invisible patterns, latent associations, industry dynamics, consumer desires, and other important business knowledge [29]. The ability to evaluate vast volumes of data can help a company cope with important knowledge that can impact the corporation [30].

The principal aim of BDA is, therefore, to assist industry organizations in strengthening their interpretation of data and thereby to make successful and knowledgeable choices. BDA allows data mineworkers and experts to scrutinize a vast amount of data that cannot be analyzed employing conventional methods [29]. BDA comprises technology and materials that can turn a vast quantity of organized, formless, and semi-organized data into an extra understandable framework for investigative procedures. The procedures employed in these computational methods have to recognize forms, tendencies, and associations in the data across several time prospects [31]. Such methods, after analyzing the results, illustrate the discoveries for effective verdict taking in tables, charts, and three-dimensional maps.

Big data processing is also a major problem for many implementations owing to the sophistication of data and the scalability of fundamental procedures facilitating these systems [32]. Obtaining useful information from big data analysis is a serious issue requiring adaptable investigative procedures and methods to report timely outcomes while existing methods and procedures are incompetent in handling BDA [33]. Therefore, there is a need for broad networks and external technologies to support parallel data. Besides, data foundations, for instance very advanced data streams obtained from various data foundations, have diverse arrangements which make it essential to incorporate multiple analytics solutions [34]. The problem is thus based on the efficiency of existing procedures employed in big data processing, which doesn't grow uninterruptedly with the exponential growth in computing capital [35]. Figure 1 displayed the big data conceptual framework for the COVID-19 Pandemic.

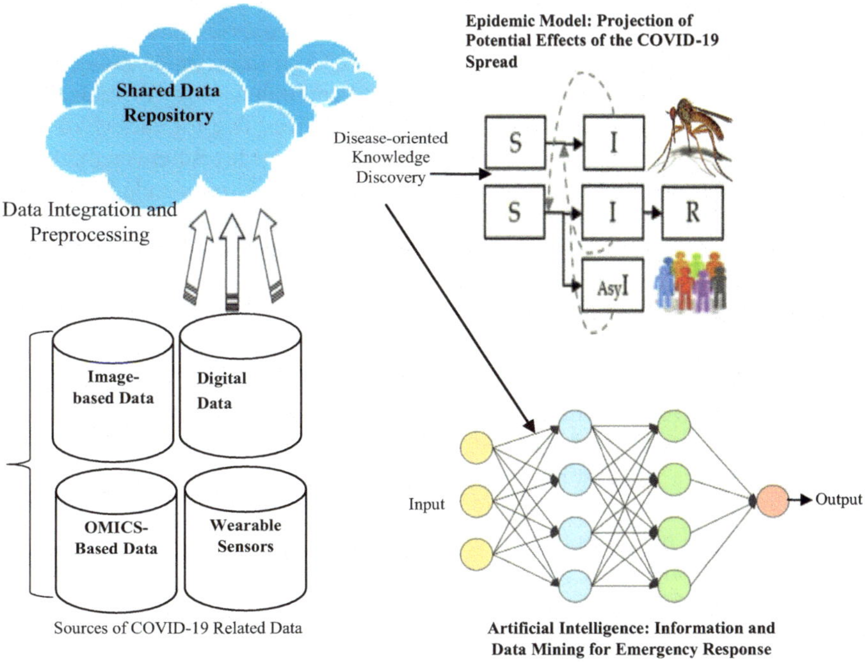

Fig. 1 An integrated big data conceptual model for COVID-19 Pandemic

BDA systems take a large amount of time to provide consumers with input and advice, although only a few applications [36] can handle massive data sets within a short processing period. By comparison, the greatest of the outstanding approaches employ a complex trial-and-error approach to tackle large volumes of data sets and data complexity [37]. There are big-data analytics platforms, for instance, the Investigative Data Examination System [38] is a big-data graphic analytics program that is employed to scrutinize complicated earth structure models of massive quantities of datasets. Big data volume is enormous and thus conventional applications for Database Management can't be used to accumulate and investigate huge data. The resolution comes from modern warehousing databases such as Apache Hadoop that support the analysis of distributed data.

Big data promises more personalized and effective medicine for patients during the COVID-19 outbreak with better precision and earlier diagnosis and tailored therapy to the specific combination of genes, environmental risk, and accurate disease phenotype in an individual. This promise comes from data obtained from various sources, ranging from molecules to cells, to tissues, to individuals and populations, and from the convergence of these data into networks that enhance understanding of health and disease. Big data-driven science could play a role in driving comparative medicine during the COVID-19 pandemic through sharing physiology, pathophysiology, and risk factor for diseases through species.

The integration of EHR data across institutions would provide for earlier unprecedented access to patient data on a scale during the COVID-19 outbreak, thereby facilitating accurate phenotype classification and objective assessment of risk factors and response to COVID-19 outbreak therapy. High-throughput molecular data will provide insight into previously unexplored pathophysiology of molecular and etiology of diseases. Big data analysis and integration from a variety of sources can lead to stronger connections drawn at the molecular level between human and animal disease, allow predictive modeling of infectious dis-ease and identifying key areas of intervention, and promote step-by-step understanding of COVID-19 disease, which can have a major effect on animal and human health. Using big data, however, comes with tremendous challenges. Therefore, in the COVID-19 pandemic, the paper discusses and includes big data opportunities, their limitations, and what's needed to capitalize on big data.

Big Data will aid in the COVID-19 pandemic handling of immense and unparalleled quantities of data from various sources such as situation briefing and updating by government entities and agencies, real-time COVID-19 monitoring and tracking outbreaks, pattern forecasting/now-casting, and health resource utilization knowledge [39]. The big data can spring from different sources: (i) image-based data obtained through radionics or data mining methods by extracting clinical and high-dimensional information from images (ii) Information derived from wearable sensors (iii) Computer and digital big data, such as smartphone, internet and other connected mobile devices (iv) molecular data that be obtained from OMICS-based methods, which includes genomics and post-genomics specialties and by wet-lab techniques [40–42].

2.1 *Big Data Analytics Life Cycle*

The BDA life cycle is demonstrated in Fig. 2, which encompasses 9 steps primarily beginning with the assessment of the market difficulty, performing an investigation on current approaches to fix the difficulty, describing the data including filtering as well as collecting the data. Established on the utilization obligation, the filtered data is extracted, validated, and cleansed. Through applying correct aggregation techniques, the collected data is suitably interpreted for further analysis. Once data is assembled out of several proveniences, the subsequent move is to perform experimental data scrutiny such that the method is selected. The concluding step in Big Data's life-cycle is to change the method developed and established into data visualization and outcomes scrutiny [43, 44].

Big Data analysis varies from conventional data analysis largely because of the data processes' length, velocity, and variety characteristics. A step-by-step approach

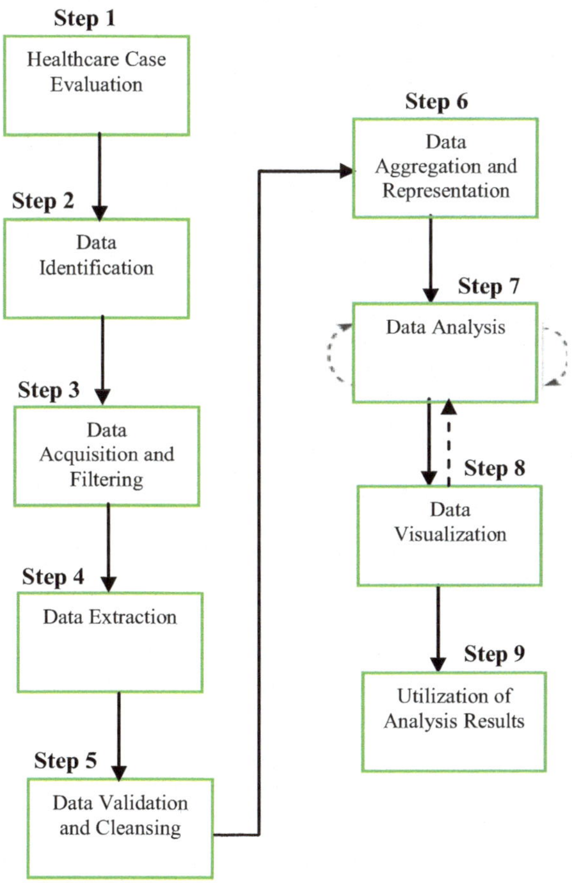

Fig. 2 The Big Data analytics lifecycle

is required to coordinate the processes and tasks involved in collecting, storing, evaluating, and repurposing data to resolve the distinct criteria for carrying out analysis of big data. From the viewpoint of Big Data acceptance and preparation, it is critical that accompanying the life span, attention is given to the matters of data processing recruiting, preparation, accomplishment, and staffing. Based on the complexity of the analytical problems being discussed, "models" that encapsulate new ideas and understandings about the existence of the dynamics and interactions that occur within the data being studied can be generated for the analytical results. A model can look like a math equation or a series of laws. Models can be used to develop the structure of the healthcare process and implementation system, so they can form the base of a new framework or software model.

3 The Opportunities of Big Data and Big Data Analytics in COVID-19 Pandemic

The possibility of fast-spreading diseases that causes uncontrolled death and a bad influence on the economies and sustainability of countries in the world has stretched the importance and needs for developing a quantitative framework to provide supports for making nearly real-time decisions in the public health system. A case study of the 2003 severe acute respiratory syndrome COVID-19 outbreak which originates from China and extends to 29 countries, which by August 2003 becomes healthcare-acquired infection in various regions [45, 46]. The Influenza (HiN1) pandemic of that originates from Mexico and spreads rapidly all over the world through airline network and infected 20 countries, with the maximum hit on the travelers coming from Mexico within a little time of the disease outbreak [47]. The socio-economic implication and outcome of the outbreak of a disease related to 2009 (influenza A(H1N1)) were projected to be a huge amount ranging between $360 billion–$4 trillion [48] been the calculation for the outbreak in the first year. Significantly, as of 28 August 2020, the SARS disease outbreaks at WUHAN in china in 2019 was calculated and projected to be 24,926,312 confirmed cases and 840,662 mortalities across the globe. Ever since the outbreak of COVID-19 in china, people that travel globally to WUHAN imported the disease to various countries of the globe.

The outbreak of severe acute respiratory syndrome disease causes trivia effects on the people and economy all over the world. This effect includes; restrictions and barns on traveling, total closure of shops and market resulting in a huge loss on earnings and proceeds, fear of contracting the disease from the infected person, unpleasant side effects on world tourism at large as many flights were canceled or suspended. Express and huge damage on government finances in various countries as agricultural activities were greatly hampered resulting in food shortage and so many other effects result from the outbreaks. Therefore it becomes imperative to make an immediate response from all angles to fight and contain the virus efficiently. Big data entails the processing of both new and existing data innovatively to proffer meaningful solutions that are of huge business benefits [49–51]. However, to process large data, or varied data will only be a mere technological solution until it is associated with business objectives and goals.

Big data promises More light to be shed on complicated facts and information on the dynamics of how infectious diseases are been transmitted with how to develop new modeling and analytical tools which have far been hidden due to lack of smooth and workable data. More progress will be made in the area of disease forecast when a huge amount of Information on epidemics required for modeling is available. Big data will be best in accomplishing this goal. Improved consistency in reporting diseases and case definition is therefore expedient within time and space. Data obtained from news media sources can give a perfect estimation and evaluation of how the disease is been transmitted. Thus, it's of high importance, especially when comprehensive and well-examined data are not available. In a country with low and middle income, and where studies on disease transmission details are scarce, resources based on internet surveys will provide an opportunity for detailed study and correct assessment on how the disease is been transmitted. For instance, in the crises of infectious diseases COVID -19 when the real-time assessment is expedient.

A well-calibrated computational model tool useful in assessing and analyzing epidemic spread signifies a potent tool to sustain the process of decision-making at a time of emergency epidemic outbreaks. Epidemic models are progressively used to generate predictions of the spatial-temporal progression of a disease outbreak at several spatial scales and for easy access to possible impacts of the various strategies of the intervention [52]. The ability to produce innovative facts or information is greatly expanded by big data. The cost applicable to answer various questions retrospectively and prospectively, by gathering ordered and structured data are exorbitant.

Acquisition of finer data in a computerized manner is achieved by analyzing unstructured data that are within EHRS using various computational techniques such as traditional language processors that extracts clinical concepts from free documents. Analyzing the unstructured data contained within EHRs using computational techniques (e.g., natural language processing to extract medical concepts from free-text documents) permits finer data acquisition in an automated fashion. For example, computerized detection within EHRS with the use of natural language processing is better used to detect complications that arise after the operation when compared to patient wellbeing indicators based on discharge coding [53].

Big data provides the possibility to generate an observable indication base for clinically related questions which may not be achievable but will be helpful with generalizability issues. Generalizability issues restrict the application of conclusions that are derived from random trials carried out on a very narrow scale of participants to patients that shows dissimilar characteristics. Big data helps disseminate knowledge. Many healthcare practitioners strive to be updated with current evidential proof and support that guides clinical practices. Figure 3 depicted the relationship between COVID-19 Pandemic and big data.

The COVID-19 outbreak can be monitored in real-time using big data. The recent pandemic outbreak has been used to create unique open-access databases containing

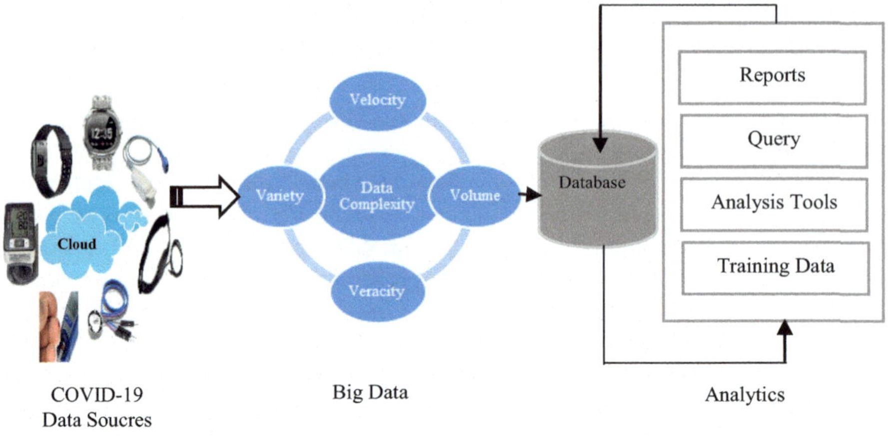

Fig. 3 The Relationship between COVID-19 Pandemic and Big Data

daily numbers of country-based infections that are widely available, and in some cases, the database contains the cities of this country. A mathematical model with AI can be combined with the knowledge having on people's movement during contact tracing to produce good results that can be used to forecast the outbreak. For example, AI-based surveillance called Blue Dot was used as a start-up based in Toronto to detect an epidemic outbreak and it appears very useful [54]. Several hours after the outbreak at Wuhan's, the system is the first to detect an epidemic outbreak [54].

Computational techniques enable us to simulate the spread of the virus in real-time, such as the framework developed at John Hopkins University, USA. Furmore, virtual Big Data, gathered from social networks and other associated non-conventional data sources, helps us to reconstruct the outbreak's early epidemiologic background. For example, between 13 January and 31 January, 2020, Sun and colleagues [55] conducted a population-level observational analysis, monitoring websites related to healthcare, social networks, and news stories in mainland China. The authors concluded that non-classical data sets will support researchers who are witnessing the spread of an epidemic in terms of health awareness, attitudes toward seeking health care, and use of health services. Non-classical datasets and data streams can inform the design and implementation of successful public health measures especially in the early stages of the outbreak.

Similarly, [56] used big data to estimate the number of new COVID-19 events, whether reported or proven. For different keywords, including COVID-19 clinical symptoms (such as dry cough, fever, chest pain, and pneumonia), the authors used a lagged sequence of "Social media search indexes" (SMSI). Authors found that new COVID-19 suspected and confirmed cases could be identified 6–9 and 10 days in advance, respectively, using techniques such as the subset selection process.

Having a reliable, responsive, and accurate diagnostic test is important in preventing and controlling infectious disorders. Scientists have managed to develop a molecular kit capable of capturing the correct diagnosis quickly and accurately and distinguishing between COVID-19 and SARS-CoV. Diagnosis of salivary seems to hold great promise in the successful diagnosis of the virus. Together with molecular assays and studies, the amplification of ether multiplex nucleic acid or microarray-based, high-resolution chest CT is important for tracking the path of the disease and its evolution in terms of intensity and reaction to care. Current research is also attempting to define early radiological prognostic predictors, which would be extremely helpful in stratifying COVID-19 patients and in their clinical management [54, 57]. Big Data will offer accurate, evidentiary forecasts to local decision-makers and policymakers. Allam and Jones [58] examined the urban outbreak of COVID-19, demonstrating how smart cities and smart networks can use high-quality, improved structured data exchange protocols to help handle such situations.

Big data seem to have huge potential for COVID-19 and other emergency management and their position is expected to grow in the future. Big data can be used to track the virus's spread in real-time, and to prepare and raise public health measures accordingly, monitor its efficacy, repurpose old com-pounds and develop new medicines, as well as identify possible candidates for vaccines and improve national and territorial response to the ongoing pandemic. Together with classical surveillance, these new methods can be exploited: while the latter allows data analysis and interpretation, the former exposes secret trends and patterns which can be used to construct predictive models.

Globally, in response to the COVID-19 virus, numerous conventional methods have been devoted to enhancing future forecasting, detection, and treatment with other alternatives. These methods, however, are usually expensive and time-consuming, have a low positive outcome rate, and require various materials, equipment, and personnel. Moreover, due to the constraint on expenditure and techniques, most countries suffer from a shortage of test kits. Thus, during the COVID-19 pandemic, these standard approaches are not sufficient to meet the requirements of rapid detection and monitoring. For COVID-19 detection, therefore, the use of connected devices along with big data is a simple and low-cost strategy. Developing successful methods for diagnosis and treatment plays a significant role in minimizing the impact of the COVID-19 virus in the COVID-19 pandemic fight.

4 Challenges of Big Data and Big Data Analytics During COVID-19 Pandemic

Many organizations have widely accepted big data and BDA. These pieces of machinery are, however, yet in its first phases. It has not yet tackled many current work challenges. Big data analysis is a crucial dispute for several utilizations owing to the nature of data and the scalability of fundamental procedures that support these methods [32]. This segment thus poses some difficulties in the BDA focused on the COVID-19 pandemic. Data security concerns occur where a network is corrupted by the utilization of BDA techniques to infer or reestablish individual information, while data is created by anonymous users. The confidentiality matter has to turn out to be a central concern in the data mining province with the advent of BDA tools employed during the COVID-19 outbreak. Consequently, most consumers are hesitant to rely on such networks, which do not have firm terms of service-level agreement (SLA) concerning abuse or misuse of personal information by customers.

Users' sensitive information must be undisclosed and safeguarded from outside intrusion. Though provisional identity, concealment, and encryption offer numerous means to implement data protection, ethical considerations for instance what to employ, how to utilize, and why employ engendered big data in COVID-19 pandemic must be determined [59]. Alternative safety jeopardy connected with the outbreak data is the variety of systems employed and the complexity of data produced, for instance, fresh computers, data formats, and procedures for communication. These systems are intended to interact with supportive utilization and can have various extents and forms external to the system. Therefore, to authenticate these devices, each unit should be issued by a system with a non-repudiable identification scheme. Besides, organizations will sustain a meta-archive of these related tools for analyzing consideration. This composite architecture of the system is innovative to safekeeping experts, resulting in elevated security risks. Any intrusion in this case thus violates network stability and disconnects interconnected equipment.

Security and privacy are crucial problems in the collection and storing of vast volumes of data in the setting of COVID-19-based BDA. Similarly, these schemes depend seriously on third party facilities and infrastructure to conduct critical processes and host secluded data. Therefore, unprecedented growth in data volume causes difficulties in obtaining every single part of vital data. There are no long-standing security mechanisms that provide full security in COVID-19-based big data scenarios [33]. Current algorithms are not meant for complex data interpretation and are thus not implemented effectually. Legacy data protection approaches are primarily designed for static data sets, while the actual data specifications dynamically alter [33]. Therefore, it is difficult to deploy these safety resolutions for energetically cumulative data. Governmental and administrative matters should also be addressed when SLAs are signed. The key disputes confronted by the layer of perception are energy optimization, node stability, entrenched functioning scheme, and multi-protocol gateway. This level also faces problems in radar expertise including procurement correctness, miniaturization, and intellect.

The ability to combine sophisticated epidemiological models and new big-data sources have been discussed [60]. For example, the use of smart-phones, social networks, or public health response satellites at different stages, mainly in the situation of disease forecasts for making a decision [60, 61]. These new sources of data include significant, real-time data on tourism visits that spread infection and spatial shifts in vulnerable residents that probably up till now were hard to report on time scales related to a rapidly fast-growing epidemic [60]. With increasing flexibility and growing universal connectivity, this information will be crucial for monitoring and containment planning strategies [62].

By principle, with correct data sharing protocols in place, accurate, up-to-date disease predictions can be generated that is guided using this data stream. The success of big data in fighting epidemics depends on various organizations public, private, and the government is needed to be in contact frequently [60, 61]. Privacy issues for daily use of new data channels need to be addressed, specifically, the most suitable way to vigorously integrate such data streams to confirm individual confidentiality. Yet even if security is tackled, the transformation of new methods into a policymaking context raises additional systemic challenges [60, 61].

Big Data mining provides many tempting opportunities [11]. Nonetheless, when investigating big data sets and mining meaning and expertise from these facts extracted, researchers and professionals face many challenges [11, 63, 64]. The complications at various levels including data collection, storing, scanning, sharing, reviewing, handling, and watching. Furthermore, security and privacy issues particularly arise in distributed applications that are powered by data. The surge of knowledge and distributed sources also surpasses our harnessing capability indeed, although the scale of big data continually grow exponentially, the actual technical ability to accomplish and explore Large Data sets is only in the comparatively lower rates of data petabytes, exabytes, and zettabytes [11]. In this chapter, we address some technical issues which are still open to research in more detail.

While working with Big Data, data scientists face a lot of obstacles. One obstacle is the compilation, integration, and storage of tremendous datasets generated from disseminated sources, with far less needed hardware and software [59, 65]. The management of big data results in another huge problem. Effective big data management is essential to promote the abstraction of accurate information to maximize investment [66, 67]. Proper management of data is the basis for BDA [68].

Another difficulty is to synchronize with an organization's internal infrastructures external data sources, and Big Data dispersed systems (sensors, apps, databases, networks, etc.) [11]. Most of the time, an analysis of the data produced within organizations is not sufficient. We need to go one step further to integrate internal data with external data sources, to gain useful insight and information. External data may include the sources from third parties, market fluctuations details, weather forecasts and traffic situations, social network data, comments from clients, and resident input. This will aid to optimize the power of analytical models used in the analysis, for example.

Big data and data stream uses the concept of collaborative and incremental learning. They deal with numerous challenges that arise during the learning of data such as data accessibility and restricted resources. They make use of User profiling and stock forecasting applications. The application of incremental learning to data produces a faster means of prediction when dealing with the new data stream. Hence, using the incremental algorithm is highly recommended when the drift concept is not available. On the other hand, it is highly recommended to use ensemble algorithms to obtain accurate outcome with large drift concept. Also, when dealing with a modest data stream or real-time processing, the incremental algorithm should be considered for use. Conversely, in the case of a complex data stream, an ensemble algorithm is considered the best.

Another big problem is analogical reasoning: fundamentally, disease forecasting is unpredictable. In the narrative on Big Data and Artificial Intelligence (AI), there is often an underlying assumption about the statistical covariates or cell phone data and difficult models of simulation that avoid the need to gather basic epidemiological details. Nevertheless, for evolving COVID-19 epidemics emphasizing this opinion still lack a reliable fact on situation counts and biotic processes that drive an outbreak of the disease, let only the behavioral reactions of infected individuals, and make it difficult to rapidly adjust or understand precise intricate prototypes on spatiotemporal scales applicable in making a verdict. Hopefully, the best effective systems would continue to be simple [69, 70] equally, out of necessity for versatile modules that provide quick responses given a great controversy surrounding emergency epidemiological studies and since simple models are available easier to interpret and communicate [71].

Clear knowledge of both the importance and weaknesses of typical outputs is a precondition for their successful implementation but is often absent. Because policymakers typically haven't yet reached in-depth modeling experience, lack of consistent message threatens two destructive results: assume that the method would be misinformed without skepticism and choices, or ignore off-hand modeling and neglect the proof that we must control the epidemics most efficiently. During epidemics, Verdicts have to be taken rapidly, on a patchy basis, and inaccurate data model could be effective tools for guiding them. Considering the above obstacles, computing capacity, novel methods, and novel data are advancing steadily sources give authentic courage for improved monitoring and valuable predicting systems. Novel database available to us comprises not only inactively experimental large data streams from cell phones but also comprehensive ecological data and local sensor information from embedded devices, internet search information, pathogenic genomic data that can be produced quickly informing response during an outbreak, [72] and crowd-sourced methods to track emergencies changing rapidly [73].

Information sharing systems and structured aggregation strategies are being established to secure personal data privacy [74], and through internet access enables rapid data transmission and collaboration between geographically distant respondent teams. Methodologically, effective modeling methods that combine multiple predictions to reduce uncertainty are being built [70, 75]. In reaction to the outbreak of COVID-19 between academic organizations, an innovative, collaborative approach has unfolded: for example, Twitter and other channels to exchange, evaluate, and publicly debate the effects of new research as it arises. (Ironically, the control of the misinformation that is now proliferating on social networking during a crisis is likely to become one of the most significant concerns for containing the disease).

Unless the above problems are resolved, these technologies will remain dislocated and impracticable. It is promising that all three problems may be strengthened by transferring most of the funding and knowledge focus to those communities most helpless to epidemics. The unpredictability of COVID-19 outbreak and the progressively technological mechanisms of these methods will require agile, dispersed groups of people covering the systematic and functioning dimensions of the epidemic response using novel Big Data methods to supplement and explain the limited spread, socio-geographical data that are necessary towards the progress of important predictions. Provincial or small groups with investigative experience and current connections with government and industry stakeholders can contribute to scalable modeling strategies that exploit broad curated and international scientific database skills, building on partnerships formed if no new or ongoing outbreaks occur. This strategy may likewise be of help to mitigate some policy concerns related to data sharing, particularly though sensitive information cannot be shared publicly.

To achieve this idea, significant continuous investment is required, develop, and finance individuals to fill what currently represents a significant void in the analytics process, especially in some countries with low and middle wages. Big data can be created from a lot of sources like social networking sites, smartphones, IoT sensors, and publicly available data [76] in different formats such as text or video. Big data applies to patient care details in the sense of COVID-19, such as medical records, X-Ray reports, case history, a list of doctors and nurses, and information about the epidemic location. Big data has proved its capability to support fighting infectious diseases like COVID-19 [77, 78].

5 Conclusion

In the healthcare industry, the new information technology has been used to address global health problems such as unequal allocation of medical services, increasing chronic illnesses, and rising medical expenses. As well, with the proliferation of intelligent and radar devices, the advanced degree of data creation in the healthcare sector has improved dramatically in current years. Big data potentially provide several promising solutions to help combat the COVID-19 epidemic. Using big data with various analytics tools can help explain COVID-19 in terms of outbreak tracking, virus growth, disease control, and vaccine manufacturing. Big data combined with smart-based applications can create complex prediction models using coronavirus data streams to estimate the outbreak, enabling health authorities to monitor coronavirus spread, and prepare successful preventive actions. Big data models also support potential COVID-19 outbreak forecasting through its ability to integrate large amounts of preventive and treatment data. Moreover, BDA from a variety of real-world sources including infected patients can help implement large-scale COVID-19 investigations to develop comprehensive treatment solutions with high reliability. This would also help healthcare providers to understand the virus development for better response to the various treatment and diagnoses. As one of the most effective solutions to combat the COVID-19 pandemic, early treatment and prediction are of importance. Hence, big data capability in the fight against the COVID-19 outbreak can be useful and distilled into four main areas of application: outbreak virus spread, monitoring forecasting, diagnosis/treatment of coronavirus, and discovery of vaccines/drugs. The relationship amid the COVID-19 outbreak and big data is presently at a point somewhere high-frequency dispensation, storage, and investigation of enormous capacities of data are needed. In this chapter, the core principles of COVID-19-based, big data, and BDA pieces of machinery in the medical sector were explored in depth. The chapter discussed the big data and BDA focusing on the COVID-19 outbreak, the opportunities, expectations, threats, and challenges during COVID-19 were presented. Data safety and confidentiality will be looked at for future research with COVID-19-based BDA with health care systems. Machine learning approaches to solve the problem related to changing data inputs should be integrated. Developing countries, particularly African hospitals, should be thinking about how big data and BDA can be deployed in hospitals to reduce costs as it is feasible and economic. Therefore, immediate analytics resolution that could offer speedy understanding would be necessary and helpful.

References

1. Guraya, S.Y.: Transforming laparoendoscopic surgical protocols during COVID-19 pandemic; big data analytics, resource allocation, and operational considerations; a review article. Int. J. Surgery (2020)
2. Ogundokun, Roseline O., Adewale F. Lukman, Golam BM Kibria, Joseph B. Awotunde, and Benedita B. Aladeitan.: Predictive modelling of COVID-19 confirmed cases in Nigeria. Inf. Dis Model. **5**, 543–548 (2020)
3. Guan, W.J., Ni, Z.Y., Hu, Y., Liang, W.H., Ou, C.Q., He, J.X., Du, B.: Clinical characteristics of coronavirus disease in 2019 in China. N. Engl. J. Med. **382**(18), 1708–1720 (2020)
4. Wang, D., Hu, B., Hu, C., Zhu, F., Liu, X., Zhang, J., Zhao, Y.: Clinical characteristics of 138 hospitalized patients with 2019 novel coronavirus–infected pneumonia in Wuhan, China. Jama **323**(11), 1061–1069 (2020)
5. Liu, Y., Gayle, A.A., Wilder-Smith, A., Rocklöv, J.: The reproductive number of COVID-19 is higher compared to SARS coronavirus. J. Travel Med. (2020)
6. Fan, C., Lei, D., Fang, C., Li, C., Wang, M., Liu, Y., … & Yu, Y.: Perinatal transmission of COVID-19 associated SARS-CoV-2: should we worry?. Clin. Infect. Dis. (2020)
7. Karimi-Zarchi, M., Neamatzadeh, H., Dastgheib, S. A., Abbasi, H., Mirjalili, S. R., Behforouz, A., …, Bahrami, R.: Vertical transmission of coronavirus disease 19 (COVID-19) from infected pregnant mothers to neonates: a review. Fetal Pediatric Pathol., 1–5 (2020)
8. Priyanka, K., Kulennavar, N.: A survey on big data analytics in health care. Int. J. Comput. Sci. Inf. Technol. **5**(4), 5865–5868 (2014)
9. Kruse, C.S., Goswamy, R., Raval, Y.J., Marawi, S.: Challenges and opportunities of big data in health care: a systematic review. JMIR Med. Inf. **4**(4), (2016)
10. Olaronke, I., Oluwaseun, O.: Big data in healthcare: Prospects, challenges and resolutions. In: 2016 Future Technologies Conference (FTC), pp. 1152–1157. IEEE (2016, December)
11. Oussous, A., Benjelloun, F.Z., Lahcen, A.A., Belfkih, S.: Big Data technologies: a survey. J. King Saud Univ.-Comput. Inf. Sci. **30**(4), 431–448 (2018)
12. Adeniyi, E. A., Ogundokun, R. O., & Awotunde, J. B.: IoMT-Based Wearable Body Sensors Network Healthcare Monitoring System. Stud. Comput. Intell. **933**, 103–121 (2021)
13. Dai, H.N., Wang, H., Xu, G., Wan, J., Imran, M.: Big data analytics for manufacturing internet of things: opportunities, challenges and enabling technologies. Enterprise Inf. Syst. 1–25 (2019)
14. Hulsen, T., Jamuar, S.S., Moody, A., Karnes, J.H., Orsolya, V., Hedensted, S., McKinney, E.: From big data to precision medicine. Frontiers in medicine **6**, 34 (2019)
15. Baro, E., Degoul, S., Beuscart, R., Chazard, E.: Toward a literature-driven definition of big data in healthcare. BioMed Research International, New York (2015)
16. Austin, C., Kusumoto, F.: The application of Big Data in medicine: current implications and future directions. J. Interventional Cardiac Electrophysiol. **47**(1), 51–59 (2016)
17. Fiske, A., Buyx, A., Prainsack, B.: Health information counselors: a new profession for the age of big data. Acad. Med. **94**(1), 37 (2019)

18. Galetsi, P., Katsaliaki, K., Kumar, S.: Values, challenges and future directions of big data analytics in healthcare: A systematic review. Social Sci. Med., 112533 (2019)
19. Krumholz, H.M.: Big data and new knowledge in medicine: the thinking, training, and tools needed for a learning health system. Health Aff. **33**(7), 1163–1170 (2014)
20. Lacroix, P.: Big Data Privacy and Ethical Challenges. In: Big Data, Big Challenges: A Healthcare Perspective, pp. 101–111. Springer, Cham (2019)
21. Riba, M., Sala, C., Toniolo, D., Tonon, G.: Big data in medicine, the present and hopefully the future. Front. Med., 6 (2019)
22. Dinh-Le, C., Chuang, R., Chokshi, S., Mann, D.: Wearable health technology and electronic health record integration: scoping review and future directions. JMIR mHealth and uHealth **7**(9), (2019)
23. McCue, M.E., McCoy, A.M.: The scope of big data in one medicine: unprecedented opportunities and challenges. Front. Veterinary Sci. **4**, 194 (2017)
24. Murdoch, T.B., Detsky, A.S.: The inevitable application of big data to health care. JAMA **309**(13), 1351–1352 (2013)
25. Tariq, N., Asim, M., Al-Obeidat, F., Zubair Farooqi, M., Baker, T., Hammoudeh, M., Ghafir, I.: The security of big data in fog-enabled IoT applications including blockchain: a survey. Sensors **19**(8), 1788 (2019)
26. Macaulay, J., Buckalew, L., Chung, G.: Internet of things in logistics. DHL Trend Research **1**(1), 1–27 (2015)
27. Hofdijk, J., Séroussi, B., Lovis, C., Sieverink, F., Ehrler, F., & Ugon, A. (2016). Transforming Healthcare with the Internet of Things. In Proceedings of the EFMI Special Topic Conference 2016
28. Mital, R., Coughlin, J., Canaday, M.: Using big data technologies and analytics to predict sensor anomalies. Amos 84 (2015)
29. Berman, E., Felter, J.H., Shapiro, J.N.: Small Wars, Big Data: The Information Revolution in Modern Conflict. Princeton University Press, Princeton (2020)
30. Raghupathi, W., Raghupathi, V.: Big data analytics in healthcare: promise and potential. Health information science and systems **2**(1), 3 (2014)
31. Teijeiro, D., Pardo, X.C., González, P., Banga, J.R., Doallo, R.: Towards cloud-based parallel metaheuristics: a case study in computational biology with differential evolution and spark. Int. J. High Performan. Comput. Appl. **32**(5), 693–705 (2018)
32. Candela, L., Castelli, D., Pagano, P.: Managing big data through hybrid data infrastructures. ERCIM News **89**, 37–38 (2012)
33. Marjani, M., Nasaruddin, F., Gani, A., Karim, A., Hashem, I.A.T., Siddiqa, A., Yaqoob, I.: Big IoT data analytics: architecture, opportunities, and open research challenges. IEEE Access **5**, 5247–5261 (2017)
34. Assuncao, M.D., Calheiros, R.N., Bianchi, S., Netto, M.A., Buyya, R.: Big data computing and clouds: challenges, solutions, and future directions. arXiv preprint arXiv:1312.472210 (2013)
35. Hashem, I.A.T., Yaqoob, I., Anuar, N.B., Mokhtar, S., Gani, A., Khan, S.U.: The rise of "big data" on cloud computing: review and open research issues. Inf. Syst. **47**, 98–115 (2015)
36. Singh, D., Reddy, C.K.: A survey on platforms for big data analytics. J. Big Data **2**(1), 8 (2015)
37. Siddiqa, A., Hashem, I.A.T., Yaqoob, I., Marjani, M., Shamshirband, S., Gani, A., Nasaruddin, F.: A survey of big data management: taxonomy and state-of-the-art. J. Netw. Comput. Appl. **71**, 151–166 (2016)
38. Steed, C.A., Ricciuto, D.M., Shipman, G., Smith, B., Thornton, P.E., Wang, D., Williams, D.N.: Big data visual analytics for exploratory earth system simulation analysis. Comput. Geosci. **61**, 71–82 (2013)
39. Awotunde, J.B., Jimoh, R.G., Oladipo, I.D., Abdulraheem, M.: Prediction of malaria fever using long-short-term memory and big data. Commun. Comput. Inf. Sci. **1350**, 41–53 (2021)
40. Bragazzi, N.L., Guglielmi, O., Garbarino, S.: SleepOMICS: how big data can revolutionize sleep science. Int. J. Environ. Res. Public Health **16**(2), 291 (2019)
41. Gianfredi, V., Bragazzi, N.L., Nucci, D., Martini, M., Rosselli, R., Minelli, L., Moretti, M.: Harnessing big data for communicable tropical and sub-tropical disorders: implications from a systematic review of the literature. Front. Public Health **6**, 90 (2018)

42. Bragazzi, N.L., Dai, H., Damiani, G., Behzadifar, M., Martini, M., Wu, J.: How Big Data and Artificial Intelligence can help better manage the COVID-19 pandemic. Int. J. Environ. Res Public Health **17**(9), 3176 (2020)
43. Erl, T., Khattak, W., Buhler, P.: Big Data Fundamentals: Concepts, Drivers & Techniques. Prentice-Hall Press (2016)
44. Gessa, A., Sancha, P.: Environmental open data in urban platforms: an approach to the big data life cycle. J. Urban Technol. **27**(1), 27–45 (2020)
45. Chowell, G., Fenimore, P.W., Castillo-Garsow, M.A., Castillo-Chavez, C.: SARS outbreaks in Ontario, Hong Kong and Singapore: the role of diagnosis and isolation as a control mechanism. J. Theor. Biol. **224**(1), 1–8 (2003)
46. Siu, A., Wong, Y.R.: Economic impact of SARS: the case of Hong Kong. Asian Econ. Pap. **3**(1), 62–83 (2004)
47. Fadel, F., Khalil El Karoui, M.D., Knebelmann, B.: Spread of a novel influenza A (H1N1) virus via global airline transportation. Nat. Rev. Immunol. **8**, 153–60 (2008)
48. McKibbin, W.J.: The Swine Flu Outbreak and its Global Economic Impact. Brookings, Brookings (2009)
49. Hurwitz, J.S., Nugent, A., Halper, F., Kaufman, M.: Big Data for Dummies. Wiley, New York (2013)
50. Yang, C., Huang, Q., Li, Z., Liu, K., Hu, F.: Big Data and cloud computing: innovation opportunities and challenges. Int. J. Digit. Earth **10**(1), 13–53 (2017)
51. Mikalef, P., Pappas, I.O., Krogstie, J., Giannakos, M.: Big data analytics capabilities: a systematic literature review and research agenda. IseB **16**(3), 547–578 (2018)
52. Liu, S., Poccia, S., Candan, K.S., Chowell, G., Sapino, M.L.: epiDMS: data management and analytics for decision-making from epidemic spread simulation ensembles. J. Infect. Dis. **214**(suppl_4), S427-S432 (2016)
53. Murff, H.J., FitzHenry, F., Matheny, M.E., Gentry, N., Kotter, K.L., Crimin, K., Speroff, T.: Automated identification of postoperative complications within an electronic medical record using natural language processing. JAMA **306**(8), 848–855 (2011)
54. McCall, B.: COVID-19 and artificial intelligence: protecting health-care workers and curbing the spread. The Lancet Digit. Health **2**(4), e166–e167 (2020)
55. Sun, K., Chen, J., Viboud, C.: Early epidemiological analysis of the coronavirus disease 2019 outbreak based on crowdsourced data: a population-level observational study. The Lancet Digit. Health (2020)
56. Qin, L., Sun, Q., Wang, Y., Wu, K.F., Chen, M., Shia, B.C., Wu, S.Y.: Prediction of number of cases of 2019 novel coronavirus (COVID-19) using social media search index. Int. J. Environ. Res. Public Health **17**(7), 2365 (2020)
57. Ai, T., Yang, Z., Hou, H., Zhan, C., Chen, C., Lv, W., …, Xia, L.: Correlation of chest CT and RT-PCR testing in coronavirus disease 2019 (COVID-19) in China: a report of 1014 cases. Radiology, 200642 (2020)
58. Allam, Z., Jones, D.S.:. On the coronavirus (COVID-19) outbreak and the smart city network: universal data sharing standards coupled with artificial intelligence (AI) to benefit urban health monitoring and management. In: Healthcare, vol. 8, no. 1, p. 46. Multidisciplinary Digital Publishing Institute (2020, March)
59. Tsai, C.W., Lai, C.F., Chao, H.C., Vasilakos, A.V.: Big data analytics: a survey. J. Big Data **2**(1), 1–32 (2015)
60. Buckee, C.: Improving epidemic surveillance and response: big data is dead, long live big data. The Lancet Digit. Health (2020)
61. George, D.B., Taylor, W., Shaman, J., Rivers, C., Paul, B., O'Toole, T., Reich, N.G.: Technology to advance infectious disease forecasting for outbreak management. Nat. Commun. **10**(1), 1–4 (2019)
62. Lai, S., Farnham, A., Ruktanonchai, N.W., Tatem, A.J.: Measuring mobility, disease connectivity and individual risk: a review of using mobile phone data and mHealth for travel medicine. J. Travel Med. **26**(3), taz019 (2019)

63. Acharjya, D.P., Ahmed, K.: A survey on big data analytics: challenges, open research issues and tools. Int. J. Adv. Comput. Sci. Appl. **7**(2), 511–518 (2016)
64. Stone, C.B., Neely, A.R., Lengnick-Hall, M.L.: Human resource management in the digital age: Big data, HR analytics and artificial intelligence. In: Management and Technological Challenges in the Digital Age, pp. 13–42. CRC Press (2018)
65. Chen, M., Mao, S., Zhang, Y., Leung, V.C.: Big data: related technologies, challenges, and future prospects (2014)
66. Wu, X., Zhu, X., Wu, G.Q., Ding, W.: Data mining with big data. IEEE Trans. Knowl. Data Eng. **26**(1), 97–107 (2013)
67. Samaraweera, G.D., Chang, M.J.: Security and privacy implications on database systems in Big Data Era: a survey. IEEE Trans. Knowl. Data Eng. (2019)
68. Gul, R., Ahsan, A.: Big Data and Analytics: Case Study of Good Governance and Government Power. In: European Conference on Intangibles and Intellectual Capital, pp. 128–XI. Academic Conferences International Limited (2019, May)
69. May, R.M.: Uses and abuses of mathematics in biology. Science **303**(5659), 790–793 (2004)
70. Viboud, C., Sun, K., Gaffey, R., Ajelli, M., Fumanelli, L., Merler, S., Vespignani, A.: The RAPIDD ebola forecasting challenge: Synthesis and lessons learnt. Epidemics **22**, 13–21 (2018)
71. Kahn, R., Mahmud, A.S., Schroeder, A., Ramirez, L.H.A., Crowley, J., Chan, J., Buckee, C.O.: Rapid forecasting of cholera risk in mozambique: translational challenges and opportunities. Prehosp. Disaster Med. **34**(5), 557–562 (2019)
72. Armstrong, G.L., MacCannell, D.R., Taylor, J., Carleton, H.A., Neuhaus, E.B., Bradbury, R.S., Gwinn, M.: Pathogen genomics in public health. N. Engl. J. Med. **381**(26), 2569–2580 (2019)
73. Schiavo, R., May Leung, M., Brown, M.: Communicating risk and promoting disease mitigation measures in epidemics and emerging disease settings. Pathogens Global Health **108**(2), 76–94 (2014)
74. De-Montjoye, Y.A., Gambs, S., Blondel, V., Canright, G., De Cordes, N., Deletaille, S., Krings, G.: On the privacy-conscientious use of mobile phone data. Sci. Data **5**(1), 1–6 (2018)
75. Ray, E.L., Reich, N.G.: Prediction of infectious disease epidemics via weighted density ensembles. PLoS Comput. Biol. **14**(2), (2018)
76. Cottle, M., Hoover, W., Kanwal, S., Kohn, M., Strome, T., Treister, N.: Transforming Health Care Through Big Data Strategies for leveraging big data in the health care industry. Institute for Health Technology Transformation. http://ihealthtran.com/big-data-in-healthcare (2013)
77. Chae, S., Kwon, S., Lee, D.: Predicting infectious disease using deep learning and big data. Int. J. Environ. Res. Public Health **15**(8), 1596 (2018)
78. Bansal, S., Chowell, G., Simonsen, L., Vespignani, A., Viboud, C.: Big data for infectious disease surveillance and modeling. J. Infect. Dis. **214**(suppl_4), S375–S379 (2016)

Application of COVID-19 Pandemic Using Artificial Intelligence

Abhishek Mehta, Trupti Rathod, and Priya R. Swaminarayan

Abstract Human services conveyance needs the help of the cutting edge innovations like registering (AI), Internet of Things (IoT), immense insights and Machine Learning to battle and appearance ahead of time against the new sicknesses. We tend to objective to check the situation of AI as an unequivocal innovation to investigate, set up us for obstruction, and battle with COVID-19 (Coronavirus) and opportunity pandemics. Gathered the most current realities with respect to AI for COVID-19, at that point broke down a simply like detect its capacity application for this sickness. We have perceived seven pivotal bundles of AI for the COVID-19 pandemic. This innovation plays a urgent situation to see the bunch of occurrences and to foresee anyplace this infection can affect in the predetermination through gathering and perusing every single past actuality. Human services organizations are a partner degree basic would cherish for dynamic advancements to deal with this infection and encourage them in acquiring right proposals in a timeframe to maintain a strategic distance from its unfurl. Artificial intelligence works in an incredibly master approach to imitate like human insight. It ought to in addition assume a significant job in comprehension and proposing the event of a vaccinum for COVID-19. This outcome driven age is utilized for right screening, breaking down, expectation, and quest for present-day victims and certain future victims. The numerous applications are applied to tracks skill of affirmed, recuperated, and demise cases.

A. Mehta (✉)
Assistant Professor, Parul Institute of Computer Application, Parul University, Vadodara, Gujarat, India
e-mail: abhishek.mehta7067@paruluniversity.ac.in

T. Rathod
Assistant Professor, Vidyabharti Trust College of MCA, Gujarat Technological University, Bardoli, Gujarat, India
e-mail: trupti123.rathod@gmail.com

P. R. Swaminarayan
Dean - Faculty of IT and Computer Science, Director - Parul Institute of Engineering and Technology - MCA, Principal - BCA - Parul Institute of Computer Application, Parul University, Vadodara, Gujarat, India
e-mail: priya.swaminarayan@paruluniversity.ac.in

D. Oliva et al. (eds.), *Artificial Intelligence for COVID-19*, Studies in Systems, Decision and Control 358, https://doi.org/10.1007/978-3-030-69744-0_3

Keywords Artificial intelligence (AI) · Applications · COVID 19 · Healthcare · Technology · Computing · Internet of things (IoT) · Machine learning · Healthcare

1 Introduction

The presence of bleeding edge PC exhibiting propels, and their appointment, in various parts all around have incited the improvement and quality peril examinations of neighborhood and overall economies. Among which, the clinical field has been particularly changed, where a development in prosperity data emphasized by availability of various advances like Big Data, Machine Learning, Internet of Things (IoT) and Artificial Intelligence (AI) and others has basically helped judicious showing limits. The openness of judicious preparing gadgets and their following use in human administrations worldwide has gotten remarkable changes clinical exercises, singular medicine and the investigation of malady transmission, and such are depended upon to continue improving precision in this field, especially in accuracy of discovering [1]. Watson [2] further notes that these progressions are offering opportunities to judicious assessment through the novel evaluation of recorded and current clinical data. Man-made knowledge perceptive devices are starting at now at use in the selection and assessment of the social protection work power, and are all around also strengthened to fuse stresses of inclusivity and meritocracy [2].

Be that as it may, the vast majority of these registering devices are moderately new and as yet developing concerning the clinical field, and there are various related issues that despite everything should be valued and comprehended. Also, wellbeing experts and related partners have not completely grasped these innovations yet. Consequently, dangerous choices are still intensely dependent upon human-based understandings that are tedious and do not have an extensiveness of information assessments. This is valid in spite of numerous advancements being much slower when contrasted with choices got from the utilization of customary figuring innovations. On this, it is noticed that lawful structures can assist with directing issues like information assortment and sharing prompting greater receptivity by the wellbeing network. Nonetheless, the absence of normalization of conventions likewise implies that the extent of information to be broke down is restricted to explicit regions. In this manner, results got specifically clinical or potentially geological areas may not make a difference in others.

The utilization of AI-driven calculations for early identification of pandemics is in its development and might be a strong course sooner rather than later to help better readiness. It is normal that as the exactness of these innovations keep on propelling, they will have an increasingly articulated job in advancing the detailing of novel wellbeing strategies. This paper studies how information and AI forms helped in the beginning phases of the identification of the COVID-19 pandemic and gives fundamental supporting proof to grandstand that upgraded information sharing conventions will add to future urban wellbeing strategy globally.

Malady episodes simply like the coronavirus as often as possible spread excessively quick for researchers to find a treatment. Be that as it may, withinside the predetermination, engineered knowledge should help specialists to make a higher showing. While it's probable excessively past due for the juvenile period to play a central position withinside the current pandemic, there's a craving for the accompanying flare-ups. Artificial intelligence is perfect at brushing by means of hills of insights to find associations that make it less difficult to choose what assortments of cures should artistic creations or which investigations to seek after in this manner.

The question is the thing that Big Data will give you while it best gets pitiful pieces of records on a recently developed tainting like Covid-19, which initially rose past due shutting yr in China and has nauseated extra than 75,000 individuals in around months. Reality that specialists controlled to flexibly the quality sequencing of the shiny new infection inside long stretches of the essential expressed examples is promising in light of the fact that it proposes there's far extra on the spot insights to be had now while episodes occur. Andrew Hopkins, pioneer government official of Oxford, England-fundamentally based absolutely startup Exscientia Ltd. Is among the ones racing to help instruct manufactured insight for tranquilize disclosure. He figures new cures should cross from hypothesis to clinical looking at in as low as 18 to two years in the resulting decade, approach to AI.

Scientia planned a fresh out of the box new compound for rewarding an over the top habitual infection that is prepared to be analyzed withinside the lab after considerably less than a yr withinside the primer examinations stage. That is around 5 occasions faster than normal, predictable with the organization. Cambridge-principally based absolutely Healx has a similar methodology, in any case, it utilizes framework concentrating to find new utilizes for present pills. The two gatherings feed their calculations with records - gathered from resources including diaries, biomedical databases, and clinical preliminaries - to help propose new solutions for infections. The gatherings each utilization a team of human analysts to compositions along the AI to help manual the framework. In Exscientia's methodology, named the Centaur Chemist, medicate creators help train the calculations procedures for searching for mixes. Healx places the AI's forecasts to scientists who analyze the results and figure out what to seek after.

Neil Thompson, Healx's pioneer innovation official, expressed the strategy may be sent contrary to torment simply like the coronavirus as protracted in light of the fact that it had adequate insights on the fresh out of the box new illness. Healx isn't running on handling the coronavirus or tweaking its period for episodes, in any case, it wouldn't be a stretch. "We're entirely close," Thompson expressed in a meeting. "We wouldn't have any desire to expel a great deal roughly the AI calculations we use. We have a take a watch coordinating medication houses to infirmity highlights." One seizes for a portion of this innovation is clinical looking at. Indeed, even pills effectively secure to be utilized to treat one issue must be analyzed once sooner than they're recommended for another. The arrangement of showing they might be secure and ground-breaking on an enormous wide assortment of people can take years sooner than going to controllers for audit.

To be amazing, AI-essentially based thoroughly medicate manufacturers could need to devise ahead of time of time, picking out a plague genome plausible to thought process issues withinside the fate and concentrated on it while there are not many impetuses to do as such. Peruse extra around how drug makers are attempting to discover ways to deal with stop the coronavirus. Another obstacle is finding ensured staff.

"It's difficult to find people who can work on the crossing point of AI and science, and it's intense for colossal gatherings to settle on brief decisions on a time this way," expressed Irina Havas, a partner at challenge capital organization Atomic and past wellbeing specialist who sits at the leading body of Healx. "It's presently not, at this point adequate to be an AI engineer, you have to capture and get into the bundles of science."

The gigantic degree real factors of COVID-19 casualties may be fused and separated with the guide of using preferred system getting over know computations to higher see the case of viral spread, likewise improve expressive pace and precision, increase novel stunning repairing methodologies, and point of fact see the best inclined individuals essentially subject to revamp innate and physiological characteristics. Motivationally, inside a short interval of time when you consider that COVID-19 scene, preferable structure getting over acknowledge frameworks had been utilized in requested kind of COVID-19 genomes (8), CRISPR-in a general sense based totally COVID-19 acknowledgment measure (6), perseverance estimate of uncommon COVID-19 casualties (11), and going over limit sedate up-and-comers towards COVID-19 (4). Modified mindful strategies can fundamentally get from excellent portrayals of the majority essentially reliant on requested COVID-19 lack of protection. The early remark that developed individuals have a better open door than COVID-19 is tried with the guide of using a latest finding that a growing number of teenagers be badgering by phenomenal COVID-19 appearances, showing a crushing need of an all out chance examination in a general sense reliant on revamp innate and physiological characteristics.

This hypothesis ought to be likewise broke down with demanding exploratory plans and dependable period clinical recognitions. As such, natural science (e.g. ACE2 explanation level) and clinical real factors (e.g. age, breath test, viral weight, and perseverance) of COVID-19 casualties with principal clinical conditions may be examined with the guide of using structure getting familiar with methods to now not, now best observe any solid limits (e.g. ACE2) for chance gauge, at any rate besides equivalently complete chance sort and desire for a not too bad planning of advancing issue fix and COVID-19 watchman (Fig. 1). ACE2 innate polymorphism, addressed with the guide of using diverse genetic interpretations in human genome, has been exhibited to influence contamination limiting development (1), proposing a possible inherited tendency to COVID-19 ailment. Along these lines, system getting familiar with appraisal of genetic adjustments from asymptomatic, moderate or crazy COVID-19 casualties may be finished to sort and are expecting individuals essentially reliant on their shortcoming or security from limit COVID-19 tainting, with the guide of using which the structure getting familiar with variation furthermore can restore the ones composed innate structures, including ACE2 polymorphism, of their dynamic

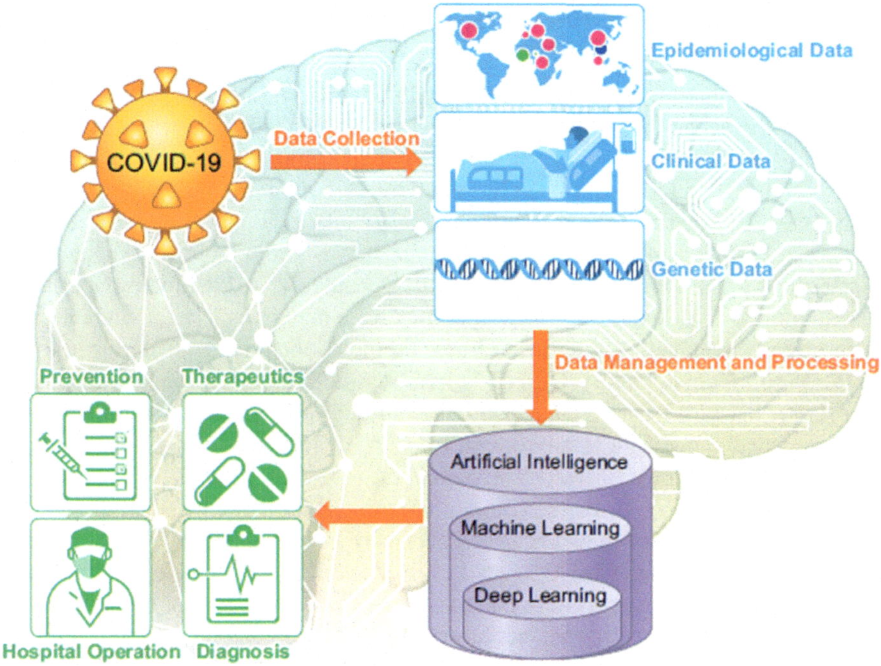

Fig. 1 Use of man-made reasoning and AI in the battle against COVID-19

path as fundamental capacities with respect to important and foolish assessments (Fig. 1).

At the present time, ceaseless undertakings had been made to fabricate novel expressive methods the utilization of system getting familiar with computations. For example, system getting progressively familiar with in a general sense based altogether screening of SARS-CoV-2 test structures the utilization of a CRISPR-mainly based totally disease distinguishing proof contraption got set up with over the top affectability and pace (6). Neural social order classifiers have been advanced for colossal degree screening of COVID-19 casualties in a general sense reliant on their amazing breath test (10). Moreover, a significant getting familiar with basically based completely evaluation contraption of thoracic CT photos got worked for modified disclosure and following of COVID-19 casualties after some time (five). Speedy improvement of modified suggestive structures basically reliant on fabricated knowledge and system getting familiar with now not, now best can make a promise to revived characteristic exactness and pace in any case will even watch social protection people with the guide of using diminishing their contacts with COVID-19 casualties (Fig. 1).

2 Premature Detection of the Coronavirus (COVID-19)

The true reprobation gave with the accommodating resource of the usage of the WHO on the scene of the offbeat coronavirus (COVID-19) create as made on the 9 January of 2020, in the wake of having gotten emotions from genuine property in its China Offices [7]. Before long, the contamination advanced beyond time (8 December 2019) at the same time as the primary pack of six patients initially exhorted proper straightforwardly into a Wuhan sanatorium wherein they were managed and discharged. From that treatment date on 31 December 2019, China prosperity real endeavored to choose if or now no longer they were managing a latest kind of disease with out advancement. Along these lines, the postponement in declaring the issue to the WHO China Country Office [3]. Among the bits of knowledge are given to prosperity masters create as that patients who had the symptoms and appearances and signs and signs were totally drawn from the Wuhan city catchment. This extra generally the lockdown of the entire Wuhan city at the 23 January 2020 [8].

Other than the lab ends on the contamination, it's far guided that AI-based counts, outer surface of China, had the alternative and give premature disclosure of the disease yet early than the WHO ascend as instructed, and with inside the end, made sense of how to alert adventurers that is probably at radical risk of being impacted. Inquisitively, the request rises concerning why the style will end up being right now not, now related to the supportive resource of the use of associations in China; head to the wisdom that information sharing principles must be barbed on this heading. Among the a victory associations is BlueDot with the intention of scoured information from records ends, transporter labeling, and animal sickness flare-ups, to predict areas which is in all probability is apparently dependent upon the scene, creating from locale in China [10]. Another business undertaking relationship with some capacities, Metabiota, used the identical system through Big Data assessment to song flight information to capably expect that domain is in all probability in peril to a coronavirus erupt days early than any case ascend as coordinated in any of those nations [6].

CT imaging is significant for finding, evaluation, and arranging COVID-19 pollution. Follow-up checks each three-five days are normally pushed for infection movement. It has been referenced that respective and fringe ground-glass opacification (GGO) without or with union are key CT discoveries in COVID-19 patients. Be that as it may, on account of lost programmed measurement instruments, best a subjective effect and a troublesome portrayal of aggravated areas are directly used in radiological reports. In this paper, profound learning (DL)- fundamentally based absolutely division machine is progressed to precisely evaluate pollution zones of premium (ROIs) and their volumetric proportions WRT The lung. The general execution of the machine transformed into assessed through assessing the precisely sectioned tainting territories with the physically portrayed ones on 300 chest CT sweeps of 300 COVID-19 patients. For quick guide outline of training tests and suitable guide mediation of electronic outcomes, a human-tuned in (HITL) approach has been followed to help radiologists for tainting area division, which significantly diminished the full division time to four mins after three cycles of variant refreshing.

The basic Dice closeness coefficient affirmed a 91.6% settlement among modernized and control infraction divisions, and the recommend estimation slip-ups of the extent of sullying (POI) transformed into 0.3% for the total lung. At long last, suitable applications, comprising of yet at this point not, at this point obliged to the assessment of follow-up CT outputs and defilement dispersions withinside the flaps and sections associated with clinical discoveries, have been talked about.

Create AI-essentially based absolutely programmed CT photo assessment gear for recognition, measurement, and checking of Coronavirus; show they can separate coronavirus victims from non-victims. Materials and Methods: Multiple overall datasets, comprehensive of from Chinese infirmity aroused districts had been incorporated. We blessing a device that utilizes solid 2D and 3-d profound acing designs, improving and adjusting current AI molds and blending them in with logical comprehension.

We performed more than one review analyses to investigate the general execution of the contraption withinside the discovery of suspected COVID-19 thoracic CT capacities and to survey the development of the sickness in each influenced individual during that time the utilization of a 3-d amount audit, delivering a Corona rating. The gander at comprises of an evaluating set of 157 overall victims (China and U.S). Results: Classification results for Coronavirus versus Non-coronavirus occurrences as indicated by thoracic CT research had been 0.996 AUC (95percentCI: 0.989-1.00); on datasets of Chinese control and aggravated victims. Conceivable working point: 98.2% affectability, 92.2% explicitness.

For the time assessment of Coronavirus victims, the device yield permits quantitative estimations for littler opacities (amount, breadth) and representation of the greater opacities in a cut basically based absolutely warmness map or a 3-d amount show. Our directed Corona rating estimates the advancement of the affliction as the years progressed. End: This fundamental gander at, that is directly being raised to a greater populace, set up that quickly advanced AI-basically based absolutely photo assessment can achieve unnecessary exactness withinside the recognition of Coronavirus notwithstanding measurement and checking of disease trouble.

A major amount of non-tainting zones improper to this look at had been also isolated the utilization of the 3-d division model, alongside the fibrotic state of aspiratory, calcification spots, or restorative zones analyzed inaccurately. In this way, an extra the class changed into brought as unseemly to-defilement with the exception of COVID-19 and Flu A-viral-pneumonia. Flu A-viral-pneumonia, and 175 refreshing cases). In this manner, a total of 3957 applicant 3D shapes had been created from the 3-d division model.

Just the domain close to the focal point of this dice contained most realities around this awareness of defilement. Subsequently, most straightforward the center photo all in all with the 2 companions of each dice changed into assembled to represent this spot for predetermination class steps. Next, all photo patches had been physically named by means of method of methods for master radiologists into types: unseemly to-defilement and pneumonia. The photos withinside the last class had been analyzed mechanically as COVID-19 or Influenza-A-viral-pneumonia fundamentally dependent on the logical investigation results.

Distinctive elements of COVID-19: ground-glass appearance, draping fringe dispersion nearby the pleura, and generally numerous fair-minded considerations of contaminations for one case. The styles have been enhanced fundamentally dependent on those discoveries. The photograph class of the adaptation got intended to separate the appearance and state of different contaminations. Besides, relatively good ways from-side as an extra weight got utilized for the variant to explore the relative district realities of the fix at the aspiratory photograph. The consideration of diseases situated close to the pleura became to be considerably more liable to be distinguished as COVID-19.

The old style ResNet-18 network shape got utilized for photograph trademark extraction. Pooling activities have been widely used for the dimensional markdown of realities to spare you overfitting and improve the difficulty of speculation. The yield of the convolution layer got leveled to a 256-dimensional trademark vector after which changed directly into a 16-dimensional trademark vector the utilization of a full-association network. For the locale intrigue network, the charge of relatively good ways from-side turned out to be previously standardized to the equivalent request of significant worth after which linked to this full-association network shape. Next, 3 full-association layers have been going with to yield the absolute last class final product all things considered with the confidence score.

The infection assortment from the ones anticipating device were transferred online to help specialists over the zone in finding an antibody, and to improve their analysis. Following purposeful coordinated efforts among splendid organizations, for the most part in measurements and data sharing, a few degrees of accomplishment in going up against the episode have just been made with the helpful asset of the utilization of a group of specialists drove with the valuable asset of the utilization. This research facility is likewise directed to boast productively positioned the infection in an open record wherein labs acquainted with the helpful asset of the utilization of the WHO can get appropriate of access to strengthen the quest for future immunizations. Also, the infection might be utilized to grow tests to help discover guardians which are conceivably contaminated and aren't by and by demonstrating any indications and side effects and signs and side effects of the infection, along these lines helping in guaranteeing that the broaden of the sickness is diminished.

3 Succinct Review on Transferable Syndrome Outburst in the Year 2020

This is of explicit essentialness because of the reality in the past endemic sicknesses right now are being planned by means of human being introduction to no endemic nations, accordingly cause epidemic episodes. Despite the fact that guidelines right now are being changed to spare you the unfurl of an infirmity to non-endemic nations,

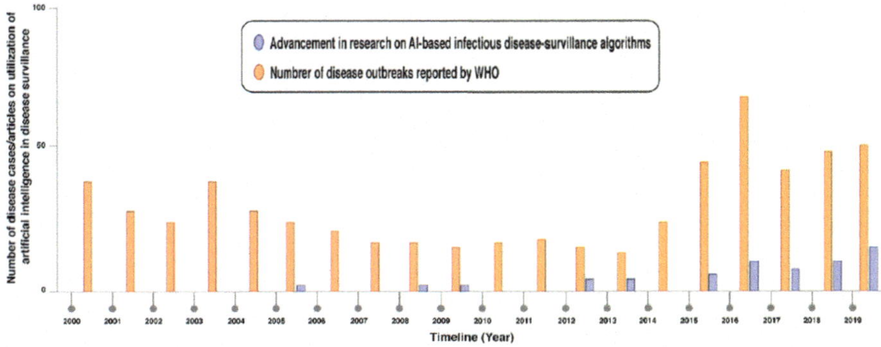

Fig. 2 AI based infectious diseases- surveillance algorithms

a decent arrangement artwork remains needed to find a scourge sooner than its genuine frequency all together that medicinal services strategies might be higher controlled and affected.

A PubMed question with the watchwords "("engineered knowledge") OR ("gadget knowledge") OR ("profound knowledge") AND ("infirmity reconnaissance"), likewise helps that present was a developing style in examines in regards to the improvement of AI-basically based absolutely calculations to higher are anticipating the consequences of present day medicinal services data, and thus to are expecting sickness flare-ups ahead of time. In spite of the fact that we do investigate that definite years do now not, at this point evidence any examinations on AI-innovation in infirmity observation, there was incredible examinations finished at the subject of AI-fundamentally based absolutely non-open human services. Figure 2 demonstrates the developing amount of AI-essentially put together thoroughly concentrates with respect to social insurance by means of a look for on PubMed the utilization of the catchphrases "("manufactured insight") AND ("pestilence") spoke to withinside the y-pivot, and the x-hub speaks to year.

4 Applications of Artificial Intelligence in COVID-19 Pandemic

4.1 Premature Detection and Diagnosis of Infection

Man-made intelligence can rapidly investigate unpredictable side effect and other 'warnings' and subsequently caution the patients and the human services specialists [4, 5]. It assists with giving quicker dynamic, which is financially savvy. It assists with building up another conclusion and the board framework for the COVID 19 cases, through helpful calculations.

4.2 Protrusion of Suitcases and Transience

This development can path and guess the possibility of the contamination from the open data, web-based life and media stages, about the threats of the sickness and its plausible spread. Supplementary, it envisions the quantity of optimistic cases and death in any territory. Computerized reasoning can lend a hand perceive the most fragile areas, people and countries and acquire checks in like way (Fig. 3).

4.3 Progress of Drugs and Vaccines

PC based knowledge is used for sedating investigate by examining available data on COVID-19. It is significant for a steady transport plan and improvement. This development is used in quickening drug testing continuously, where standard testing takes a ton of time and consequently helps with animating this technique through and through, which may not be possible by a human [6, 7]. It can help with perceiving accommodating meds for the handling of COVID-19 people. It has become an unfathomable resource for suggestive test plans and vaccination headway [9, 10]. Man-made brainpower helps in making inoculations and meds at a ton of snappier rate than anticipated and is furthermore valuable for clinical fundamentals during the improvement of the immune response.

4.4 Tumbling the Work of Healthcare Employees

Because of an abrupt and monstrous increment quantities of people through COVID-19 deadly disease, social insurance experts encompass an extremely elevated outstanding burden. Here, AI is utilized to decrease the outstanding burden of human services laborers. It help in early judgment and giving treatment at a beginning phase utilizing advanced methodologies and choice knowledge, offer the greatest preparing to understudies and specialists in regards to this new infection. Artificial intelligence can affect expectations unwearied consideration and address increasingly budding difficulties which diminish the outstanding task at hand of the specialists.

5 The Original AI Capability of Bluedot and Metabiota

5.1 Bluedot

For BlueDot to complete expectations on flare-up with respect to irresistible sicknesses, it is predicated intently on AI and device becoming more acquainted with

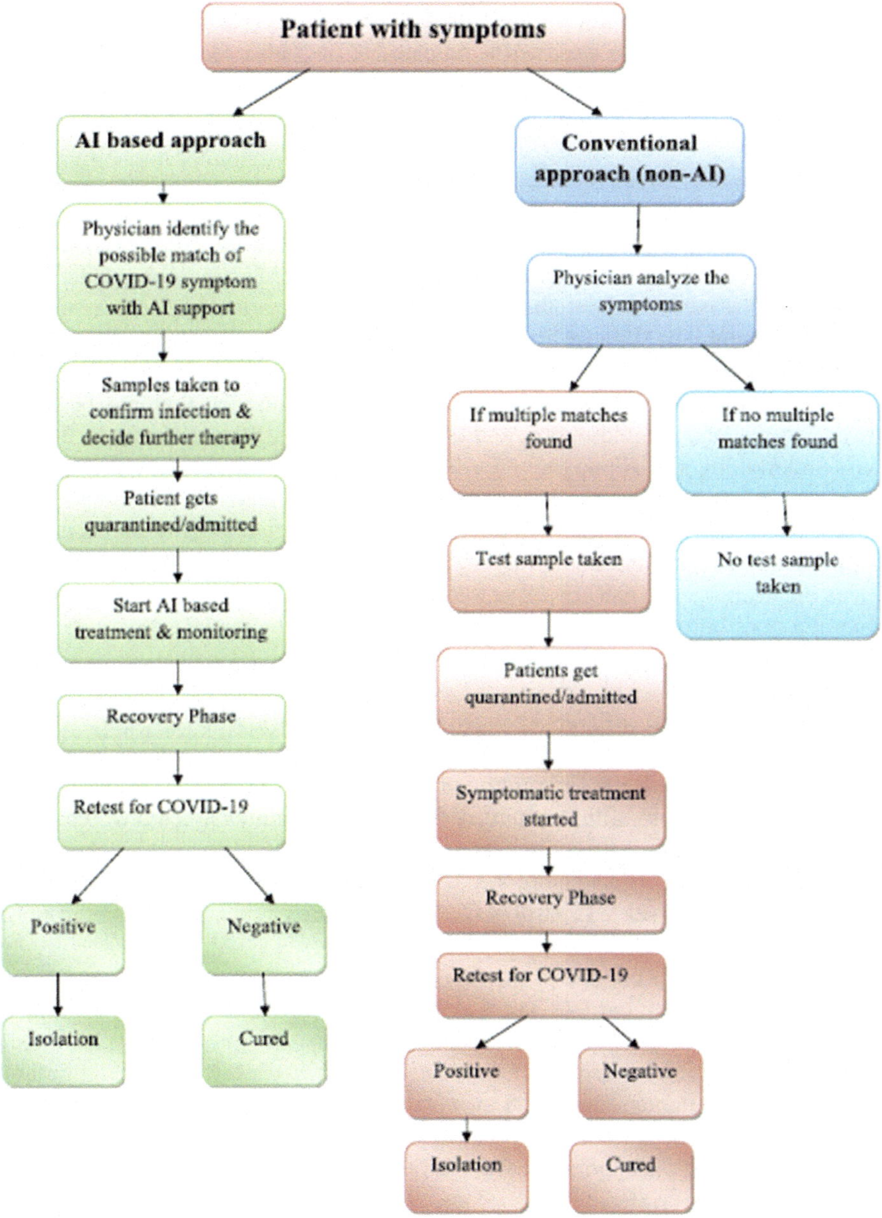

Fig. 3 General technique for AI applications that assist specialists to recognize the COVID-19 reactions

innovation. With these, and the use of different home-grown language handling calculations, the business endeavor is prepared to do gather records from a gigantic assortment of reasserts along with data retailers and overall aircraft tagging records. Beginning its site, this beginning up helps that it techniques enormous proceedings sourced from more than 10,000 representative and medium reasserts consistently, beginning more than sixty dialects. It's records place also comprises of realities on masses thickness; questioned from reasserts like nationwide censuses, World Factbook and nationwide records reports.

Different reasserts of records that BlueDot is predicated on incorporate the overall Infectious Disease Alert, continuous climate circumstances and bug vectors and creatures' issue supplies. With realities from these kinds of datasets, the business undertaking at that point utilizes sifting apparatus to slim down areas of intrigue and recruit viable grouping rigging to allow the short disclosure of districts that may be showed up as warm spots, bloodless spots and spatial anomalies. With the records, the business undertaking at that point applies device becoming acquainted with and home-grown language handling innovation to show the machine, and it's far subsequently equipped for transport ordinary markers to its customers, explicitly on occurrences of atypical issue and the possibility stressed and the anticipated areas particularly plausible to appreciate flare-ups. The tutoring of the machine incorporates the utilization of a possibility assessment form that uses the enormous datasets sourced from differing area names to recognize, banner and explain portraying capacity expect the unfurl flare-ups. Crafted by this web-essentially based absolutely fire up had been built up at some phase wherein changed into able to do productively craft forecasts the use of worldwide air visit records to anticipate the overall pathway of the episode.

BlueDot is restrictive programming program-as-a-supplier intended to find, tune and expect irresistible affliction unfurl. The BlueDot motor assembles records on more than one hundred fifty ailments and conditions round the part looking every 15 min, 24 h per day. This comprises of genuine records from partnerships simply like the Center for Disease Control or the World Health Organization. Yet, the gadget furthermore depends on substantially less based records.

A lot of BlueDot's prescient limit originates from records it gathers out of entryways genuine wellness care resources along with, for instance, the worldwide moves of more prominent than 4 billion travelers on business flights every year; human, creature and bug masses records; climate records from satellites; and neighborhood records from columnists and social insurance laborers, pouring through 100,000 on line articles each day spreading over sixty five dialects.

BlueDot's specialists physically named the records, developed a scientific classification so appropriate key expressions might be filtered proficiently, after which executed framework examining and home grown language handling to instruct the gadget. Subsequently, it says, most straightforward a bunch of occasions are hailed for human experts to dissect.

BlueDot conveys customary signs to wellness care, government, business, and open wellness customers. The signs offer short outlines of abnormal illness episodes that its AI motor has found and the risks they'll present.

On account of COVID-19, the gadget hailed articles in Chinese that articulated 27 pneumonia occurrences identified with a commercial center that had fish and stay creatures in Wuhan. Notwithstanding the alarm, BlueDot viably perceived the towns that had been somewhat identified with Wuhan the utilization of such things as universal aircraft tagging records to help expect in which the aroused is most likely voyaging. The worldwide areas that BlueDot anticipated may have the best degree of travelers from Wuhan had been: Bangkok, Hong Kong, Tokyo, Taipei, Phuket, Seoul, and Singapore. At long last, eleven of the towns on the apex in their posting had been the essential areas to look COVID-19 occasions.

COVID-19 become now not, at this point BlueDot's previously hit. The motor has been utilized to proficiently expect that the Zika infection may unfurl to Florida in 2016, six months sooner than it occurred. The product program furthermore concluded that the 2014 Ebola episode would withdraw West Africa.

5.2 Metabiota

Metabiota depends on innovation calculations to make expectations around irresistible confusion episodes, spreads, intercessions, and event seriousness. Utilizing Neuro-Linguistic Programming (NLP) calculations, this San Francisco basically based absolutely manager assembles monstrous amounts of realities from each true and informal reassets, similar to the ones from organic, financial, political and ecological outskirts, and through unrivaled scientific and perception of frequencies, seriousness, and time of episodes, it might deliver right forecasts. Dissimilar to BlueDot, which scarcely ever depends upon via web-based networking media for realities, Metabioita is situated to here and there, as withinside the current instance of the COVID-19 flare-up, to aggregate and utilize online life realities to make its forecasts.

Other than inclusion offices, Metabiota's artworks also points of interest legislative offices, non-income associations, temporary workers, and establishments among various elements who depend upon such records to settle on better-educated decisions in exercises of irresistible issue episodes. It is a result of this that the business delayed its degree to take into account inclusion offices, and these days it has gathered a total issue database. It is currently utilizing present day, prescient innovation like concentrating to make forecasts. subsequent this, while COVID-19 transformed into stated, from beginning to end the utilize of this innovation, it transformed into on the front in foreseeing the accompanying affected wards, aside from Wuhan in which the infection transformed into above all else encountered; this forecast arrived each week ahead of time sooner than the essential examples have been said during the ones goals. This transformed into did through the use of home grown language handling; in which the business transformed into capin a situation to utilize online networking realities from outstanding reassets to tune the unfurl of the infection; henceforth, render considerably more noteworthy right expectations.

6 Conclusion

The situation of Artificial Intelligence (AI) with inside the late identification radical coronavirus is archived on this document from end to end the works as a art of organizations, BlueDot and Metabiota, it shows AI-pushed calculations can deliver additional specific expectations and readings with inside the fate through improved records sharing. The paper helps that improved records sharing activity should be authorized inside the city wellness region simultaneously as standing through the size of privateers and assurance as a result of the sensitive idea of insights happening engineering. happening this, AI techniques illustration beginning well-dressed records reasserts furthermore commencing well-dressed city innovation and that related mechanical ideas, combined with wearable advances, can and should be energized, in light of the fact that it will deliver huge datasets and subsequently extra right forecast and discovery. For this completion, there's a need for the normalization of conventions to rouse verbal trade among devices and all through structures without bargaining records assurance and halting records oversight. The innovative upheaval upon us will see a developing utilization of registering strategies, and as their exactness will increment higher control choices can be delivered; as with inside the instance of pandemics, and could hence bring about its extraordinary situation in city wellness strategy.

References

1. Brickwood, B.: The power of AI in providing rapid at-home assessments of the coronavirus, The Health Europa, 6th March 2020
2. Suthaharan, S.: Machine learning models and algorithms for big data classification. Integr. Series Inf. Syst. **36**, 183–206. Springer
3. Tryfona, N., Price, R., Jensen, C.S.: Conceptual Models for Spatio-Temporal Applications, vol. 2520, pp. 79–116. Springer
4. Thampi, S., Gelbukh, A., Mukhopadhyay, J.: Advances in signal processing and intelligent recognition systems. Adv. Intell. Syst. Comput. **264**, 439–450. Springer
5. Zin, T.T., Takahashi, R., Hama, H.: Innovative computing, information and control. In: Second International Conference on, Sept 2007, pp. 310–310
6. Maddah, E., Beigzadeh, B.: Use of a smartphone thermometer to monitor thermal conductivity changes in diabetic foot ulcers: a pilot study. J. Wound Care **29**(1), 61–66 (2020)
7. Story, A., Aldridge, R.W., Smith, C.M., Garber, E., Hall, J., Ferenando, G., Abubakar, I.: Smartphone-enabled videoobserved versus directly observed treatment for tuberculosis: a multicentre, analyst-blinded, randomised, controlled superiority trial. The Lancet **393**(10177), 1216–1224 (2019)
8. Ghoshal, B., Tucker, A.: Estimating uncertainty and interpretability in deep learning for coronavirus (COVID-19) detection. arXiv preprint arXiv:2003.10769 (2020)

9. Mirza, M., Osindero, S.: Conditional generative adversarial nets. arXiv preprint arXiv:1411.1784. In: Nguyen, T., Khosravi, A., Creighton, D., Nahavandi, S.: Epidemiological dynamics modeling by fusion of soft computing techniques. In: The 2013 International Joint Conference on Neural Networks (IJCNN), pp. 1–8. IEEE (2014)
10. Khan, A., Sohail, A., Zahoora, U., Qureshi, A.S.: A survey of the recent architectures of deep convolutional neural networks. Artif. Intell. Rev. (2020). https://doi.org/10.1007/s10462-020-09825-6

Application of Artificial Intelligence for COVID-19 Epidemic: An Exploratory Study, Opportunities, Challenges, and Future Prospects

Joseph Bamidele Awotunde, Sakinat Oluwabukonla Folorunso, Rasheed Gbenga Jimoh, Emmanuel Abidemi Adeniyi, Kazeem Moses Abiodun, and Gbemisola Janet Ajamu

Abstract The occurrence of coronavirus (COVID-19) is greater than that of 2003 representing respiratory infections syndrome (SARS). As of 12 August 2020, the reported cases are more than 73,435 deaths and more than 2000 deaths worldwide, and both COVID-19 and SARS are distributed across regions, infecting living beings. By contrast, in 2003, SARS claimed 774 lives but in the shortest time, COVID-19 claimed more than that. But the major difference among them is that since 17 years of SARS others power new tool has emerged, which could be used as an instrument in fighting this virus and keeping it within reasonable limits. Artificial intelligence (AI) is one of those tools. Recently, AI is causing a paradigm shift in the healthcare sector, and the applicability it in the COVID-19 outbreak might yield profit especially in predicting the location of the next outbreak. The application of AI in COVID-19 can be expediting the diagnoses and monitoring of COVID-19 and minimizes the burden of these processes. Therefore, this chapter discusses the areas of applicability of AI during the COVID-19 pandemic. Discusses several extraordinary opportunities brought by AI in the COVID-19 outbreak and the research challenges of AI during

J. B. Awotunde (✉) · R. G. Jimoh
Department of Computer Science, University of Ilorin, Ilorin, Nigeria
e-mail: awotunde.jb@unilorin.edu.ng

R. G. Jimoh
e-mail: jimoh_rasheed@unilorin.edu.ng

S. O. Folorunso
Department of Mathematical Science, Olabisi Onabanjo University, Ago-Iwoye, Nigeria
e-mail: sakinat.folorunso@oouagoiwoye.edu.ng

E. A. Adeniyi · K. M. Abiodun
Department of Department of Computer Science, Landmark University, Omu Aran, Nigeria
e-mail: adeniyi.emmanuel@lmu.edu.ng

K. M. Abiodun
e-mail: moses.abiodun@lmu.edu.ng

G. J. Ajamu
Department of Agricultural Extension and Rural Development, Landmark University, Omu Aran, Nigeria
e-mail: ajamu.gbemisola@lmu.edu.ng

D. Oliva et al. (eds.), *Artificial Intelligence for COVID-19*, Studies in Systems, Decision and Control 358, https://doi.org/10.1007/978-3-030-69744-0_4

the outbreak. In medical detection, the use of AI has increased tremendously. This has been commonly used to achieve relatively precise recognition accuracy and to reduce the burden on health systems by reducing the time of evaluation associated with conventional approach detection procedure. The AI techniques are seen as a major aspect in identifying the risk of infectious diseases in enhancing the forecasting and identification of potential world health threats. The continued expansion of AI for the Covid-19 disease outbreak has dramatically improved monitoring, diagnosis, monitoring, analysis, forecasting, touch trailing, and medications/vaccine production process and minimized human involvement in nursing treatment.

Keywords Artificial intelligence · Coronavirus · COVID-19 epidemic · Diagnosis · Prediction · Healthcare system

1 Introduction

The outbreak of Coronavirus (COVID-19) infection at Wuhan, Chain in December 2019 spreading widely across the world. Globally, as stated to the WHO as of 1 September 2020, there were 25,328,298 identified COVID-19 cases, with 850,926 global deaths at 10:50 am CEST in 213 countries/regions [1]. Since it is a new pandemic, real drug strategies were not anticipated to be ready for any time soon; meanwhile, community-based control methods such as stay home policy and lock-outs were effectively applied by affected countries to flatten the pandemic curve affecting an estimated 3 billion people worldwide [2].

COVID-19 is extremely infectious and can spread complications before and after the onset. Monitoring and lockdown have to encompass anyone with symptoms and properly isolate persons who have been infected from those who are not, to allow good containment. Patients carrying the virus could either be minor symptomless (like fever, sore throat, and sneezing) or have serious clinical signs (such as pneumonia, respiratory failure, and eventually death) [3]. The transmittable SARS-CoV-2 condition is called "coronavirus disease" (COVID-19) [4]. Gratitude to the recent developments in analytical techniques and information and communication technologies (ICTs), artificial intelligence (AI) and big data will aid manage the immense, unparalleled volume of data generated from patient monitoring, real-time tracking of disease outbreaks, now-casting/ predicting patterns, daily situation briefings and public updates [5].

The use of machine learning and statistical methods to forecast uncertain or potential effects is referred to as predictive analysis [6, 7]. It responds to the question as to what is the next step? It also uses past and present data to predict actions, patterns, and activity in the future. The prediction is rendered using quantitative questions, automated machine learning, and statistical analysis [7]. Experts need to construct predictive models that are used for forecasting in predictive analytics [7]. Artificial Intelligence (AI) is an umbrella word that depicts various tools for knowledge and control. Without an AI instrument, the data from a wearable would be without any worth to the merchant as well as the consumer. For this purpose, wearable app inventors are progressively adding AI engine inside wearable medical apps. Furthermore, AI aided data mining is also fundamental to the attainment of an intellectual medical care platform that connects many smartphones, website, IoT gadgets, and wearables together to congregate data and benefit fascinating medical comprehensions of an individual [8, 9].

Health professionals are in desperate need of technology for decision-making to tackle this epidemic and allow them to get timely feedback in real-time to prevent its transmission. AI works to simulate the human intellect competently. This may also play a crucial role in interpreting and recommending the creation of a COVID-19 vaccine. This result-driven engineering is used to better scan, evaluate, forecast, and monitor current clinicians and patients expected to be future. The relevant technologies relate to the monitoring of verified, recovered, and death cases.

The scientific research centered on generating new data through the performing of basic experiments to answer specific questions related to any infectious diseases. The collection and storing of a huge amount of data digitally are growing exponentially. This may require patients to receive care at various hospitals within a region, thus underrepresent or over-represent key clinical feature studies single-site. The 2019 outbreak of coronavirus infection (COVID-19) represents an increasing global threat. People are more bonded than ever, our towns are extremely highly populated and in previous years most people have seen successive waves of the fresh severe acute respiratory syndrome (SARS), Ebola virus, Zika virus, and recently COVID-19 and influenza viral infections threatening worldwide epidemics.

The data science analysis using AI is newly evolving, intending to empower health care systems and organizations to connect to harness information and convert it to usable knowledge and preferably personalized clinical decision making. Utilizing deep learning, the implementation of AI in the field of infectious diseases has implemented a range of improvements in the modeling of knowledge generation. Big data can be interpreted, stored, and collected in healthcare through the constantly emerging field of AI models, thereby allowing the understanding, rationalization, and use of data for various reasons. Therefore, this chapter discusses the concept of AI techniques to guaranteeing better expansion and research against the COVID-19. The hope of using AI in COVID-19 will have a great impact on the quality of outbreak diagnosis, prediction, and treatment and can be delivered quality care to patients across socioeconomic and geographic boundaries.

2 Artificial Intelligence (AI) Techniques in COVID-19 Outbreak

During this global health emergency, the healthcare profession is pursuing technological innovations to track and regulate the spreading of outbreak Coronavirus. AI is one of those tools that can quickly monitor the rapid spreading of the diseases, classify high-risk patients, and is important for real-time monitoring of this outbreak. It can also forecast mortality risk by an appropriate review of the clinicians' previous results. AI can help us combat this epidemic through mass screening, medical support, warning, and recommendations about managing infections [10–12]. This innovation can enhance COVID-19 patient preparation, medication, and reporting performance, as a reliable medical method.

Figure 1 displays the systematic process for AI-based applications that help general practitioners recognize COVID-19 symptoms. The flowchart advises and describes a patient's diagnosis and treatment with AI-based COVID-19. The flowchart illustrates AI's role in substantial high precision treatment processes and decreases uncertainty and time taken. The health personnel focuses not only on the patient's condition but also on infection prevention with the implementation of AI. Significant indications and test analyzes are performed with the best classification with the assistance of AI. It also shows the series of phases taken during the entire method is reduced, making them more procurable.

Artificial Intelligence (AI) centers on complications that hypothetically only individuals and animals can unravel, difficulties needing intelligence. It is a section of computer science considering complications for which there are no operational computational algorithms. The term acts as patronage under which further approaches have been added over time [13]. Methods of artificial intelligence have produced an increased focus level within the research community. As defined in many recent findings, machine learning approaches offer valuable detection accuracy in comparison with different data classification techniques [14–16]. Accomplishing conspicuous correctness in forecasting is significant because it could lead to an appropriate precaution programmer. Forecasting correctness may differ varying on diverse studying systems methodologies. Hence, it is fundamental to recognize devices proficient in offering extreme accuracy of projection in COVID-19 outbreaks and outbursts.

Artificial Intelligence approaches are the best successful policymaking methods aimed at the genuine world and systematic difficulties. The intention is also to examine the performance of diverse AI approaches for the categorization of COVID-19 samples. Diverse categorization performance capacities have been employed for the assessment of the performance of AI approaches. Six commonly used Artificial Intelligence approaches are as follows: Artificial Neural Network (ANN), Support Vector Machine (SVM), linear regression, K-Nearest Neighbor (KNN), multilayer perceptron, and classification algorithm.

In previous research works, Machine Learning was put to application in the biomedical field [15–19], for the involvement of heart disease and diabetes [21], in the investigation of diabetes proteins [20] among others. The best significant AI techniques that have been utilized by academics are ANN, SVM, Fuzzy Logic systems, K-means classifier, and many others [15, 16, 22–24].

An alternative type of AI techniques that had been applied by scholars to classify COVID-19 cases is the fuzzy logic classifier method [25]. Al-Qaness et al. [25] Unveil a novel predictive method for estimating and predicting the number of reported COVID-19 instances over the next ten days, due to the previous cases

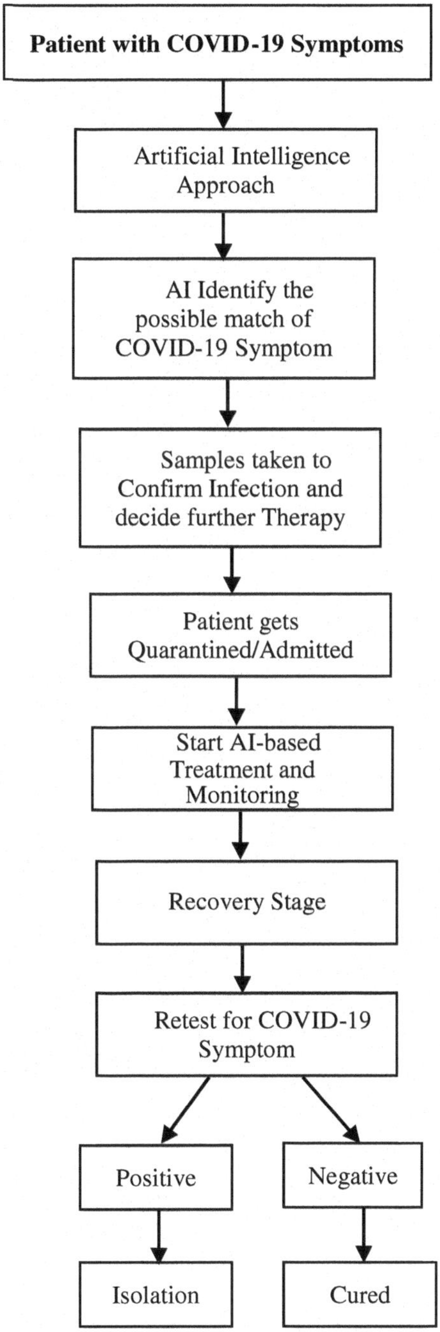

Fig. 1 An AI-based general technique in recognizing the COVID-19 symptoms

reported observed in China. The suggested framework is an enriched adaptive neuro-fuzzy inference system (ANFIS) using a greatly improved flower pollination algorithm (FPA) using the algorithm Salp swarm (SSA). The accuracy of their studies was examined in contradiction to the rate of misclassified instances, and it gives a promising performance concerning Mean Absolute Percentage Error (MAPE), root - mean - square Relative Error (RMSRE), Root Mean Squared Relative Error (RMSRE), Determination Coefficient (R2), and Computation Time. Also, we evaluated the proposed framework utilizing two separate datasets of reported cases of weekly influenza in two nations, namely the USA and China. The results showed an even strong performance.

Numerous techniques and algorithms were also utilized to extract confidential information from biomedical datasets to predict the COVID-19 outbreak. The Adaptive Neuro-Fuzzy Inference Method (ANFIS) [26] is commonly used in analyzing and modeling issues in the time series and has shown strong success in several current applications. It provides versatility in evaluating time series data non - linearity, as well as incorporating the features of both artificial neural networks (ANN) and fuzzy logic systems. It has been used in different applications for prediction. An AI is the capacity of systems that are normally in the computer hardware and software format to imitate or surpass individual intelligence in daily engineering and systematic undertakings connected with identifying, intellectual, and performing. AI is multifaceted since individual intelligence is multifaceted, hence including objectives that vary from knowledge representation and intellectual to acquiring, to ophthalmic observation and language understanding.

Hitherto, the implementations of AI methods have shown positive results in numerous commercial and tourism environments to discover new behavior and identify the potential for the future. The recent modern systems, like machine learning, ANN techniques, have shown positive outcomes in the extraction from a massive dataset of nonlinear dynamic structures. Recent findings using AI techniques to monitor rodent reservoirs of future zoonotic diseases within a disease-related framework [27], Predict Extended-spectrum β-lactamase (ESBL) generating species [28], and regulation of outbreaks of tuberculosis (TB) and gonorrhea [5]. It can be hard to forecast public response to infectious diseases. However, we are progressively able to compare population behavior with deadly diseases with the accessibility of Big Data and the emergence of AI methods. For example, dedicated studies employed a psychosocial informatics and data science method [29–31]. During the outbreak era, examined infection control outbreaks correlated with digital activity trends through search engine trends (such as Google Trend). It is envisaged that the development of AI technologies for infection control data analytics will boost our opportunity to actively monitor social interaction to infectious diseases and effectively forecast infectious spread, which can help policymakers take timely steps to respond to any pandemic. Applications of AI can be useful tools in assisting diagnoses and decision making in COVID-19 treatment.

3 The Applicability of Artificial Intelligence During COVID-19 Pandemic

Artificial Intelligence is a revolutionary technology that can be used to tackle disease outbreak COVID-19. This innovation helps to better scan, monitor, and forecast current and potential patients. The key implementation of AI is to identify and diagnose the infection early on. An AI can be used to produce medicines and vaccines, and to reduce the strain of medical personnel. The techniques of AI may be outlined in two groups based on two separate styles of learning: supervised and unsupervised machine learning. Supervised learning is the process of introducing a feature from the training samples, including SVM, Decision Tree, Random Forest, Naïve Bayes (NB), Artificial Neural Network (ANN), Bootstrap Aggregating, AdaBoost, that could easily manage the regression and classification problem in health information [32, 33].

All these approaches may be beneficial in assessing diagnostic accuracy and in recommending effective care for patients with COVID-19. In particular, the predictive results from these approaches may be used to alert authorities and the populace in anticipation and recommend suitable strategies for prevention and management. Unattended learning techniques such as Principal Component Analysis (PCA) may be used to minimize data proportions, making it possible for scientists to recognize some primary COVID-19 disease outbreak causes [34]. Some unsupervised principles of learning, like K-means, might classify COVID-19 victims and identify suspicious patients which might direct scientists to concentrate on these medical situations. Furthermore, topic models like the Latent Dirichlet Allocation (LDA) may be used to remove the issues from the medical book record. Recently, deep learning models were widely used in prediction and diagnosis, filtering social networks, and computational biology and are considered effective techniques for analyzing infectious diseases.

AI can scrutinize the abnormal symptoms as well as other 'obvious signs' swiftly and alerts patients and medical officials [35, 36]. It provides great quicker policy-making, which is cost-effective. It tends to help, through valuable techniques, establish a new treatment and monitoring skills for the COVID 19 cases. Using diagnostic imaging innovations such as Computed Tomography (CT), Magnetic Resonance Imaging (MRI) scanning of human organs, AI helps diagnose highly contagious cases.

AI will provide relevant information with the aid of real-time analysis, which is useful in preventing this infection. It could be used to forecast possible sites of an outbreak throughout this epidemic, the proliferation of the epidemic, the need for spaces, and health care providers. AI is useful for the potential detection of viruses and illnesses, with the aid of prior coached data over data that are present at various times. It describes the features, sources, and factors why infection has dispersed. This will be a promising technique in the future for fighting other outbreaks and infectious diseases. It can provide precautionary action and tackle various illnesses.

In the future, AI can play a crucial role in making healthcare more informative and reactive.

AI will create a smart framework to automatically track and forecast the spreading of this outbreak. [10, 38, 39]. A genetic algorithm may also be built to remove the visual characteristics of this infection. It has the potential to provide patients with daily alerts and also to offer better options for COVID-19 epidemic follow-up.

AI can easily determine this virus' level of transmission by recognizing the fragments and 'hot spots' and can effectively track the individuals' contacts and even monitor them. It can foresee this spread of the disease's future path, and possibly reoccurrence. These technologies can also monitor and predict the existence of the epidemic from the data, social media, and broadcasting channels present, about the threats of the outbreak and its probable spreading. It can also forecast the number of use cases and deaths in any area. AI will help recognize the areas, citizens, and communities most affected and take effective measures.

Analysis of available data on COVID-19 allows the use of AI for drug testing. It's suitable for the production and creation of therapeutics. This innovation is used to expedite drug screening in real-time, where normal screening takes a lot of time and thus enables to greatly achieve a better result, which a person would not be able to accomplish [37–39]. Identifying useful drugs for treating COVID-19 patients can help. This has become a strong instrument for designing diagnostic tests and improving vaccinations [40–42]. AI helps to produce vaccines and therapies much quicker than normal and is also effective in clinical trials during vaccine production.

Healthcare workers have such a heavy workload because of a rapid and unprecedented rise in the number of patients during the COVID-19 outbreak. Here AI is being used to minimize health professionals' duties [43–48]. It assists with initial screening and effective medication using digital methodologies and decision-making skills, provides the best exercise for students and health professionals on this new virus [49–51]. AI can greatly impact clinical outcomes and address more future problems that reduce the physicians' burden.

4 The Challenges Applying Artificial Intelligence During COVID-19 Pandemic

AI can become an instrument in fighting COVID-19 and related infectious diseases. Conversely, AI programs are only at a foundational level, and the effects of such AI interventions will take some time to be evident [52]. In its analysis of the use of AI toward COVID-19, [53] concluded that at this point, very little of the [AI] programs tested are operationally mature. In reality, AI is limited by the lack of data and by much more data. There are (yet) inadequate available data to train AI models, inadequate open datasets and approaches to work on, yet also possible problems of big data hubris, non-adjustment of methods, and outer data and a deluge of scientific results, all of which have to be switched.

Valuable as these are, the concern is that after the epidemic is over, data protection degradation will not be pushed back and policymakers will continue to help their increased capacity to monitor their populations- and use the data collected for other purposes in the battle with COVID-19. As [54] advises "though if coronavirus diseases are almost being eliminated, some information-hungry policymakers may claim they wanted to keep biometric tracking mechanisms in place because they are afraid of a second wave of the diseases, or because a new Ebola outbreak is emerging in the central region of Africa, or because … you have the concept". The use of AI for COVID-19 prediction and diagnosis is hindered by a deficiency of relevant training samples, AI resources such as image recognition and automation are not.

While it has been stated that several Chinese clinics have implemented "AI-Based" radiology innovation, the promise of AI is still not implemented. Radiologists elsewhere have raised concerns that inadequate data are available to train AI models, that most of the accessible COVID-19 samples emerge from Chinese medical centers and may suffer from sample preference, and that the use of CT scans and X-rays may pollute instruments and further transmit the infection. The use of CT scans in European medical centers has progressively decreased after the disease outbreak has ended.

Owing to a lack of evidence, crowded social platforms and outlier data, big data hubris, and computational complexities, COVID-19 spread AI predictions are still not very reliable and valid [55]. The majority of frameworks used for monitoring and forecasting so far do not use AI approaches. Rather, most analysts consider epidemiologically proven models, the so-called SIR models. The Robert Koch Institute in Berlin, for example, uses an immunological SIR method that captures into account government control steps, such as lockdowns, quarantines, and social distancing recommendations. This method was established in China to demonstrate that containment would succeed in limiting the incidence to slower than the [56] exponential value. Table 1 presents overviews of AI problems in the COVID-19 epidemic.

The latest outbreak of COVID-19 has brought the difficulty of securing personal data to a head in a transnational sense [57], this is because COVID-19 spreads fast with the international travel of people [58]. Many countries require international travelers to disclose their personal information such as the name, gender, date of birth, travel history, the purpose of travel, and residence, among others, and impose quarantine requirements accordingly [59]. Using a genuine case where Chinese media secretly published the sensitive information of a foreign traveler, the article describes that multiple patterns for LEX cause emerged at each point of dispute-of-law analysis: (1) the EU, the US, and China vary in characterizing the right to personal data; (2) The expanding centralized approach to relevant legislation lies in the fact that all three territories either find the law on personal information privacy to be a contractual law or follow linking factors leading to the law of the forum, and (3) actively support the de-Americanization of meaningful data privacy legislation. The patterns and their mechanisms have important consequences in the application of regulations for transnational information [57].

Evolving contagious diseases like HIV/ AIDS, SARS, and pandemic influenza, and the 2001 anthrax attacks, have proven that we appear vulnerable to risks to

Table 1 Limitations of artificial intelligence

S/No	Challenges of AI	Explanations
1	Requires proper supervision	It doesn't have any other information like a person to represent the exact result It needs serious monitoring and data collection; else, practitioners and physicians are not producing accurate findings
2	Not provide creative thinking	Only precise information will yield enough performance It can not satisfy the definition of innovative thinking in COVID-19 like a human being, because a human being can feel, learn to make a valuable decision about the computer system This new technology does not allow for new decision without any data
3	Only learns from the given data	AI always operates from the patient's provided data Precise diagnosis and forecasting of COVID-19 relies on the data collected
4	Crucial for treatment by AI algorithm used	One of the major drawbacks is the proportion of accuracy of the estimation used by the AI algorithm, which is quite important for the care and even more so The potential scenario of the predictions would be whether an AI's function is an absolute way or whether it requires more data and train over time
5	Does not understand the emotion	AI approaches do not grasp the feelings, human reasoning, and motives for making the right decision AI computers do just what they are configured to do

health from contagious diseases [60–62]. The key expert recommendation for 2 decades has been the value of improving global public health surveillance to provide an early warning [61, 62]. Based on digital information sources, including data from smartphones and other digital equipment, the outbreaks triggered by new findings are of special importance infectious diseases [60, 61, 63], the survey data and accurate predictions for which are indeed limited. Recent research shows the likelihood of predicting the spreading of COVID-19 by integrating Government Aviation Guide data with WeChat App data on human accessibility and other digital platforms run by Chinese technology giant Tencent [64].

Smartphone data also demonstrated possibilities for modeling regional cholera erupted in Haiti during the 2010 outbreak [65], while using Big Data analysis demonstrated efficacy during the Ebola crisis in the year 2014–2016 [66]. Moreover, the big data gathering of cellular data from users around the world, particularly mobile data archives and social network accounts, also raised questions about security and data integrity during those recent epidemics. In 2014, the GSM organization (a sector body that serves the benefits of major mobile network operators) urged privacy issues to issue privacy rules for the use of cell phone data to respond to an Ebola outbreak [67].

In the information-intensive world of 2020, these issues can easily be compounded by pervasive data points and automated surveillance devices. China is the area hardest hit with COVID-19, has reportedly used omnipresent transmitter data and safety monitoring software to avoid disease spread [68]. The New York Times reports [69], how these data are reviewed and recycled for monitoring reasons is not clear. For instance, the document said that Alipay Health Code, an Alibaba-backed government-run app that helps decision on who is to be isolated for COVID-19, also seemed to share details with the police [63]. The European republic, in Italy with the highest figure of COVID-19 incidents, the remote data-privacy agency was advised to issue a statement [70], on 2 March 2020 to explain the requirements of permissible data usage for containment and prevention. In its declaration, the expert cautioned against data gathering and analysis by a non-institutional body that violates privacy [70].

5 Conclusion

Coronavirus is a disease that has spread globally after it was reported in Wuhan, China. Smart medical technology has played a significant role in the battle against COVID-19. This chapter explores how AI in combating the COVID-19 epidemic offers secure, reliable, and efficient responses. New technology in the field of medicine, artificial intelligence has successfully contributed to combating COVID-19. AI allows safer, more reliable, and more effective medical technologies compared to the conventional procedure of the public health system, which relies primarily on human labor. Current AI-enhanced implementations in COVID-19 include especially the specialized new methodology, the differentiation of the respiratory and infection area, clinical evaluation, and evaluation, as well as groundbreaking preclinical and applied research. Besides, several commercial applications were already produced which clearly show the functionality of this innovation to fully implement AI to tackle COVID-19. These illustrate the global community's enthusiasm for AI-enhanced developments in the medical sector, especially during the COVID-19 outbreak. Given the significance of AI across all aspects of COVID-19's health-based assessment, this chapter seeks to discuss thoroughly the position of AI in combating the COVID-19 disease outbreak, which will motivate future real-world applications and methodological study. In the following, we first introduce smart AI for COVID-19 and then discussed the overview of common machine learning techniques in COVID-19 global battle, including early detection and prevention, monitoring patient care, vaccine, and drug growth, prediction of confirmed and mortality cases, and contract tracking of individual cases. The chapter finally, discuss several challenges and open problems of the application of AI for COVID-19. Patients suspicious of COVID-19 are in desperate need of diagnosis and adequate care in epidemic areas and thus AI is an important technology in this direction.

References

1. COVID-19 Dashboard by the Center for Systems Science and Engineering (CSSE) at Johns Hopkins University (JHU) (2020).https://coronavirus.jhu.edu/map.html. Accessed September 2020
2. Dunford, D., Dale, B., Stylianou, N. Lowther, Ahmed, M., Arenas, IdIT:. Coronavirus: The world in lockdown in maps and charts. BBC News. https://www.bbc.com/news/world-521 03747
3. Perrella, A., Carannante, N., Berretta, M., Rinaldi, M., Maturo, N., Rinaldi, L.: Editorial–Novel Coronavirus 2019 (Sars-CoV2): a global emergency that needs new approaches. Eur Rev Med Pharmaco **24**, 2162–2164 (2020)
4. Kannan, S., Ali, P.S.S., Sheeza, A., Hemalatha, K.: COVID-19 (Novel Coronavirus 2019)-recent trends. Eur. Rev. Med. Pharmacol. Sci **24**(4), 2006–2011 (2020)
5. Wong, Z.S., Zhou, J., Zhang, Q.: Artificial intelligence for infectious disease big data analytics. Infect. Dis. Health **24**(1), 44–48 (2019)
6. Brown, D.E., Abbasi, A., Lau, R.Y.: Predictive analytics: predictive modeling at the micro level. IEEE Intell. Syst. **30**(3), 6–8 (2015)
7. Jayanthi, N., Valluvan, K.R.: A review of performance metrics in designing of protocols for wireless sensor networks. Asian J. Res. Soc. Sci. Hum. **7**(1), 716–730 (2017)
8. Ahmed, M.B., Boudhir, A.A., Santos, D., El Aroussi, M., Karas, İ.R. (Eds.): Innovations in Smart Cities Applications Edition 3: The Proceedings of the 4th International Conference on Smart City Applications. Springer Nature (2020)
9. Rodgers, W.: Artificial Intelligence in a Throughput Model: Some Major Algorithms. CRC Press (2020)
10. Haleem, A., Javaid, M., Vaishya, R.: Effects of COVID 19 pandemic in daily life. Curr. Med. Res. Pract. (2020)
11. Bai, H.X., Hsieh, B., Xiong, Z., Halsey, K., Choi, J.W., Tran, T.M.L., …, Jiang, X.L.: Performance of radiologists in differentiating COVID-19 from viral pneumonia on chest CT. Radiology (2020)
12. Hu, Z., Ge, Q., Jin, L., Xiong, M.: Artificial intelligence forecasting of covid-19 in china. arXiv preprint arXiv:2002.07112 (2020)
13. Bravo, C.E., Saputelli, L.A., Rivas, F.I., Perez, A.G., Nikolaou, M., Zangl, G., …, Nunez, G.: State-of-the-art application of artificial intelligence and trends in the E&P industry: A technology survey. In: SPE Intelligent Energy International. Society of Petroleum Engineers (2012, January)
14. Dey, R., Bajpai, V., Gandhi, G., Dey, B.: Application of artificial neural network (ANN) technique for diagnosing diabetes mellitus. In: 2008 IEEE Region 10 and the Third international Conference on Industrial and Information Systems, pp. 1–4. IEEE (2008, December)
15. Karegowda, A.G., Punya, V., Jayaram, M.A., Manjunath, A.S.: Rule based classification for diabetic patients using cascaded k-means and decision tree C4. 5. Int. J. Comput. Appl. **45**(12), 45–50 (2012)
16. Liberti, L., Lavor, C., Maculan, N., Mucherino, A.: Euclidean distance geometry and applications. SIAM Rev. **56**(1), 3–69 (2014)
17. Caballero-Ruiz, E., García-Sáez, G., Rigla, M., Balsells, M., Pons, B., Morillo, M., … Hernando, M.: Automatic blood glucose classification for gestational diabetes with feature

selection: decision trees vs. neural networks. Paper presented at the XIII Mediterranean Conference on Medical and Biological Engineering and Computing (2014)
18. Kurd, Z., Kelly, T., Austin, J.: Developing artificial neural networks for safety-critical systems. Neural Comput. Appl. **16**(1), 11–19 (2007)
19. Samarasinghe, S.: Neural networks for applied sciences and engineering: from fundamentals to complex pattern recognition: Auerbach publications
20. Berglund, E., Sitte, J.: The parameterless self-organizing map algorithm. IEEE Trans. Neural Netw. **17**(2), 305–316 (2006)
21. Feizollah, A., Anuar, N.B., Salleh, R., Wahab, A.W.A.: A review on feature selection in mobile malware detection. Digit. Investig. **13**, 22–37 (2015)
22. Amato, F., López, A., Peña-Méndez, E.M., Vaňhara, P., Hampl, A., Havel, J.: Artificial Neural Networks in Medical Diagnosis: Elsevier (2013)
23. Baldwin, J.F., Xie, D.W.: Simple fuzzy logic rules based on fuzzy decision tree for classification and prediction problems. Paper presented at the International Conference on Intelligent Information Processing (2004)
24. Kumari, V.A., Chitra, R.: Classification of diabetes disease using a support vector machine. Int. J. Eng. Res. Appl. **3**(2), 1797–1801 (2013)
25. Al-Qaness, M.A., Ewees, A.A., Fan, H., Abd El Aziz, M.: Optimization method for forecasting confirmed cases of COVID-19 in China. J. Clin. Med. **9**(3), 674 (2020)
26. Jang, J.S.: ANFIS: adaptive-network-based fuzzy inference system. IEEE Trans. Syst. Man Cybern. **23**(3), 665–685 (1993)
27. Han, B.A., Schmidt, J.P., Bowden, S.E., Drake, J.M.: Rodent reservoirs of future zoonotic diseases. Proc. Natl. Acad. Sci. **112**(22), 7039–7044 (2015)
28. Goodman, K.E., Lessler, J., Cosgrove, S.E., Harris, A.D., Lautenbach, E., Han, J.H., Tamma, P.D.: A clinical decision tree to predict whether a bacteremic patient is infected with an extended-spectrum β-lactamase–producing organism. Clin. Infect. Dis. **63**(7), 896–903 (2016)
29. Bragazzi, N.L., Alicino, C., Trucchi, C., Paganino, C., Barberis, I., Martini, M., Icardi, G.: Global reaction to the recent outbreaks of Zika virus: Insights from a Big Data analysis. PLoS ONE **12**(9), (2017)
30. Alicino, C., Bragazzi, N.L., Faccio, V., Amicizia, D., Panatto, D., Gasparini, R., Orsi, A.: Assessing Ebola-related web search behaviour: insights and implications from an analytical study of Google Trends-based query volumes. Infect. Dis. Poverty **4**(1), 54 (2015)
31. Mahroum, N., Adawi, M., Sharif, K., Waknin, R., Mahagna, H., Bisharat, B., Watad, A.: Public reaction to Chikungunya outbreaks in Italy—Insights from an extensive novel data streams-based structural equation modeling analysis. PLoS ONE **13**(5), (2018)
32. Kononenko, I.: Machine learning for medical diagnosis: history, state of the art and perspective. Artif. Intell. Med. **23**(1), 89–109 (2001)
33. Foster, K.R., Koprowski, R., Skufca, J.D.: Machine learning, medical diagnosis, and biomedical engineering research-commentary. Biomed. Eng. Online **13**(1), 94 (2014)
34. Wang, Y., Fan, Y., Bhatt, P., Davatzikos, C.: High-dimensional pattern regression using machine learning: from medical images to continuous clinical variables. Neuroimage **50**(4), 1519–1535 (2010)
35. Ai, T., Yang, Z., Hou, H., Zhan, C., Chen, C., Lv, W., …, Xia, L.: Correlation of chest CT and RT-PCR testing in coronavirus disease 2019 (COVID-19) in China: a report of 1014 cases. Radiology, 200642 (2020)
36. Luo, H., Tang, Q.L., Shang, Y.X., Liang, S.B., Yang, M., Robinson, N., Liu, J.P.: Can Chinese medicine be used for prevention of corona virus disease 2019 (COVID-19)? A review of historical classics, research evidence and current prevention programs. Chin. J. Integr. Med., 1–8 (2020)
37. Haleem, A., Vaishya, R., Javaid, M., Khan, I.H.: Artificial Intelligence (AI) applications in orthopaedics: an innovative technology to embrace. J. Clin. Orthopaedics Trauma **11**, S80–S81 (2020)
38. Biswas, K., Sen, P.: Space-time dependence of corona virus (COVID-19) outbreak. arXiv preprint arXiv:2003.03149 (2020)

39. Stebbing, J., Phelan, A., Griffin, I., Tucker, C., Oechsle, O., Smith, D., Richardson, P.: COVID-19: combining antiviral and anti-inflammatory treatments. The Lancet Infect. Dis. **20**(4), 400–402 (2020)
40. Sohrabi, C., Alsafi, Z., O'Neill, N., Khan, M., Kerwan, A., Al-Jabir, A., …, Agha, R.: World Health Organization declares global emergency: a review of the 2019 novel coronavirus (COVID-19). Int. J. Surgery (2020)
41. Chen, S., Yang, J., Yang, W., Wang, C., Bärnighausen, T.: COVID-19 control in China during mass population movements at New Year. The Lancet **395**(10226), 764–766 (2020)
42. Bobdey, S., Ray, S.: Going viral–Covid-19 impact assessment: a perspective beyond clinical practice. J. Marine Med. Soc. **22**(1), 9 (2020)
43. Gozes, O., Frid-Adar, M., Greenspan, H., Browning, P.D., Zhang, H., Ji, W., …, Siegel, E.: Rapid ai development cycle for the coronavirus (covid-19) pandemic: Initial results for automated detection & patient monitoring using deep learning ct image analysis. arXiv preprint arXiv:2003.05037 (2020)
44. Pirouz, B., Shaffiee Haghshenas, S., Shaffiee Haghshenas, S., Piro, P.: Investigating a serious challenge in the sustainable development process: analysis of confirmed cases of COVID-19 (new type of coronavirus) through a binary classification using artificial intelligence and regression analysis. Sustainability **12**(6), 2427 (2020)
45. Whitelaw, S., Mamas, M.A., Topol, E., Van Spall, H.G.: Applications of digital technology in COVID-19 pandemic planning and response. The Lancet Digit. Health (2020)
46. Wan, K.H., Huang, S.S., Young, A.L., Lam, D.S.C.: Precautionary measures needed for ophthalmologists during pandemic of the coronavirus disease 2019 (COVID-19). Acta Ophthalmol. **98**(3), 221–222 (2020)
47. Li, L., Qin, L., Xu, Z., Yin, Y., Wang, X., Kong, B., …, Cao, K.: Artificial intelligence distinguishes COVID-19 from community acquired pneumonia on chest CT. Radiology (2020)
48. Smeulders, A.W., Van Ginneken, A.M.: An analysis of pathology knowledge and decision making for the development of artificial intelligence-based consulting systems. Anal. Quantit. Cytol. Histol. **11**(3), 154–165 (1989)
49. Gupta, R., Misra, A.: Contentious issues and evolving concepts in the clinical presentation and management of patients with COVID-19 infectionwith reference to use of therapeutic and other drugs used in Co-morbid diseases (Hypertension, diabetes etc). Diabetes Metabolic Syndrome: Clin. Res. Rev. (2020)
50. Hussain, A., do Vale Moreira, N.C.: Clinical considerations for patients with diabetes in times of COVID-19 pandemic. Diabetes Metabol Syndrome **14**(4), 451 (2020)
51. Gupta, R., Ghosh, A., Singh, A.K., Misra, A.: Clinical considerations for patients with diabetes in times of COVID-19 epidemic. Diabetes Metabol Syndrome **14**(3), 211 (2020)
52. Petropoulos, G.: Artificial intelligence in the fight against COVID-19. Bruegel (23 March) (2020)
53. Bullock, J., Pham, K.H., Lam, C.S.N., Luengo-Oroz, M.: Mapping the landscape of artificial intelligence applications against COVID-19. arXiv preprint arXiv:2003.11336 (2020)
54. Harari, Y.N.: The world after coronavirus. Financial Times **20** (2020)
55. Naudé, W.: Artificial Intelligence against COVID-19: an early review (2020)
56. Maier, B.F., Brockmann, D.: Effective containment explains subexponential growth in recent confirmed COVID-19 cases in China. Science **368**(6492), 742–746 (2020)
57. Huang, J.J.: COVID-19 and Applicable Law to Transnational Personal Data: Trends and Dynamics. Sydney Law School Research Paper, (20/23) (2020)
58. Chen, B.: Historical foundations of choice of law in fiduciary obligations. J. Private Int. Law **10**(2), 171–203 (2014)
59. Douglas, M.: Characterisation of breach of confidence as a privacy tort in private international law. UNSWLJ **41**, 490 (2018)
60. Bloom, D.E., Cadarette, D.: Infectious disease threats in the 21st century: strengthening the global response. Front. Immunol. **10**, 549 (2019)
61. Morse, S.S.: Public health surveillance and infectious disease detection. Biosecurity Bioterrorism: Biodefense Strategy, Pract. Sci. **10**(1), 6–16 (2012)

62. Paules, C.I., Eisinger, R.W., Marston, H.D., Fauci, A.S.: What recent history has taught us about responding to emerging infectious disease threats. Annals Intern. Med. **167**(11), 805–811 (2017)
63. Ienca, M., Vayena, E.: On the responsible use of digital data to tackle the COVID-19 pandemic. Nat. Med., 1–2 (2020)
64. Wu, Z., McGoogan, J.M.: Characteristics of and important lessons from the coronavirus disease 2019 (COVID-19) outbreak in China: summary of a report of 72 314 cases from the Chinese Center for Disease Control and Prevention. JAMA (2020)
65. Bengtsson, L., Gaudart, J., Lu, X., Moore, S., Wetter, E., Sallah, K., Piarroux, R.: Using mobile phone data to predict the spatial spread of cholera. Sci. Rep. **5**, 8923 (2015)
66. Bates, M.: Tracking disease: Digital epidemiology offers new promise in predicting outbreaks. IEEE Pulse **8**(1), 18–22 (2017)
67. Cinnamon, J., Jones, S.K., Adger, W.N.: Evidence and future potential of mobile phone data for disease disaster management. Geoforum **75**, 253–264 (2016)
68. Mor, N.: Resources for primary care providers to meet patients needs during the COVID-19 epidemic (2020)
69. Mozur, P., Zhong, R., Krolik, A.: In coronavirus fight, China gives citizens a color code, with red flags. New York Times **1** (2020)
70. Mathur, A.N.: Strategies for solving wicked problems of true uncertainty: Tackling pandemics like Covid-19 (Version: April 13, 2020) (No. WP 2020-04-03). Indian Institute of Management Ahmedabad, Research and Publication Department (2020)

Diagnosing COVID-19 Virus in the Cardiovascular System Using ANN

Palanisamy Satheesh Kumar, Jeevitha, and Manikandan

Abstract The novel corona virus disease (COVID-19) is a deadly SARS- COV-2 communicable virus causing the world economy to crash. COVID-19, which causes interstitial pneumonitis and severe acute respiratory distress syndrome (ARDS), primarily affects the lungs multiple organs, especially the cardiovascular system. The ability of this virus to spread through human-to - human and surface-to-human transmission contributes to a devastating process in the world Biological signal analysis based on computer system allows medical officers to manage Covid-19 tasks such as intensive care ECG monitoring, fatal ventricular fibrillation, etc. The most common complications include heart dysfunctions such as tachycardia, bradycardia, ventricular fibrillation, cardiac arrhythmias, heart injury [highly responsive troponin I (hs-cTnI) elevation and creatine kinase, fulminant myocarditis, heart failure, pulmonary embolism, and disseminated intravascular coagulation (DIC). Mechanistically, SARS-CoV-2 binds to transmembrane angiotensin-converting enzyme 2 (ACE2), a homologue of ACE, after proteolytic cleavage of its S protein by a serine protease, to join type 2 pneumocytes, macrophages, perivascular pericytes, and cardiomyocytes. This can result in myocardial dysfunction and injury, endothelial dysfunction, plaque instability, microvascular dysfunction, and myocardial infarction (MI). In this research, for classification purposes, the heart pulse base signal and characteristics such as spectral entropy, largest lyapunov exponent, Poincare plot and detrended fluctuation analysis are extracted and presented. The Poincare plot RR intervals summarise the RR time series obtained in one image from an ECG, and the quantity of a time interval derives the HRV information length. The prediction of heart rate fluctuation due to Covid or other heart problems is made simpler by this study.The better accuracy level in diagnosing heart pulse irregularity using Artificial

P. Satheesh Kumar (✉) · Jeevitha · Manikandan
Coimbatore Institute of Technology, Coimbatore, Tamil Nadu, India
e-mail: satheeshkumar.p@cit.edu.in

Jeevitha
e-mail: jeevivijaya19@gmail.com

Jeevitha · Manikandan
Government College of Technology, Coimbatore, Tamil Nadu, India

D. Oliva et al. (eds.), *Artificial Intelligence for COVID-19*, Studies in Systems, Decision and Control 358, https://doi.org/10.1007/978-3-030-69744-0_5

Neural network(ANN) is an integer value (0 to 4).The processing time for analyzing heart dysfunctionalties is 0.05 s using ANN.

Keywords COVID-19 · First return maps · Artificial neural network · ECG · Spectral entropy · Lyapunov exponent

1 Introduction

Nowadays, without symptoms suggestive of infection, the predominant symptoms of the patients were cardiac in nature [1, 2]. A standard diagnostic algorithm for acute coronary syndrome is followed, although the initial ECG results of diffuse ST elevations and elevated cardiac enzymes increased the possibility of myopericarditis, as this remains a more frequent cause of this presentation. As experience with the COVID-19 pandemic increases, the treatment pathway for cardiac presentations can also develop rapidly.

One area of uncertainty is whether in response to ECG changes and positive troponin, to proceed to coronary angiography, which risks exposure Additional infection healthcare staff [3]. Similarly, the role of endomyocardial biopsy in the detection of myocarditis is uncertain. Hemodynamic evaluation played a crucial role in the detection of profound cardiogenicity in this case [4].

On 11 March 2020, the World Health Organization (WHO) named the novel outbreak of COVID-19 coronavirus, first identified on 8 December 2019 in Hubei province in China, as a pandemic. This outbreak, recognised by Dr. Zhang Jixian of the Hubei Provincial Hospital of Integrated Chinese and Western Medicine as a new beta-coronavirus infection, has spread exponentially in almost all countries around the world. Current statistics providing information on international case numbers and case fatality are provided by the Johns Hopkins University (JHU) Coronavirus Resource Center. Despite lung tropism, where it induces interstitial pneumonitis, multi-organ failure occurs in the most serious cases [5]. It appears that the cardiovascular (CV) system has complex interactions with COVID- 19. The planet suffered from epidemic and pandemic issues periodically. The wake of epidemic destroyed millions of lives. With the spread of COVID-19 this year, the whole planet has practically halted and the world is constantly struggling against the destruction of the virus. The covid targets the respiratory organs and contributes to heart malfunctioning due to serious problems.

1.1 Electrocardiography

17% of patients with COVID-19 hospitalised have concomitant arrhythmia [7], and electrocardiographic abnormalities may occur in those with myocardial injury, such as myocardial ischaemia, even in the absence of significant epicardial coronary stenosis due to Microcirculatory function impairment, myocarditis, or as a side effect of treatment with COVID-19 [8]. Of the COVID-19, 41% sighted ST-T modifications and 13% QT prolongation, patients have an irregular electrocardiogram (ECG). In patients with HF, Serial ECGs must be performed either with or without concomitant azithromycin in hospitalised patients with elevated levels of troponin and in those at higher risk of receiving drugs with pro-arrhythmic effects, including chloroquine or hydroxychloroquine. Unique protocols for ECG surveillance has been developed.

The "natural pacemaker" of the heart produces electric pulses at the top of the right atrium (RA) originating from the Sino Atrial node (SA). This electrical signal branches through the atria, induces contractions and dilates to pump blood to the ventricles. The heart, beating at an elevated rate, affects the irregular distribution of blood if the pacemaker is affected. The heart beat is a sequence of electrical waves characterised by positive and negative peaks, each of which is calculated by an electrocardiogram (ECG) with two distinct data. Second, the cumulative electrical wave time from the heart can be detected by calculating time intervals and can determine if the electrical activity is irregular or normal. Secondly, the heart muscle is determined by the volume of electrical pulse. A paediatric cardiologist who can assess whether or not the heart pumping is overworked. The standard ECG signal rate ranged from [.05–100] Hz and its pulse level is [1–10] mV [9, 10]. Successive alphabetical letters such as P, Q, R, S and T derive the characterization of the ECG from positive and negative peaks.

1.2 Cardiovascular Risk Factors Associated with the Worse Outcomes of COVID-19

COVID-19 was associated with a variety of primary comorbidities. This relationship seems to be dominated by association with age [12] and may influence the actual significance of other variables reported in univariate analyses. Compared with younger patients, older patients (mean age 63 years; range 53–71) are more likely to experience the composite outcome of ICU admission, mechanical ventilation, or death (mean age 46 years, range 35–57) [13]. An instance of electron microscopy image of a betacoronavirus is shown in Fig. 1. After gain-of-function mutations within the receptor-binding domain (RBD) and the acquisition of a furinprotease cleavage site, COVID-19 is caused by a novel beta-coronavirus, possibly originating from bats. The WHO has called it Coronavirus 2 Extreme Acute Respiratory Syndrome (SARS-CoV-2) [14].

Males tend to be more vulnerable to complications associated with COVID-19, comprising between 50% and 82% of hospitalized patients in the four publications documenting such data [5, 14, 16, 17] and the most recent Italian study.

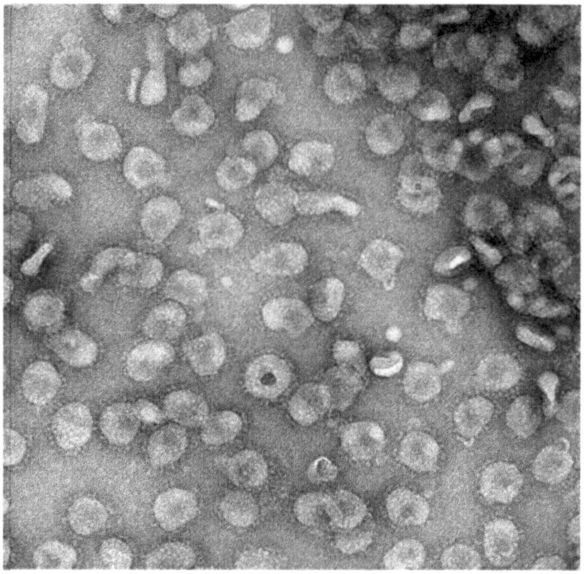

Fig. 1 Characteristic structure of betacoronavirus. Negative stain electron microscopy showing a betacoronavirus particles with clubshaped surface projections surrounding the periphery of the particle, a characteristic feature of coronaviruses. The photograph depicts a murine coronavirus. Kindly provided by Professor David Bhella, Scottish Centre for Macromolecular Imaging; MRC Centre for Virus Research; University of Glasgow

2 COVID-19 Cardiovascular Manifestations

Rapidly developing systemic inflammation, a pro-inflammatory cytokine storm, and sepsis are associated with extreme COVID-19, leading to multiorgan failure and death.

2.1 COVID-19 and Cardiac Arrhythmia

Metabolic dysfunction, myocardial inflammation, and activation of the sympathetic nervous system are associated with viral infections, all of which are predisposed to cardiac arrhythmia. In a new study on 138 patients hospitalised for COVID-19,21 16.7% of patients experienced arrhythmias, which ranked second only to severe complications following ARDS. In 7% of patients who did not need ICU treatment and in 44% of subjects who were admitted to an ICU, arrhythmia was found. Atrial fibrillation, conduction obstruction, ventricular tachycardia, and ventricular fibrillation remained elusive but included more descriptions of these manifestations [15, 16].

In viral myocarditis, these arrhythmias are also observed. It is estimated that some patients mainly reported CV symptoms during the initial outbreak, such as palpitations and chest tightness, rather than respiratory symptoms. The heartbeats in the sino atrial node start as an electrical impulse, and the sequence of heartbeats is called the sinus rhythm. Arrhythmia in the heartbeat is nothing but an abnormality. Cardiac arrhythmia is associated with electrical pulse dysfunction and irregular mechanical activity of the heart. Arrhythmias classified according to the origin of irregular electrical activity, typically from the atria, ventricles, or atrio ventricular node, are abnormal heart beats [19].

2.2 COVID-19 Myocardial Injury and Heart Failure

Most reports suggest that virtually all hospitalised patients with COVID-19 exhibit elevated levels of serum creatine kinase (CK) and lactate dehydrogenase (LDH).6,43,44 Additionally, a number of studies indicate that possible outcomes of SARS-CoV-2 infection are cardiac complications, including fulminant myocarditis.

In a new study by in-hospital Chinese subjects in 23% of COVID subjects. In comparison to 12% of survivors, approximately 52% of non-survivors had heart failure. In 5 of the first 41 patients diagnosed with COVID-19, evidence of myocardial injury, such as an increase in high-sensitivity cardiac troponin I (cTnI) levels (> 28 pg/mL), was detected. Spectral entropy, H (from an ECG.), determines the complexity of the HRV signal.

2.3 COVID-19 and Myocarditis

Well-recognized symptoms of acute viral infections are heart injury and acute myocarditis. In cardiac muscle autopsy specimens, myocyte necrosis and mononuclear cell infiltrates are reported in a recent report of the National Health Commission of the PRC. This finding, together with case reports of fulminant myocarditis, suggests that myocarditis has been reported in COVID-19 patients, acute cardiac injury may be an important causeThe incidence, clinical meaning, and mechanism(s) of myocardial inflammation in COVID-19 disease, however, remain unclear [16, 17], Clinically, myocarditis with COVID-19 may only manifest as mild chest pain and palpitations, which in most patients may be difficult to differentiate from other causes. However, in others, myocarditis results in fulminant illness. There are common transient ECG changes that can help to diagnose the presence and severity of myocardial injury. Myocarditis can advance to block of conduction, tachyarrhythmias, and left ventricular function dysfunction. Myocarditis is also suspected in other clinical settings when heart damage is observed in the absence of an ACS. If cardiac magnetic resonance imaging (MRI) detects traditional acute myocardial injury signals, the diagnosis can also be confirmed [18]. Myocyte necrosis and mononuclear cell infiltrates can be specifically shown by endomyocardial biopsy (EMB), long considered the gold standard diagnostic test.

In some cases, EMB can detect evidence of a viral origin, while in others it is suspected of an immunologically autoimmune-mediated origin of myocarditis. Biopsy findings of patients with acute myocarditis in Europe suggest that viral aetiology is suspected. At the moment, this evidence is scarce in COVID-19 and is focused on individual case series, stressing the need for systematic evaluation. Although several studies highlight that fulminant myocarditis can be a significant clinical presentation of the disease, the exact incidence of this complication remains uncertain. During the current COVID-19 pandemic and related health crisis, cardiac MRI and EMBs as diagnostic instruments are likely to be inappropriate, but should be considered in the future. Animal models of viral myocarditis indicate distinct pathological phases starting with viral-mediated myocyte lysis. This cardiac injury contributes to the activation of the innate immune response with the release of proinflammatory cytokines. Proteins released by cell lysis can show viral antigen-like epitopes and may be presented via the Main Histocompatibility Complex (MHC). Myosin heavy chain, a cardiac sarcomere protein, appears to be a prime example of molecular mimicry. At this point, due to the clearance of the virus by the innate immune response, EMBs may display inflammatory changes but no detectable viral particles. The predominant characteristic demonstrated by activation of antibodies and T lymphocytes is an acquired immune response.

2.4 *Variability in Heart Rate*

Heart beats are caused by relaxation and dilation of the heart muscle is nothing but electrical depolarization which can be observed on an electrocardiogram. The depolarization of the heart chambers are visualized by the P-wave. The Q, R and S waves generates the QRS complex, which represents the depolarization lower portion of heart chambers.

The analysis of Poincare plots of nonlinear dynamics is very much useful in HRV analysis. The Poincare plot is defined for a vectors, x1, x2, ... xN. In the medical perspective, the interval between the successive RR isRRin and RRin+ 1 respectively (Fig. 2).

2.5 *COVID-19 and Ischemic Heart Disease*

Although little is known about the effects of COVID-19 on ACS, many pathways associated with viral diseases can lead to plaque destabilisation in patients with COVID-19.57 Patients with heart failure are at increased risk of acute events or exacerbation; atherosclerotic plaques can potentially be destabilised by viral disease through systemic inflammatory responses, cytokine storm. In COVID-19, all of these were observed. Acute MI was reported in two out of five deaths in early reports in the case of SARS and MERS. It is important to consider that type 2 MI is the most prevalent subtype in viral conditions, thus limiting the utility of invasive management for coronary revascularization (especially type 2 MI). Invasive versus non-invasive treatment choices for patients with ACS and COVID-19 disease should be carefully

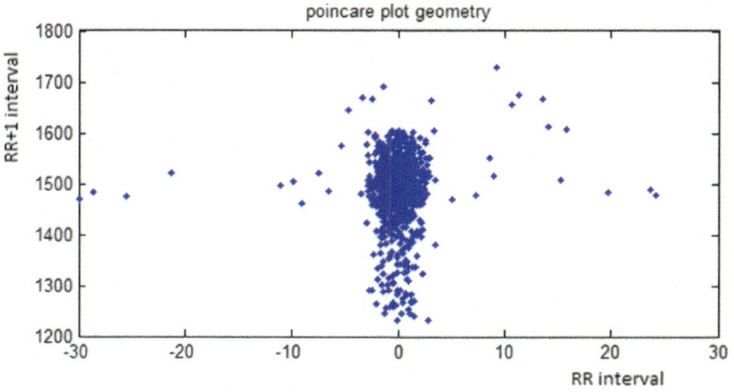

Fig. 2 The Poincare plot for normal ECG

considered. In addition, a recent single-cell human heart atlas found that pericytes express particularly high levels of ACE2 in the heart. One of the consequences of this finding is potential local microvascular inflammation during pericyte SARS-CoV-2 infection, leading to serious microvascular dysfunction and contributing to non-obstructive coronary artery (MINOCA) myocardial infarction. Recent studies of the clinical course of MI cases during COVID-19 may clarify this. In addition, the cytokine storm can contribute to development of endothelial dysfunction through well-characterized mechanisms.

3 Results and Discussion

This chapter presents the discussion on results obtained from the proposed algorithm. A sample ECG signal was obtained from the database.

The results are shown for the following cases:

(i) Normal ECG
(ii) Ventricular fibrillation
(iii) Cardiac arrhythmia

The user selects the input signal from the ECG database. The input signal is then filtered using discrete wavelet transform. The discrete wavelet transform used is daubechies wavelet(db4). The compression ratio of db4 is 1.1363. The discrete wavelet transform produces approximation coefficient and the detailed coefficient. The approximation coefficient is used for extraction of certain parameters like detrended fluctuation analysis, spectral entropy, largest lyapunov exponent, Poincare plot and the fuzzy classifier classifies the disease according to the output range. In the Artificial neural network, training of the neural network is done prior classifying the disease.

4 Results from Artificial Neural Network

The simulation results of classification and analysis of cardiac waves using artificial neural network have been obtained as follows:

The network is trained first and then the classification of cardiac diseases is done. The performance, epoch, time and gradient of the training network can be calculated using ANN. The normal ECG signal selected by the user from the database after training the neural network has the ANN's combined parameter value of 4. The input signal after discrete wavelet transform produces the approximation coefficient and detailed coefficient. Figure 3 shows the input signal, approximation coefficient, detail coefficient for a normal ECG. Figure 4 shows detrended fluctuation analysis, spectral entropy, largest lyapunov exponent, Poincare plotand the message box which indicates that the selected signal is normal ECG.

The ventricular fibrillation ECG signal selected by the user from the database after training the neural network has the ANN's combined parameter value of 1. The input signal after discrete wavelet transform produces the approximation coefficient and detailed coefficient. Figure 5 shows the input signal, approximation coefficient, detail coefficient for a diseased signal. Figure 6 shows detrended fluctuation analysis, spectral entropy, largest lyapunov exponent, Poincare plot and the message box which indicates that the selected signal is ventricular fibrillation.

The cardiac arrhythmia ECG signal selected by the user from the database has the fuzzy classifier's combined parameter value is 3. The four parameters in this fuzzy classifier are detrended fluctuation analysis, spectral entropy, largest lyapunov exponent, Poincare plot. The input signal after discrete wavelet transform produces the approximation coefficient and detailed coefficient. Figure 7 shows the input signal, approximation coefficient, detail coefficient for a diseased signal. Figure 8

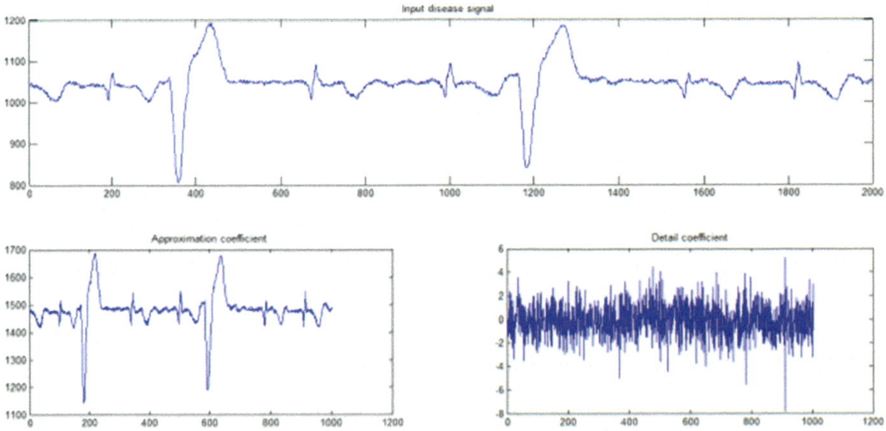

Fig. 3 Input signal, approximation coefficient, detail coefficient of normal ECG

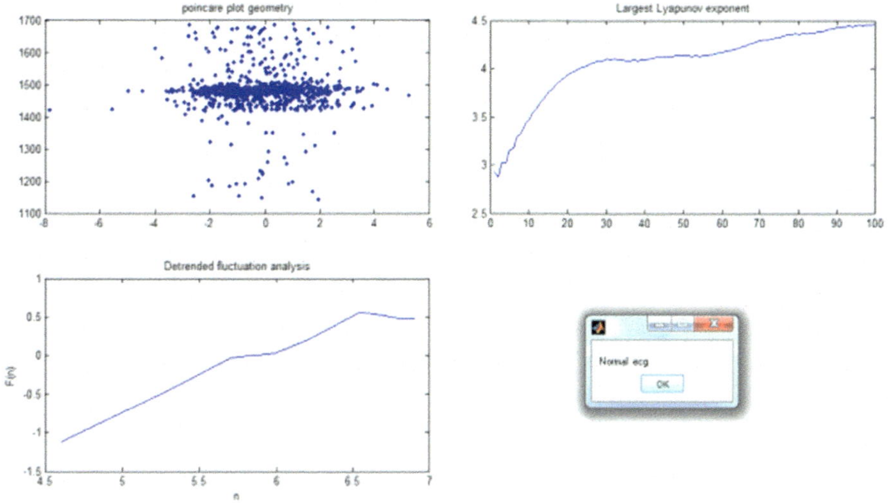

Fig. 4 Poincare plot, LLE, DFA of normal ECG

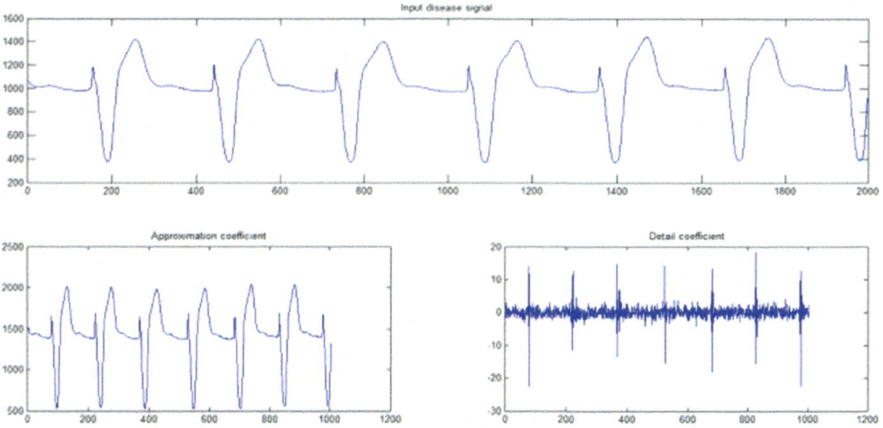

Fig. 5 Input signal, approximation and detail coefficient of ventricular fibrillation

shows the detrended fluctuation analysis, spectral entropy, largest lyapunov exponent, Poincare plotand the message box which indicates that the selected signal is cardiac arrhythmia.

If myocarditis is diagnosed with SARS-CoV-2, a comprehensive clinical assessment, including CMR, should be conducted. In patients with myocarditis, intensive post-discharge monitoring and a sport restriction for at least 3–6 months is recommended on the basis of general recommendations for myocarditis. A return to sports should be assessed by a multidisciplinary, expert team, and include input from sports cardiology and sports medicine.

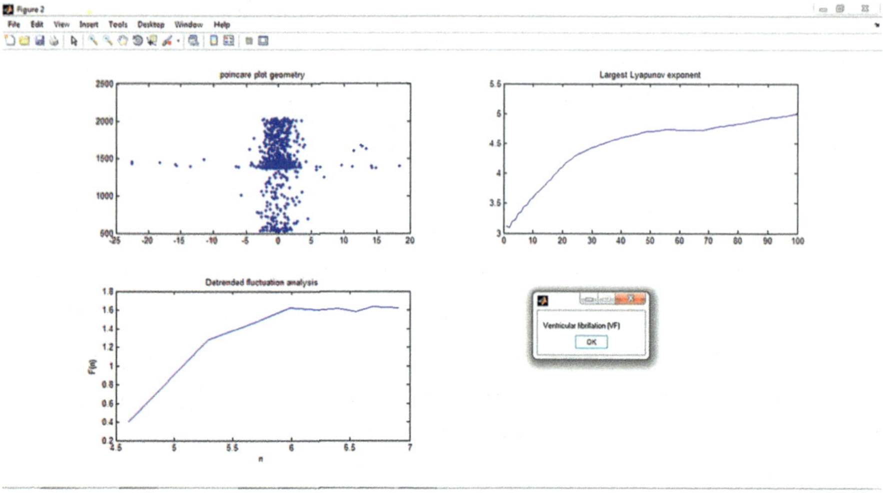

Fig. 6 Poincare Plot, LLE and DFA of ventricular fibrillation

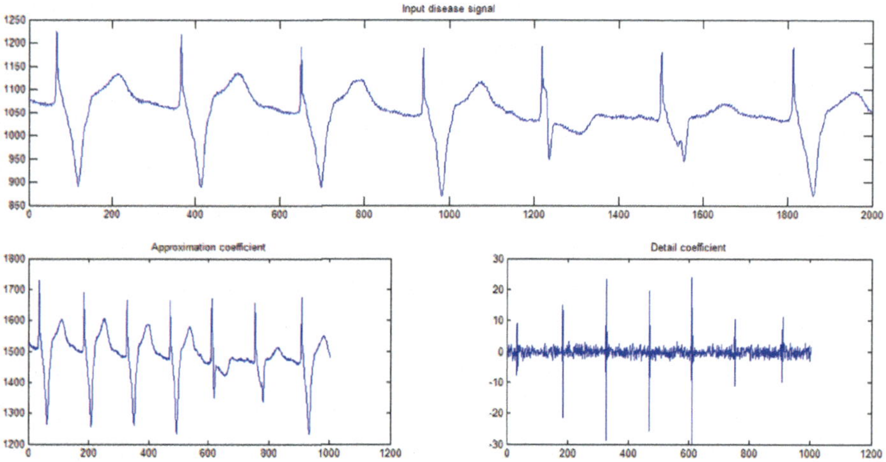

Fig. 7 Input signal, approximation and detail coefficient of cardiac arrhythmia

5 Conclusion

For clinicians worldwide, the COVID-19 epidemic faces significant challenges. It is therefore important for outpatient HF patients to take strict preventive measures to reduce the risk of exposure to infection. Moreover, HF patients are also at higher risk of serious complications once they acquire the infection. It is critical to rule out COVID-19 in any patient with HF who is hospitalised as symptoms may overlap significantly. As COVID-19 is a worldwide outbreak of a new infectious disease

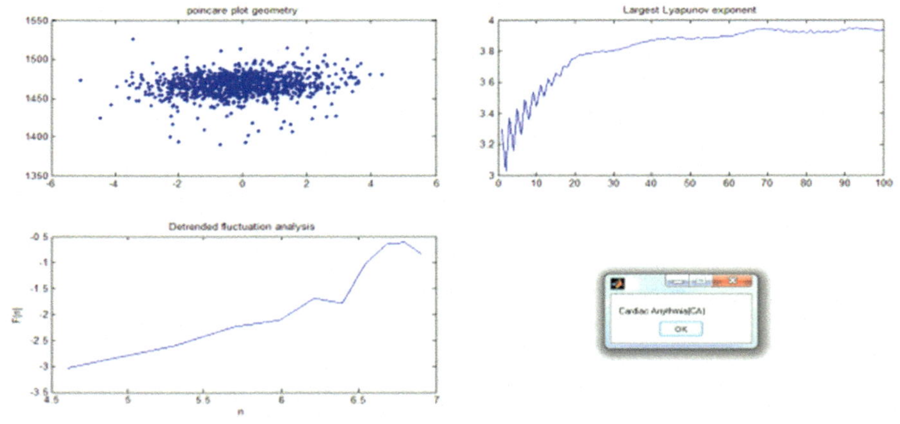

Fig. 8 Poincare plot, LLE and DFA of cardiac arrhythmia

with insufficient data regarding concomitant HF, this position paper will be beneficial for clinicians worldwide Taking care of HF patients with suspected or overt concomitant COVID-19 as well as patients who are at risk of this infection. It is important to emphasise that these expert recommendations are mainly based on the current pandemic situation and will need to be revised according to the shifts around the globe. COVID-19 is associated with a range of cardiovascular complications, including myocardial injury and myocarditis, AMI, heart failure, dysrhythmias and VTE, respectively. Some of the drugs used for the treatment of COVID-19 may also have heart problems. It is critical for emergency clinicians to be aware of these complications when treating a COVID-19 patient.

References

1. Dong, E., Du, H., Gardner, L.: An interactive web-based dashboard to track COVID-19 in real time [published online February 19, 2020]. The Lancet Infectious Diseases. https://doi.org/10.1016/s1473-3099(20)30120-1
2. Shi, S., Qin, M., Shen, B., Cai, Y., Liu, T., Yang, F., Gong, W., Liu, X., Liang, J., Zhao, Q., et al.: Association of cardiac injury with mortality in hospitalized patients with COVID-19 in Wuhan, China [published online March 25, 2020]. JAMA Cardiol. https://doi.org/10.1001/jamacardio.2020.0950
3. Welt, F.G.P., Shah, P.B., Aronow, H.D., Bortnick, A.E., Henry, T.D., Sherwood, M.W., Young, M.N., Davidson, L.J., Kadavath, S., Mahmud, E., et al.: Catheterization laboratory considerations during the coronavirus (COVID-19) pandemic: from ACC's Interventional Council and SCAI. J. Am. Coll. Cardiol. **75**, 2372–3275. doi:10.1016/j.jacc.2020.03.021
4. Clerkin, K.J., Fried, J.A., Raikhelkar, J., Sayer, G., Griffin, J.M., Masoumi, A., Jain, S.S., Burkhoff, D., Kumaraiah, D., Rabbani, L., et al.: Coronavirus disease, (COVID- 19) and cardiovascular disease [published online March 21, 2020]. Circulation (2019). https://doi.org/10.1161/circulationaha.120.046941

5. MacLaren, G., Fisher, D., Brodie, D.: Preparing for the most critically ill patients with COVID-19: the potential role of extracorporeal membrane oxygenation JAMA. 2020;323:1245–1246. https://doi.org/10.1001/jama.2020.2342
6. Shastri, S., Singh, K., et. al.: Time series forecasting of COVID-19 using deep learning models: India-USA compaitive case study. Chaos, Solit. Fract. **140** (2020)
7. Shinde, G.R., Kalamkar, A.B., Mahalle, P.N., et al.: "Forecasting models for coronavirus disease(COVID-19): a survey of the state-of-the art. SN Comp Sci. **1**, 197 (2020)
8. Wang, D., Hu, B., Hu, C., Zhu, F., Liu, X., Zhang, J., Wang, B., Xiang, H., Cheng, Z., Xiong, Y., Zhao, Y., Li, Y., Wang, X., Peng, Z.: Clinical characteristics of 138 hospitalized patients with 2019 novel coronavirus-infected pneumonia in Wuhan, China. JAMA **323**, 1061–1069 (2020)
9. Huang, C., Wang, Y., Li, X., Ren, L., Zhao, J., Hu, Y., Zhang, L., Fan, G., Xu, J., Gu, X., Cheng, Z., Yu, T., Xia, J., Wei, Y., Wu,W., Xie, X., Yin, W., Li, H., Liu, M., Xiao, Y., Gao, H., Guo, L., Xie, J., Wang, G., Jiang, R., Gao, Z., Jin, Q., Wang, J., Cao ,B.: Clinica features of patients infected with 2019 novel coronavirus in Wuhan, China. Lancet 395:497–506
10. Ponikowski, P., Voors, A.A., Anker, S.D., Bueno, H., Cleland, J.G., Coats, A.J., Falk, V., Gonzalez-Juanatey, J.R., Harjola ,V.P., Jankowska, E.A., Jessup, M., Linde, C., Nihoyannopoulos, P., Parissis, J.T., Pieske, B., Riley, J.P., Rosano, G.M., Ruilope, L.M., Ruschitzka, F., Rutten, F.H., van der Meer, P.: ESC Guidelines for the diagnosis and treatment of acute and chronic heart failure: The Task Force for the diagnosis and treatment of acute and chronic heart failure of the European Society of Cardiology (ESC). Developed with the special contribution of the Heart Failure Association (HFA) of the ESC. Eur J Heart Fail 18:891–975 (2016)
11. Crespo-Leiro, M.G., Metra, M., Lund, L.H., Milicic, D., Costanzo, M.R., Filippatos, G., Gustafsson, F., Tsui, S., Barge-Caballero, E., De Jonge, N., Frigerio, M., Hamdan, R., Hasin, T., Hulsmann, M., Nalbantgil, S., Potena, L., Bauersachs, J., Gkouziouta, A., Ruhparwar, A., Ristic, A.D., Straburzynska-Migaj, E., McDonagh, T., Seferovic, P., Ruschitzka, F.: Advanced heart failure: a position statement of the Heart Failure Association of the European Society of Cardiology. Eur. J. Heart Fail. **20**, 1505–1535 (2018)
12. Xu, Z., Shi, L., Wang, Y., Zhang, J., Huang, L., Zhang, C., Liu, S., Zhao, P., Liu, H., Zhu, L., Tai, Y., Bai, C., Gao, T., Song, J., Xia, P., Dong, J., Zhao, J., Wang, F.S.: Pathological findings of COVID-19 associated with acute respiratory distress syndrome. Lancet Respir. Med **8**, 420–422 (2020)
13. Inciardi, R.M., Lupi, L., Zaccone, G., Italia, L., Raffom M., Tomasoni, D., Cani, D.S., Cerini, M., Farina, D., Gavazzi, E., Maroldi, R., Adamo, M., Ammirati, E., Sinagra, G., Lombardi, C.M., Metra, M.: Cardiac involvement in a patient with coronavirus disease 2019 (COVID-19). JAMA Cardiol 2020 Mar 27. https://doi.org/10.1001/jamacardio.2020.1096 [Epub ahead of print]
14. World Health Organization. Clinical management of severe acute respiratory infection (SARI) when COVID-19 disease is suspected: interim guidance, 13 March 2020. https://apps.who.int/iris/handle/10665/331446. Accessed 3 June 2020
15. Li, Y.L.T., Liu, M., Wu, M., Tao, L.: Electrocardiogram abnormalities in patients with COVID-19. Chin. J. Cardiac. Arrhyth. (2020). https://doi.org/10.3760/cma.j.cn.113859-20200302-00044
16. Naksuk, N., Lazar, S., Peeraphatdit, T.B.: Cardiac safety of off-label COVID-19 drug therapy: a review and proposed monitoring protocol. Eur. Heart. J. Acute Cardiovasc. Care **9**, 215–221 (2020)
17. Chorin, E., Wadhwani, L., Magnani, S., Dai, M., Shulman, E., Nadeau-Routhier, C., Knotts, R., Bar-Cohen, R., Kogan, E., Barbhaiya, C., Aizer, A., Holmes, D., Bernstein, S., Spinelli, M., Park, D.S., Stefano, C., Chinitz, L.A., Jankelson, L.Q.T.: interval prolongation and torsade de pointes in patients with COVID-19 treated with hydroxychloroquine/azithromycin. Heart Rhythm 2020 May 11. https://doi.org/10.1016/j.hrthm.2020.05.014 [Epub ahead of print]
18. Giudicessi, J.R., Noseworthy, P.A., Friedman, P.A., Ackerman, M.J.: Urgent guidance for navigating and circumventing the QTc-prolonging and torsadogenic potential of possible pharmacotherapies for coronavirus disease 19 (COVID-19). Mayo Clin. Proc. **95**, 1213–1221 (2020)

19. Abishek, M., Ezio, B., Flavio, H., Fenton, J., Glimm, J., Gray, R.A., Cherry, E.M., Smolka,S.A., Grosu, R.: Curvature analysis of cardiac excitation wavefront. IEEE Trans. Comput. Biol. Bioinformat. **10**(2) (2013)
20. Carro, J., Rodriguez, J.F., Laguna, P., Peuyo, E.: Analysis and improvement of a human ventricular cell model for investigation of cardiac arrhythmias. Comput. Cardiol. **2**(2) (2010)
21. Demir, B.E., Yorulmaz, F., Guler, I.: Microcontroller controlled ECG simulator. In: National Biomedical Engineering Conference (BIYOMUT' 10), Antalya, Turkey (2010)
22. Adams, R.J.: Heart disease and stroke statistics 2010 update: a report from American Heart Association. Circulation **121**, e46-e215 (2009)
23. Pelliccia, A., Solberg, E.E., Papadakis, M., Adami, P.E., Biffi, A., Caselli, S., et al.: Recommendations for participation in competitive and leisure time sport in athletes with cardiomyopathies, myocarditis, and pericarditis: position statement of the Sport Cardiology Section of the European Association of Preventive Cardiology (EAPC). Eur. Heart J. **40**(1), 19–33 (2019)

An Efficient Mixture of Deep and Machine Learning Models for COVID-19 and Tuberculosis Detection Using X-Ray Images in Resource Limited Settings

Ali H. Al-Timemy, Rami N. Khushaba, Zahraa M. Mosa, and Javier Escudero

Abstract Clinicians in the frontline need to assess quickly whether a patient with symptoms indeed has COVID-19 or not. The difficulty of this task is exacerbated in low resource settings that may not have access to biotechnology tests. Furthermore, Tuberculosis (TB) remains a major health problem in several low- and middle-income countries and its common symptoms include fever, cough and tiredness, similarly to COVID-19. In order to help in the detection of COVID-19, we propose the extraction of deep features (DF) from chest X-ray images, a technology available in most hospitals, and their subsequent classification using machine learning that do not require large computational resources. We compiled a five-class dataset of X-ray chest images including a balanced number of COVID-19, viral pneumonia, bacterial pneumonia, TB, and healthy cases. We compared the performance of proposed pipelines combining 14 individual pre-trained deep networks for DF extraction with machine learning classifiers. A novel pipeline consisting of ResNet-50 for DF computation and ensemble of subspace discriminant classifier was the best performer in the classification of the five classes, achieving a detection accuracy of $91.6 \pm 0.57\%$ ($\pm$ Confidence Interval, CI) at 95% confidence level). Furthermore, the same pipeline

A. H. Al-Timemy (✉)
Biomedical Engineering Department, al-Khwarizmi College of Engineering, University of Baghdad, Jaderiyah, Baghdad, Iraq
e-mail: ali.altimemy@kecbu.uobaghdad.edu.iq

Centre for Robotics and Neural Systems, Cognitive Institute, Plymouth University, Plymouth, UK

R. N. Khushaba
Australian Centre for Field Robotics, the University of Sydney, 8 Little Queen Street, Chippendale, NSW 2008, Australia
e-mail: Rami.Khushaba@sydney.edu.au

Z. M. Mosa
College of Pharmacy, Uruk University, Baghdad, Iraq
e-mail: zahraa.ma.alkhafaji@uruk.edu.iq

J. Escudero
School of Engineering, Institute for Digital Communications, the University of Edinburgh, Edinburgh King's Buildings, EH9 3JL, UK
e-mail: Javier.Escudero@ed.ac.uk

D. Oliva et al. (eds.), *Artificial Intelligence for COVID-19*, Studies in Systems, Decision and Control 358, https://doi.org/10.1007/978-3-030-69744-0_6

achieved accuracies of 98.6 ± 0.34% (± CI) and 99.9% in three-class and two-class problems focused on distinguishing COVID-19, TB and healthy cases; and COVID-19 and healthy images; respectively. The pipeline was computationally efficient requiring just 0.19 s to extract DF per X-ray image and 2 min for training a classifier on a CPU machine. The results suggest the potential benefits of using our pipeline in the detection of COVID-19, particularly in resource-limited settings as it relies in accessible X-rays and limited computational resources. The final constructed dataset, named COVID-19 five-class dataset and codes, are available from https://drive.google.com/drive/folders/1toMymyHTy0DR_fyE7hjO3LSBGWtVoPNf?usp=sharing.

Keywords COVID-19 · Deep features · Machine learning · Pneumonia · ResNet-50 · Tuberculosis

1 Introduction

During December 2019, the world witnessed the outbreak of a new, previously unknown, virus and disease in Wuhan, China, resulting in an infectious disease known as Coronavirus Disease (COVID-19),[1] which is caused by a recently discovered coronavirus. Coronaviruses are a large family of viruses which may cause respiratory infections ranging from the common cold to more severe diseases such as Middle East Respiratory Syndrome (MERS) and Severe Acute Respiratory Syndrome (SARS). The most common symptoms of COVID-19 include fever, cough, difficulty in breathing, and tiredness, which may develop to pneumonia and potentially lead to death [1, 2]. The symptoms of pulmonary diseases may be confused and there might be a misdiagnosis of COVID-19 cases with that of other pulmonary diseases, such as other types of viral pneumonia, bacterial pneumonia, and Tuberculosis (TB). This complicates the doctor's task to detect COVID-19 quickly to manage the disease, isolate the patient, and trace recent contacts if relevant.

In the current situation of the COVID-19 crisis, there are more than 34 million cases around the world and the numbers are rising at a rate of new 250000 cases per day[2]. Multiple countries are experiencing an increase in the number of patients admitted to hospital, which may compromise their healthcare systems. The situation is even more precarious in low-income countries that may have difficulties in accessing some of the most recent testing technology.

The current testing method utilized to confirm COVID-19 cases is the Reverse Transcription Polymerase Chain Reaction (RT-PCR) [3]. The accuracy of the test is around 60–70% and it takes few hours to 2 days to get the results [4]. Other tests recommended by the World Health Organization (WHO), but not in mass use

[1] https://www.who.int/emergencies/diseases/novel-coronavirus-2019/question-and-answers-hub/q-a-detail/q-a-coronaviruses#:~:text=symptoms.

[2] https://www.worldometers.info/coronavirus/

yet, include the *Cobas SARS-CoV-2 Qualitative assay*[3]. Due to the high number of cases affected every day, the waiting time to obtain the results may be longer. Furthermore, tests are difficult to access, expensive and are unavailable to certain hospitals or regions.

TB is a very serious and deadly pulmonary disease. In 2018 alone, 10 million people had TB worldwide and it caused 1.5 million deaths. It is regarded as a major cause of death from a single infectious agent worldwide [5]. Low-middle income countries account for 2/3 of the TB cases, including India which has the largest number of TB cases, followed by China, Indonesia, Philippines, Pakistan, Nigeria and Bangladesh [5]. Multidrug Resistant (MDR) TB, a severe type of TB which requires chemotherapy and expensive toxic medications for treatment, remains a crisis and threat for public health. MDR-TB mainly appears in three countries: India, China and the Russian Federation. In the current COVID-19 pandemic, TB is major issue. Both TB and COVID-19 spread by close contact between people and the symptoms may be similar to COVID-19, such as fever, cough, tiredness [6]. Thus, low-income countries may face a health crisis where the COVID-19 crisis is compounded by the presence of TB. Large number of COVID-19 cases[4] are reported in India (6500000), Pakistan (313984) and Bangladesh (367565), which results in less attention given to TB. In such cases, there is a need to achieve fast TB and COVID-19 detection. The COVID-19 pandemic may cause a global reduction of 25% in the detection of TB. This could lead to an increase of 13% in TB deaths due to disruption to TB detection and treatment [7].

Radiology can be utilized to help in the detection of COVID-19 in images of Computerized Tomography (CT) [3, 8–10] or X-rays [4, 11–13] since darkened spots and also opacities that looks like ground glass, can be observed [3]. Thus, it is suggested that X-ray and CT scans can help to select and quantify COVID-19 and aid doctors to detect this disease quickly [13, 14]. CT is relatively complex modality, and it is not available in all clinics. On the other hand, an X-ray scan is a simple imaging system, and it can be available in all hospitals and in small clinics. Hence, it has been proposed for Computer Aided Diagnosis (CAD) for aiding COVID-19 detection [15–18] and TB screening [19, 20].

In the healthcare field, a new subbranch of artificial intelligence algorithms denoted as Deep Learning (DL) is being increasingly developed as a CAD tool to help doctors achieve better clinical decisions with high precision [21]. Therefore, achieving good performance on disease detection problems. Similarly, DL methods can be an aid to the doctors for improving the quality of the detection of COVID-19 [4, 12, 13, 22] and TB [19, 20]. Moreover, automatic screening of TB has been proposed with deep learning [19, 20, 23]. However, deep learning typically requires Graphical Processing Units (GPUs), which may not be available in limited resource settings.

---

[3]https://www.who.int/news-room/detail/07-04-2020-who-lists-two-covid-19-tests-for-emergency-use.

[4]https://www.worldometers.info/coronavirus/

A convolutional neural network (CNN), one of the most widespread DL methods, has been applied to the medical field [24–26] to tackle a variety of problems such as COVID-19 detection with CT and X-ray images [9, 10, 15, 16, 18, 27–29]. Several new CNN designs have been proposed for COVID-19 detection such as COVID-Net [22], CovidxNet [15], CoroNet [13], DarkCovidNet [4], COVIDiagnosis-Net [30], and nCOVNet [31]. Despite this remarkable research, the main challenges with CNN include its need for a large number of images for training the network in addition to the long training time, even with GPU support.

On the other hand, Transfer Learning (TL) is proposed to deal with the challenge of the need for a large set of images and long training times of CNN. A pretrained CNN such as ResNet-50 [18], VGG-19 [18], DenseNet-201 [32] and MobileNet-v2 [33] can be utilized to learn a new task by fine tuning of the last fully connected layers. The pretrained networks are trained on a dataset of ImageNet [34] which has more than million images with 1000 classes. Despite its simplicity, this approach still requires a significantly long training time. TL has been applied to COVID-19 detection from X-ray images [4, 13, 15–19, 22, 23, 27–29, 35–38] where pretrained networks such as ResNet-50 [27, 35, 39], VGG-19 [17, 40], DenseNet-201 [41] and Xception [39] has been used for COVID-19 detection with X-ray images.

Inspiring research has been done to tackle the COVID-19 detection with X-ray images. Panwar et al. proposed nCOVNet [31] for COVID-19 detection for 2-class dataset (142 normal and 142 COVID-19 images). A detection accuracy of 88% was obtained with 30% holdout. Wang and Wong [22] developed COVID-Net and validated it on a dataset of 358 COVID-19, 5538 normal and 8066 pneumonia images with 91% sensitivity for COVID-19 cases with 30% holdout. It should be noted that the 3-class images were not balanced. DarkCovidNet was proposed in [4] to detect COVID-19 for 3-class dataset including 125 COVID-19 cases, 500 pneumonia and 500 normal images with an accuracy of 87.2%, utilizing the 5-fold cross validation to avoid overfitting. However, only 125 cases were included in their model. Khan et al. [13] proposed CoroNet CNN to detect COVID-19 from X-ray images of 4-class dataset of 284 COVID-19, 310 normal 330 pneumonia bacterial and 327 pneumonia viral. Their dataset represents the largest balanced 4-class COVID-19 dataset so far. Detection accuracy of 89.6% was obtained with 4-fold cross validation with Google Collaboratory Ubuntu server and Tesla K80 graphics card.

Deep Feature (DF) extraction is a process in which the features are directly acquired from the last fully connected layer of a pretrained deep learning network (e.g., AlexNet, ResNet-50 and VGG-19) without the need for re-training the networks. The main advantage of employing a pretrained model is huge savings in the computational time required to train these models from scratch, and hence the possibility of running these models on a CPU machine without the need for expensive GPU enabled computational power. An initial attempt by Sethy et al. [35], utilized 127 images of 3-class of COVID-19, pneumonia (viral and bacterial) and normal, 80–20% data split of training and testing was used to evaluate the model. An accuracy of 95.33% was obtained with ResNet-50 deep features and Support Vector Machines (SVM) classifier. However, it is not known how the performance of ResNet-50 compares to other pre-trained DL models, especially given that the dataset contained a small number of images. In [36], ResNet1523 and XGBoost classifiers were evaluated on a 3-class dataset (normal 1341 images, pneumonia 1345 images and only 62 COVID-19) with 30% holdout. From previous two studies, DF have been proposed for COVID-19 detection, but it was not investigated in depth.

The main challenges with the previous literature are related to one or more of the following:

(1) the small number of COVID-19 images, in comparison to other diseases considered, included in the datasets thus leading to unbalanced dataset;
(2) the need for GPU resources to train the newly proposed CNN or the pretrained CNNs.
(3) the class separability of COVID-19 DF is not known in problems where a larger number of diseases is considered.
(4) the detection of COVID-19 in the presence of TB in the same study has not been previously investigated, to the best of our knowledge.

In this chapter, we harvest the power of the good feature presentation of 14 state-of-the-art pretrained deep networks and the simplicity of machine learning classifiers for COVID-19 detection on a CPU machine in just under ten minutes for the whole training and testing, something that makes the proposed CAD suitable for low computational power settings. In addition, the proposed DF pipeline is evaluated on a balanced 2186 X-ray images of 5 classes including COVID-19, normal, bacterial pneumonia, viral pneumonia and TB.

The main contributions of the current study are:

(1) We constructed a five-class COVID-19 dataset, named COVID-19 five-class balanced dataset, including a large number of COVID-19 and TB images, which was not investigated before to the best of our knowledge.
(2) A pipeline of features from 14 individual state-of-the-art pretrained deep networks combined with machine learning classifier are investigated using a five-fold cross validation scheme to avoid overfitting, without the need to train the pretrained networks.
(3) The proposed pipeline can run on a CPU machine, which makes it simple and efficient, and suitable for low-middle income countries.
(4) Five-class separability analysis of COVID-19 DF using Silhouette criterion clustering evaluation and high dimensional t-SNE visualization were investigated to understand the separation of the 2186 5-class images.

2 Methodology

2.1 COVID-19 5-Class Balanced Dataset

The 5-class COVID-19 dataset, constructed in this study, consists of 3 main sources. The COVID-19 cases are acquired from Cohen et al. dataset [37] which is collection

Table 1 The details of the COVID-19 5-classes dataset

Class	Number of x-ray images
COVID-19	435
Normal	439
Pneumonia-bacterial	439
Pneumonia-viral	439
Tuberculosis	434 (394 + 40 augmented)
All 5-class dataset	2186

of X-ray and CT images of variety of pulmonary diseases, including COVID-19, SARS and MEARS, compiled from many sources. The dataset is updated on a regular basis to include more cases. Until 15/6/2020,[5] it had 752 X-ray images, among them 435 COVID-19 X-ray images which were utilized in this study. This dataset has the largest number of X-ray images of COVID-19 cases. The CT and lateral X-ray images were excluded from this study. The average age of the COVID-19 patients is 54.6 ± 16.7 years (mean ± standard deviation), including 256 males and 136 females, and the gender for 43 images was not provided, since the metadata accompanying the dataset is not complete.

The second source of images is the pneumonia and normal dataset [38] which has 5863 X-ray images[6] of 3-class including normal, pneumonia bacterial and pneumonia viral. We randomly selected 439 images of each class from the pneumonia dataset to be included in the study, to construct the COVID-19 balanced 5-class dataset.

The last source of X-ray images is TB dataset from U.S. National Library of Medicine, consisting of two datasets of chest X-ray. TB dataset were made available to expedite research in CAD of pulmonary diseases specially TB[7] [19, 23]. The TB dataset includes 394 images from 2 sources (336 images from China set and 58 images from Montgomery County set) [19, 23]. The TB X-ray images have a slightly less number than other classes in this study which may have an influence on the detection performance due to unbalanced classes [42]. To balance the TB class, augmentation [43] of random images has been done by rescaling 40 random X-ray images. The details of the constructed COVID-19 5-class balanced dataset is illustrated in Table 1. The current COVID-19 5-class dataset has a larger number of COVID-19 X-ray images, than previous studies [4, 12, 13, 35]. Ethical approvals of the datasets used were obtained by the corresponding publications. Samples of X-ray images of the 5 classes included in this study, with their labels, are shown in Fig. 1.

[5]https://github.com/ieee8023/covid-chestxray-dataset.

[6]https://www.kaggle.com/paultimothymooney/chest-xray-pneumonia.

[7]https://www.kaggle.com/kmader/pulmonary-chest-xray-abnormalities?select=ChinaSet_All Files.

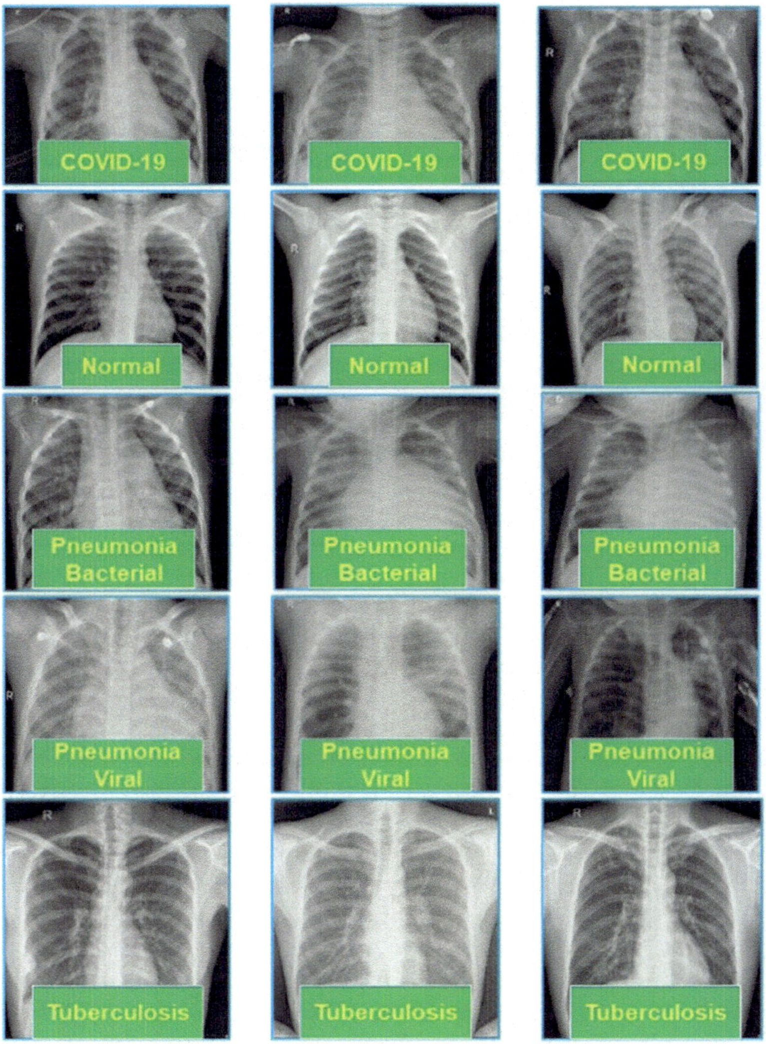

Fig. 1 Samples of the five-class X-ray images for the COVID-19, normal, pneumonia bacterial, pneumonia viral and TB

2.2 The Pipeline of Deep Feature Extraction from Pretrained Networks and Machine Learning Classification

In this section, the details of the proposed COVID-19 detection method will be presented. Figure 2 presents the block diagram of the proposed pipeline for COVID-

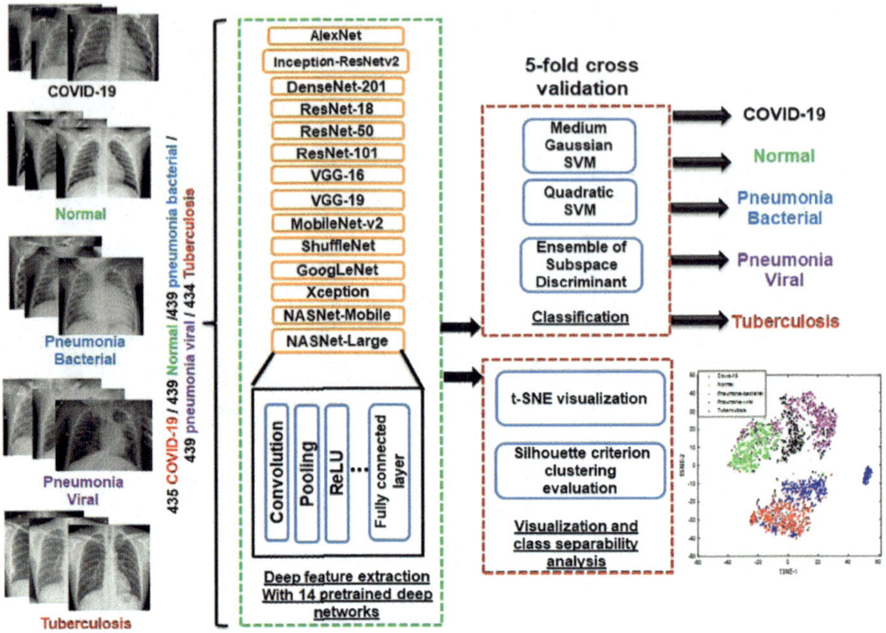

Fig. 2 The block diagram of the proposed 5-classes COVID-19 detection method

19 detection with deep features and machine learning classifiers on 5-class COVID-19 balanced dataset. The details of each part of the methodology will be presented in the next paragraphs.

To perform the classification of the extracted features for each of the 14 networks, we utilized machine learning classifiers. Classification Learner (CL) App in Matlab 2019b was used to perform the classification. We utilized five-fold Cross Validation (CV) for analysis in this study to avoid overfitting, as done in [4, 13, 27]. To select the best classifier for the COVID-19 5-class dataset, we carried out a pilot study with multiple classifiers in the CL App, including *k*-Nearest Neighbors (KNN), Linear Discriminant Analysis (LDA), Support Vector Machines (SVM), and variety of ensemble classifiers including boosting, bagging and subspace discriminant. The best three classifiers in the pilot study were quadratic SVM, medium Gaussian SVM and ensemble of subspace discriminant classifiers. The setting for the SVM classifiers utilized in this study are as follows (1) quadratic SVM (kernel function: quadratic, box constraint level = 1, one vs one classification); (2) medium Gaussian SVM (kernel type: Gaussian, kernel scale = 32, box constraint level = 1, one versus one classification). As for the ensemble of subspace discriminant classifier, random subspace ensembles [53] of a group of discriminant analysis classifier was used. Subspace ensembles have been utilized with the following settings (learner: discriminant. learning rate = 0.1, number of learners = 30, subspace dimension = 500).

In order to extract the DFs from the pretrained networks, 14 individual state-of-the-art pretrained networks were included in this study ranging from the networks with simple designs such as AlexNet and ShuffleNet to the advanced complex designs such as VGG-19 and NASNet-Large which requires large GPU power for training. This study investigated 14 networks larger than previous studies, where 11 and 13 networks were investigated in [35, 44], respectively. These networks are pretrained on ImageNet dataset [34] which has one million images for 1000 classes. In this study, we will input the X-ray images to each individual pretrained network and extract the feature vectors directly at the fully connected layer, without the need for training the network on the X-ray images. The full details of the 14 pretrained networks utilized in this study for feature extraction, with their input size, number of layers the name of the fully connected layer as well as the number of parameters are illustrated in Table 2. Preprocessing was performed to change the input size of the X-ray images to match the input of the targeted pretrained network (Table 2). The size of the extracted feature vector for each network was equal to 2186 × 1000 (number of X-ray images × number of DF), for each of the 14 networks.

2.3 Performance Evaluation of the Proposed COVID-19 Detection Pipeline

The performance of the proposed COVID-19 detection was evaluated with the following classification performance measures including accuracy, precision, recall, specificity, and *F*-score, given by

$$\text{Accuracy} = \frac{Number\ of\ correctly\ classified\ images}{Total\ number\ of\ images} \tag{1}$$

$$\text{Precision} = \frac{Sum\ of\ all\ TP}{Sum\ of\ all\ TP + FP} \tag{2}$$

$$\text{Recall} = \frac{Sum\ of\ all\ TP}{Sum\ of\ all\ TP + FN} \tag{3}$$

$$\text{Specificity} = \frac{TN}{TN + FP} \tag{4}$$

$$F - \text{score} = 2 * \frac{\text{Precision*Recall}}{\text{Precision} + \text{Recall}} \tag{5}$$

where TP (True Positive), TN (True Negative), FN (False Negative) and FP (False Positive). We also estimated the Area Under the Receiver Operating Characteristics (ROC) Curve (AUC) in the CL App in MATLAB 2019b.

To estimate the Confidence Interval (CI), we used Monte Carlo simulations by running random 5-fold cross-validation 200 times on the 5- and 3- class dataset, with

Table 2 The details of the 14 pretrained deep networks utilized in this study

Network name	Reference	Input size	Fully connected layer	No. of layers	No. of parameters in Million
AlexNet	Krizhevsky et al. [45]	227 × 227 × 3	fc8	25	61
Inception-ResNet-v2	Szegedy et al. [46]	299 × 299 × 3	predictions	824	23.2
DenseNet-201	Huang et al. [32]	224 × 224 × 3	fc1000	708	20
ResNet-18	He et al. [47]	224 × 224 × 3	fc1000	71	11.7
ResNet-50	He et al. [47]	224 × 224 × 3	fc1000	177	25.6
ResNet-101	He et al. [47]	224 × 224 × 3	fc1000	347	44.6
VGG-16	Simonyan and Zisserman [48]	224 × 224 × 3	fc8	41	138
VGG-19	Simonyan and Zisserman [48]	224 × 224 × 3	fc8	47	144
MobileNet-v2	Sandler et al. [33]	224 × 224 × 3	Logits	154	3.5
ShuffleNet	Zhang et al. [49]	224 × 224 × 3	node_202	172	1.4
GoogLeNet	Szegedy et al. [50]	224 × 224 × 3	Loss3-classifier	144	7
Xception	Chollet et al. [51]	299 × 299 × 3	Predictions	170	22.9
NASNet-Mobile	Zoph et al. [52]	224 × 224 × 3	Predictions	913	5.3
NASNet-Large	Zoph et al. [52]	331 × 331 × 3	Predictions	1243	88.9

the best performed network. Then, we report the computational 95% CI by discarding the top 5 and bottom 5 values.

In order to verify the statistical significance of the achieved classification results, we started first by verifying the distribution of the classification results using a Kolmogorov-Smirnov (KS) goodness-of-fit hypothesis test; this is to justify the selection of any parametric/nonparametric significance test. Based on the KS test results, a Friedman's test was then employed as a nonparametric test for data having a two-way layout (data grouped by two categorical factors). The first factor being related to the selected DL models with 14 levels (14 models) and the second being related to the selected 3 traditional classifiers (quadratic SVM, medium Gaussian SVM, and ensemble of subspace discriminant classifiers). We have also studied other class combinations, including 3-classes (COVID-19 vs. normal vs. TB) and 2 -classes (COVID-19 vs. normal) to show the robustness of the proposed method with different number of COVID-19 classes.

To investigate class separability of the COVID-19 features, we utilized *t*-Distributed Stochastic Neighbor Embedding (*t*-SNE) data visualization [54, 55] to reduce dimensions of the deep features computed with the pretrained networks. This was done for the 5-class, 3-class and 2-class COVID-19 features. In addition, The Silhouette criterion—a clustering evaluation measure—[56] was used to evaluate the quality of the 5-class COVID-19 features.

3 Results

In this section, we will present the results of the analysis of the five-class COVID-19 balanced dataset with the proposed deep feature extraction and machine learning classification pipeline. Figure 3 shows the results of the classification accuracy with the 14 state-of-the-art deep feature learning methods integrated with three classifiers (quadratic SVM, medium Gaussian SVM and ensemble of subspace discriminant). ResNet-50 and ResNet-101 were the best DF, with all classifiers, compared to the

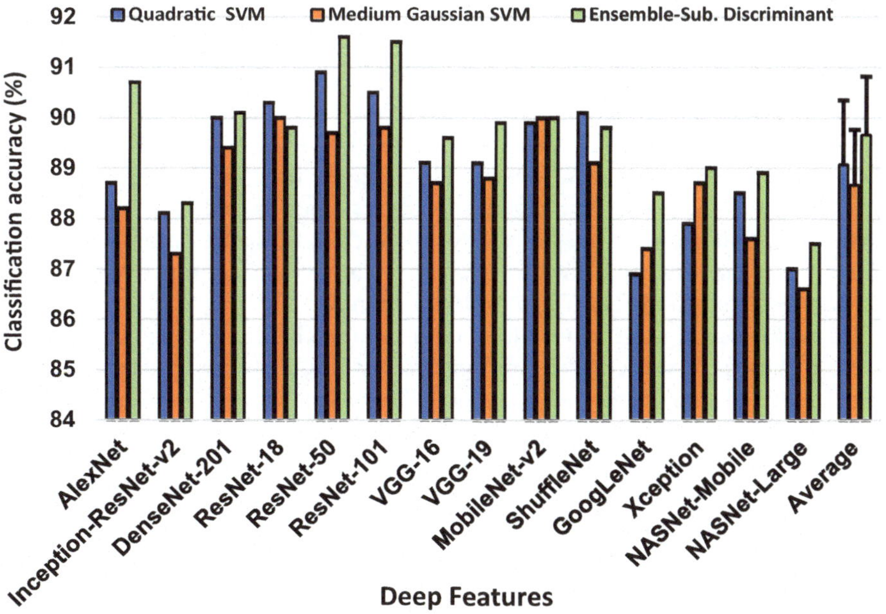

Fig. 3 Classification accuracy for DF extracted from the 14 deep networks investigated in this study with 5-class COVID-19 images with 3 machine learning classifiers. The average of all classifiers is also shown with error bars representing standard deviation

Table 3 The time needed to extract deep features from all pretrained networks for all 2186 images. Time estimated for 5-fold CV on Core *i5* CPU computer with 16 GB RAM

No.	Network Name	Time for deep feature extraction (minutes) for 2186 images
1	AlexNet	3.25
2	Inception-ResNet-v2	33.54
3	DenseNet-201	20.79
4	ResNet-18	6.50
5	ResNet-50	6.90
6	ResNet-101	11.60
7	VGG-16	31.85
8	VGG-19	38.72
9	MobileNet-v2	5.37
10	ShuffleNet	4.62
11	GoogLeNet	7.16
12	Xception	24.75
13	NASNet-Mobile	8.07
14	NASNet-Large	94.05

other networks. In addition, ensemble of subspace discriminant classifier was the best on average among the other classifiers. To show the effectiveness of the proposed method, we calculated the time for feature extraction of all 2186 images, with all pretrained networks (Table 3), which ranges from few minutes for simple networks (AlexNet and ResNet-50) to > 30 min for big networks such as VGG-19 and NASNet-Large. On average, 0.09 s is needed to extract the DFs with AlexNet for a single image. This time was calculated on a Core *i5* CPU computer with 16 GB RAM. It is worth noting that the time to perform the classification of the whole dataset with five-fold cross-validation was equal to 0.5 min for SVM classifiers and 2 min for ensemble of subspace discriminant classifier. In addition, all classification performed in this study, was done with 5-fold CV to avoid overfitting.

Using Friedman's test, a p-value < 0.001 returned by this test indicated that the average classification accuracies are significantly different across the three levels of the classifiers factor (three traditional classifiers). This was followed by a multiple comparison of means with Bonferroni choice for the *critical value* which further indicated that, across all DL models, no significant differences existed between the quadratic SVM and ensemble of subspace discriminant classifier and quadratic and medium Gaussian SVM (p-value > 0.05 for all tests) while significant differences existed between medium Gaussian SVM and ensemble of subspace discriminant classifiers (p-value < 0.001). Similarly, Friedman's test also indicated statistically significant differences across the 14 levels of the DL models factor, with a p-value $=$ 0.001. Overall, the combination of ResNet-50 with the ensemble of subspace discriminant classifiers achieved the highest classification accuracy, followed by ResNet-101 with the ensemble of subspace discriminant classifiers. However, ResNet-101 required almost double the computational time of ResNet-50, per the results from Table 3.

While the pipeline consisting of ResNet-50 and ensemble of subspace discriminant classifier showed as the best performer among all networks and classifiers (detection accuracy $91.6 \pm 0.57\%$, accuracy ± CI), it was also very efficient (6.9 min for DF and 2 min for classification, see Table 3). It will be chosen to perform the subsequent analysis in this study.

The confusion matrix for the 5-class COVID-19 detection dataset with ResNet-50 and ensemble of subspace discriminant classifier is shown in Fig. 4. COVID-19 and TB achieved the best performance compared to the other classes, where less than 1% of the COVID-19 cases were mis-detected as normal and TB (Fig. 4), while the lowest performance was for pneumonia bacterial and viral. In addition, classification measures for each class in terms of precision, recall, specificity, *F*-score and AUC were also calculated (Table 4). The highest specificity was for COVID-19, normal and TB classes, which shows the potential use of our proposed method to aid for quick COVID-19 and TB detection.

The second part of the analysis was to investigate the class separability with the state-of-the-art high dimensional *t*-SNE visualization to understand how the features are distributed in the feature space (Fig. 5). Clear separation of the COVID-19 and TB classes compared to that of normal can be observed, while there is an area of overlap

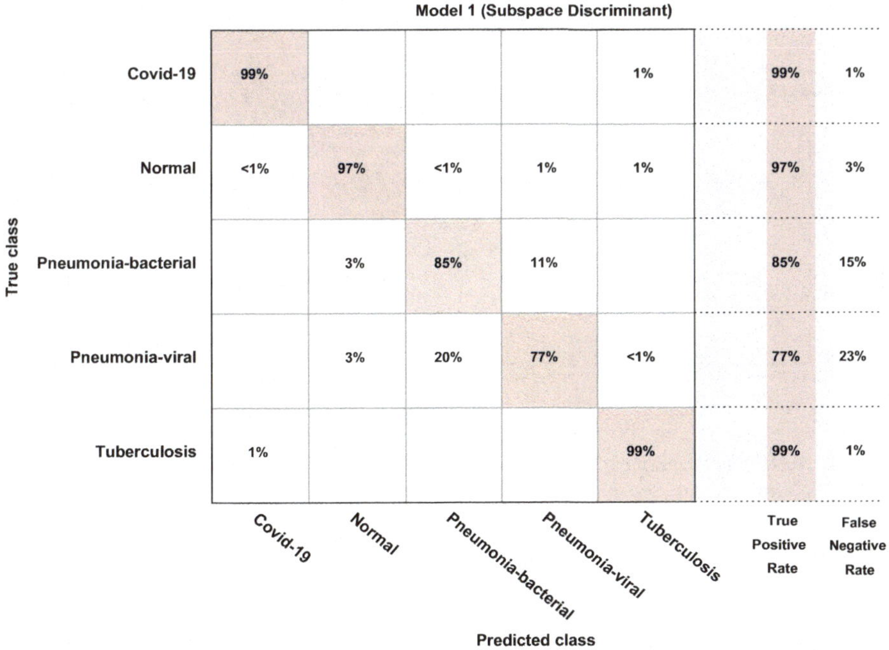

Fig. 4 Confusion matrix for ResNet-50 for 5-class COVID-19 classification with ensemble of subspace discriminant classifier (5-fold CV)

Table 4 The classification performance including precision, recall, specificity, *F*-score and AUC for ResNet-50 and ensemble of subspace discriminant classifier. The overall detection accuracy is equal to 91.6 ± 0.57% (accuracy at 95% confidence level)

Class	Precision	Recall	Specificity	*F*-score	AUC
COVID-19	99	98.6	99.8	98.8	1
Normal	94	97.2	98.5	95.6	0.99
Pneumonia-bacterial	81	85.4	95	83.1	0.97
Pneumonia-viral	86.3	77.2	97	81.5	0.97
Tuberculosis	97.3	99.3	99.3	98.3	1

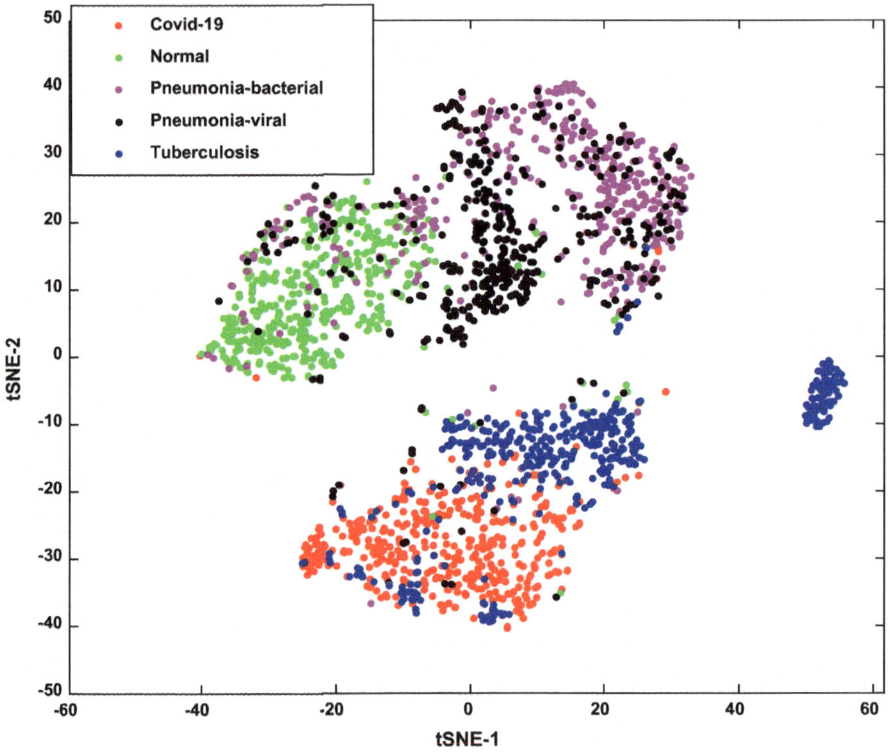

Fig. 5 *t*-SNE visualizations of five-class balanced COVID-19 features extracted from ResNet-50 for 2186 X-ray images. See corresponding confusion matrix in Fig. 4

of bacterial and viral pneumonia. Silhouette criterion values illustrated in Table 5, where the higher the values, the better the class separation, showed that COVID-19 and normal have a high Silhouette criterion values whereas pneumonia-bacterial has the lowest value (Table 5).

Table 5 Silhouette criterion values for 5-class COVID-19 balanced dataset

Class	Silhouette criterion values
COVID-19	0.5345
Normal	0.5843
Pneumonia-bacterial	−0.7114
Pneumonia-viral	0.3220
Tuberculosis	−0.3190

Table 6 The classification performance for 3-class (COVID-19 vs. normal vs. TB) with ResNet-50 and ensemble of subspace discriminant with 5-fold CV. The overall detection accuracy is equal to 98.6 ± 0.34% (accuracy ± CI at 95% confidence level)

Class	Precision	Recall	Specificity	F-score	AUC
COVID-19	98.39	98.39	99.20	98.39	1
Normal	100	98.86	100	99.43	1
Tuberculosis	97.49	98.62	98.74	98.05	1

Since there is an area of overlap between the 2-class of COVID-19 and TB to that of normal, we investigated three-class of COVID-19 versus normal versus TB due to the relevance of TB to some low- and middle-income countries [5]. Table 6 shows classification performance matrices for the three-class problem and the corresponding confusion matrix is illustrated in Fig. 6. The overall accuracy for the three-class problem was 98.6 ± 0.34% (accuracy ± CI). The t-SNE visualization displayed in Fig. 7 shows clear area of separation between normal and COVID-19 and also TB. There are some TB cases that are overlapped with COVID-19 cases.

Finally, to investigate the performance of our proposed COVID-19 detection method for 2-class COVID-19 versus normal, similar to [4, 12, 13]. The results are shown in Fig. 8 and t-SNE visualization is shown in Fig. 9. High detection accuracy rate of 99.9 was obtained on 847 images of COVID-19 and normal with five-fold CV.

We then ran a test with our proposed method on the four-class COVID-19 dataset [13] with four-fold CV for a straightforward comparison with that study. Our detection accuracy was equal to 90.2% (Fig. 10) which outperformed their accuracy (89.6%) [13]. Notably, our approach only required a CPU computer while their work needed a Tesla GPU machine.

4 Discussion

We presented in this chapter an efficient approach employing existing and pretrained DL models for the classification of five-class COVID-19 images with three traditional machine learning classifiers. The main power of the features produced by these models is attributed to the fact that these networks learned the most discriminant

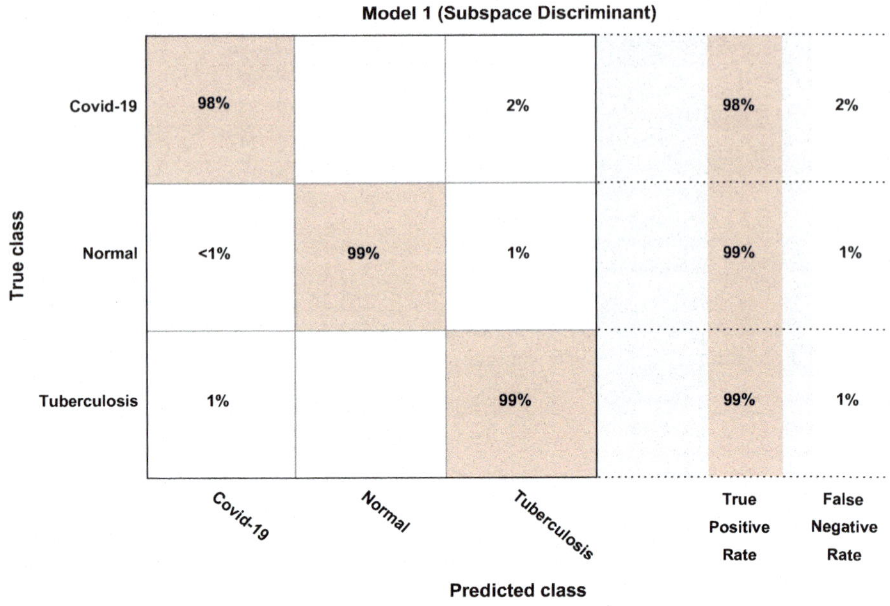

Fig. 6 Confusion matrix for the 3-class (COVID-19 vs. normal vs. TB)

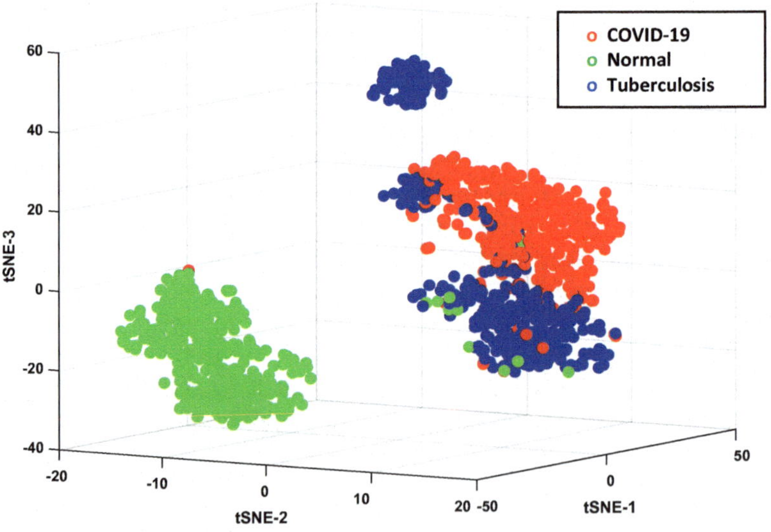

Fig. 7 *t*-SNE visualization in 3 dimensions for the 3-class DF of ResNet-50 for COVID-19 versus normal versus TB. See corresponding confusion matrix in Fig. 6

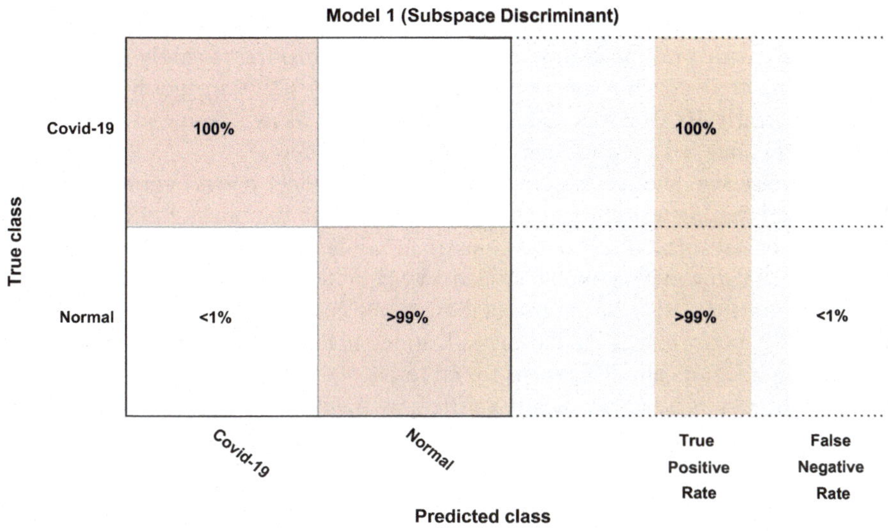

Fig. 8 Confusion matrix for 2-class of COVID-19 versus normal. The detection accuracy is equal to 99.9%

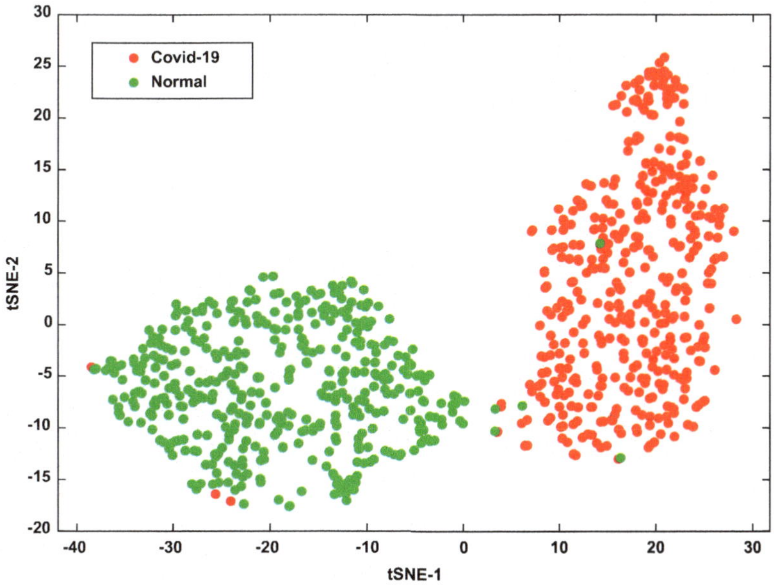

Fig. 9 2-class *t*-SNE visualization for COVID-19 vs. normal. See corresponding confusion matrix in Fig. 8

parameters to classify the original images, upon which these models were developed, without any hand crafting feature extraction algorithms. Interestingly, the DF were extracted from models not specifically trained on COVID-19 images but on general images of nearly 1000 classes and each model learned its own features or descriptors that best separate between the considered classes of images.

When observing the accuracy of the utilized DL models, it was found that ResNet-50 [47] had the highest classification accuracy across the quadratic SVM and the ensemble of subspace discriminant classifier, while being close to the best model results when using the medium Gaussian SVM classifier. The employed Friedman's test supported the statistical analysis of these results indicating a significant difference between the performance of the classification models across the 14 utilized DL models, with significant differences for all tests.

Once the results were statistically verified, we then studied the computational time requirements needed to extract deep features from all pretrained 14 networks for 2186 images, with the results indicating that AlexNet took only 3.25 min on average across several runs to extract the important features from 2186 images. ResNet-50, being the best performing model on the current set of images, took approximately 0.19 s per image, run on standard Core *i*5 CPU computer (6.90 min for the whole dataset of 2186 images, Table 3). On the other hand, the worst performing model in terms of the computational cost was the NASNet-Large as it took around 94 min to extract the features. Other models had their computational costs ranging across those

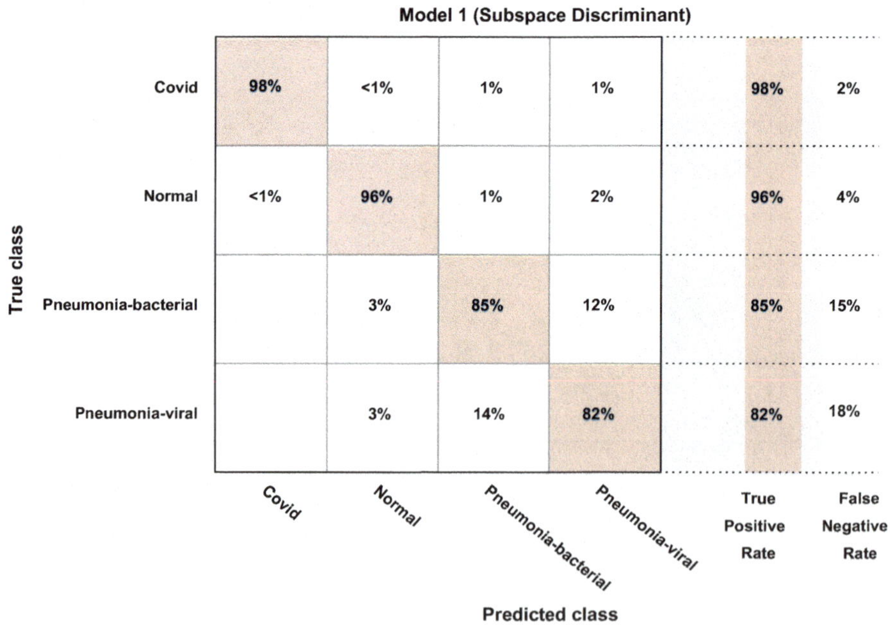

Fig. 10 The confusion matrix of our proposed method on the four-class dataset used in [13]

values. This in turn supports the first finding regarding the best performing model as ResNet-50 took only around a quarter of the average time for all models considered in Table 3.

COVID-19 and TB are two classes that are best detected among the five classes investigated in this study, specificity is equal to 99.8% and 99.3%, respectively (Table 4). This may be clinically important, especially for some low and middle income countries, to detect both TB and COVID-19 since TB has a higher mortality rate more than COVID-19. The proposed pipeline can run on low resource settings (CPU computer instead of GPU).

The silhouette criterion values for the TB cases were low (Table 5), despite having a good detection accuracy (Table 4). This may be attributed that TB has two distinct clusters (Figs. 5 and 7), which increase the distance between the samples belonging to TB class, despite being distinct from normal and other types of pneumonia.

The subsequent analysis focused on ResNet-50, as we decided to further understand the performance of this DL network across each of the individual classes in the five-class dataset considered here. The importance of this step in the analysis can be appreciated when considering the similarity between some of the symptoms of the considered diseases, specially fever, tiredness and cough, for TB and COVID-19. Interestingly, the trained ResNet-50 model showed only 1% errors when it comes to the proper identification of COVID-19 and TB, while most of the confusion took a place between pneumonia bacterial and viral, with pneumonia viral being the most confused about class of diseases. These results were further supported by all the precision, recall, specificity, *F*-score and AUC measures for ResNet-50. These measures support the potential use of the proposed model as a quick and reliable CAD in COVID-19 and TB detection.

When inspecting the *t*-SNE visualizations of five-class balanced COVID-19 features extracted from ResNet-50 for 2186 X-ray images, it was found that COVID-19 and TB were completely separated from normal and Pneumonia bacterial and viral. However, there was some degree of overlapping between COVID-19 and TB when visually inspecting the *t*-SNE feature projections across the first two dimensions. However, this visual overlapping was tackled with the power of our nonlinear classification models, in a 3D *t*-SNE visualization.

We also investigated the classification performance for three-class (COVID-19 vs. normal vs. TB) with ResNet-50 and ensemble of subspace discriminant and the two-class (COVID-19 vs. normal). In both set of tests, COVID-19 is shown to be completely separated from normal, and clearly separated from TB.

As we quantified the performance of our proposed combination of DL and machine learning models, we then analyzed the reported performance results from several other research groups as shown in Table 7 in comparison to our model results. Our proposed COVID-19 detection pipeline outperformed the state-of-the-art-literature, illustrated in Table 7. It should be noted that each model tested a different dataset, different testing split and also different classes. Hence, the comparison between these models here is for illustrative purposes but it shows the potential of our approach combining DF and simple classifiers in this task.

Table 7 Comparison to the previous literature on COVID-19 detection with X-ray images

Study	Dataset	Evaluation method	Techniques used	Detection accuracy
Narin et al. [27]	**2-class:** 50 COVID-19/50 normal	5-fold CV	Transfer learning with Resnet50 and InceptionV3	98%
Panwar et al. [31]	**2-class:** 142 COVID-19/142 normal	Holdout 30%	nCOVnet CNN	88%
Chowdhury et al. [12]	**3-class:** 423 COVID-19 1579 normal 1485 pneumonia viral	5-fold CV	Transfer learning with ChexNet	97.7%
Wang and Wong [22]	**3-class:** 358 COVID-19/5538 normal/8066 pneumonia	Holdout 30%	COVID-Net	93.3%
Kumar et al. [36]	**3-class:** 62 COVID-19/1341 normal/1345 pneumonia	Holdout 30%	Resnet1523 features and XGBoost classifier	90%
Sethy and Behera [35]	**3-class:** 127 COVID-19/127 normal/127 pneumonia	Holdout 20%	Resnet50 features and SVM	95.33%
Ozturk et al. [4]	**3-class:** 125 COVID-19/500 normal 500 pneumonia	5-fold CV	DarkCovidNet CNN	87.2%
Khan et al. [13]	**4-class:** 284 COVID-19/310 normal/330 pneumonia bacterial/327 pneumonia viral	4-fold CV	CoroNet CNN	89.6%%

(continued)

Table 7 (continued)

Study	Dataset	Evaluation method	Techniques used	Detection accuracy
This study	**5-class:** 435 COVID-19/439 normal/439 pneumonia bacterial/439 pneumonia viral/434 Tuberculosis **3-class:** 435 COVID-19/439 normal/434 Tuberculosis	5-fold CV	Resnet50 features and ensemble of subspace discriminant classifier	$91.6 \pm 0.57\%$[a] $98.6 \pm 0.34\%$[b]

[a]Detection accuracy (Acc.) with 95% Confidence Interval (CI)
[b]The CI for the previous literature is not provided

The study has a potential limitation of relatively small number of COVID-19 and TB images, despite being the largest compared to previous literature so far. More COVID-19 and TB images are needed to improve the robustness of the proposed pipeline in a future research. The separation of the TB cases in two clusters in the *t*-SNE visualization should also be investigated in the future.

5 Conclusion

We proposed a combination of deep and machine learning models for the classification of X-ray chest images into five classes including COVID-19, in contrast with viral pneumonia, bacterial pneumonia, and TB, and in comparison, to the normal healthy subjects. Our work was motivated by the challenging conditions in low resource environments, where TB and COVID-19 can be a major healthcare problem. A key characteristic of our study is that the pre-trained networks can be utilized without GPU support as no (re-) training of the deep networks is required. Thus, we are able to extract DF of the X-ray images efficiently with a CPU-enabled computer. Our developments were tested using five-fold cross-validation, achieving $91.6 \pm 0.57\%$ accuracy (accuracy $\pm$ CI) with a pipeline consisting of ResNet-50 for DF computation and ensemble of subspace discriminant classifiers in the distinction of the five groups or classes of diseases. In addition, we explored the classification accuracy in three- and two-class problems (COVID-19, TB and healthy cases; and COVID-19 and healthy cases; respectively) and obtained accuracies over 98% on both cases. Our study is limited by the relatively small number of COVID-19 and TB images, but it shows the promise of a pipeline requiring low computational resources to contribute to the detection of COVID-19 and TB using X-ray images where other more advanced or computationally demanding techniques may not be available.

Acknowledgements The authors are grateful for the research groups who provided the X-ray images. We would like also to thank all medial staff around the world who are in the first line of defense against COVID-19.

References

1. Rothan, H.A., Byrareddy, S.N.: The epidemiology and pathogenesis of coronavirus disease (COVID-19) outbreak. J. Autoimmun. 102433 (2020)
2. WHO) WHO (2020) Coronaviruses (COVID-19)
3. Xie, X., Zhong, Z., Zhao, W., et al.: Chest CT for typical 2019-nCoV pneumonia: relationship to negative RT-PCR testing. Radiology 200343 (2020)
4. Ozturk, T., Talo, M., Yildirim, E.A., et al.: Automated detection of COVID-19 cases using deep neural networks with X-ray images. Comput. Biol. Med., 103792 (2020)
5. (WHO) WHO Tuberculosis. https://www.who.int/news-room/fact-sheets/detail/tuberculosis. Accessed 1 Jul 2020
6. (WHO) WHO (2020) Tuberculosis and COVID-19. https://www.who.int/news-room/q-a-detail/tuberculosis-and-the-covid-19-pandemic. Accessed 28 Jun 2020
7. Glaziou, P.: Predicted impact of the COVID-19 pandemic on global tuberculosis deaths in 2020. medRxiv (2020)
8. Butt, C., Gill, J., Chun, D., Babu, B.A.: Deep learning system to screen coronavirus disease 2019 pneumonia. Appl. Intell. **1** (2020)
9. Pathak, Y., Shukla, P.K., Tiwari, A., et al.: Deep Transfer Learning based Classification Model for COVID-19 Disease. IRBM (2020)
10. Ardakani, A.A., Kanafi, A.R., Acharya, U.R., et al.: Application of deep learning technique to manage COVID-19 in routine clinical practice using CT images: results of 10 convolutional neural networks. Comput. Biol. Med., 103795 (2020)
11. Perumal, V., Narayanan, V., Rajasekar, S.J.S.: Detection of COVID-19 using CXR and CT images using Transfer Learning and Haralick features. Appl. Intell., 1–18 (2020)
12. Chowdhury, M.E.H., Rahman, T., Khandakar, A., et al.: Can AI help in screening viral and COVID-19 pneumonia? arXiv Prepr arXiv200313145 (2020)
13. Khan, A.I., Shah, J.L., Bhat, M.M.: Coronet: A deep neural network for detection and diagnosis of COVID-19 from chest x-ray images. Comput. Methods Progr. Biomed., 105581 (2020)
14. Lalmuanawma, S., Hussain, J., Chhakchhuak, L.: Applications of Machine Learning and Artificial Intelligence for Covid-19 (SARS-CoV-2) pandemic: a review. Chaos, Solit. Fract., 110059 (2020)
15. Hemdan, E.E.D., Shouman, M.A., Karar, M.E.: Covidx-net: a framework of deep learning classifiers to diagnose covid-19 in x-ray images. arXiv Prepr arXiv:200311055 (2020)
16. Minaee, S., Kafieh, R., Sonka, M., et al.: Deep-covid: Predicting covid-19 from chest x-ray images using deep transfer learning. arXiv Prepr arXiv200409363 (2020)
17. Apostolopoulos, I.D., Mpesiana, T.A.: Covid-19: automatic detection from x-ray images utilizing transfer learning with convolutional neural networks. Phys. Eng. Sci. Med., 1 (2020)
18. Hammoudi, K., Benhabiles, H., Melkemi, M., et al.: Deep learning on chest X-ray images to detect and evaluate pneumonia cases at the era of COVID-19. arXiv Prepr arXiv200403399 (2020)
19. Jaeger, S., Karargyris, A., Candemir, S., et al.: Automatic tuberculosis screening using chest radiographs. IEEE Trans. Med. Imaging **33**, 233–245 (2013)

20. Cao, Y., Liu, C., Liu, B., Brunette, M.J., Zhang, N., Sun, T., Zhang, P., Peinado, J., Garavito, E.S., LLG, et al.: Improving tuberculosis diagnostics using deep learning and mobile health technologies among resource-poor and marginalized communities. In: IEEE International Conference on Connected Health: Applications, Systems and Engineering Technologies (CHASE), pp 274–281 (2016)
21. Rav, D., Wong, C., Deligianni, F., et al.: Deep learning for health informatics. IEEE J. Biomed. Heal Inform. **21**, 4–21 (2017)
22. Wang, L., Wong, A.: COVID-Net: A tailored deep convolutional neural network design for detection of COVID-19 cases from chest X-Ray Images. arXiv Prepr arXiv200309871 (2020)
23. Candemir, S., Jaeger, S., Palaniappan, K., et al.: Lung segmentation in chest radiographs using anatomical atlases with nonrigid registration. IEEE Trans. Med. Imaging **33**, 577–590 (2013)
24. Alzubaidi, L., Fadhel, M.A., Oleiwi, S.R., et al.: DFU_QUTNet: diabetic foot ulcer classification using novel deep convolutional neural network. Multimed. Tools Appl., 1–23 (2019)
25. Chen, H., Ni, D., Qin, J., et al.: Standard plane localization in fetal ultrasound via domain transferred deep neural networks. IEEE J Biomed. Heal inform. **19**, 1627–1636 (2015)
26. Norouzifard, M., Nemati, A., GholamHosseini, H., et al.: Automated glaucoma diagnosis using deep and transfer learning: proposal of a system for clinical testing. In: 2018 International Conference on Image and Vision Computing New Zealand (IVCNZ). IEEE, pp. 1–6 (2018)
27. Narin, A., Kaya, C., Pamuk, Z.: Automatic detection of coronavirus disease (covid-19) using x-ray images and deep convolutional neural networks. arXiv Prepr arXiv200310849 (2020)
28. Loey, M., Smarandache, F., Khalifa, M.N.E.: Within the lack of chest COVID-19 X-ray dataset: a novel detection model based on GAN and deep transfer learning. Symmetry (Basel) **12**, 651 (2020)
29. Luz, E., Silva, P.L., Silva, R., Moreira, G.: Towards an efficient deep learning model for covid-19 patterns detection in x-ray images. arXiv Prepr arXiv200405717 (2020)
30. Ucar, F., Korkmaz, D.: COVIDiagnosis-Net: deep bayes-squeezenet based diagnostic of the coronavirus disease 2019 (COVID-19) from X-ray images. Med. Hypotheses 109761 (2020)
31. Panwar, H., Gupta, P.K., Siddiqui, M.K., et al.: Application of Deep Learning for Fast Detection of COVID-19 in X-Rays using nCOVnet. Chaos, Solit. Fract., 109944 (2020)
32. Huang, G., Liu, Z., Van Der Maaten, L., Weinberger, K.Q.: Densely connected convolutional networks. In: Proceedings of the IEEE Conference on Computer Vision and Pattern Recognition, pp. 4700–4708 (2017)
33. Sandler, M., Howard, A., Zhu, M., et al.: Mobilenetv2: Inverted residuals and linear bottlenecks. In: Proceedings of the IEEE Conference on Computer Vision and Pattern Recognition, pp. 4510–4520 (2018)
34. Russakovsky, O., Deng, J., Su, H., et al.: Imagenet large scale visual recognition challenge. Int. J. Comput. Vis. **115**, 211–252 (2015)
35. Sethy, P.K., Behera, S.K., Ratha, P., Biswas, P.: Detection of coronavirus Disease (COVID-19) based on deep features and support vector machine. Int. J. Math. Eng. Manag. Sci. **5**, 643–651 (2020)
36. Kumar, R., Arora, R., Bansal, V., et al.: Accurate Prediction of COVID-19 using Chest X-Ray Images through Deep Feature Learning model with SMOTE and Machine Learning Classifiers. medRxiv (2020)
37. Cohen, J.P., Morrison, P., Dao, L.: COVID-19 image data collection. arXiv Prepr arXiv200311597 (2020)
38. Kermany, D.S., Goldbaum, M., Cai, W., et al.: Identifying medical diagnoses and treatable diseases by image-based deep learning. Cell **172**, 1122–1131 (2018)
39. Rahimzadeh, M., Attar, A.: A modified deep convolutional neural network for detecting COVID-19 and pneumonia from chest X-ray images based on the concatenation of Xception and ResNet50V2. Inf. Med. Unlocked 100360 (2020)
40. Brunese, L., Mercaldo, F., Reginelli, A., Santone, A.: Explainable Deep learning for pulmonary disease and coronavirus COVID-19 detection from X-rays. Comput Methods Programs Biomed 105608 (2020)

41. Chowdhury, A., Shankaran, R., Kavakli, M., Haque, M.M.: Sensor applications and physiological features in drivers' drowsiness detection: A review. IEEE Sens. J. **1748**, 3055–3067 (2018). https://doi.org/10.1109/JSEN.2018.2807245
42. Issarti, I., Consejo, A., Koppen, C., et al.: Computer aided diagnosis for suspect keratoconus detection. Comput. Biol. Med. **109**, 33–42 (2019). https://doi.org/10.1016/j.compbiomed.2019.04.024
43. Johnson, J.M., Khoshgoftaar, T.M.: Survey on deep learning with class imbalance. J. Big Data **6**, xx (2019). https://doi.org/10.1186/s40537-019-0192-5
44. Karar, M.E., Hemdan, E.E.D., Shouman, M.A.: Cascaded deep learning classifiers for computer-aided diagnosis of COVID-19 and pneumonia diseases in X-ray scans. Complex Intell. Syst., 1–13 (2020)
45. Krizhevsky, A., Sutskever, I., Hinton, G.E.: Imagenet classification with deep convolutional neural networks. In: Advances in Neural Information Processing Systems, pp. 1097–1105 (2012)
46. Szegedy, C., Ioffe, S., Vanhoucke, V., Alemi, A.A.: Inception-v4, inception-resnet and the impact of residual connections on learning. In: Thirty-First AAAI Conference on Artificial Intelligence (2017)
47. He, K., Zhang, X., Ren, S., Sun, J.: Deep residual learning for image recognition. In: Proceedings of the IEEE Conference on Computer Vision and Pattern Recognition, pp. 770–778 (2016)
48. Simonyan, K., Zisserman, A.: Very deep convolutional networks for large-scale image recognition. arXiv Prepr arXiv14091556 (2014)
49. Zhang, X., Zhou, X., Lin, M., Sun, J.: Shufflenet: An extremely efficient convolutional neural network for mobile devices. In: Proceedings of the IEEE Conference on Computer Vision and Pattern Recognition, pp 6848–6856 (2018)
50. Szegedy, C., Liu, W., Jia, Y., et al.: Going deeper with convolutions. In: Proceedings of the IEEE Conference on Computer Vision and Pattern Recognition, pp. 1–9 (2015)
51. Chollet, F.: Xception: Deep learning with depthwise separable convolutions. In: Proceedings of the IEEE Conference on Computer Vision and Pattern Recognition, pp. 1251–1258 (2017)
52. Zoph, B., Vasudevan, V., Shlens, J., Le Q V (2018) Learning transferable architectures for scalable image recognition. In: Proceedings of the IEEE conference on computer vision and pattern recognition. pp 8697–8710
53. Ho, T.K.: The random subspace method for constructing decision forests. IEEE Trans. Pattern Anal. Mach. Intell. **20**, 832–844 (1998)
54. Van Der Maaten L (2013) Barnes-hut-sne. In: Proceedings of the International Conference on Learning Representations,
55. van der Maaten, L., Hinton, G.: Visualizing data using t-SNE. J Mach Learn Res **9**, 2579–2605 (2008)
56. Rousseeuw, P.J.: Silhouettes: a graphical aid to the interpretation and validation of cluster analysis. J. Comput. Appl. Math. **20**, 53–65 (1987)

Understanding Role of Information and Communication Technology Application in Vietnam's Prevention and Control of COVID-19 Pandemic

Nguyen Le Thy Thuong, Thuy T. Dang, and Tran Ngoc Diem

Abstract Information and communication technology (ICT) is a combination stressing the important role in the prevention of COVID-19 in Vietnam. This article shows that the communication has greatly contributed towards the success of anti-pandemic propaganda campaign encouraging the spread of message "Fighting the pandemic is like fighting against the enemy" and getting enthusiastic response nationwide. Additionally, a wide variety of applications for warning and detecting new cases has been created. Information technology also has great significance for digital transformation in some public services that previously required the direct participation and contact of the people, thereby helping alleviate the risk of infection with corona virus. However, certain negative impacts of a strong and drastic propaganda strategy of the media on people's psychology are readily visible. At the same time, any low efficiency of ICT applications for digitizing public services and detecting new cases is another constraint that needs improvement if Vietnam desires to maintain a good performance in the fight against COVID-19 as in the first stage.

Keywords Coronavirus · COVID-19 · Propaganda · Vietnam

1 Introduction

The COVID-19 pandemic has cast a shadow over all continents and most parts of the world bringing to the forefront the importance of disease prevention. Vietnam shares a long border with China not only driving a huge flow of people and goods back and forth between the two sides but also owning high degree of international exchange and openness, hence since the first start of COVID-19 outbreak, Vietnam ranks among countries categorized with best anti-pandemic performance globally. According to Politico's ranking of 30 leading countries in COVID-19 fight published on May 21 2020, Vietnam lands number one with numerous indicators showing the

N. Le Thy Thuong · Thuy T. Dang (✉) · T. N. Diem
Vietnam Institute for Indian and Southwest Asian Studies, Hanoi, Vietnam
e-mail: thuy0183@gmail.com

Vietnam Academy of Social Sciences, Hanoi, Vietnam

D. Oliva et al. (eds.), *Artificial Intelligence for COVID-19*, Studies in Systems, Decision and Control 358, https://doi.org/10.1007/978-3-030-69744-0_7

best community health and economic status [1]. The shared border line of 1.450 km with China—the country, where the pandemic originated, Vietnam recorded the first case of COVID 19 infection on January 23. As of November 2020, Vietnam now reports a total of 1,213 cases, of which 1,070 recoveries and 35 deaths and no severe COVID-19 cases. The cure rate is high (up to 96.4%) with the high rate of severe cases; controlling to the utmost death rate and cross-infection rate may be acquired in health-care facilities [2]. It is noteworthy that there are three rather extended periods which Vietnam confirms no new community transmission case: the first lasts 22 days, the second last 99 days. Until the end of the 99-day period mentioned above, there was no death due to COVID-19. After this time, new cases were recorded in Da Nang, first discovered at Da Nang Hospital C on July 25. The pandemic then spread rapidly and all had link to three hospital where curing lots critically ill patients with existed illness and extremely low resistance. Up to now all cases dying with corona virus have existed illnesses, most of them suffered from severe underlying diseases such as heart failure, chronic kidney failure, diabetes … In the third time period, taking into account on November 8, 2020, Vietnam has detect no new community transmission case for 66 days.

The evolution of COVID-19 pandemic in Vietnam shows that the number of community transmission cases has been kept to a minimum and remained zero cases for an entirely long time. So, along with medical measures and quarantine, what other methods has Vietnam's government used to prevent and combat the pandemic? Obviously, to limit the risk of community transmission, several tools that are capable of supporting effective social management should be used, thus they have not only wide coverage capabilities but also overall effectiveness and quick and prompt processing speed. Through researching, the authors find out that regarding Vietnam's prevention of pandemic, the ICT application plays a very important role reflecting its key role in the following areas: (1) anti-pandemic propaganda campaign; (2) case detection and warning; (3) digital transformation in public services to reduce the risk of infection and ensure the normalization of all activities at state agencies during times maintaining social distancing.

2 Literature Review

Due to the undeniable effects of ICT application in information dissemination about infectious diseases, various researches on the role of ICT in disease prevention have been conducting worldwide. Through studying many important information technology innovations to develop early warning capabilities, global health governance capabilities and impact of the technology on World Health Organization (WHO)'s capacity to handle disease, Galaz [3] shows that the explosion of the Internet and other information technology play a crucial role in increasing international organizations' capacity to cope with infectious diseases. The author argues that WHO's increasingly effective response to emerging infectious diseases has revealed that in an era of technological changes, towards sustainable governance, we should consider the wide range of challenges in information management faced by states, organizations and international partnerships. Shirky [4] argued that the spread of social media such as Twitter and Facebook, web-based surveillance systems and online collaboration had a distinct impact on collective action, political behavior and social movements on an international scale. O'Leary [5] records and analyzes the strengths and weaknesses of numerous applications for detecting infections used during COVID-19 pandemic. Authors' detailed analysis of the applications provides us important information to compare and clarify the strengths and weaknesses of the applications issued by the Government of Vietnam. Moreover, O'Leary also lists and reviews the shortcomings of online education remaining it unable to replace traditional education, so it is not an effective method in normalizing the operation of the education industry during COVID-19 outbreak. Regarding the negative impacts of ICT, Laato et al. [6] points out that the rapid spread of misinformation is amplified by social media and has may lead to lack of compliance with public health measures or participation in non-recommended behaviors. Identified as fake or inaccurate information, especially intentionally deceptive information [7], Fake news poses a serious threat to public health in pandemics such as COVID-19 [8].

As Vietnam has become one of the typical examples of success in fighting against COVID-19, there have been certain papers on the role of information technology and propaganda in the prevention of COVID-19 pandemic in Vietnam. Coronavirus (COVID-19) is an infectious disease that causes a respiratory infection turning from common cold to more severe breathing difficulty. The outbreak is believed to spread from the Hunan seafood market in Wuhan, China in December 2019, where sells live bats, snakes, pandas and many other wildlife animals (Shereen et al. 2020: 91–98). Currently, the number studies on Vietnam's prevention and control strategy of COVID-19 is limited. According to few studies we have collected, Hanks [9] evaluated Vietnam as a typical example in controlling COVID-19. One of the remarkable points in Vietnam's prevention and control is the very effective use of social media and information technology to propagate against COVID-19 because nearly 90% of the population owns smart phone or mobile phone. The government uses a variety of applications and channels to quickly alert citizens of suspected COVID-19 cases and areas; help people be tested and keep up to date with accurate scientific information aiming at minimizing risk for exposure to corona virus. A study by Viet-Phuong La et al. [10] highlights the effectiveness of communication on anti-pandemic outcomes in Vietnam. The authors note the emergence of the word—"war" in Vietnam's propaganda messages. Meanwhile, a study by Hong Kong Nguyen [11] shows that the initial success in slowing the spread of the virus is due to the government's focus on communication and propaganda for people to be aware of prevention mainly through technology and actively track pathogens. Transparent communication and cooperation between the government and the people have helped Vietnam to control small number of infections. Even when dealing with a wave of cases "imported" from abroad, Vietnam handled the crisis effectively and avoided the risk of becoming a COVID-19 hot spot.

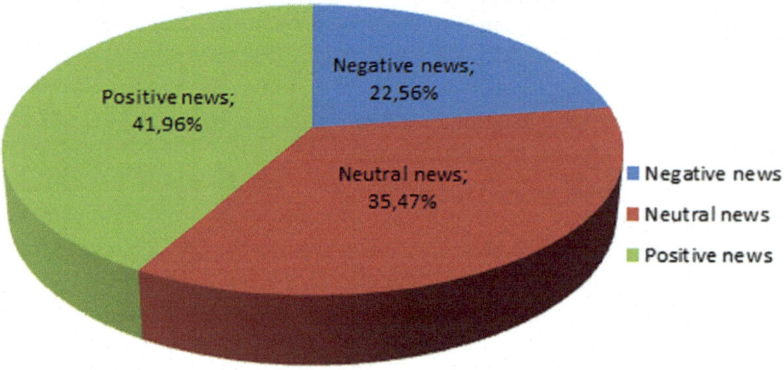

Fig. 1 Proportion of articles on COVID-19 in Vietnam classified by nuance. *Source* Ministry of Information and Communications, Vietnam

3 The Role of the Communication in Propagating Against COVID-19 in Vietnam

In May 2020, a global consumer audience data and research group—YouGov (United Kingdom) publish a poll of readers indicating the level of media's credibility in coronavirus coverage in different countries globally. In which, Vietnam ranked first, with 89% of the respondents saying that they believe media coverage. The analysis again showed that up to 94% of Vietnamese people believe that their Government has been very good at handling COVID-19 pandemic [12]. These figures partly reveal the correctness and effectiveness of communication on prevention and control of COVID-19 pandemic in Vietnam (Fig. 1).

> During the pandemic, the Vietnamese media system conveyed a consistent message—"fight pandemic as anti-enemy"—affirming that Vietnam's pandemic prevention campaign was a war, over that promotes nationalism, maximizing the participation of people in the campaign.

On January 28, 2020, the Prime Minister issued Directive No. 05/CT-TTg stating: "Ministries, branches and localities should not be nonchalant to encourage the spread of pandemic and must consider the fight against pandemic as "fight against the enemy". The mass mobilization of the entire political system is applied in order to protect health and life of the people, minimize death toll due to the pandemic". The "Fighting the pandemic is like fighting against the enemy" order mentioned in an official government document implicitly asserts that the Vietnamese government indeed considers the prevention campaign of COVID-19 pandemic to be definitely a war (Only No. 05/CT-TTg). Shortly, the message of "Fighting the pandemic is like fighting against the enemy" has emerged repeatedly in many official statements of the leaders and government officials,[1] emphasizing that the whole political system,

---

[1]Some typical articles:

On August 2, 2020, speaking at a meeting of the Government's Standing Board with provinces and cities nationwide on COVID-19 prevention, Prime Minister Nguyen Xuan Phuc emphasized from the government to each Vietnamese citizen, has all entered into the spirit of war.

The statistical results of our group (using Google search engine and Python code) show that the message "Fighting the pandemic is like fighting against the enemy" appears about 483,000 times on e-newspapers, of which 8 times on official website of the Vietnam People's Army. "Fighting the pandemic is like fighting against the enemy" becomes a big topic of the official website of Vietnamese Government.[2] Other language in wartime such as white-shirted soldier (those working in the medical field—about 184,000 times), anti-pandemic frontline (about 2,210,000 times), battle, date of return, triumph, victory, front, enemy—us, rear—frontline, great solidarity… appears dense on the mass media of Vietnam.

The purpose of the propaganda message "Fighting the pandemic is like fighting against the enemy" first and foremost is to reflect the seriousness and danger of COVID-19 pandemic by comparing its devastation with wars, thereby enhancing vigilance of the people and indirectly demonstrates the government's choice to "sacrifice economic benefits to protect people's health". However, if only emphasizing the dangerous nature of pandemic, it will cause excessive anxiety, social stigma towards people at high risk of getting severe COVID-19 disease, the production and business operations suspensions, etc. Thus, the propaganda with regard to war of Vietnam aims to convey positive, confident, cheer up, encouraging messages. Along with "Fighting the pandemic is like fighting against the enemy", the message "Leave no one behind" is also actively communicated through articles and music production. This message is intended to affirm that all domestic residents including all persons, citizens or foreigners living in Vietnam, will be protected against disease and undergone treatment for coronavirus infection. According to data collected from Google Search Engine and Python code, the message "Leave no one behind" appears about 325 times in e-articles about fight against COVID-19 in Vietnam and about 12,400 times on e-newspaper regarding music and digital music service such as Google, Zing, Nhacuatui …

---

that all levels and sectors must not neglect the prevention of COVID-19 pandemic. "Every citizen is a soldier in the fight against the Covid-19 pandemic". See at https://laodong.vn/thoi-su/moi-nguoi-dan-la-1-chien-si-moi-nha-thon-ban-la-1-phao-dai-chong-dich-824591.ldo.

Deputy Prime Minister Vu Duc Dam, Head of the Steering Committee for Covid-19 prevention and control, repeatedly mentioned the message of "Fighting the pandemic is like fighting against the enemy". These news are widely spread by Vietnamese media. See at https://moh.gov.vn/hoat-dong-cua-dia-phuong/-/asset_publisher/gHbla8vOQDuS/content/chung-ta-moi-thang-tran-au-nen-van-phai-e-cao-canh-giac.

[2]Some typical articles:

http://vpcp.chinhphu.vn/Home/Pho-Thu-tuong-Vu-Duc-Dam-chu-tri-cuoc-hop-BCD-phong-chong-dich-benh-Covid19/20203/27441.vgp

http://baochinhphu.vn/Chong-dich-nhu-chong-giac/519.vgp

During a meeting on undertaking unexpected tasks related to the management of cross-border exits and entries and the case of foreigners entering Vietnam illegally on July 29, 2020, Deputy Minister of National Defense Le Chiêm emphasizes that Fighting the pandemic is a fight during peacetime. See at http://baochinhphu.vn/Hoat-dong-Bo-nganh/Chong-dich-la-nhiem-vu-chien-dau-trong-thoi-binh/402437.vgp.

One of the most important missions of propaganda with regard to war is to build war "symbols" that have been effectively implemented by Vietnamese media. Numerous impressive images of military officers and soldiers, border guard services; stories about doctors fighting at the heart of the pandemic, soldiers who could not attend his own father's funeral or could not come visit his newborn baby have been released by the press and media.[3] These images are repeatedly promoted through articles, reports, propaganda posters and become powerful symbols. They appear dense in order to reach people anytime, anywhere; increase motivation and strength for those who directly participate in the anti-pandemic fight and encourage people to be calm and proactive. These symbols are of great significance in activating the national spirit and fighting will of the people.

Vietnam waged two wars against France and the US by mobilizing participation of all the people. Not only the soldiers but also the people in the rear also participate in the war by contributing money, in the propaganda campaign, protests, and even fight to protect revolutionary bases area. "All-People's War" is the key for Vietnam to win these wars. During the COVID-19 pandemic, the model of " All-People's war" was once again repeated in propaganda messages. On March 30, 2020, General Secretary and President Nguyen Phu Trong's call urged *all Vietnamese compatriots, comrades and soldiers across the country and compatriots abroad to unite with one heart, one mind and one practice; to actively and effectively apply the Party and State's guidelines and the direction and administration of the Government and the Prime Minister*. The message "Every citizen is a soldier in the fight against the COVID-19 pandemic" was echoed regularly on the official websites of state agencies.[4] The Vietnam Fatherland Front (VFF) of many provinces and cities has issued a call for "The participation of all people supporting the prevention and control of COVID-19 pandemic" in order to advocate common agencies, organizations, businesses and individuals

[3] Some typical articles:

Bach Mai Hospital (2020a). Tâm sự xúc động của bác sĩ mùa dịch: 'Bệnh viện là chiến trường, không phải ổ dịch' [The doctor's emotional words during the pandemic: 'Hospital is a battlefield, not an outbreak of infection']. Retrieved Aug 3, 2020 from http://bachmai.gov.vn/tin-tuc-va-su-kien/tin-trong-nganh-menuleft-34/6160-tam-su-xuc-dong-cua-bac-si-mua-dich-benh-vien-la-chien-truong-khong-phai-o-dich.html

Vu Phuong (2020). Xúc động hàng trăm bác sĩ tình nguyện vào 'rốn dịch' Đà Nẵng. Thanh Niên online 31/07/2020. Retrieved Aug 3, 2020 from https://thanhnien.vn/doi-song/xuc-dong-hang-tram-bac-si-tinh-nguyen-vao-ron-dich-da-nang-1258692.html

Bach Mai Hospital (2020b). Những chiến sĩ thầm lặng nơi "đầu sóng" [The soldiers silently at the "front of the wave"]. Retrieved Jul 21,2020 from http://bachmai.gov.vn/tin-tuc-va-su-kien/tin-trong-nganh-menuleft-34/6322-nhung-chien-si-tham-lang-noi-dau-song.html.

[4] Some typical articles:

Thien Lam (2020). Mỗi người dân là một chiến sĩ trong cuộc chiến chống dịch Covid-19 [Every citizen is a soldier in the fight against the Covid-19 pandemic]. Báo Nhân dân điện tử [Nhan Dan Online] 01-04-2020. Retrieved Jul 25, 2020 from https://nhandan.com.vn/tin-tuc-y-te/moi-nguoi-dan-la-mot-chien-si-trong-cuoc-chien-chong-dich-Covid-19-453906/

Phong Thu (2020). Cuộc chiến chống dịch COVID - 19 của Việt Nam [The fight against COVID - 19 of Vietnam]. Báo ảnh Việt Nam [Vietnam Pictorial] 28/04/2020. Retrieved Jul 25, 2020 from https://vietnam.vnanet.vn/vietnamese/cuoc-chien-chong-dich-Covid-19-cua-viet-nam/444583.html.

joining hand supporting state in the fight against pandemic.[5] The involving of Vietnamese people in financial support for the government's Anti-COVID 19 campaign is a considerable achievement in propaganda. From the date of its launch to April 29, 2020, the total amount of cash and in-kind contributions of agencies, units, organizations, businesses and individuals at home and abroad supporting and pledging the prevention and fight against pandemics was 1,900 billion VND, of which, through the Vietnam Fatherland Front, nearly 914 billion VND; in 63 provinces and cities, the total amount estimated reached more than 1,025 billion VND, including 150 billion VND via text message through the National Humanitarian Portal No. 1407 launched by the Standing Committee in collaboration with the Ministry of Information and Communications, the Vietnam Red Cross and the Ministry of Health since 19th March 2020 to now [13]. This reflect the fact that the message of war in Vietnam's anti-pandemic propaganda demonstrates the effectiveness of promoting nationalism, calling for the solidarity and response of all Vietnamese people to the infection-prevention campaign of COVID-19 pandemic.

Thanks to the transparency, consistency, and pervasiveness, the message of "Fighting the pandemic is like fighting against the enemy"—anti-pandemic propaganda in Vietnam has achieved certain successes. However, in order for this message to be disseminated, the government needs to fully mobilize the participation of all forces and all propaganda tools. The propaganda about the prevention and control of the pandemic has been effectively deployed in all forms of communication such as press, SMS messages and all types of social networks, Internet platforms, direct communication in the community …

The press plays a very important role in the anti-pandemic propaganda of Vietnam. The Government considers the communication to be a direct force to engage with the army, medical team and police in the prevention and control of pandemic. According to Project Syndicate, since January 3, Vietnamese media has described a strange disease originating from Wuhan (China). In the period from January 9 to March 15, an average of 127 articles on this topic per day published on 13 of Vietnam's most popular online newspapers, overwhelming fake news [11]. The press agencies all have categories, columnist for propagating against the pandemic. According to the statistics of the Ministry of Information and Communications, from February 1 to May 31, 2020, the press has published a total of 560,048 news and articles on COVID-19 pandemic, of which, in terms of posture, 3 kinds of positive, neutral and negative news accounting for 41.96%, 35.47% and 22.56% respectively. When Vietnam entered the "new normal" post COVID-19 the rate of news articles relating COVID-19 pandemic is still remaining at 28-40% of news and articles about economic recovery and growth but not neglecting prevention and control of COVID-19 infection [14].

[5]The call for the entire people's support for the prevention of COVID-19 pandemic of the Vietnam Fatherland Front in Hai Phong city has a paragraph that reads: With the motto "Fighting the pandemic is like fighting against the enemy", all for the people's lives, The Vietnam Fatherland Front Committee calls on all levels, branches, business communities, organizations and individuals with a high spirit and responsibility to the city and people to contribute and unanimously actively support for the prevention and control of COVID-19 pandemic. See at https://haiphong.gov.vn/tin-tuc-su-kien/Loi-keu-goi-toan-dan-tham-gia-ung-ho-phong-chong-dich-COVID-19-41695.html.

Due to the detection of patient no. 17, the bewilderment increased and commodity market was in danger of chaos, *"Vietnam promptly directed and its fellow press reported that Vietnam assured sufficient goods along with a reserve to cope with all situations"* (Speech of Prime Minister Nguyen Xuan Phuc at the preliminary conference on information and propaganda about prevention and control of COVID-19 pandemic). For the Vietnamese government, the press front plays a very important role in shaping public opinion, reflecting reality and criticizing errors and inadequacies in the society; commending organizations and individuals who do well; spreading images of people participating in anti-pandemic campaign with a weighty spirit and responsibility.

According to Quach [15], one of the most effective tools that Vietnam uses to propagate about the spread of the SARS-CoV-2 virus is community education which is largely deployed through the popular media. The pandemic has been becoming complicated, people using the internet and social networks have sharply increased, and all topics related to prevention and control of pandemic have been capturing rapt attention. Social networks have become a communication channel to update the pandemic progress, as well as an effective way to prevent and control disease. The fact that 65% of the approximately 96 million Vietnamese people have access to the internet, mainstream information channels and social media (60% of which use Facebook) has effectively helped share information about the disease.

Many social networks of Vietnam have closely cooperated with the authorities to provide the fastest and most accurate reports on the pandemic progress and prevention recommendations to user accounts, such as: Lotus, Gapo, Zalo … Typically, the Ministry of Health officially launched its official information channel on the Lotus social network called "Ministry of Health" to convey the instructions of the Government, the National Steering Committee, Ministry of Health; advise prevention and control of COVID-19, publish information about COVID-19 outbreak progression in Vietnam and worldwide. Gapo, a community partner of the Ministry of Health ran a music project known as "Viet Nam Oi! Beat Bay COVID". The project consists of lyrics that spread positive energy and call for all people not only to join hands and together overcome difficulties but also to express gratitude to everyone especially the team of nurses and doctors working day and night for the sick. The project received strong response of more than 3 million Gapo users by posting self-recorded clips such as: singing cover, lip sync, dancing, acting … on the chorus music background. Similarly, the social network Zalo also offered health recommendations to users, and at the same time released a sticker set related to messages such as frequent washing hand, wearing a mask in public.

Additionally, each citizen using social networks is also an communication and propaganda channel to contribute to the fight against the COVID-19 pandemic in Vietnam. In the first 5 months of 2020, on Vietnam's social networks, nearly 17 million status and comments mentioning COVID-19 pandemic in Vietnam [14]. Saying no to bad news, fake news, lots of people have shared positive information affirming Vietnam's achievements in the fight against COVID-19 pandemic; spread examples of selfless service to the community, beautiful actions and shared to ease difficulties for vulnerable groups imbued with human love in the pandemic.

Activities of propaganda against the pandemic by different types of culture have also been strengthened and spread by social media. Many poems and songs were written with the spirit of "Fighting the pandemic is like fighting against the enemy" as the main idea. On February 23, 2020, the Ministry of Health of Vietnam collaborated with national artists such as Khac Hung, Min, Erik to release the song encouraging hand wash "Ghen Co Vy" on YouTube, thereby propagating about how to prevent disease. This music production with hash tag #GhenCoVyChallenge then attracted 37.7 million views. Later, this song featuring the "Handwashing Dance" by Quang Dang (for the purpose of guiding proper hygiene to prevent corona virus) became famous when praised by John Oliver on the show Last Week Tonight with John Oliver of HBO on March 1, 2020. Furthermore, various songs have been released to the public such as: The song "Ti˜ên COVID" ("Bye, COVID") by the Department of Communications (Ministry of Health), Health & Life Newspaper collaborated with Le Thien Hieu to record "Việt Nam ơi, đánh bay COVID"("My Vietnam, take away COVID"), "Ông bà anh thời COVID-19" ("My granparents during COVID-19 pandemic"), "Khúc hát đôi bàn tay" ("Song of hands") … and especially a song set—"Faith" includes 60 songs of 52 musicians which were selected by the Art Council (of Vietnam Musicians Association) from more than 100 songs of professional and amateur musicians nationwide written during the period of social distancing in the first half of April 2020.

In general, the promotion of propaganda through the media has formed the top and daily concern of Vietnamese people is how the pandemic has spread; How many cases of SARS-COV -2 virus infection are reported in Vietnam?; how many COVID-19 patients are cured?; How is life in isolation zones?… The people also use social media and information technology applications to update information about pandemics, medical reports, and express their feelings for people participating in the fight against pandemics, make material contributions as well as support the anti-pandemic campaign. Moreover, they have shared materials and spirit with each other to be together ready when the war against the pandemic enters the most difficult period.

4 The Role of Information Technology Application in Warning and Detecting COVID-19 Patients

Aiming at enhance the effectiveness of pandemic warning and detection, Vietnamese residents regularly receive updates on the pandemic via SMS or text messages via online applications. As of March 21, 2020, telecom companies have sent more than 13 billion propaganda messages about prevention and control measures of COVID-19 to their mobile subscribers [14].

Applications tracking COVID -19 suspected infected people have been applied in many countries around the world to detect cases quickly. Along with the US,

Singapore, Australia, Vietnam is one of the first countries to apply technology to track suspected infected cases. Below are the applications being designed in Vietnam:

Name of Application	Provider/Developer
The management system for quarantine people and COVID-19 patients (Vietnamese name: Hệ th´ông quản lý người cách ly và người bệnh COVID-19)	Smart Medical center, Ho Chi Minh City's Department of Health
Vietnam Health declaration	Department of Information Technology, Ministry of Health
Bluezone	Ministry of Health and Bkav Corporation
NCOVI	Department of Information Technology, Ministry of Information and Communication
COVID-19	Department of Information Technology, Ministry of Health
Vietnamese Health (Vietnamese name: Sức khỏe Việt Nam)	Ministry of Health and Viettel Group
FAMILY-COVID19	Family Hospital (Da Nang)

Source The Authors

In addition, the new feature of nCOV pandemic prevention is further added to applications for smart city management of some localities such as Hanoi, Quang Ninh …

On March 9, 2020, the Ministry of Information and Communications and the Ministry of Health launched the NCOVI Application for Vietnamese people. The application includes many functions such as: "Risk Factor" (for people traveling from areas that are experiencing high levels of COVID-19 spread; having contact with patients or suspected of being infected) help them to receive timely support from health authorities; "All-people medical declaration" (for people to update health status for themselves and their family members). There is also a health monitoring function, an information reflection (allowing users to report suspicious cases or people who need to be under health monitoring) and alert function. This application gives people update on pandemic, health recommendations and support of health authorities and alerts areas with reported cases of COVID-19. Furthermore, the user can proactively report information about the pandemic to the Ministry of Health. On the same day, the Vietnam Health Declaration Application was officially launched by the Ministry of Information and Communications for the newly imported citizens to fill medical declarations aiming at monitoring and preventing COVID -19 pandemic. Up to 00:00 on July 27, 2020, the total number of NCOVI app downloads reached over 7.2 million. In addition, 837,300 compulsory medical declarations for guest entry through the tokhaiyte.vn website and the Vietnam Health Declaration app have been filled [14]. These are significantly practical contributions to help authorities to grasp epidemiological information of all people, thereby quickly localizing and tracing new positive cases.

The most strongly deployed application in recent times is Bluezone. This is a solution that applies Bluetooth low energy. Smartphones installed Bluezone can communicate with each other for a distance of 2 m, recording close contact for 14 days. If there is an F0 (COVID-19 positive cases/infected cases), the health authority (the Provincial Center for Disease Control) will enter the data of F0 into the system. The system sends F0 data to all phones in the Bluezone community. The history of exposure to F0 (exposed to F0 (called F1) or persons exposed to F1 (called F2)) will be compared by Bluezone on an analyzer. If there is a match, the application will immediately alert the user to the risk for severe COVID-19. The phone screen immediately appears instructions to contact the competent health authorities to get help. Bluezone can also help warn people on group F2. The principles of Bluezone are confidentiality, anonymity and transparency because the application only saves data on the user's phone without transferring to the system or collecting the user's location.

The Ministry of Health and the Ministry of Information and Communication have piloted the Bluezone App in Da Nang—a high risk infection area first, then expand vastly into others. These two ministries have deployed a massive communication campaign through the press compelling Da Nang's residents to install and use Bluezone; through all telecommunications subscriptions supplying installation instructions and through organizations and unions mobilizing members to install applications.

Moreover, the Da Nang Department of Education and Training directs all training institutions located in Da Nang city so that students who have smartphones install Bluezone for themselves and their relatives; Restaurants, hotels, offices, businesses … in Da Nang are required to disseminate Bluezone to everyone; Local radio system (commune and ward) reports and periodically reminds about installing Bluezone app, turning on Bluetooth … Local authorities visit each family distribute leaflets and guide residents to install and use Bluezone; Da Nang Youth Union launches a movement to install Bluezone and support people to install this application.

In early August, when the pandemic became complicated and spread to other provinces outside Da Nang, the Government asked the entire residents to install Bluezone including foreigners meeting the deadline before August 8. On August 1, following the directions of the Prime Minister, the Ministry of Information and Communications issued Document No. 2841/BTTTT-THH identifying 10 propaganda measures to widely deploy the Bluezone within 63 provinces and cities nationwide. All Vietnamese mobile subscribers have received text messages from the Ministry of Health asking to install Bluezone. Vietnam Television's News has also again and again broadcasted information about this application.

Data from the Department of Informatics, Ministry of Information and Communications shows that as of 11 a.m. on August 2, total number of Bluezone app download reached 1,851,827, an increase of 1,644,000 downloads compared to July 25. By the end of August 2, the Bluezone users exceeded 2 million [16]. The news program on the evening of August 7 of Vietnam Television announced that according to the data of the Department of Informatics, the Ministry of Information and Communications, as of 11:00 on August 7, the number of Bluezone downloads was approximately 10 million.

4.1 The Role of Information Technology in Digitizing Public Services Towards Reducing Risk of Infection

With the aim of minimizing the risk of infection, ensuring the operation of State administrative agencies and meeting urgent requirements related to production and business activities of enterprises and people's lives, The Government issued Directive No. 16/CT-TTg dated March 31, 2020 of the Prime Minister on the implementation of urgent measures to prevent and control the COVID-19 pandemic, including focusing on information technology (IT) application to take full advantage of the e-government. On the government's informational websites, ministries and provincial people's committees have boosted propaganda, guidance and encouragement for people and businesses to use online public services at level 3 and level 4 on National Online Public Service Portal, Ministry-level and Province-level online Public Service Portal targeted for reduction of travel and direct contact. Ministries and localities are required to prioritize resources, complete the integration, and provide 30% of online public services at level 3 and level 4 according to "2020 Plans" of ministries and localities on the National Public Service Portal and initially serve people and businesses. The Government also suggested ministries and localities to thoroughly implementing electronic data interchange; ensure the completion of electronic data at 4 levels of authorities before June 30, 2020 and quota for processing data (except for confidential documents) via computer network (80% for ministerial level; 60% at the provincial level and 30% at the district level) [17].

The Government also connects and integrates online payment system into the National Public Service Portal to promote online payment regarding various fees, charges, taxes, penalties for administrative violations, voluntary insurance, health insurance and other financial obligations in settling administrative procedures and providing public services on the National Public Service Portal, at ministerial and provincial level public service portals. In addition, it is necessary to organize meetings and work online at ministries, agencies, and provincial People's Committees according to the Prime Minister's Decision defining meeting regime in management and administration activities of the agencies not joining the state administrative system.

The statistics results of the Government in April 2020 show that 226 online public services at level 3 and level 4 are provided on the National Public Service Portal, of which over 103 thousand registered accounts; 4.3 million status synchronization records and 27.5 million visits searching for information and services on the National Public Service Portal are estimated. These initial results reflect the warm welcome of people and businesses to those which are provided on the National Public Service

Portal. In terms of electronic data interchange on the National Document Axis, after one year of operation, about 1.6 million electronic documents are transferred between Governments and ministries and localities [17].

5 Discussion and Conclusion

In the prevention of the COVID-19 pandemic in Vietnam, there is a close connection between information technology and communication. Communication is a propaganda tool for people to adapt to the use of information technology applications in work and life. In contrast, digital technology is one of the means for the government to promote communication, especially through the internet. The use of information technology and communication to fight pandemics in Vietnam has some of the following characteristics:

Firstly, the government's strict involvement and control over all anti-pandemic information and communication technology activities: All applications for COVID-19 case detection are developed by either the Ministry of Health or the Ministry of Information and Communication in cooperation with private sector. During the propaganda campaign, the government has ensured the massive coverage and domination of mainstream media. *One of the downsides of the media boom, especially internet and social media, is that it can create "mazes" of fake information that distract readers. The Government implements a wide range of measure tackling this serious problem such as criminal sanctions for spreading fake news, "mutation" of official news about pandemic to overwhelm fake news and provide "no living land"*. Right from the first days of anti-pandemic campaign, almost all news agencies, press, official radio and television stations at both central and local level of Vietnam have actively involved, increased broadcasting length, created more Television Program Categories, arranged more reporters and editors to exploit all aspects of pandemics. They are not afraid of hot spots, COVID-19 outbreaks pursuing goals of information update 24/7, the latest and most up-to-date information about *pandemic* preparedness and *management*, prevention recommendations to serve the needs of the public. Thanks to that, official and accurate information about the prevention and control of COVID-19 pandemic is in the mainstream of communication. Therefore, due to the rising of people's confidence in Party's leadership, Government's administration the participation of all levels and sectors has been encouraged.

Secondly, the openness and transparency without hiding bad news being a significant crucial factor for the success of Vietnam: Since the very beginning, the deep transparency of communication about coronavirus and the government's prevention strategy has been established. All symptoms, prevention measures and nearest testing points were spread widely through the media, governmental websites and on-site units, as well as through posters at the site, hospitals, offices, apartments and marketplaces, via text message and voice message to each mobile subscriber. Information technology application plays an important role in alerting user new infection.

Thirdly, the drastic and radical participation of information and communication technology units in prevention of pandemic: In order to increase the propaganda's effectiveness, the media attention does not merely focus on infected patients. It means, along with reporting, the press make lots of in-depth analysis and news report on Vietnam's anti-pandemic campaign. The media also boosts reporting acceptable behavior and advises against discrimination towards infected and isolated people. The press has also specifically directed towards humanistic news and articles combating stigma, defined long-term and quality categories and conveyed message of a good, safe, meaningful, caring life and full attention to the elderly, family and being introverted. Many press agencies have promptly reported and published articles on the dual goals of both successful prevention of pandemic and socio-economic development, reflecting overcoming patterns of enterprises, organizations and effective, innovative solutions in the difficult economic context... During the days when Vietnam regularly detected infected cases in the community, the mainstream media operates at full capacity. The activities of other industries may be halted, but the news media is always maintained. Nevertheless, when Vietnam temporarily confirms no new cases in the community, the mission of the media has not accomplished. The propaganda apparatus still operates frequently so that the residents keep sufficient attention, meanwhile, strives to perform the task of socio-economic development, proactively performs information for foreign purposes, propagates Vietnamese successful efforts building the image of Vietnam as a safe, attractive, dynamic and potential destination in the eyes of foreign investors and friends.

Fourthly, the Vietnam's information and communication technology application in anti-pandemic campaign is helping set the trend in using new technology for consumers. The Vietnamese people will gradually adapt to the installation and use of health monitoring and disease control applications. In the context of the constantly genetically modified virus, the COVID-19 pandemic is at risk of becoming a common disease that humankind has lived in the fear of potent infectious. Therefore, the tendency to install and use health monitoring applications may explode in upcoming time. In addition, official websites that used to have limited number of visitors, such as the Government of the Socialist Republic of Vietnam Portal, Official website of the Ministry of Health, have significantly advanced since the pandemic occurred in Vietnam. This fact shows that Vietnamese people have turned to the official pages to update the most accurate information and avoided being manipulated by hearsay.

Fifthly, the level of using the two information technology and communication tools is different from time to time: Before Vietnam discovered an outbreak in Da Nang and there were no deaths, the pandemic was accessible to control, the communication campaign has been conducted with the aim of raising awareness of the people, and preventing all disease transmission. Thus, at this time the propaganda campaign of smartphones' APPs for COVID 19 management has not been strongly promoted. However, after the 99-day without active cases in the community, the Da Nang outbreak appeared accordingly a number of deaths, pushing the pandemic to a higher level of complexity and speed of spread. More than that, the task of information technology applications with the goal of finding and tracing the infection is on top priority. Up to now, the government has used a variety of measures to ensure that all residents owning smartphone are aware of the disease alert and prevention via Apps.

Finally, the ICT application is not an independent activity but is a part of Vietnam's rapid response chain every time a new case is confirmed: whenever any patient is reported, not only the health sector but also the information sites simultaneously update and call on those at risk of infection to be tested. Along with that, almost all applications (App) update the new disease status to help localize and warn the people. A quick response is the key to Vietnam's anti-pandemic successes, and the ICT application is the tool to make that rapid response chain has worked effectively.

In general, Vietnam's prevention and control strategy of COVID-19 pandemic leaves its own mark through mobilizing the power of the media and social networks; efficiently promoting scientific and technical advances, information technology applications, and dynamic forces, means; combining tradition and modernity; making full use of forms. The communication method is diversified and lively, ensuring information discipline, not provoking society especially in big cities, but still maintaining residents' sufficient attention and compliance with prevention of the pandemic. The campaign was highly appreciated by the international media: *"Vietnam has shown that, thanks to its creativity, information about the spread of corona virus can be provided without underestimating the dangerous situation"*. [13]. The communication and information work has contributed to achieve social consensus and people's beliefs, arousing the national spirit and patriotism for successful pandemic's prevention and control.

However, the downside of anti-pandemic communication campaign in Vietnam is that it fuels an overwhelming fear of the pandemic and undue stigma towards people at risk for coronavirus infection. The message of war in the anti-pandemic propaganda deepens the impression that the COVID-19 pandemic is a fearsome and dangerous enemy like the enemy of war. Thus, when a case of infection occurs in the community, all places relating to the patients even at the position with extremely low chance of spread leads to a period of stagnation which seriously affects production and business activities. When the pandemic broke out in Da Nang at the end of July 2020, some videos showing alienation to Danang's citizens were posted on social media [18]. This proves that excessive stigma against people at risk for infection becomes a reality that should be divorced. In order to ensure the effectiveness of the propaganda, the media has actively reported recovered cases, patients under treatment, however, this effort is not enough for people to feel secure and trusting. This provides evidence that propaganda of war is really a "double-edged sword". On the one hand, it promotes nationalism, uphold the spirit of solidarity to fight against pandemics, on the other hand, it mainly causes the stagnation of production and business leading to bad consequences for the economy.

In terms of information technology applications, although the authorities at all levels have used many different propaganda tools urging people to install IT applications, the number of user is still much lower than the total population. This low usage rate is due to a wide variety reasons mostly caused by the low efficiency of these applications. Synthesizing the opinions of people who download NCOVI apps on Apple's App Store indicates that approximately 26% of users complain about the slow update speed, 17% are not satisfied with the power consumption of the App and 32% worry about the cyber security capabilities. Similarly, even though Bluezone only uses "file access" permission to record "close contact" history on device memory, 18% of users irritate provider using application access to their own photos, media, and files and using customer information, nearly 20% of users review that the app is difficult to use or the installation is difficult, and other features are still limited. Moreover, owing to special technology of Bluezone, this software will prove effective if high usage rate rises. In Vietnam, approximately 75–80 million adults using mobile phones, therefore, the App will only be effective in case that about 60% of people (equivalent to 45–50 million people) download Bluezone. Moreover, this app can only be installed on smartphones. However, in the context that Vietnam is facing a new COVID-19 pandemic wave and the considerable number of cases without detecting the source of infection in the community, this app is still an appropriate solution to promptly warn and detect case of infection. Moreover, a wide range of applications having similar functions at the same time has shown inconsistency and waste of resources but not as effective as expected, especially it cause people to get confused about selection. Regarding the digitalization of public services, because of the lack of implementation time and synchronous among localities, this cannot replace the traditional forms of public service.

In Vietnam, the complicated pandemic situation today requires the government, ministries and agencies to coordinate with private sector to further accomplish the existing information technology applications. The quality of apps, especially the processing and updating speed, needs to be improved, so that they become the fastest source of up-to-date information. In addition, when promoting propaganda through mainstream media and social media, the government needs to give reasonable instructions to create a sense of peace of mind among the people, especially to seek and promptly handle fake news.

6 Study Limitations and Contributions

The above are only small number of prominent aspects, not all contribution of information and communication technology to the prevention of COVID-19 pandemic in Vietnam. In fact, the presence of information and communication technology in other fields such as education, banking, e-commerce … is also greatly crucial, especially in the context that Vietnam must take advantage of all tools, measures and time to reduce the risk of community infection. However, due to limited resources, the authors only focus on the three main aspects mentioned above. We hope that our analysis will offer agencies, organizations seeking to learn from Vietnam's experience in preventing COVID-19 pandemic helpful suggestions. As concerns assessments of the ICT's role in the fight against COVID-19 in Vietnam, we prove that in order to control the pandemic, it is impossible not to mark propaganda by communication and pandemic alert via smartphone applications. Based on analysis in this article, we believe that we can open up more long-term research directions on information technology application, coordination between information technology and communication, the application of Artificial Intelligence in prevention of COVID-19.

References

1. Heat, R., Jin, B.: Ranking the global impact of the coronavirus pandemic, country by country. Politico (2020). https://www.politico.com/interactives/2020/ranking-countries-coronavirus-impact/. Accessed 03 Aug 2020
2. Ministry of Information and Communications Portal: Đã có trên 17,6 triệu lượt khai báo y t´ê tự nguyện qua ứng dụng NCOVI [Over 17.6 million voluntary medical reports through the NCOVI application]. MIC (2020). https://www.mic.gov.vn/Pages/TinTuc/143650/da-co-tren-17-6-trieu-luot-khai-bao-y-te-tu-nguyen-qua-ung-dung-NCOVI.html. Accessed 03 Aug 2020
3. Galaz, V.: Pandemic 2.0: can information technology help save the planet?. Environ.: Sci. Policy Sustain. Dev. **51**(6), 20–28 (2010)
4. Shirky, C.: Here Comes Everybody: The Power of Organizing without Organizations. Penguin Books, New York (2008)
5. Oleary, D.E.: Evolving information systems and technology research issues for COVID-19 and other pandemics. J. Organ. Comput. Electron. Commerce **30**(1), 1–8 (2020)
6. Samuli Laato, A.K.M., Islam, Najmul., Islam, Muhammad Nazrul, Whelan, Eoin: What drives unverified information sharing and cyberchondria during the COVID-19 pandemic? J. Eur. J. Inf. Syst. **29**(3), 288–305 (2020)
7. Lazer, D.M., Baum, M.A., Benkler, Y., Berinsky, A.J., Greenhill, K.M., Menczer, F., Nyhan, B., Pennycook, G., Rothschild, D., Schudson, M., Sloman, S.A., Sunstein, C.R., Thorson, E.A., Watts, D.J., Zittrain, J.L., Metzger, M.: The science of fake news. Science **359**(6380), 1094–1096 (2018)
8. Zarocostas, J.: How to fight an infodemic. The Lancet **395**(10225), 676 (2020)
9. Hanks, J.: How Vietnam contained the pandemic. Workers World **62**(15), 9 (2020)
10. La, Viet-Phuong., Pham, Thanh-Hang., Ho, Manh-Toan., Nguyen, Minh-Hoang., Nguyen, Khanh-Linh P., Vuong, Thu-Trang., Nguyen, Hong-Kong T., Tran, Trung., Khuc, Quy., Ho, Manh-Tung, Vuong, Quan-Hoang: Policy response, social media and science journalism for the sustainability of the public health system amid the COVID-19 outbreak: The Vietnam lessons. Sustainability **12**(2931), 20 (2020)
11. Hong Kong Nguyen: Vietnam's Low-Cost COVID-19 Strategy. Project Syndicate (2020). https://www.project-syndicate.org/commentary/vietnam-low-cost-success-against-covid19-by-hong-kong-nguyen-2020-04?barrier=accesspaylog. Accessed 02 Aug 2020
12. Smith, M.: International COVID-19 tracker update: 18 May. YouGov (2020). https://yougov.co.uk/topics/international/articles-reports/2020/05/18/international-COVID-19-tracker-update-18-may?utm_source=twitter&utm_medium=website_article&utm_campaign=covid_article_8. Accessed 02 Aug 2020
13. Vietnam veröffentlicht animiertes Video übers Händewaschen – es wird zum Hit im Internet. Stern. https://www.stern.de/gesundheit/coronavirus–vietnams-lied-uebers-haendewaschen-wird-zum-hit-9167582.html. Accessed 04 Aug 2020
14. Ministry of Information and Communications. 2020. Báo cáo Sơ k´êt Công tác thông tin, tuyên truy`ên v`ê phòng, ch´ông dịch COVID-19 ngày 16/06/2020" [Preliminary report on propaganda campaign of the prevention and control of COVID-19 dated 16/06/2020]
15. Quach, G.: Vietnam's Coronavirus Death Toll Is Zero. The Cost? Total Surveillance. One Zero (2020). https://onezero.medium.com/vietnams-coronavirus-death-toll-is-zero-the-cost-total-surveillance-1cf3d0c6172b. Accessed 02 Aug 2020
16. Thao, L.: Toàn dân cài ứng dụng Bluezone để phòng, ch´ông dịch COVID-19 [All people install Bluezone App to prevent and combat COVID-19]. Nhân dân Điện tử [Nhan

Dan Online] (2020). https://nhandan.com.vn/thong-tin-so/toan-dan-cai-ung-dung-bluezone-de-phong-chong-dich-COVID-19-611288/. Accessed 06 Aug 2020

17. Government Office: Ứng dụng CNTT trong công việc để phòng, ch´ông COVID-19 [Information technology application in the prevention and control of COVID-19]. Vietnam Government Portal (2020). http://vpcp.chinhphu.vn/Home/Ung-dung-CNTT-trong-cong-viec-de-phong-chong-COVID19/20204/27506.vgp. Accessed 03 Aug 2020
18. Viet Anh: Xử phạt một cá nhân có hành vi kỳ thị người Đà Nẵng [Sanction an individual who discriminates against Da Nang's people]. Nhân dân Điện tử [Nhan Dan Online] (2020). https://nhandan.com.vn/thoi-su-phap-luat/xu-phat-mot-ca-nhan-co-hanh-vi-ky-thi-nguoi-da-nang-610794/. Accessed 04 Aug 2020

Robotics and Automation: The Rescuers of COVID Era

Abhishek Chauhan

Abstract Today, when whole world is fighting against novel coronavirus and some countries are struggling to control this pandemic, robotics and automation can play a significant role not only by saving people but can also aid in controlling and preventing the spread of the virus. These advanced technologies are not only being applied widely to pharmaceutical and medical device manufacturing processes but are also helping the doctors and nurses in identifying and diagnosing the COVID patients. In the era of science and technology, people have realized the importance of robotics and automation and are using these technologies exclusively in field of education, grocery stores, restaurants and food delivery outlets etc. to maintain the norm of social distancing. Due to rapid increase in the number of epidemics and now this corona pandemic, demand for robotics and automation has increased manifold in healthcare, medical and pharmaceutical sectors due to shortage of medical staff and equipments and fear of spreading the disease from one person to another. Moreover, robots can also be used by the manufacturing industries to revive their production and to reduce the impact of present and future epidemic challenges. Although the use of robots and automation is not new, but people still have certain apprehensions of using these technologies on large scale. Some of the problems associated with robotics and automation are lack of funding, high initial cost, reduction in job, adaptability, lack of human interaction, regular updation, cyber virus threats etc. To deal with coronavirus robots and automation are being used in different forms and types such as telerobots for interaction and communication with patients, medical robots for disinfection purpose, drones and patrol robots for public safety, robot vans for delivering food and other essential items, 3D printing for manufacturing medical equipments etc. We cannot predict how long this coronavirus will last, but these cutting-edge technologies can be used for the revival of industrial production, and it's high time for manufacturing industries to upgrade their production and assembly lines with automation tools and digital technologies for safe and continuous operations. These technologies can be used with aim to decrease the workload of existing workforce and not to replacing them. Existing robots can be repurposed to save time and money and there is no need for stockpile the robots which can make them outdated. It is

A. Chauhan (✉)
Panjab University SSG Regional Centre, Hoshiarpur, Punjab, India
e-mail: abhishek_chauhan@pu.ac.in

D. Oliva et al. (eds.), *Artificial Intelligence for COVID-19*, Studies in Systems, Decision and Control 358, https://doi.org/10.1007/978-3-030-69744-0_8

very well known that resources cannot be developed in one day. It takes number of years to build them so that they can be used in case of emergency. So, it is high time that governments and agencies all over the world should come up with a proper plan to integrate robotic and automation with the existing workforce for the fight against the next pandemic and enhancing the efficiency.

Keywords Coronavirus · Robotics · Automation · Social distancing · Workload

1 Introduction

World Health Organization in March, 2020 declared coronavirus a global pandemic: a disease prevalent in the whole world affecting large number of people. This virus transmits through respiratory droplets and human contact [1]. In such a situation robotics and automation can play a very important role by allowing people to maintain social distance during COVID-19 as it spreads through human to human contact. But there has always been resentment among human beings over the increasing automation of labor due to robots, but the COVID-19 has proved that both humans and robots can work together to save lives during pandemics. Scientists and researchers have also outlined areas where robots and automation can be used in future global health outbreaks. These areas are health care, logistics, investigation and continuity of work and maintenance of socioeconomic functioning [2], remote handling, transportation, inspection, surveillance, and operation in hazardous environments [3]. During the spread of different diseases like SARS in 2002 in China, Ebola epidemic in West Africa in 2015, Nipah virus outbreak in Kerala in 2018, it was seen that these viruses are very risky for healthcare workers and contact less operations were needed at that time to avoid the spread of virus. So, people all over the world quickly adapted the use of robots during COVID-19 pandemic. As on 19 July 2020, there have been 14,043,611 confirmed cases of COVID-19, including 597,583 deaths, reported to World Health Organisation [4]. As globally the numbers of corona cases are increasing as shown in Fig. 1, robots and automation technologies like UVD robots,

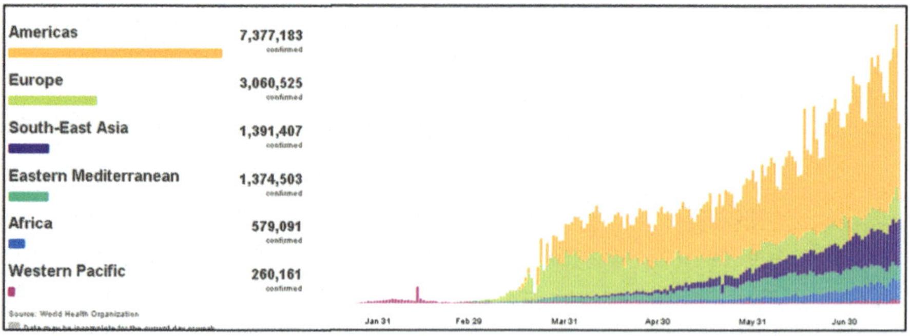

Fig. 1 Number of Corona cases in different part of the world as on 18 July, 2020 [4]

drones, and telerobots are widely applied due to high risk of infection involved for health workers. Robots and automation are also helping to remain safe and to supply things that humans need due to remote working and home learning during this virus spread.

In America The Robot Institute defined a robot as "a reprogrammable, multifunctional manipulator designed to move tools, parts, material, or specialized devices through various programmed motions for the performance of a variety of tasks [5]. Therefore, robots are widely used in hospitals, grocery shops, restaurants and other important services in the fight against the coronavirus which is promoting the concept of workplace automation. The automation is being applied in the form of software and hardware. Companies are using robots and automation to maintain their efficiency and operations during Covid-19. In hospitals due to high risk involved in treating with corona patients along with increased workload many hospitals are adapting to such technologies.

Even before the outbreak of corona pandemic robots and automation technology have been widely used commercially as service robots for performing work which were dirty and unsafe for human beings like detonation of bombs and investigation of uncharted and potentially dangerous environments. In future, robots and automation technology will become an integral part of our economy. It was also predicted that nearly four million industrial robots will be in use by 2021 as shown in Fig. 2. It can also be seen that South Korea has highest density of robots installed against per 10,000 employees and minimum robot density per 10,000 employees is in Asia as shown in Fig. 3.

Nowadays, robots are also being used widely in this pandemic as they reduce human exposure to viruses and can quickly adapt with in every situation. The use of robots and automation in current scenario is to keep people safe, patient care, produce products in demand and to provide essential services as per situation and robots are performing jobs of disinfecting hospitals and public places, checking temperatures of people in public areas, helping isolated patients, collecting COVID

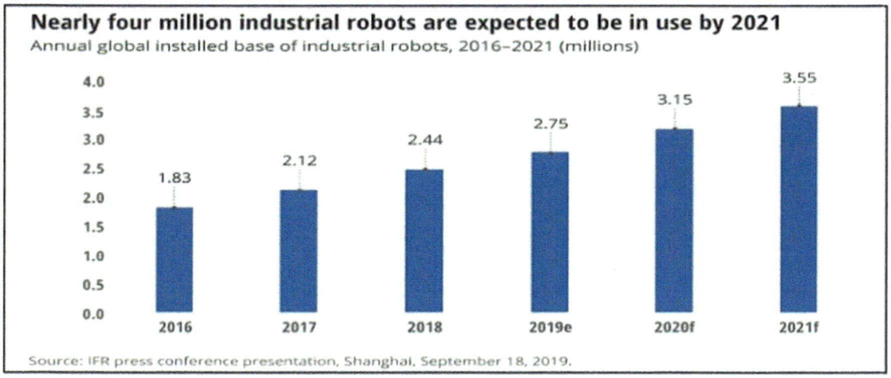

Fig. 2 Expected Industrial Robots by 2021 [*Source* International Federation of robotics]

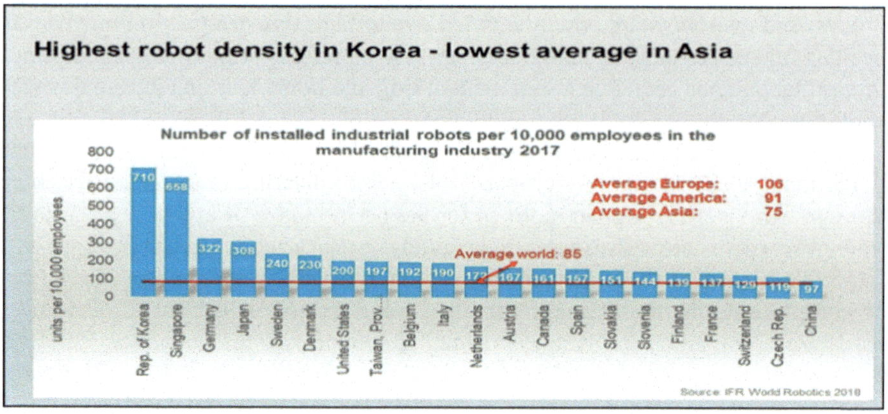

Fig. 3 Robot density per 10,000 employees country-wise [*Source* International Federation of robotics]

samples for testing, and helping people to attend conferences and exhibitions virtually. With limited healthcare capacity worldwide like hospital beds, medical staff, doctors etc. and shortage of critical medical equipment like test kits, personal protective equipment (PPE), ventilators etc. it is very much clear that robots and automation technologies are one of the unsung heroes of humans fight against coronavirus. They are need of the hour as well as of future and it is expected that industrial robots market size will increase from USD 44.6 billion in 2020 to USD 73.0 billion by 2025 which is shown in Fig. 4.

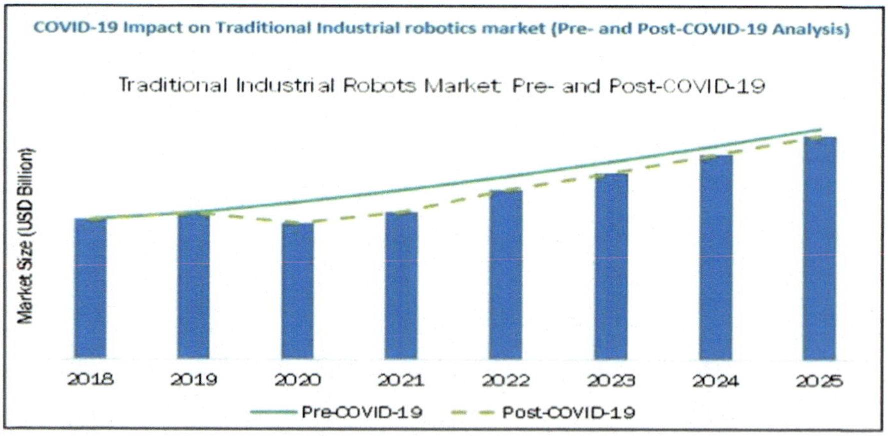

Fig. 4 COVID-19 Impact on the Industrial Robots Market Size [*Source* Markets and Markets, Credit: Sachin Garg, Associate Vice President, Semiconductor & Electronics, Markets and Markets Research Pvt Ltd]

Therefore, governments and industries must come up with mundane robots in future so that they will be ready to work with the front line health care workers when the next pandemic arrives [6]. This pandemic is biggest threat for humans and it is totally up to us how we can use these technologies for the benefit of the mankind. As there is no vaccine and effective treatment for COVID-19 disease the best way to deal with it is to stop and minimize transmission and execute personal shielding measures [7].

2 Importance of Robotics and Automation During Coronavirus

Importance of robots and automation in different sectors such as medical, service, delivery, industry etc. can be seen from the growth of different robots market over the years. The expected growth of different robots market i.e. medical robots, delivery robots, service robots, industrial robots is shown in Fig. 5, 6, 7 and 8.

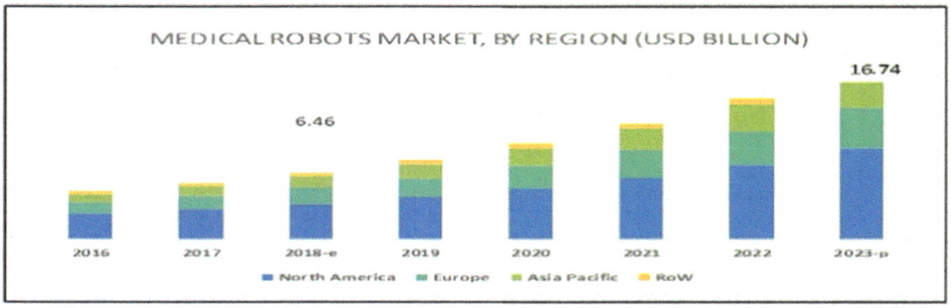

Fig. 5 Expected Medical Robots market by 2023 [*Source* Markets and Markets, Credit: Sachin Garg, Associate Vice President, Semiconductor & Electronics, Markets and Markets Research Pvt Ltd]

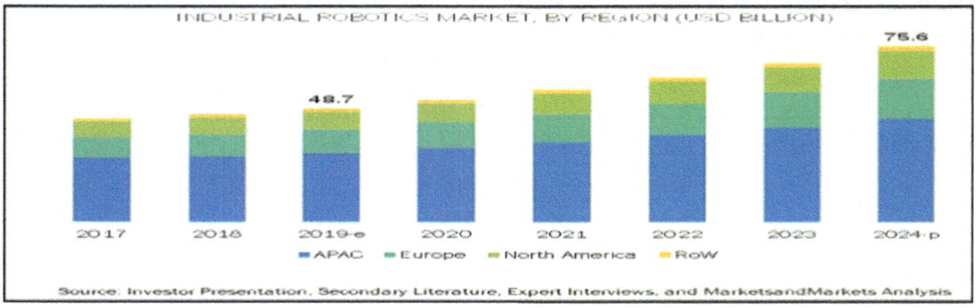

Fig. 6 Expected Industrial Robots market by 2024 [*Source* Markets and Markets, Credit: Sachin Garg, Associate Vice President, Semiconductor & Electronics, Markets and Markets Research Pvt Ltd]

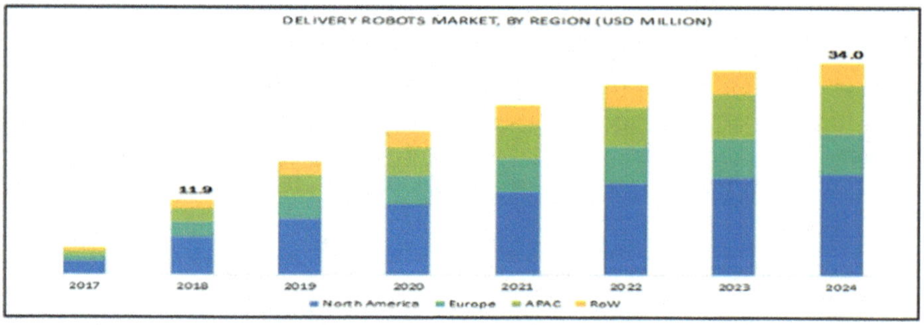

Fig. 7 Expected Delivery Robots market by 2024 [*Source* Markets and Markets, Credit: Sachin Garg, Associate Vice President, Semiconductor & Electronics, Markets and Markets Research Pvt Ltd]

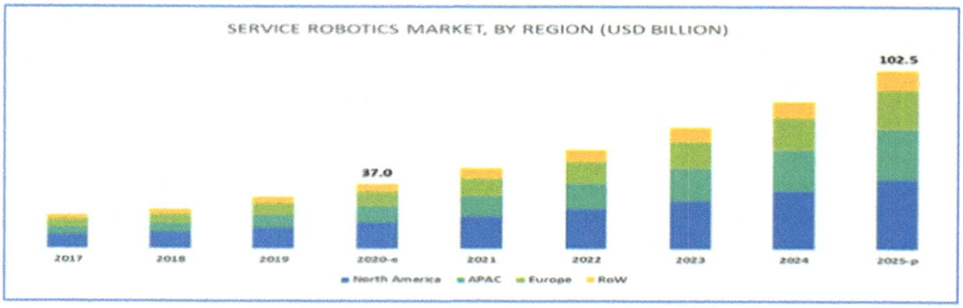

Fig. 8 Expected Service Robots market by 2025 [*Source* Markets and Markets, Credit: Sachin Garg, Associate Vice President, Semiconductor & Electronics, Markets and Markets Research Pvt Ltd]

These figures clearly show that there is clear trend of increase in use of robots in different sectors and there will be tremendous growth in the robotics market in coming future. Due to availability of robots in different sectors, robots are widely used and there are several advantages of using robots and automation during coronavirus. The robots have emerged as rescuers and warriors for the fight against coronavirus where workload in health care sector has increased manifold and maintaining distance amongst each other is an essential criteria due to shortage of manpower. Further, robots do not get tired, become inattentive, suffer human fragilities like jittering or shaking and are more accurate than human beings in performing the task allotted to them [5]. Some of the benefits are mentioned in the Fig. 9 and are explained point wise below:

2.1. Maintaining Social Distancing: The one metre policy for social distancing has been suggested by World Health Organization based on the assumption that SARS-CoV-2 is transmitted in big isolated droplets [8]. Further secondary infection at high rate is reported among members of a house and in people who are in close contact with the patient of COVID-19 [9]. The rules for social distancing have

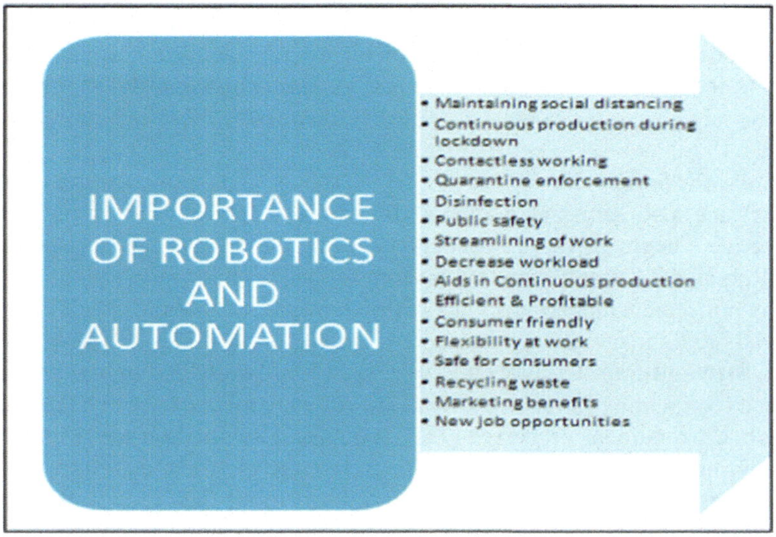

Fig. 9 Importance of Robotics & Automation

been implied to reduce the risk of transmission of COVID-19 in many countries as it can aid in reducing the incidences of COVID-19 [10, 11] and the timings of social distancing and adherence level had a major effect on COVID-19 occurrence [12]. Use of automation and robotics can reduce contact in hospitals, grocery stores, manufacturing floor etc. and allow the health workers and other staff to maintain social distancing [13] and also reduce the number of workers to physically come to workplace. Robots are doing jobs of workers which workers cannot do as they are working from home for their safety.

2.2. Continuous Production during Lockdown: Lockdown has been imposed in many countries throughout the world to suppress the corona curve but it had a large social and economic cost with problem of massive unemployment [14]. Due to coronavirus, manufacturers are not able to produce things due to lack of labor force and in lieu of following norms of social distancing. Robotics and automation are playing important role by running production lines for continuous supply of essential items like masks, ventilators, PPE kits etc.

2.3. Contactless Working, Quarantine Enforcement & Disinfection: The earliest legislation in India regarding provisions related to safety of public health was The Indian Penal Code, 1860 which was supplemented by special law known as Epidemic Diseases Act, 1897 and has two major parts: first part dealing with quarantine rule and other with public nuisance. The law was for the first time enacted in former British India to tackle bubonic plague in Mumbai and nationwide lockdown from March 25, 2020 to April 14, 2020 due to COVID-19 outbreak in India is covered under Disaster Management Act, 2005 [15]. During coronavirus, robots like drones are mainly used for quarantine enforcement, isolation checking and disinfecting of hospitals and public places. They are also helping health workers to take care of patients suffering from the coronavirus. Robots are safe as there is no human to human contact, they are used to supply medicines to patients in hospitals, delivering things to individuals who order online and to those who are isolated at home. This way they are promoting contactless delivery, decreasing cross-infection and spread of virus.

2.4. Public Safety: During this pandemic, robots are not only helpful in hospitals but they are also acting as a support for public safety as well as public works. Co-operative teams of service robots have been a research target for several years [16]. Robots are not only assisting doctors and nurses in hospitals but they are also helping policemen, industrialists etc. In this way they are making general public safe and ready to fight against any disaster.

2.5. Streamlining: The cost effectiveness and the quality of shared services can be enhanced by creating workforce virtually of software robots that can help companies streamline operational processes [17]. Robots and automation are also helpful in streamlining of work at places where there is surge in orders due to high demand. Warehouses are using robots to automate and streamline their order fulfillments and grocery stores for streamlining of different works at different counters.

2.6. Decrease Workload: Robots are supporting front line workers during COVID-19. They are not replacing them but they are reducing the workload of the workers like in hospitals where workload has been increased due to increase in number of patients and chances of spread virus are so high. They are helping in doing work safely and helping health workers to handle the increased workload. Further, the Amazon Company has been using Kiva robots for increasing the efficiency of order fulfillment process. By using robots Amazon did not replaced human workers, humans now stand on platforms while an army of social robots brings the right package to them at the right time and thus Amazon's employees now take 15 min to fulfill some orders instead of 90 min, an increase of 20% in efficiency [17]. Thus, robots and automation has decreased the work pressure on humans and enhanced the efficiency manifold.

2.7. Savings in Long Run & Continuous Production: The importance of robots is widening due to rapid development of Artifical Intelligence (AI) [18]. The coronovirus has resulted in massive disruption of production of goods by affecting supply chains which forced the industrialists to automate their production lines. No doubt, initial investment in robots and automation is high but they are useful in long run and can save lots of money. They help in continuous supply without any disruption and do not demand any salary, holidays and other benefits. They do not demand masks, sanitizers and other medical equipments to work in conditions like coronavirus. They can be used anywhere as per choice to increase the production anytime under any conditions.

2.8. Efficient & Profitable: Robots and automation helps the companies to do their work more efficiently under conditions like in coronavirus. The companies who are adopting automation at workplaces during coronavirus and are using these technologies for their daily work are preferred by the customers. This is definitely going to increase their profit in coming times. Investments in robotics benefit the human factor positively [19].

2.9. Consumer Friendly: Robots are becoming common at hospitals, nursing homes, school and at place of work and are evolving from task oriented focus to the one who can act as a companion and is social [20]. Use of robots and automation at any place for human purpose during coronavirus makes it consumer friendly, as use of technology is reducing personal contact which is the main reason for spread of deadly virus.

2.10. Flexibility at Work: One of the major advantages of automation is the flexibility it provides at work during COVID-19. These technologies are mainly based on digital approach and cloud capabilities which make them more flexible. Companies are providing automatic system which requires minimal amount of interaction. These systems are able to work without having people on site.

2.11. Long Lasting Impact & New Normal: It is clear that coronavirus is not going to end soon and social distancing will be new normal once we all get back to our daily routine. We all are going to change the ways we work even after the pandemic is over. Organizations are moving towards automation and use of robots to get things done. This trend of automation is likely to be continued in future because of its great advantages. They will also help us to get prepared for any future pandemic. They are going to be new normal at our workplaces. They will be the preferred areas of investments by different companies for maintaining continuity of their supply chains.

2.12. Safe: Robots and automation are looked upon as a means for contactless delivery which promote safety. Therefore, robots are widely applied in food services due to health concerns in COVID-19. Food chains are also testing robots as cooks and servers for safety of their consumers. Warehouses and grocery stores are already using robots to increase safety and efficiency. Many companies are using robots for sorting, shipping and packing to ensure safety of their customers. In hospitals the primary use of robots is to decrease the personal contact and ensure sterilization, cleaning and support reducing the threat of transmission among doctors and medical staff [21].

2.13. Recycling: During coronavirus, people are using masks and PPE kits as a personal protection against viruses which becomes medical waste after use. So, it is very important to dispose such waste as it can further spread the virus. Therefore waste should be disposed or recycled properly. Robots can be used to recycle waste or dispose it much more safely than humans.

2.14. Marketing benefits: Use of robots in pandemic like COVID-19 can also be used as marketing strategy by companies. People will prefer places which have few workers and more machines because of low risk of getting contaminated with virus at these places. Convenience, availability, flexibility, efficiency are some of the benefits provided by Service robots [22].

2.15. Reorganization: During coronavirus, the demand of certain equipments like ventilators, masks etc. for health care has increased drastically while demand in certain sectors like car manufacturing is almost nil. So, the situation like coronavirus has helped many industries to transform and reorganize their factories into ventilator builders. Robots and automation is helping such industries to reorganize their production lines to produce health care components like ventilators etc.

2.16. New Job Opportunities: People have apprehensions that use of technology always reduces jobs. But this is not true everywhere and in every situation. Technology use requires adaptability which means that there is need to upgrade our skills for smooth functioning of the work and to keep our job secure. Use of automation and robots will results in new job opportunities as people will be required to make new robots, install them, for their programming, protection from cyber viruses and for their maintenance and service.

3 Applications of Robotics & Automation

The market for robots and automation is expanding at a rapid pace due to vide applicability at different areas of work like hotels, restaurants, hospitals, retail stores and also at home. By 2023, market for consumer robots is expected to reach 14.9 billion [23]. Robots are being used in the field of education as a teaching aid in a flexible and intensive manner [24], in cardiac surgery as a safe alternative over the traditional techniques [25], in food industry to perform various processes like food processing and packing, handling and serving [26], in construction to reduce accidents on construction sites and perform difficult tasks [27]. Automation has brought a lot of convenience in people's life and production which has made manufacturing and mechanical design improve in recent years [28], in armed forces for surveillance of border areas [29] and many more.

3.1 Applications (Pre- COVID)

Use of Robots and automation is not something new during coronavirus. They were widely used in Pre-COVID in different sectors to make work easier, safer and faster. Some of the areas in which they were used before coronavirus are given below and briefly shown in Fig. 10.

a. Military and Intelligence operations: In armed forces robots and automation are used in different forms like drone which is used by military personnel's for surveillance and intelligence purpose at border areas. They are also used for disposal of bombs and land mines. Unmanned aerial vehicles have the most versatile use in modern warfare and with advancement in technology the day is not far when the future battles and wars will be fought by robots [29]. Figure 11 (a) and (b) is showing the talon robot which is light weight robot and daksh robot which is remote controlled. Both are used for the military applications.
b. Heavy engineering and Manufacturing: Robots and automation has speeded the process of manufacturing in industries with production of equipments with high quality.

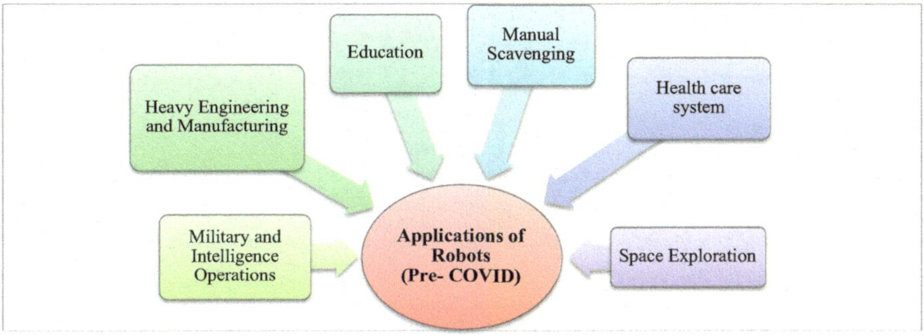

Fig. 10 Applications of Robots (Pre- COVID)

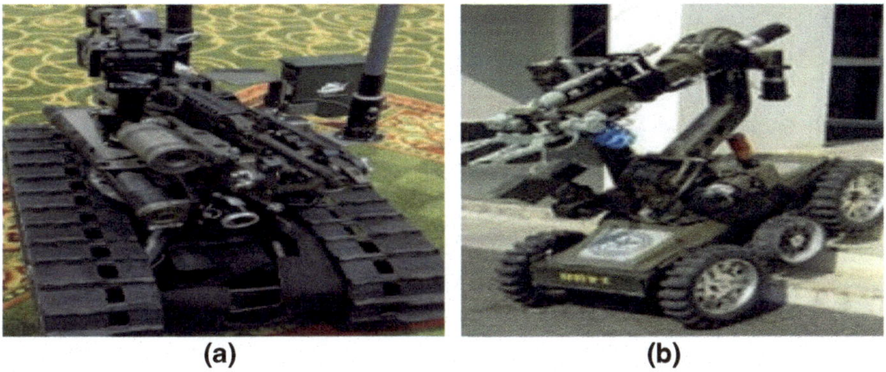

Fig. 11 **a** Talon robot, unmanned military robot and, **b** Daksh made by DRDO to handle hazardous objects [30] *Source* https://iopscience.iop.org/article/10.1088/1742-6596/1172/1/012035/pdf, http://creativecommons.org/licenses/by/3.0

c. Education: Social robots enhance affective and cognitive outcomes in the field of education as peer learners or tutors analogous to those of human tutoring [31]. Example is virtual conferencing tools or apps like Skype etc.
d. Manual scavenging: Scavenging by man has been declared illegal in 2013 as hundreds of people die performing the task, so mechanical driven device and electronic automation is used for the purpose of cleaning and inspection of sewage. Robot like BhrtyArtana is a sewer robot that cleans any blockage in the sewage pipeline by conducting an inspection first for cracks, obstacles, corrosion etc. with the help of a camera atop which are viewed in a software by the operator [32].
e. Health care system to perform complicate surgeries: The robots have now entered the operation theatres in the hospitals as the technology is progressing in subjects such as actuators, mechatronics and sensors [33].The task of a surgeon can be accomplished and improved by using computer assisted strategies and robots can perform with precision and safety like orthopaedic surgery, spine

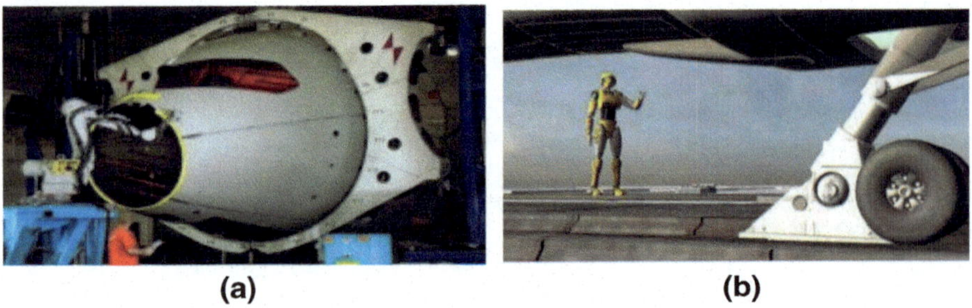

Fig. 12 **a** Assembling of Aircraft done by Robot and **b** Air traffic control robots [30] *Source* https://iopscience.iop.org/article/10.1088/1742-6596/1172/1/012035/pdf, http://creativecommons.org/licenses/by/3.0

surgery and anthroplasty [34, 35]. The task which are dangerous, repetitive and requires accuracy and force are being performed by robots in commercial industry [35].

f. Space navigation and exploration: The exploration of space has become easy with advancement in robotics and automation as tasks like rescue missions, search, surveillance require that the robots move efficiently in the environment, avoiding obstacles during motion and keeping under consideration the robots' physical constraints [36]. It is also widely used for aeronautical and aerospace industries like assembly of aircrafts, air traffic control etc. as shown in Fig. 12 (a) and (b) respectively.

3.2 Applications (Post- COVID)

Robotics in present time is of great importance because of their wider applications and promoting virus free environment. Robots and automation is helping people in battling the virus. Robots are used by different countries in different sectors to deal with the situation of coronavirus which is shown in Fig. 13 [6].

Therefore, depending upon the requirement and situation robots can be used anywhere to save and protect the human life from coronavirus. Some of the important applications of robots and automation in current situation are as follows:

3.2.1 Healthcare: Health care workers have suffered mortality and morbidity along with other patients in COVID-19 pandemic. All specialties physicians may die due to COVID. In a recent research on 278 physicians it was reported that the countries with the most reported physician deaths were Italy (121/278; 44%), Iran (43/278; 15%), Philippines (21/278; 8%), Indonesia (17/278; 6%), China (16/278; 6%), Spain (12/278; 4%), USA (12/278; 4%) and UK (11/278;4%) [37]. Use of robots in hospitals is not new and due to coronavirus, robots are widely used in hospitals for disinfection, delivery, lifting bed of patients etc. They are being used to control the spread of corona virus as well as other epidemic diseases and to reduce

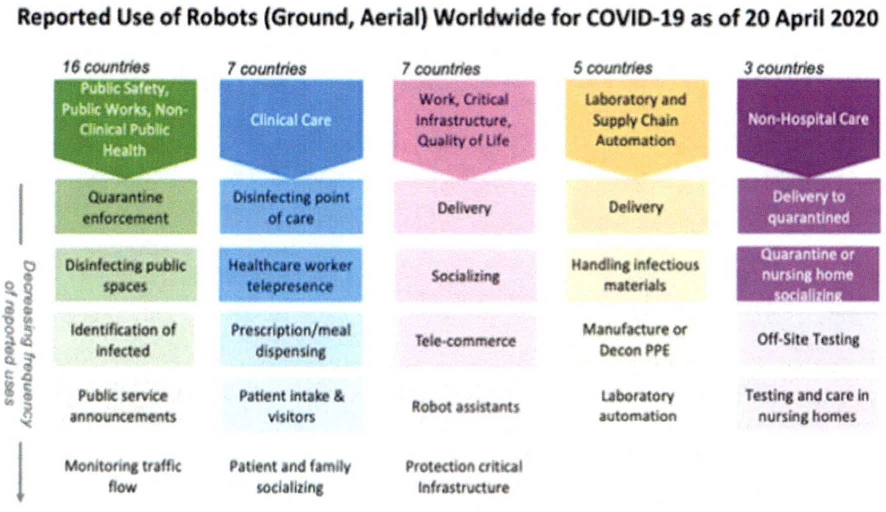

Fig. 13 Application of Robots worldwide for COVID-19 [6] *Source* https://www.weforum.org/agenda/2020/05/robots-coronavirus-crisis, Credit: R. Murphy, V. Gandudi, Texas A&M; J. Adams, Center for Robot-Assisted Search and Rescue

the workload of medical workers. Some of the areas of healthcare where they are being used are:

Corona Testing: Robots are used for automatic testing of COVID-19 patients. As they are immune to virus, they are used to collect sample of patients. They can be used for mass testing when there is shortage of medical staff. Robots are performing these tests quickly and efficiently. The areas and the ways in which they are used for testing purpose are given below:

Drive Through Concept: The concept of Drive-through restaurant is also used by automation companies to test drivers for coronavirus. Example is the Bavarian automation company called Boka Automatisierung which is using fully automated system similar to concept of drive-through restaurant for testing any car driver who wants to have corona test. In this concept, a tablet is used to identify the driver through the side window of the car and a robot arm provides the test tube to driver. A video tutorial guides sample collection and test tube is returned back. Then test results are informed telephonically [38].

Sorting Blood Samples: Testing procedures of coronavirus requires collection of blood samples and due to increase in number of patients day by day there is too much load on the lab technicians to perform the tests quickly and correctly. COVID test is very time consuming also. Therefore robots are being used to collect blood samples of the patients so that workload of lab technicians gets reduced and they can concentrate on preparing reports. Example is the Aalborg University Hospital in Denmark which have fully automated laboratory. KUKA robots are sorting around three thousand blood samples daily leading to decrease in workload of technicians [38] (Fig. 14).

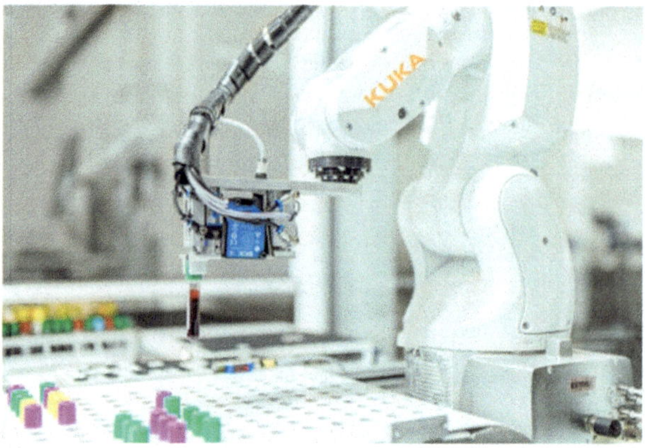

Fig. 14 Kuka Robot sorting blood samples [38] *Source* https://assets.kuka.com/web/53001dd4365b475a/bloodsamples © KUKA

Test Results: Processing and sorting of test results takes lot of time manually as they are done on spreadsheets. Therefore, hospitals are also using software robots to get Covid-19 test results. Example is the Mater Misericordiae University Hospital in Dublin which is using software applications which replies automatically to data inputs and helps in getting test results for Covid-19 [39]. Robots do this job in minutes which helps the medical staff in controlling infection properly because they are able to spend more time with patients. It makes medical staff to use existing resources in better way to control the infection. Hospitals are also using software robots to automate their appointments, claims settlement and other lab testing [39].

Manufacturing of Masks: Robots are being applied to manufacture masks due to increase in demand as well as shortage of labor during coronavirus. Example is machine manufacturer PIA Automation of Germany, who deals in production of automotive and consumer goods. They have reorganized their existing production lines for the production of masks and have started producing 140,000 protective masks per day [38].

Disinfection: Nowadays, robots are being used in hospitals for disinfection purpose. Some of the examples are:

a. UVD Robots which helps in disinfecting different areas of the hospitals using ultraviolet light without exposing medical workers to the virus. Examples are:

i. Kochi-based Asimov Robotics made KARMI-Bot [40] (Fig. 15).
ii. Xenex's LightStrike Germ-Zapping Robots which is based on UV light concept and takes very less time to disinfect any room and reduce the infection rate up to 80 percent [41] (Fig. 16).
iii. Delhi firm Persapien developed Minus Corona UV Bot, which helps in disinfection of corridors and wards of hospitals, ICUs etc. to prevent the spread of virus [40].
iv. Blue Ocean Robotics developed UVD robot which uses UV-C light to remove harmful bacteria and microorganisms [41] (Fig. 17).

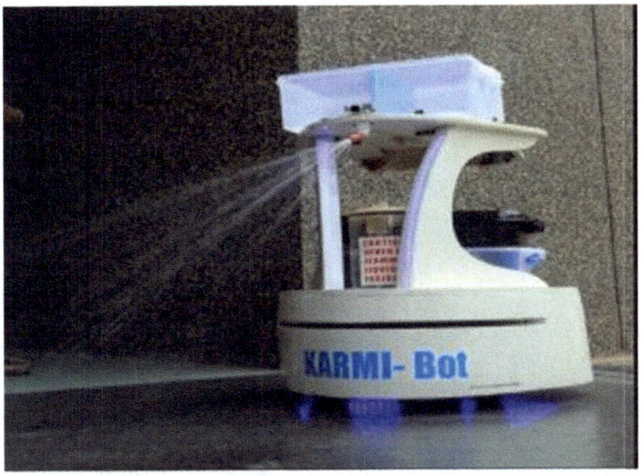

Fig. 15 KARMI-Bot developed by Asimov robotics [40] *Source* https://www.thehindu.com/profile/photographers/Special-Arrangement/

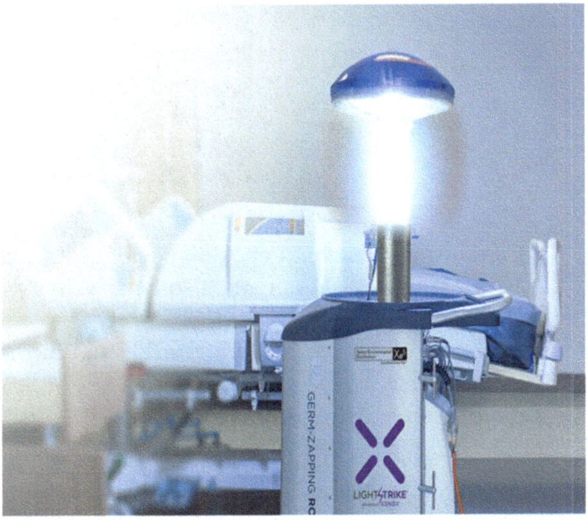

Fig. 16 Xenex's LightStrike Germ-Zapping Robot [41] *Source* https://www.xenex.com © Xenex Germ Zapping Solution

Tracing Patients: Robots are also doing important tasks like flagging of patients at the entrance of the hospitals which have flu like symptoms and have low oxygen level. Example is a cylindrical robot which is rolled in room of the corona patient to measure his temperature, blood pressure and oxygen level [6].

3.2.2. Patient Care: Robots and automation are not only used for disinfection but also used for patient care in several forms. The use of robots in patient care not only reduce the entry of medical staff in patients room but reduce the demand of personal protective equipments required for staff in dealing with COVID patients. Some of the uses of robots in patient care are as follows:

Interaction: Robots are used by doctors, nurses, and receptionists etc. to interact with patients by maintaining social distancing. Examples are:

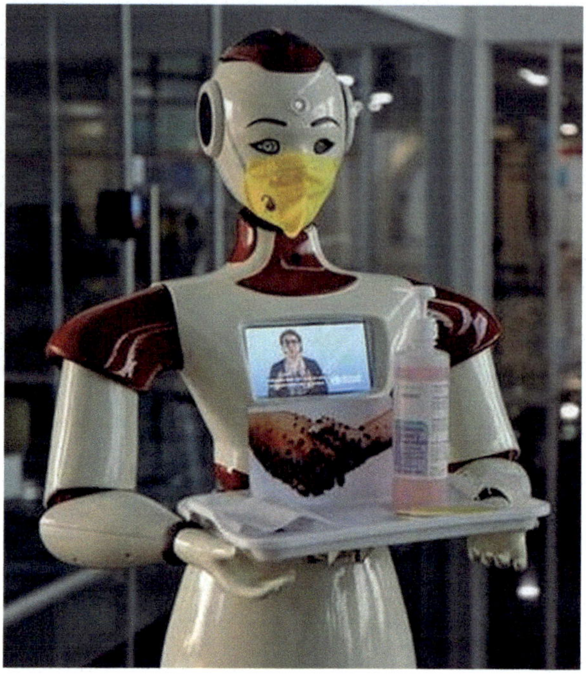

Fig. 17 Medical Robots [40] *Source* https://www.thehindu.com/sci-tech/technology/gadgets

i. Carts which have high-end audio and visual connections to communicate with COVID-19 patients. These carts also have a digital stethoscope and other tools to assist the medical team [2].

Delivery: Robots are delivering meals and medicines to share the workload of medical workers.

Examples are:

i. The robot named Sona 2.5 was used in Sawai Man Singh Government Hospital, Jaipur, to deliver food and medicines to virus infected patients [40] (Fig. 18).
ii. The tiruchi software company made robots Zafi and Zafi Medic were used in Mahatma Gandhi Memorial Government Hospital to deliver food and medicines to patients which were quarantined [41] (Fig. 19).
iii. KARMI-Bot robot which can perform jobs like delivering food and medicines on time, remote monitoring of the wards, video-conferencing with doctors etc. [40].

Physiotherapy: Robots like cobots i.e. collaborative robotic arms are used by physiotherapists for their work. These robots help the patients without having physically contact. Example is the Reha-Robot which helps physiotherapists by maintaining social distancing. The Life Science Robotics Company has also developed ROBERT, which is used for mobilizing patients [38, 41].

3.2.3. Education: Automation and software technologies are also used in education field due to closure of educational institutes in different parts of world due to

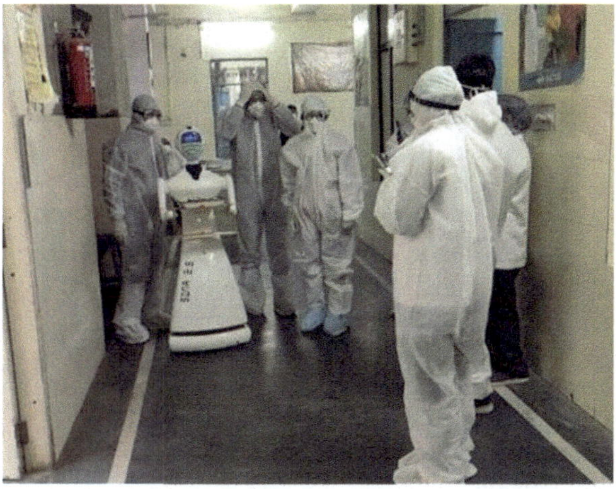

Fig. 18 Sona 2.5 was used in Sawai Man Singh Government Hospital, Jaipur [40] *Source* https://www.thehindu.com/sci-tech/technology/gadgets

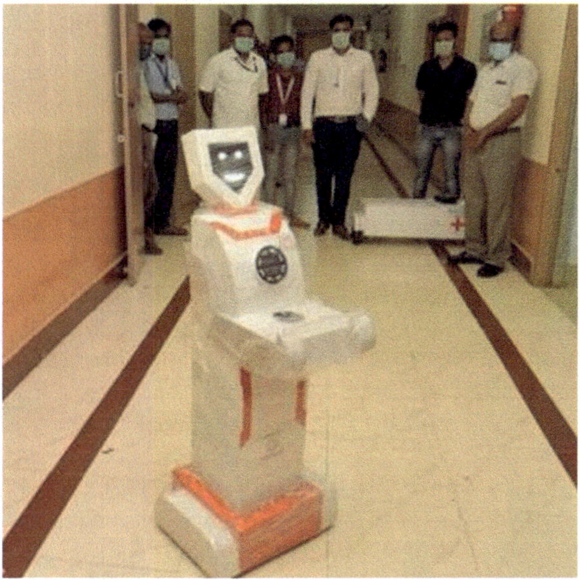

Fig. 19 Zafi Robot [40] *Source* https://www.thehindu.com/sci-tech/technology/gadgets

coronavirus. Due to frequent lockdowns humans are more comfortable to connect remotely. Many video conferencing apps like Zoom, Webex etc. are gaining popularity due to work from home option during COVID 19. Use of artificial intelligence has also increased and it is used to develop technologies which can replace tutors and trainers. Artificial intelligence is also being used by Facebook and Google to remove more inappropriate posts which are creating panic in society about COVID 19 [39]. YouTube is also using automatic system for content moderation without human review [43]. Using robots in education impact students positively [44].

3.2.4. Prison and Old Age Homes: The UVD robots are also being used to disinfect other places where there is high possibility of spreading coronavirus due to lack of space. So, they are also used to disinfect prisons and old age homes due to high chance of virus spreading in these areas due to population and risk of getting infected due to old age.

3.2.5. Networking: Automation is also being used in networking due to increase in demand of cloud storage platform due to work from home option given by several companies due to coronavirus. Automated software and chatbots are developed to improve communication and interaction of workers who are working from home [39].

3.2.6. Restaurants and food industry: Robots are being used for harvesting, spraying water, seeding, packaging, meat processing, detecting the quality of the final products, cleaning of bottles in beverage and food industries [25]. Robots are not only delivering food to people in hospitals or those who are under isolation due to coronavirus but they are also ensuring supply of fresh food and goods to people at their homes. Unmanned vehicles and other mobile robots are delivering cooked food at different locations. They are also helping in taking orders and serving food in the restaurants eliminating the human to human touch. The concept of dark kitchens is coming up where cooking and handling of food is totally done by robots. Some of the examples of robots that are helpful in preparing food are Miso Robotics that can grill and fry the hamburger, CafeX which can make coffee and other drinks and Picnic which can prepare pizza [45].

3.2.7. Retail: Nowadays many retail stores are using technology to deliver things at homes to prevent their workers and customers from coronavirus. Robots are used to keep stores clean so that their employees and customers remain safe from the virus. Examples are the cleaning robots which are doing jobs like disinfection of surfaces, customer support, re-stocking etc. so that workers can focus on other tasks that are essential during the COVID-19 outbreak. They also provide input to retail workers on areas that need to be cleaned immediately and information to manage stores properly [10]. The Walmart, Retail Company is also using robots to clean their floors [42].

3.2.8. Public Work: Robots are also used for public safety and to perform public works during COVID-19.Goverment departments are using robots for spraying disinfectants to disinfect the public places. They are also broadcasting messages about coronavirus and social distancing at public places to aware the public [2]. Small robots are also used to disinfect streets and houses where cases of coronavirus have been reported. Drones are also being used in many residential areas to see whether people are following norms of social distancing or not.

3.2.9. Grocery Stores: During coronavirus, there is increase in online orders as customers prefer online delivery to avoid contamination of virus. So, grocery stores are adopting technologies which provide contactless options. They are using mobile payment services instead of cash payments. Robots are helping the store owners by removing supply chain problems like delivering and stocking of items. Robots are performing tasks like preparing orders, checking inventory, gathering items, bagging and delivering of groceries [43].

3.2.10. Vaccine & Medicine Development: Pharmaceutical companies are working to develop vaccine or medicines for treatment of the virus. The robotics companies are providing automated solutions to the different companies so that they can speed up manual and repetitious tasks required in the production of vaccination and medicines. Examples are:

a. The Hamilton Company has developed automated workstations which can be used for testing of novel coronavirus [9].

b. ABB robots help the medical lab to produce Covid-19 testing kits [9].

Other Areas: Other areas of application of robots during coronavirus are:

a. Cleaning of office spaces.
b. Production floors.
c. Disinfection of airplanes, airports, lodgings and cafes.
d. Delivering of meals to quarantined people in hotels.
e. Enforcement of curfews.
f. Scanning of visitors to check fever, oxygen level etc.
g. Distribution of hand sanitizer.
h. Real estate sector where teleoperating robots are showing properties to customers by keeping them stay at home.
i. Drones are being used as lighting purpose at night to carry out construction activities in case of emergency situations.
j. In some countries students are using robots by fixing their photograph on the face of robot to walk the stage for collecting their degrees of graduation.
k. In some countries, people are using drones to walk their dogs by maintaining isolation norms during lockdowns [2].
l. Sanitization of train compartments and stations.

k. e-commerce companies to fulfill online orders.

4 Problems Associated with Robotics & Automation

No doubt robots and automation are helping the people in fight against coronavirus and will become an integral part at different workplaces in future because of their benefits and applications. But there are certain problems and drawbacks of using robots and automation initially as well as in long term. Some of them are:

4.1. Funding: There has not been sufficient funding for infectious disease-related robotics research in recent years. Lack of interest and lack of funding once the emergency situation gets over is one of the reasons for the same. We will not be ready for next pandemic without sustained and continuous research efforts in the field of robotics and automation.

4.2. Costly: In general, robots and automation are very expensive to purchase, install and maintain which in turn increases the labor cost which limits their wide-spread use. The cost of robots and automation directly depends upon the volume. They are affordable when prepared and purchased in bulk. Life of some of machines is very less and availability of spare parts is also an issue in case of breakdown. There is also need of skilled labor for programming of robots.

4.3. Adaptability: Sometimes it is difficult to adapt the things when you are not in such situation before. Integrating robots and automations immediately into existing system as happening during COVID-19 can lead to many problems. People working in the system are not familiar with automatic environment as they are used to and comfortable with their daily routine. This can lead to workflow problems and faults. During an emergency, people are busy and under stress that they are not able to learn new things. They are not able to adapt certain tasks like frequent reboot or change of batteries that comes with new technology [2].

4.4. Lack of Human Touch: Robots and automation lacks in human touch and interaction. Like in hospitals, people need human touch and connection during their recovery or in restaurants customers need human interaction which lacks with robots and automation. Moreover problems faced by the customers cannot be heard by robots. So sometimes, customers need more human interaction rather than technology for their grievances.

4.5. Harmful for Human Beings: Some of the robots which are using UVD technology for disinfection are dangerous as ultraviolet light can be damaging for the health of humans. Use of technology for their daily work will also make people and lazy which can impact their health and efficiency.

4.6. Unemployment: It is also observed that most of the industries are automating their production lines to limit the workers on job floor and most of the work is being carried out remotely [7]. This pandemic has resulted in replacing humans with robots. The main reason of replacement of human with robots is the norm of social distancing as all workers cannot do the work together due to space constraints. When some company replaces a worker with a robot, most of the time company is not going to hire anyone for same work. Robots are very costly to make and to integrate into workplace but once they are installed and in use, they are less costly as compared to human workers as they do not take leave, salary etc. [11]. No doubt, automation in retail, services, and manufacturing will result in decrease in jobs now and in future as well.

4.7. Breakdowns: Sometime automated systems don't work properly due to technical problems and breakdowns [11]. Therefore, customers try to avoid using them. For example people prefer cash counters at grocery stores etc. because sometime automated system gets down due to some technical reason or sometimes money gets deducted without actual payment.

4.8. Updation: Another problem associated with robots and automation is that they require continuous updation as technology keeps on changing frequently, which makes them more costly. Lack of updates will make them outdated easily. Due to increase in demand, changes in technology and their wider applications in current scenario, there is need of robots which are environment friendly, multi-purpose, updated and adaptable so that they can be used in long term [38].

4.9. Limited Applications: Before COVID-19, robots were mainly used in discrete manufacturing sectors like in automobile and electronics industries [12]. Now, with the decrease in production in these industries due to COVID-19, the industrial robots segment has witnessed nil growth this year. Therefore, need of the hour is to implement automation in other sectors to increase their applications and usage.

4.10. The problem with automation cannot be done at once as it takes lots of investment and time. In current scenario, when demand of products are low, it will be very difficult for industries to implement it at one go.

4.11. It is not an easy job to automate everything. Some jobs are easier to automate than others. So it will take some time to get some automation done in every segment of the life due to lack of funds.

4.12. Technological change also results in new kind of jobs but these jobs are likely to be in two sectors i.e. digital-age jobs and service jobs. It is also observed that these sectors do not provide good packages as other sectors do.

4.13. The automation will worsen inequality in wealthy countries. People with skills suited for digitized workplace will have a much easier time than the people who are expected to learn these skills from start. This can intensify inequality which will result in populism and destabilization of political establishments in many countries.

4.14. The companies are turning towards robots in order to safeguard their production and supply chains against any future disruptions. Therefore, robots have created a challenge in emerging markets. Millions of jobs are at stake in developing countries which are factories of textiles and light manufacturing industries in the world.

4.15. The governments of countries should get ready to face challenges as people are losing their jobs and there is increase in inequality so governments should help people to learn new skills and create new jobs otherwise displaced people will create trouble for system in future.

The robots are also prone to viruses. These cyber viruses are also very dangerous. If companies want automation, they should invest massively in cyber security to protect it against hackers.

5 Types of Robotics and Automation

During coronavirus, everyone is looking towards robots and automation as a means to do their work efficiently along with safety. Different applications of robots have come up during this pandemic and depending upon the purpose for which it has to be used different types of robots and automation technologies are developed. Some of them are explained below:

5.1. Telerobotics: These are the robots used to check the condition of patients without the need for a physical presence by the doctor, only using the tablet that incorporates the robot. There is shortage of medical equipments like PPE kits and there is risk of transfer of virus for health workers so telerobots are proving very useful in this crisis. Telerobotic system provides robotic arm to healthcare workers by which they can control and check medical equipment remotely used for patient care. A manipulator which is remote controlled and has virtual buttons and dials on a touch screen so that healthcare staff can work on medical equipment present in

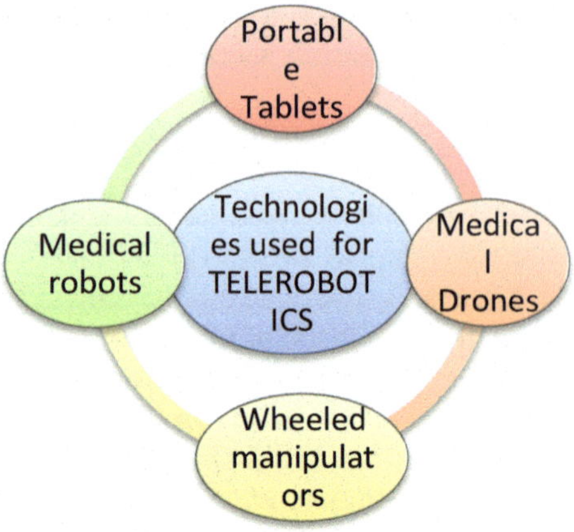

Fig. 20 Technologies used for Telerobotics

patients room without any PPE [13]. Example is the voice-interactive Zafi robot that was developed as explainer of school subjects and is repurposed for medical purpose. Zafi has a payload of eight kilograms and can work as medical attendant without any contact. Zafi Medic robot can deliver things up to 20 kilograms, and have working range of one kilometre with live coverage [39]. There is also increase in demand of virtual meeting tools like Zoom, Microsoft (Skype) and others as people prefers to work from home due to lockdowns.

Another example is wheeled mobile manipulator which is used to test patients before they enter in hospitals. These manipulators consists of standard instruments for measuring fever, oxygen level etc. of patient without any help of frontline worker. Such telerobots can be used for isolation of patients and keep them away from other high-risk patients [13]. Some of the technologies used for telerobotics during COVID-19 are given in Fig. 20.

5.2. Medical Robots or Cleaning Robots: The pandemic like coronavirus has integrated many technologies such as predictive diagnostics, Artificial Intelligence and telemedicine [39] to develop medical robots. Example is the UVD Robots, which are self driven to sterilize hospitals and other areas using ultraviolet light [9]. These robots prevent the spread of coronavirus without exposing medical staff to the virus. Groceries and restaurants offering delivery are also using these robots. Schools or offices are also using these robots for cleaning their premises.

5.3. Drones: The coronavirus has also developed the need to check whether patients are following the norms of isolation and public is following the norm of social distancing. Therefore drones are being used more frequently in the fight against coronavirus. Example is the quadcopter who can carry test samples to testing centers and can supervise whether people are following isolation norms [2]. Drones are providing thermal images to detect fever in people and other respiratory ailments in public. Drones are also helpful in education and provide instruction to the public to make them aware about this disease. Other roles of the drones are the transportation of medical and other consumer supplies, and aerial spray disinfection. DBCMS

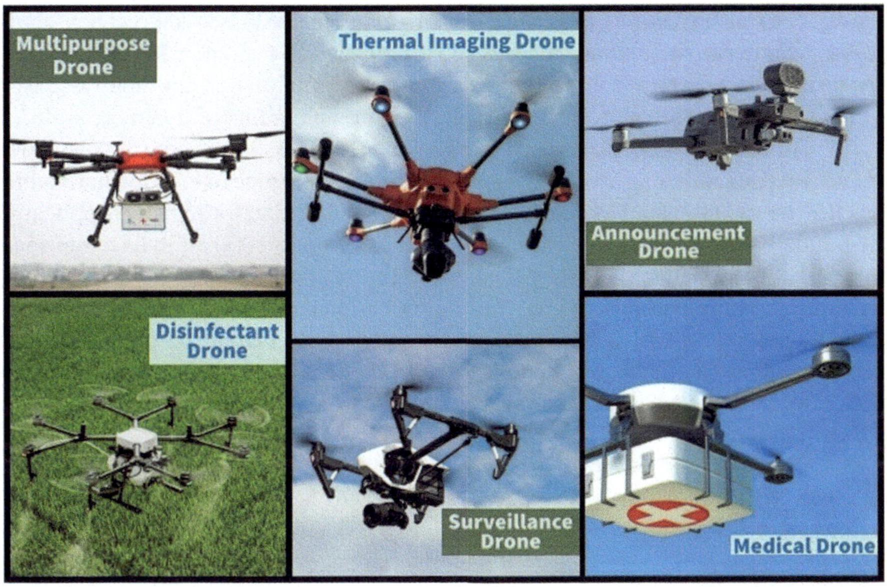

Fig. 21 Applications of drones for COVID-19 management [46] *Source* https://ieeexplore.ieee.org/stamp/stamp.jsp?tp=&arnumber=9086010, https://creativecommons.org/licenses/by/4.0/

i.e. Drone Based Covid-19 Medical Service mechanism has been proposed for the safety of medical staff who are at risk to coronavirus infection as they are directly exposed to it in hospitals. This mechanism can be used to improve the process used for treatment of Covid-19 patients [14]. Various applications of drones are given in Fig. 21.

5.4. Brain-Powered Robots: These robots are based on cloud to identify digital commands and send them to the physical world. These robots can work in public spaces to reduce number of people and can manage data with minimum interaction with customers. Brain-powered robots are very helpful in maintaining low human interaction [8].

5.5. Chatbots: The chatbots are basically software application which helps in conducting online-chat and avoid direct human contact. So these chatbots are very helpful during coronavirus. Example is the PayPal which is using chatbots for customer inquiries through message during coronavirus. They are also providing automatic translation services so that English-speaking associates can talk to their customers who are not familiar with English [8]. In coronavirus, people want to avoid going to hospitals due to fear of contamination. So these chatbots helps in symptom detection and reduce mental stress by enabling people to assess their health at regular intervals [47]. Aarogya setu has a chabot which enables people to assess their health as and when required.

5.6. Patrol Robots: These are the robots which are mainly used in shopping malls, public places and airports. These robots remind people to wear face masks and wash hands. They also monitor mask-wearing and helps the police to keep check on the public to prevent the spread of virus [15]. Guangzhou Gosuncn Robot Company has manufactured patrol robot consisting of high-resolution cameras and IR sensors which can scan temperature of ten people who are in a radius of five meters [48].

5.7. Robot Vans: They are also called logistics robots. These are the robots who deliver food and other logistics to people at their locations due to lockdown. Example is self-driven robot van, Hercules, developed by UDI, China for logistics application [15]. It delivers food and other things and can carry up to 1000 kg in its cargo space using light detection and ranging method, stereo vision cameras and deep-learning algorithms. Many companies are working on automatic systems having vision and navigation controls which can move on ground as well as in air to deliver items to people at home in situations like today due to coronavirus [13]. US-based Starship Technologies has developed battery-powered, six-wheeled robot for delivery services [48] and is shown in Fig. 22.

5.8. Disinfectant Robots: Disinfectant robots demand is increasing due to outbreak of the coronavirus. Example is the UVD Robots [48] and shown in Fig. 23

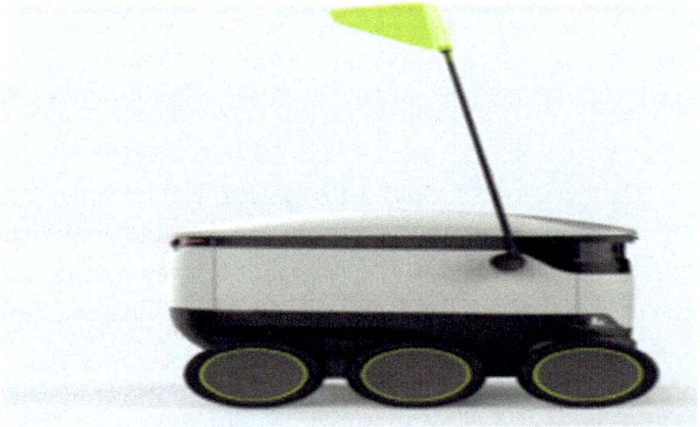

Fig. 22 Delivery Robot [48] *Source* https://www.emerald.com/insight/content/doi/10.1108/IR-05-2020-0101/full/html?skipTracking=true

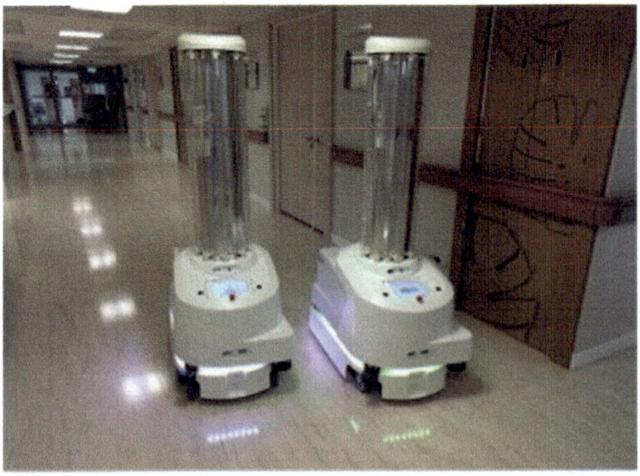

Fig. 23 UVD Robots [48] *Source* https://www.emerald.com/insight/content/doi/10.1108/IR-05-2020-0101/full/html?skipTracking=true

which are used for disinfecting places to fight the coronavirus. These robots are helpful in disinfecting and killing diseases, viruses, bacteria etc. present in the system by breaking down their molecular structure with help of UV light system. Siemens and Aucma are also working on prototype of an intelligent disinfection robot that will be available soon for fight against virus [15].

5.9. Our global supply chains is heavily dependent upon human operators like truck drivers, cargo workers and crane operators of the port to maintain continuous supply of things and other essential goods from one part to other part of world. Therefore use of automation in trucking, ships, and cranes [13] are being developed and used to come out of the crisis due to coronavirus.

5.10. Several mobile apps are being developed and used for ordering food at home by people to protect them from getting exposed to virus at restaurants. Several food and drink apps are used by people to get delivery services. DoorDash and Instacart are providing services which are helping people to remain isolated and maintain social distance. DoorDash is also providing contactless delivery options due to COVID-19. It has option of delivery instructions as per choice like leaving the order outside the door to avoid any contact with the driver [49].

5.11. Automation technologies such as video conferencing [39] are being used for virtual work from home for maintaining social distancing and self isolation due to coronavirus. Example is the zoom app which is widely used for office meetings and socializing with people due to lockdowns due to COVID-19 [50].

5.12. During coronavirus, the 3D printing technology has been used by many industries to develop prototypes and preparation of medical equipments. This technology is used to produce face shields [51], masks, goggles, and gloves. Now this technology has been applied to prepare affordable ventilators also [13].

Autonomous Robots or Mechanical Design Robots: Autonomous robotic systems are able to do work without interacting with human worker. Some of the types of autonomous robots are:

Fixed-base manipulators: These manipulators are formed by attaching links in a sequence which form joints. They have one part fixed to the ground and the other part free to do the task. These skilled manipulators can be used to work easily and efficiently in current conditions of coronavirus [13].

Wheeled mobile robots: These are the systems which are like self driving cars. They are not fixed. Therefore, they can be easily used to deliver medicines and other essential items to patients of coronavirus in the hospitals or quarantine centers [13].

Flying mobile robots: These are mobile robots which can fly also. Example is quadcopters. These can be used to check whether people are following norms of isolation and social distancing at quarantine centers [13].

Mobile manipulators: It is combination of mobile robot and fixed base manipulator. They can move materials, equipments, medications, PPE kits and other essential items when required in hospital [13].

5.14. Wearable Robots: These are devices which are worn by humans which can read signals from the human's body and display output to the user in the form of audio or video to improve the capabilities of the user. This information can be related to body or physical activity. An example of consumer wearable robots is the tracker

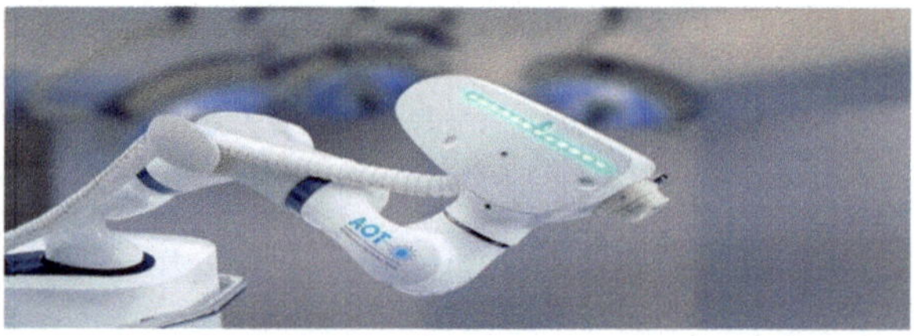

Fig. 24 CARLO: A Collaborative Robot who assists laser system for bone surgery *Source* https://www.kuka.com/en-in/industries/solutions-database/2019/02/aot-ag © AOT AG

that provides feedback to people on their workout. Wearable also helps to monitor heart rate, brain waves etc. Another example is the augmented reality/virtual reality displays by which healthcare workers can do diagnosis and planning of treatment remotely. Exoskeleton robots are also one kind of wearables used to enhance motor skills or to restore abilities of user [13]. A machine is developed at Tsinghua University in Beijing having robotic arm on wheels which can do ultrasounds and mouth swab tests and listen to lung sounds [52].

5.15. Collaborative Robots: Collaborative robotic systems are used to enhance the abilities of human operator. These robots have a handle on its manipulator which is manually controlled by the user. They are very helpful in dynamic and changing tasks or conditions. These robots act as mediator between a patient and doctor, which eliminate the use of PPE kit. A collaborative robot reduces fatigue of the worker during repetitive tasks. A collaborative manipulator helps in maintaining proper posture, sufficient distance while taking swab of COVID patients [13] (Fig. 24).

5.16. Social Robots or Physical Robots: They are also called companion robots. Social robots can interact and communicate with users keeping in view user's mood, temperature, stress etc. using inbuilt sensors [13]. They are used to check mental health of people who are under isolation so that they do not feel lonely and stressed up being away from their family members. They also provide emotional support and remove anxiety [53].They are designed keeping in view elderly care and children with disabilities as these people are most affected due to coronavirus as their family members cannot visit to see them due to lockdowns. Technologies like video-chat apps are being used to make senior citizens to interact with their families and doctors. They also help in delivering items in their rooms and maintaining social distancing between them.

5.17. Reprogrammable Robots: These are the robots which are developed for different purpose and are repurposed keeping in view the emergent requirement. Example is the Zafi robot which was originally an explainer for school subjects but is repurposed as Zafi medic for medical scenario due to coronavirus [39]. Governments are promoting manufacturers to repurpose their factories to make ventilators which are very important for treatment of critical patients of coronavirus. Manufacturers like JCB, Rolls Royce and others are repurposing their production lines and training workers for making ventilators in short time [54].

5.18. Mobile Apps: The software developers are developing different mobile apps in a fight against coronavirus. They are based on data collected by the governments for testing programme. This app warns the user when he is 100 metres away from the location of infected person. It also provides information of coronavirus patient like gender, age, nationality etc. An example is Aarogya Setu app which is used for contact tracing and self assessment by the user [41].

5.19. Smart Technologies: The coronavirus has lead to development of smart technologies. Example is smart helmet developed by the Shenzhen-based company who has a range of 5 meters to detect person with a fever. It gives a sound when person having a fever is nearby. Some of the features of helmet are temperature detection, AR visor, camera to read QR codes, wifi, Bluetooth, 5G etc. which can transmit data to the hospital. The helmet has face recognition technology which displays the subjects name on the AR visor along with medical history. It needs only few minutes to examine a queue of 100 people approximately [41].

6 Different Applications for Which Robots Are Used All Over World During Coronavirus

Different robots have been used by different countries for their fight against coronavirus based upon requirements of current situations. Some of them are given below:

Germany: Robots are advising customers at grocery stores to avoid panic while buying things and overcrowding.

Italy: Robots are placed in a room at Circolo Hospital, Varese, who check condition of patients and send information to the doctors. These robots have touch-screen facility through which patients record messages to send to doctors.

USA: Delivery service Postmates are using robots to deliver meals to customers.

China: Robots are used to provide hand sanitizer, food, groceries and disinfection of streets.

Belgium: Video-conferencing robots like ZoraBots are used at nursing homes to make aged people to stay in touch with their relatives.

South Africa: Tech Company Netcare is using robots based on UV light to sanitise hospitals [5].

India & France: The police are using drones to check lockdown, monitor parks and public places so that people do not go out of their homes for non-essential work [41].

7 Future Development and Investment on Robotics

Some companies have developed robots and automation which are already in use to fight COVID-19 and companies from all over the world are working day and night to produce robots and automation which can further strengthen the fight against this deadly virus and any future pandemic. Some of the companies have shown their determination to develop automotive technologies for betterment of mankind. Some future developments on robots and automation are given below:

- FANUC has said that the production of ROBOT, ROBODRILL, ROBOSHOT and ROBOCUT will carry on.
- KUKA has mentioned that its new KRIONTEC robots will be best in terms of energy requirements, running costs, and maintenance requirements.
- Service robotics manufacturer named PAL robotics in collaboration with EU project, SPRING will develop social humanoid robots.
- Yaskawa Electric has mentioned that it will continue to develop innovative products which will help in a fight during COVID-19. The company's robots are very useful for laboratory automation in current scenario [12].

Investment in Robotics: Robotics R&D programs are basically run by government of the country. Different countries are doing investments in the development of robotics through various projects and programs. Some of the investments done by different countries in their robotics R& D programs are given below:

China: China is looking to upgrade their capabilities in manufacturing by 2025 and to use advanced robots in 10 core industries. They have Robot Industry Development plan through which they are working on developing global robot manufacturers, creating industrial clusters, targeting domestic market share of 45% for high-end robots and increasing their robot density per 10,000 workers in 2020. They have invested 577 million USD in robot development in 2019.

Japan: Japan is number one in manufacturing of robots and delivered 52% robots globally in 2018. Japan is working on Abenomics Growth Strategy. Japan has increased its budget in 2019 for robot innovation. Japan is working on manufacturing and other important areas like healthcare, infrastructure and agriculture for robotics.

Korea: Korea has Intelligent Robot Development and Supply Promotion Act to develop the robot industry. This plan promotes robotics in these sectors like manufacturing, healthcare, logistics and robot software. The budget of korea for robot development is 126 million USD in 2020.

European Union: European Union has Robotics projects funded by Horizon 2020 and is working on the development of robotics in manufacturing, healthcare, commercial, transportation and agri-food robotics. This project has budget of 780 million USD for seven years.

Germany: Germany is promoting the use of new digital technologies with the help of "PAiCE" program having funding of 55 million USD for five years.This will be spent on creation of platforms for service robotics solutions in the areas including service, manufacturing and logistics.

USA: The National Robotics Initiative (NRI) is supported by the US Government for robotics development. This program focuses on use of science and technology with aim to create collaborative robots which can assist humans. The budget of NRI was 35 million dollars in 2019. USA is also providing funding to robotics in defense and space areas through and the Mars Exploration Program the Department of Defense [55].

8 Conclusions and Suggestions

No doubt, use of robotics and automation for work automation is need of hour due to crisis that world is facing for its existence due to coronavirus but there are also apprehensions of using these technologies by human beings. So here are some suggestions which can be helpful so that there is balance while integrating automation at workplace. Some of them are:

8.1. It is very much clear that robots and automation are for the benefits of workers and cannot be replaced with them. Robots are mainly used for the jobs that workers cannot do due to some reasons or due to safety reasons. They only help the workers to reduce their workload and make them do some other important activities. These robots are teleoperated which enable them to apply their expertise and compassion to sick and isolated patients remotely [2]. They only reduce the disinfection time so that PPE kits, masks and other aides can be used by the hospital staff and shortage of these equipments can be avoided.

8.2. It is human nature to show resistance to change or to adapt any new things with difficulty. Same is happening during COVID- 19, when robots and automation has become part of our new normal. So some research agencies and other institutes must come with data and research that how robots could help reduce infection risks for front-line health care workers so that they adopt this easily. Research laboratories and startups are working on creating robots that will help health workers to collect blood samples and mouth swab remotely. These robots which are under development are not going to help now but they will make a difference in future disasters definitely. So momentum of robotics research should continue for the benefit of the mankind [2].

It is also seen that robots cannot be used everywhere. So, proper areas should be located where robots and automation can be implemented easily without disrupting the workflow and displacing the existing workers.

8.4. It is also happening most of the time that whenever there is emergency, we are quick enough to adopt new technologies but we quickly forget the things once the disaster gets over and get back to our old working. This leads to decrease in interest and funding for development of robotics and automation.

8.5. It is better to repurpose the existing robots than going for new robots and also to convert existing manufacturing/assembly lines for building the same as building a new and specialized robot takes lots of time and resources.

It is better not to stockpile robots as they gets outdated easily and when need comes to use them operators using them get rusty or may get retired.

8.7. The government and other industries should learn a lesson from the present situation and should start working in such a way that simple robots will be integrated with the existing workforce so that same can be used during next pandemic.

8.8. Robots working at different workplaces do not bring human touch especially at places like hospitals, restaurants etc. Customers want more human interaction than technology. So robots and technology can be best used during unique and uncertain times like COVID-19 [42].

8.9. Evolvement of robotics and technology during COVID era have made employees to reevaluate and question their job and there is urgent need for them get re-skilled to ensure that they can easily adapt with the automation at their workplace. On the same time organizations must think to re-train their workforce to find new ways of getting them to work.

8.10. Development of automation and robots and due to COVID- 19 for maintaining social distancing, a mindset have been developed at higher levels that humans should be replaced with machines but it has been found that automation of the workplace can increase labor cost because robots require person to install it, to operate it as well as to maintain it which can prove to be more costly.

8.11. Organizations and manufacturers must start preparing them for post-pandemic. As due to COVID-19 they have time now to prepare them for automation and get ready once the lockdown gets over. Else they have to wait for many months to get the things done from the suppliers of their choice due to number of automation projects starting at the same time.

8.12. Robotics main purpose is to keep medical workers safe and share workload so that they can help the sick protect as many people as possible. There is need of flexible manufacturing and automation during this crisis time rather than traditional manufacturing as it helps in developing products which are responsive to needs. Robotics development needs time and money before it can be used for situations like coronavirus. Research and investment in these technologies are need of hour to make our systems safe and to protect important life's of people. But if we want to save our future from any pandemic, then these new technologies require continuous research, development and integration. It is to be realized that these technologies are critical for the development of safe, vigorous and capable system which can fight not only coronavirus but future pandemics if any, properly.

References

1. World Health Organization. Coronavirus disease 2019 (COVID-19): situation report, 72 (2020)
2. Wise, C.: How robots and other tech can make the fight against coronavirus safer. Retrieved from https://www.pbs.org/newshour/science (2020)
3. Nehmzow, U., Recce, M.: Scientific methods in mobile robotics. Robot. Auton. Syst. **24**(1), 1–4 (1998)
4. WHO Coronavirus Disease (COVID-19) Dashboard. Retrieved from covid19.who.int
5. Kurfess, T.R. (ed.).: Robotics and Automation Handbook. CRC Presas (2018)
6. Murphy, R.R., Adams, J., Gandudi, V.B.M.: Robots have demonstrated their crucial role in pandemics - and how they can help for years to come. Retrieved from https://www.weforum.org/agenda/2020/05/robots-coronavirus-crisis (2020)
7. Tavakoli, A., Vahdat, K., Keshavarz, M.: Novel. Coronavirus Disease 2019 (COVID-19): An Emerging Infectious Disease in the 21st Century. Iran South Med. J. **22**(6), 432–450 (2020)
8. Coronavirus disease (COVID-19) advice for the public: World Health Organisation; 2020. Retrieved from https://www.who.int/emergencies/diseases/novel-coronavirus-2019/advice-for-public. Accessed 18 July 2020

9. Qureshi, Z., et al.: What is the evidence to support the 2-metre social distancing rule to reduce COVID-19 transmission? The Centre for Evidence-Based Medicine develops, promotes and disseminates better evidence for healthcare (2020)
10. Alagoz, O., et al.: Impact of Timing of and Adherence to Social Distancing Measures on COVID-19 Burden in the US: A Simulation Modeling Approach." *medRxiv* (2020)
11. Du, Z., Xu, X., Wang, L., Fox, S.J., Cowling, B.J., Galvani, A.P., Meyers, L.A.: Early Release-Effects of Proactive Social Distancing on COVID-19 Outbreaks in 58 Cities, China
12. Alagoz, O., Sethi, A., Patterson, B., Churpek, M., Safdar, N. Impact of Timing of and Adherence to Social Distancing Measures on COVID-19 Burden in the US: A Simulation Modeling Approach. medRxiv (2020)
13. Qureshi, D., Salim, M., Singh, P., Swarnkar, P., Goud, H.: Robotics solutions to combat novel corona virus disease-2019 (COVID-19). In: Pushpendra, Swarnkar, P., Goud, H.: Robotics Solutions to Combat Novel Corona Virus Disease-2019 (COVID-19)(June 2, 2020) (2020)
14. Karin, O., et al.: Adaptive cyclic exit strategies from lockdown to suppress COVID-19 and allow economic activity. medRxiv (2020)
15. Nomani, M.Z.M., Rauf, M., Ahmed, Z., Faiyaz, T., Khan, S.A., Tahreem, M.: Quarantine Law Enforcement & Corona Virus (COVID-19) Pandemic in India. J. X'idian Univ. **14**(4), 536–542 (2020)
16. Thiel, S., Häbe, D., Block, M.: Co-operative robot teams in a hospital environment. In: 2009 IEEE International Conference on Intelligent Computing and Intelligent Systems, vol. 2, pp. 843–847. IEEE (2009, November)
17. Zarkadakis, G., Jesuthasan, R., Malcolm, T.: The 3 ways work can be automated. Harvard Business Review.[online]. https://hbr.org/2016/10/the-3-ways-work-can-beautomated (2016)
18. Liu, J., Ren, L., Gong, D.: The Effects of Robots on the Long-Run Economic Growth. Tehnički vjesnik **27**(1), 73–80 (2020)
19. Arslan, U., Akkuş, N., Temiz, İ.: The Effects of Offline Simulation on Return on Investment for Robotic Investments. Umut Arslan J. Eng. Res. Appl. 10(01) (Series -III):18–22. ISSN: 2248-9622 (2020)
20. Lum, H.C.: The role of consumer robots in our everyday lives. In: Living with Robots, pp. 141–152. Academic Press (2020)
21. Khan, Z.H., Siddique, A., Lee, C.W.: Robotics utilization for healthcare digitization in global COVID-19 management. Int. J. Environ. Res. Public Health **17**(11), 3819 (2020)
22. Van Pinxteren, M.M., Wetzels, R.W., Rüger, J., Pluymaekers, M., Wetzels, M.: Trust in humanoid robots: implications for services marketing. J. Serv. Market. (2019)
23. Castelo, N., Schmitt, B., Sarvary, M.: Human Or Robot? the Uncanny Valley in Consumer Robots. In: NA - Advances in Consumer Research Volume 46, eds. Andrew Gershoff, Robert Kozinets, and Tiffany White, Duluth, MN: Association for Consumer Research, Pages: 183–187. http://www.acrwebsite.org/volumes/2411700/volumes/v46/NA-46 (2018)
24. Kubilinskiene, S., Zilinskiene, I., Dagiene, V., Sinkevièius, V.: Applying robotics in school education: a systematic review. Baltic J. Modern Comput. **5**(1), 50 (2017)
25. Doulamis, I.P., Spartalis, E., Machairas, N., Schizas, D., Patsouras, D., Spartalis, M., Dimitroulis, D.: The role of robotics in cardiac surgery: a systematic review. J. Robot. Surgery **13**(1), 41–52 (2019)
26. Iqbal, J., Khan, Z.H., Khalid, A.: Prospects of robotics in food industry. Food Sci. Technol. **37**(2), 159–165 (2017)
27. Llale, J., Setati, M., Mavunda, S., Ndlovu, T., Root, D., Wembe, P.: A review of the advantages and disadvantages of the use of automation and robotics in the construction industry. In: Construction Industry Development Board Postgraduate Research Conference, pp. 197–204). Springer, Cham (2019, July)
28. Jianbo, Y.: Development direction of mechanical design, manufacturing and automation. In: 2019 3rd International Conference on Education Technology and Economic Management (ICETEM 2019) (2019)
29. Szegedi, P., Koronváry, P., Békési, B.: The use of robots in military operations. Sci. Res. Educ. Air Force-AFASES **1**. https://doi.org/10.19062/2247-3173.2017.19.1.25 (2017)

30. Kumar, J.A., Srinivas, G.: Recent trends in Robots smart material and its application in aeronautical and aerospace industries. J. Phys.: Conf. Series **1172**(1):012035. IOP Publishing. https://doi.org/10.1088/1742-6596/1172/1/012035 (2019, March)
31. Belpaeme, T., Kennedy, J., Ramachandran, A., Scassellati, B., Tanaka, F.: Social robots for education: a review. Sci. Robot. **3**(21) (2018)
32. Vaani, I., Sushil, S.J., Kunjamma, U.V., Ramachandran, A., Bai, V.T., Thyla, B.: BhrtyArtana (A pipe cleaning and inspection robot). In: 2017 Third International Conference on Sensing, Signal Processing and Security (ICSSS), pp. 422–425. IEEE (2017, May)
33. Casals, A.: Robots in surgery. In: Autonomous Robotic Systems, pp. 222–234. Springer, London (1998)
34. Casals, A., Hernansanz, A., Sayols, N., Amat, J.: Assistance strategies for robotized laparoscopy. In: Iberian Robotics Conference, pp. 485–496. Springer, Cham (2019, November)
35. Shenoy, R., Nathwani, D.: Evidence for robots. Sicot-j **3** (2017)
36. Arvanitakis, I., Tzes, A., Giannousakis, K.: Synergistic exploration and navigation of mobile robots under pose uncertainty in unknown environments. Int. J. Adv. Robot. Syst. **15**(1), 1729881417750785 (2018)
37. Ing, E.B., Xu, Q., Salimi, A., Torun, N.: Physician deaths from corona virus (COVID-19) disease. Occup. Med. **70**(5), 370–374 (2020)
38. Schwarzkopf, P.: Robotics and automation against COVID-19. Retrieved from https://rua.vdma.org/en/viewer/-/v2article/render/48069235 (2020)
39. Loten, A.: Calling All Robots: Businesses Automate the Battle Against Coronavirus. Retrieved from https://www.wsj.com/articles (2020)
40. Nahla, N.: Medical Robots to the Rescue in the Battle Against Coronavirus. Retrieved from https://www.thehindu.com/sci-tech/technology/gadgets (2020)
41. ways robots fight against the COVID-19 pandemic. Retrieved from https://www.eu-robotics.net/eurobotics/newsroom/press/robots-against-covid-19.html (2020)
42. Thomas, Z.: Coronavirus: Will Covid-19 speed up the use of robots to replace human workers. Retrieved from https://www.bbc.com/news/technology-52340651 (2020)
43. Morgan, B.: 10 Examples of Robots Helping To Fight COVID. Retrieved from https://www.forbes.com/sites/blakemorgan/2020/04/22 (2020)
44. Alsoliman, B.S.H.: The utilization of educational robotics in Saudi Schools: potentials and barriers from the perspective of Saudi Teachers. Int. Educ. Stud. **11**(10), 105–111 (2018)
45. Shaw, K.: A3 Special report: how robots and automation are fighting Covid-19. Retrieved from https://www.robotics.org/content-detail.cfm/Industrial-Robotics-Industry-Insights (2020)
46. Chamola, V., Hassija, V., Gupta, V., Guizani, M.: A comprehensive review of the COVID-19 pandemic and the role of IoT, Drones, AI, Blockchain, and 5G in managing its impact. IEEE Access **8**, 90225–90265 (2020). https://doi.org/10.1109/ACCESS.2020.2992341
47. Miner, A.S., Laranjo, L., Kocaballi, A.B.: Chatbots in the fight against the COVID-19 pandemic. npj Digit. Med. **3**:65 (2020). https://doi.org/10.1038/s41746-020-0280-0
48. Bogue R. Robots in a contagious world. Industrial Robot: the international journal of robotics research and application. Vol. 47 No. 5, pp. 673-6429 (2020). https://doi.org/10.1108/IR-05-2020-0101
49. Banskota, S., Healy, M., Goldberg, E.M.: 15 smartphone apps for older adults to use while in isolation during the COVID-19 pandemic. Western J. Emergency Med. **21**(3), 514 (2020)
50. Chawla, A.: Coronavirus (COVID-19)–'Zoom' Application Boon or Bane. Available at SSRN 3606716. 2020 May 20
51. Flanagan, S.T., Ballard, D.H.: 3D printed face shields: a community response to the COVID-19 global pandemic. Acad. Radiol. **27**(6), 905 (2020)
52. Behar, J.A., Liu, C., Tsutsui, K., Corino, V.D., Singh, J., Pimentel, M.A., Karlen, W., Warrick, P., Zaunseder, S., Andreotti, F., Osipov, M.: Remote health monitoring in the time of COVID-19. arXiv preprint arXiv:2005.08537. 18 May 2020
53. Aymerich-Franch, L., Ferrer, I.: The implementation of social robots during the COVID-19 pandemic. arXiv preprint arXiv:2007.03941. 8 Jul 2020

54. Malik, A.A., Masood, T., Kousar, R.: Repurposing factories with robotics in the face of COVID-19 (2020)
55. International Federation of Robotics. How Nations Invest in Robotics research. Press release Jun 5, 2020

Nonparametric Tests for Comparing COVID-19 Machine Learning Forecasting Models

Dmitriy Klyushin

Abstract The rapid spread of the COVID-19 pandemic has revealed an acute problem associated with forecasting the development of epidemics in different countries and assessing the accuracy of these forecasts. The most widely used models for predicting viral outbreaks are the SIR and SEIR models and their modifications. The complexity of predicting the development of epidemics using these models is associated with the large uncertainty of the parameters included in these models; therefore, many researchers have attempted to apply machine learning methods for forecasting. The objects of our study were the Grey Wolf Optimizer (GOW) methods, as well as two machine learning models (MLP multilayer perceptron and ANFIS adaptive network fuzzy inference system). Ranking the models in increasing order of their accuracy is not difficult, but in many cases it makes no sense, since the model predictions in the statistical sense differ little from each other (homogeneous) and therefore such models can be considered equivalent. The chapter describes an effective nonparametric tests both traditional and new for comparing the results of time series prediction, which makes it possible to assess their homogeneity and identify groups of forecasting methods whose forecast results differ statistically significantly from each other. The results of comparison of forecasting machine learning models for different countries are presented. The effectiveness of the applied method of nonparametric testing of the homogeneity of models is shown.

Keywords COVID-19 · Machine learning · Time series · Forecasting · Nonparametric test

1 Introduction

COVID-19 is rapidly spreading around the planet, infecting more and more people (according to the Johns Hopkins Institute, as of August 25, 2020, it was 24 million people, of which more than 820 thousand people died). These numbers highlight

D. Klyushin (✉)
Department of Computer Science and Cybernetics, Taras Shevchenko National University of Kyiv, Prospect Akademika Glushkova, 4D, 03680 Kiev, Ukraine
e-mail: dokmed5@gmail.com

D. Oliva et al. (eds.), *Artificial Intelligence for COVID-19*, Studies in Systems, Decision and Control 358, https://doi.org/10.1007/978-3-030-69744-0_9

the importance of accurately predicting the development of COVID-19 epidemics in different countries, allowing their governments make the right decisions. The problem of uncertainty in the parameters of standard models is complicated by new factors unpredictable mobility of the population in the modern world, a variety of measures to reduce the infectiousness of the virus in different countries through the introduction of a mask regime, social distancing, and full, partial or adaptive quarantine, etc. In such circumstances, the accuracy of standard epidemiological models has questioned. As an alternative to standard models for simulation of epidemic such as SIR and SEIR it was proposed to use novel methods of machine learning. These methods do not use assumptions on parameters describing an epidemic situation and are based only on observations.

In either case, using any of the above mentioned models we obtain some forecasts of time series and must compare them by some tests. The most widely used tests are accuracy measures: MSE (mean square error), MAPE (mean absolute percentage error) and MAD (mean absolute deviation). When comparing one method of forecasting a time series with another, we must take into account not only the indicators of their accuracy, but also the statistical homogeneity of their errors. If there is no significant statistical difference between the errors of different forecasting methods, then they can be considered as equivalent ones although they may differ in accuracy. If there is such a difference, then the choice of the best forecasting method with the minimum error rate becomes statistically justified.

The purpose of this chapter is to describe the effective nonparametric methods for testing homogeneity of two samples and apply it for estimation of forecasting effectiveness of several models used for prediction of COVID-19 outbreak in various countries.

The purpose of this chapter is to describe effective nonparametric methods for testing the homogeneity of two samples and apply them to assess the forecasting performance of multiple models used to predict the COVID-19 outbreak in different countries.

Section 2 describes the main challenges in predicting the COVID-19 outbreak. Section 2.1 provides a brief overview of work that used standard and machine learning models to predict the COVID-19 outbreak. Section 2.2 describes nonparametric methods for comparing forecast models. Section 3 contains a description of the nonparametric Klyushin–Petunin test used to assess the statistical homogeneity of errors for each model under consideration. Section 4 describes the results of applying this method, along with the Kolmogorov-Smirnov and Wilcoxon signed-rank tests, to evaluate the effectiveness and rank predictive models for the COVID-19 outbreak in Italy, Germany, Iran, China, and the United States. Section 5 summarizes considerations and describes future work.

2 Challenges of Forecasting of COVID-19 Outbreak

The main challenges of forecasting of COVID-19 outbreak are complexity, validations and usefulness of the forecasting models [10]. The validity and reliability of the results of forecasting models in the context of the Covid-19 pandemic are of paramount importance as they are used by governments to make decisions about the entire population of a country. Consequently, assessing the quality of the results obtained becomes an extremely important issue.

2.1 Forecasting Models for COVID-19 Outbreak

There are many deterministic and stochastic models for infectious diseases forecasting. The most popular are compartment models SIR and SEIR that have various modifications such as SIRS, SEI, SEIS, SI, SIS, SEIRS, MSEIRS and LISEIR [16]. The abbreviations SIR and SEIR means than the model consists of class S of susceptible to infection part of population, class I of infected part of population, class R of removed part of population (recovered, immunized, died), and class E of exposed part of population. The models SIR [23] and SEIR (Aaron and Shwartz 1984) are the systems of ordinary differential equations using parameters that describe the death rate and the rate of new infections.

The standard models SIR and SEIR, and their modifications were widely used for prediction of COVID-19 outbreak in various countries [2, 5, 12, 15, 20, 27, 32]. Mathematically, these models are very nice and accurate but the main problem is that their parameters depend on many unpredictable factors. The curves constructed using these methods are mathematically justified but often they occurs far from the true epidemical curves.

Currently, the most popular among epidemiologists are the models SIR, SEIR, and their modifications, which have become de facto standard in this field of science [37]. The disadvantages of these models noted above, associated with the high uncertainty of the parameters, often stimulate investigators to switch from direct forecasting of time series to modeling scenarios according to the "what if" principle. Unlike modeling based on solving systems of ordinary differential equations (both deterministic and stochastic), machine learning methods use only training data and therefore can theoretically give more accurate results based on real data.

The machine learning methods applied for prediction of COVID-19 outbreak are survey in [13]. Also, it should been noted the papers [3, 9, 18, 19, 25, 26, 28, 34–36, 39] where problem of the forecasting of COVI-19 outbreak was solved.

The variety of mathematical models for predicting the COVID-19 epidemic requires efficient model evaluation tools. Such a toolkit should take into account both the accuracy of the models and the statistical nature of their errors. Nonparametric methods are widely used in predictive analytics [8, 11], biostatistics (Wiel 2009), and weather forecasting [6] to estimate prediction error difference between predictors. These methods do not impose any requirements on error distributions (only absence of ties) and do not use preconditions for their analysis.

We will apply the Klyushin–Petunin test, Kolmogorov–Smirnov test and Wilcoxon signed-rank test to results of the methods described in [3]. In this paper variants of the method of smart optimization Grey Wolf Optimizer (GWO) and two machine learning methods for prediction time series are considered: multilayer perceptron (MLP) and adaptive network fuzzy inference system (ANFIS).

Grey Wolf Optimizer is so-called nature-inspired optimization algorithm imitating the behavior of the wolf pack in the hunting [31]. For estimation we will use the results of forecasting with the help of logistic, linear, logarithmic, quadratic, and power equations published in [3].

From the category of machine learning methods Ardabili et al. selected the multilayered perceptron MLP and adaptive network-based fuzzy inference system ANFIS [21] as the most frequently used. For our aims it is not important what algorithms was used for prediction COVID-19 outbreak as far as we shall compare the statistical homogeneity of their results using nonparametric methods.

2.2 Nonparametric Methods for Comparing Forecast Models

The main question when comparing the accuracy of the two models of time series prediction is formulated as follows: does the observed difference in predictions reflect the actual difference between the models, or is random sample variability prevailing, which strongly depends on the samples on the basis of which the time series is built?

The main idea of comparison of prediction error difference of two forecasting models consists is the following. Suppose that we have two forecasting models generating two predictions of the time series $x_i^{(1)}$ and $x_i^{(2)}$, $i = 1, \ldots n$.. Let $x_i, i = 1, \ldots, n$ be true values of time series. Compute residuals $d_i = x_i^{(1)} - x_i^{(2)}$, $i = 1, \ldots, n$. Null hypothesis about equal accuracy of models 1 and 2 is equivalent to the hypothesis that the mathematical expectation of d_i is equal to zero, i.e. $E(d_i) = 0$. Thus, the problem may be reduced to testing the hypothesis that $E\left(x_i^{(1)}\right) = E\left(x_i^{(1)}\right)$. Usually, to test this hypothesis the Wilcoxon signed-rank test or its modifications are used [8, 11]; Wiel 2009; [6] that is very effective for testing the hypothesis of distribution location shift. We proposed the alternative method that effectively tests not only the hypothesis of distribution location shift but also the hypothesis about equivalence of distributions when the mathematical expectation is zero but the standard deviations are different [24]. It tests whether distributions of forecasts generated by two forecasting models are the same. Similar idea but grounded on the Kolmogorov–Smirnov statistics is described in [14].

The advantage of the Klyushin–Petunin test is that it does not put forward any assumptions about the distribution functions of the general populations from which the samples are drawn (except for their absolute continuity, i.e., the absence of ties), and is also insensitive to autocorrelation, which may be observed in the forecast results. The numerous experiments with samples from various distributions shown that test statistics is more stable and sensitive than Kolmogorov–Smirnov and Wilcoxon statistics and more robust to possible outliers.

3 Klyushin–Petunin Nonparametric Test for Homogeneity

According to Hill's assumption $A_{(n)}$ [17] for exchangeable random values $x_1, x_2, \ldots, x_n \in G$ with absolutely continuous distribution:

$$P\left(x \in \left(x_{(i)}, x_{(j)}\right)\right) = \frac{j-i}{n+1}, \quad j > i \tag{1}$$

where $x \in G$ is a sample value, and $\left(x_{(i)}, x_{(j)}\right)$ is an interval constructed on the i-th and j-th order statistics. Based on this assumption, in [36] a nonparametric test for estimation the homogeneity of samples from populations with absolutely continuous distribution functions was developed. Let we have two samples $x_1, x_2, \ldots, x_n$ and $y_1, y_2, \ldots, y_n$ from distributions F_1 and F_2. Suppose that $F_1 = F_2$ and construct the variational series $x_{(1)}, x_{(2)}, \ldots, x_{(n)}$. Denote as $A_{ij}^{(k)}$ an event $\left\{y_k \in \left(x_{(i)}, x_{(j)}\right)\right\}$. If $j > i$ then

$$P\left(y_k \in \left(x_{(i)}, x_{(j)}\right)\right) = p_{ij} = \frac{j-i}{n+1}. \tag{2}$$

Then, compute the confidence interval for binomial proportion of the event $A_{ij}^{(k)}$ in Bernoulli trials (for example the Wilson interval but this is not unique choice):

$$\begin{aligned} p_{ij}^{(1)} &= \frac{h_{ij}^{(n,k)} n + g^2/2 - g\sqrt{h_{ij}^{(m,k)}(1 - h_{ij}^{(m,k)})n + g^2/4}}{n + g^2}, \\ p_{ij}^{(2)} &= \frac{h_{ij}^{(n,k)} n + g^2/2 + g\sqrt{h_{ij}^{(m,k)}(1 - h_{ij}^{(m,k)})n + g^2/4}}{n + g^2}, \end{aligned} \tag{3}$$

where $h_{ij}^{(n,k)}$ is the relative frequency of the event $A_{ij}^{(k)}$ in n trials. Then, construct the confidence interval $I_{ij}^{(n)} = \left(p_{ij}^{(1)}, p_{ij}^{(2)}\right)$ with a significance level depended on the parameter g. If g is equal to 3 than the significance level of $I_{ij}^{(n)}$ is less than 0.05 [24]. Denote by B an event $\left\{p_{ij} = \frac{j-i}{n+1} \in I_{ij}^{(n)}\right\}$. Put $N = (n-1)n/2$ and calculate the frequency L of the event B. The value $h = L/N$ is a homogeneity measure of samples x and y which we shall call *p-statistics*.

Let us put $h_{ij}^{(n)} = h$, $n = N$ and $g = 3$, and construct the confidence interval $I_n = (p_1, p_2)$ for $p(B)$. The confidence intervals $I_{ij}^{(n)} = \left(p_{ij}^{(1)}, p_{ij}^{2}\right)$ and $I = (p_1, p_2)$ are called *intervals based on the 3 s-rule.* If the hypothesis that distributions are identical holds, this scheme called the *generalized Bernoulli scheme* [22, 29, 30]. If the hypothesis is false, this scheme is called the *modified Bernoulli scheme.* In general case, when the null hypothesis can be either true or false, the trial scheme is called *MP-scheme* (Matveichuk–Petunin scheme). If $F_1 = F_2$, $\lim\limits_{n\to\infty} \frac{j-i}{n+1} \in (0, 1)$, and $\lim\limits_{n\to\infty} \frac{i}{n+1} \in (0, 1)$, then the asymptotic significance level β of a sequence of confidence intervals $I_{ij}^{(n)}$ based on the 3 *s*-rule, is less than 0.05 [24].

Let $B_1, B_2, \ldots$ be a sequence of in a random experiment E, $\lim\limits_{n\to\infty} p(B_k) = p^*$, $h_{n_1}(B_1), h_{n_2}(B_2), \ldots$ be a sequence of relative frequencies of $B_1, B_2, \ldots$, respectively, and $\frac{k}{n_k} \to 0$ as $k \to \infty$. The random experiment E is *strong* if $h_{n_k}(B_k) \to p^*$ as $k \to \infty$. In a strong random experiment the asymptotical significance level of the Wilson confidence interval I_n when $g = 3$ is less than 0.05. The test for the null hypothesis $F_1 = F_2$ with a significance level which is less that 0.05 is following: if I_n contains 0.95, the null hypothesis is accepted, else the null hypothesis is rejected.

4 Estimation of Forecast Model Using the P-Statistics

Let us consider the results of comparisons of the results of prediction COVID-10 outbreak by the modifications of GWO and MLP, and ANFIS.

The training data in [3] were drawn from the cite www.woldometers.com for Italy, Germany, Iran, USA, and China. These data describe total cases of decease in these countries over 30 days since the start moment (for example, for China authors selected January 22 and for other countries February 15).

The prediction was made for 150 days. In [3] the results for 20th, 40th, 60th, 80th, 100th, 120th, 140th, and 150th days were provided. Thus, we have predictions for 8 times moments. Using these data we can compare the models for statistical significance.

In the Klyushin–Petunin test the samples are considered as drawn from different populations if the upper boundary of the confidence interval for p-statistics is more than 0.95. In the Kolmogorov–Smirnov test and Wilcoxon signed-rank test the null hypothesis about equivalence of the distribution functions is rejected if p-value of the test is less than 0.05. The results of comparisons are provided in Tables 1, 2, 3, 4, 5, 6, 7, 8, 9, 10, 11, 12, 13, 14 and Table 15. Here, we used the following notation for the methods: 1—Logistic GWO, 2—Linear GWO, 3—Logarithmic GWO, 4—Quadratic GWO, 5 –Power GWO, 6—MLP, 7—ANFIS.

The analysis of Tables 1, 2 and 3, 4 and 5 shows that according to the Klyushin–Petunin test he models are similar (upper bound exceeds 0.95) only in 6 cases from 21 comparisons (28.5%) for Italy, in 11 cases for Germany (52.4%), 8 cases (38.1%) for Iran, 6 cases (28.5%) for China, and 11 cases (52.4%) for Germany. It is interesting

Table 1 Upper bound of the confidence intervals for the p-statistics for the forecast models of COVID outbreak in Italy

Method	1	2	3	4	5	6	7
1	1.000	0.977	0,786	0.964	0.948	0.977	1.000
2	–	1.000	0.930	0.977	0.977	0.948	0.948
3	–	–	1.000	0.930	0.948	0.930	0.930
4	–	–	–	1.000	1.000	0.930	0.930
5	–	–	–	–	1.000	0.911	0.911
6	–	–	–	–	–	1.000	1.000
7	–	–	–	–	–	–	1.000

Table 2 Upper bound of the confidence intervals for the p-statistics for the forecast models of COVID outbreak in Germany

Method	1	2	3	4	5	6	7
1	1.000	0.911	0.977	0.977	0.930	1.000	0.977
2	–	1.000	0.930	0.977	1.000	0.930	0.930
3	–	–	1.000	0.930	0.977	0.977	0.977
4	–	–	–	1.000	0.964	0.930	0.930
5	–	–	–	–	1.000	0.948	0.948
6	–	–	–	–	–	1.000	0.977
7	–	–	–	–	–	–	1.000

Table 3 Upper bound of the confidence intervals for the p-statistics for the forecast models of COVID outbreak in Iran

Method	1	2	3	4	5	6	7
1	1.000	0.977	0.930	0.948	0.930	0.930	0.964
2	–	1.000	0.930	0.989	0.947	0.964	0.948
3	–	–	1.000	0.930	0.930	0.930	0.930
4	–	–	–	1.000	1.000	0.930	0.930
5	–	–	–	–	1.000	0.911	0.911
6	–	–	–	–	–	1.000	0.977
7	–	–	–	–	–	–	1.000

that MLP and ANFIS for all countries gave statistically similar results (see entries 6–7). Also, both these methods in the prevalence majority of cases produce results that significantly differ from the results of GOW modifications for Italy, Germany, China, Iran, and USA. The variants of GOW have more variability.

The analysis of Tables 6, 7, 8, 9 and 10 shows that according to the Kolmogorov–Smirnov test the models are similar (p-value exceeds 0.05) only in 7 cases from 21

Table 4 Upper bound of the confidence intervals for the p-statistics for the forecast models of COVID outbreak in China

Method	1	2	3	4	5	6	7
1	1.000	0.930	0.930	0.930	0.930	1.000	0.997
2	–	1.000	0.930	1.000	1.000	0.911	0.911
3	–	–	1.000	0.930	0.930	0.930	0.930
4	–	–	–	1.000	1.000	0.911	0.911
5	–	–	–	–	1.000	0.911	0.911
6	–	–	–	–	–	1.000	0.997
7	–	–	–	–	–	–	1.000

Table 5 Upper bound of the confidence intervals for the p-statistics for the forecast models of COVID outbreak in USA

Method	1	2	3	4	5	6	7
1	1.0000	0.911	0.964	0.977	0.911	0.997	1.000
2	–	1.000	0.930	0.977	1.000	0.930	0.930
3	–	–	1.000	0.930	0.964	0.977	0.997
4	–	–	–	1.000	0.964	0.930	0.930
5	–	–	–	–	1.000	0.930	0.930
6	–	–	–	–	–	1.000	0.964
7	–	–	–	–	–	–	1.000

Table 6 P-value of the Kolmogorov–Smirnov test for the forecast models of COVID outbreak in Italy

Method	1	2	3	4	5	6	7
1	1.000	0.519	0.000	0.008	0.008	0.188	0.188
2	–	1.000	0.000	0.008	0.008	0.520	0.520
3	–	–	1.000	0.000	0.000	0.000	0.000
4	–	–	–	1.000	0.519	0.008	0.008
5	–	–	–	–	1.000	0.008	0.008
6	–	–	–	–	–	1.000	0.188
7	–	–	–	–	–	–	1.000

comparisons (33.3%) for Italy, in 6 cases for Germany (28.5%), 6 cases (28.5%) for Iran, 6 cases (28.5%) for China, and 2 cases (9.5%) for Germany. Note, that MLP and ANFIS were statistically different in 2 cases (Iran and USA). Also, according to the Kolmogorov–Smirnov test both these methods almost in all cases produce results that significantly differ from the results of GOW modifications for Italy, Germany, China, Iran, and USA. The GOW modifications have more variability.

Table 7 P-value of the Kolmogorov–Smirnov test for the forecast models of COVID outbreak in Germany

Method	1	2	3	4	5	6	7
1	1.000	0.001	0.001	0.059	0.001	0.520	0.188
2	–	1.000	0.000	0.008	0.906	0.049	0.001
3	–	–	1.000	0.000	0.001	0.049	0.001
4	–	–	–	1.000	0.008	0.049	0.050
5	–	–	–	–	1.000	0.049	0.001
6	–	–	–	–	–	1.000	0.520
7	–	–	–	–	–	–	1.0000

Table 8 P-value of the Kolmogorov–Smirnov test for the forecast models of COVID outbreak in Iran

Method	1	2	3	4	5	6	7
1	1.000	0.008	0.000	0.001	0.001	0.049	0.049
2	–	1.000	0.000	0.049	0.008	0.008	0.008
3	–	–	1.000	0.000	0.000	0.000	0.000
4	–	–	–	1.000	0.188	0.001	0.001
5	–	–	–	–	1.000	0.001	0.001
6	–	–	–	–	–	1.000	0.049
7	–	–	–	–	–	–	1.000

Table 9 P-value of the Kolmogorov–Smirnov test for the forecast models of COVID outbreak in China

Method	1	2	3	4	5	6	7
1	1.000	0.001	0.000	0.001	0.001	0.520	0.188
2	–	1.000	0.000	0.188	0.188	0.001	0.001
3	–	–	1.000	0.000	0.000	0.000	0.000
4	–	–	–	1.000	1.000	0.001	0.001
5	–	–	–	–	1.000	0.001	0.001
6	–	–	–	–	–	1.000	0.188
7	–	–	–	–	–	–	1.000

The analysis of Tables 11, 12, 13, 14 and 15 shows that according to two-sample Wilcoxon signed-rank test the models are similar (p-value exceeds 0.05) only in 6 cases from 21 comparisons (28.5%) for Italy, in 7 cases for Germany (33.3%), 4 cases (19.0%) for Iran, 1 case (4.76%) for China, and 7 cases (28.5%) for Germany. Note, that MLP and ANFIS were statistically different in 2 cases (Iran and USA). Also, according to the Kolmogorov–Smirnov test both these methods almost in all cases

Table 10 P-value of the Kolmogorov–Smirnov test for the forecast models of COVID outbreak in USA

Method	1	2	3	4	5	6	7
1	1.000	0.001	0.001	0.049	0.001	0.049	0.188
2	–	1.000	0.000	0.008	0.906	0.001	0.001
3	–	–	1.000	0.000	0.001	0.001	0.001
4	–	–	–	1.000	0.009	0.049	0.049
5	–	–	–	–	1.000	0.001	0.001
6	–	–	–	–	–	1.000	0.049
7	–	–	–	–	–	–	1.000

Table 11 P-value of comparison by the Wilcoxon signed-rank test the forecast models of COVID outbreak in Italy

Method	1	2	3	4	5	6	7
1	1.000	0.547	0.008	0.023	0.038	0.844	0.400
2	–	1.000	0.008	0.016	0.016	0.547	0.547
3	–	–	1.000	0.008	0.008	0.008	0.008
4	–	–	–	1.000	0.039	0.023	0.023
5	–	–	–	–	1.000	0.039	0.039
6	–	–	–	–	–	1.000	0.547
7	–	–	–	–	–	–	1.000

Table 12 P-value of comparison by the Wilcoxon signed-rank test for the forecast models of COVID outbreak in Germany

Method	1	2	3	4	5	6	7
1	1.000	0.016	0.008	0.148	0.008	0.742	0.742
2	–	1.000	0.008	0.016	0.844	0.016	0.016
3	–	–	1.000	0.008	0.008	0.008	0.008
4	–	–	–	1.000	0.008	0.148	0.147
5	–	–	–	–	1.000	0.008	0.008
6	–	–	–	–	–	1.000	0.547
7	–	–	–	–	–	–	1.000

produce results that significantly differ from the results of GOW modifications for Italy, Germany, China, Iran, and USA. The variants of GOW have more variability, while the machine learning methods MLP and ANFIS produced statistically similar results in 4 cases from 5 (excluding USA).

Comparisons of results of COVID-19 forecasting for Italy, Germany, Iran, China, and USA using GOW models and multilayer perceptron MLP, and adaptive network

Table 13 P-value of comparison by the Wilcoxon signed-rank test for the forecast models of COVID outbreak in Iran

Method	1	2	3	4	5	6	7
1	1.000	0.008	0.008	0.008	0.016	0.674	0.148
2	–	1.000	0.008	0.016	0.016	0.008	0.008
3	–	–	1.000	0.008	0.008	0.008	0.008
4	–	–	–	1.000	0.016	0.008	0.008
5	–	–	–	–	1.000	0.016	0.016
6	–	–	–	–	–	1.000	0.742
7	–	–	–	–	–	–	1.000

Table 14 P-value of comparison by the Wilcoxon signed-rank test for the forecast models of COVID outbreak in China

Method	1	2	3	4	5	6	7
1	1.000	0.016	0.008	0.016	0.016	0.043	0.068
2	–	1.000	0.008	0.016	0.016	0.016	0.016
3	–	–	1.000	0.008	0.008	0.008	0.008
4	–	–	–	1.000	0.148	0.016	0.016
5	–	–	–	–	1.000	0.016	0.016
6	–	–	–	–	–	1.000	0.068
7	–	–	–	–	–	–	1.000

Table 15 P-value of comparison by the Wilcoxon signed-rank test for the forecast models of COVID outbreak in USA

Method	1	2	3	4	5	6	7
1	1.000	0.016	0.008	0.148	0.016	0.195	0.195
2	–	1.000	0.008	0.016	0.008	0.016	0.016
3	–	–	1.000	0.008	0.008	0.008	0.008
4	–	–	–	1.000	0.008	0.145	0.148
5	–	–	–	–	1.000	0.016	0.016
6	–	–	–	–	–	1.000	0.195
7	–	–	–	–	–	–	1.000

fuzzy inference system ANFIS with three nonparametric tests for testing the hypothesis on statistical homogeneous of two samples shown that these models produce generally similar results. However, the tests have different degree of optimism, i.e. more often accept the null hypothesis about the absence of statistically significant differences between the prognoses provided by different models. The most optimistic was the Klyushin–Petunin test (average of the acceptance of the null hypotheses is

40%) followed by the Kolmogorov–Smirnov (25.7%), and the Wilcoxon signed-rank test (23.8%). The results of GOW modifications are more variable and than machine learning. The Klyushin–Petunin test differs GOW models from the machine learning models in 52.0% of cases (26 from 50), the Kolmogorov–Smirnov in 82% (41 from 50), and the Wilcoxon test % (from 50). The Klyushin–Petunin test differs various GOW modifications from one another in 72% of cases (26 from 50), the Kolmogorov–Smirnov in 72% (36 from 50), and the Wilcoxon test in 90.0% (45 from 50). Thus, the Wilcoxon test is the most sensitive. It distinguishes almost all GOW models. The Kolmogorov–Smirnov test is less sensitive, and the Klyushin–Petunin test is the most conservative. In general, all three tests did not determine the significance differences between the results produced by MLP and ANFIS (except for two cases). The exceptions were the results of application of the Kolmogorov–Smirnov tests to the Iran and USA data.

5 Conclusion and Scope for the Future Work

Before ranking the models by their accuracy it is necessary to compare the statistical homogeneity of their results. This problem may be solved either by paired comparisons and by using corresponding two–sample tests of null hypothesis about the equivalence of sample distributions (Kolmogorov–Smirnov, Wilcoxon etc) or multiple tests like Kruskal–Wallis test. We choose the paired comparisons because they allow recognizing what models are statistically differs but not just the fact that all samples in total are heterogeneous. The chapter describes application of three nonparametric tests for comparing the results of time series prediction (Klyushin–Petunin test, Kolmogorov–Smirnov test an Wilcoxon signed-ranked test), which makes it possible to assess their homogeneity and identify groups of forecasting methods whose forecast results differ statistically significantly from each other. The results of comparison of forecasting machine learning models for different countries shows high homogeneity varying from 60 to 77%. It means at least two facts: 1) the machine learning methods are consistent; 2) nonparametric tests of the models homogeneity considered in chapter are effective and robust tools for statistical analysis of forecasting models.

While the GOW variants have more variability due to the different analytical dependencies used, MLP and ANFIS are slightly differs from the statistical point of view thus the choice one of these models may be made at the basis of accuracy measure and computational complexity. As far as MLP was the most accurate method and its results do not significantly differ from ANFIS statistically, it may be considered as the most effective tool for prediction of COVID-10 outbreak

Future work to be done relates to the development of our test to compare the accuracy of time series forecasting, allowing for ties, and applying this method to study the future evolution of the COVID-19 pandemic, taking into account new factors.

References

1. Aron, J., Schwartz, I.: Seasonality and period-doubling bifurcations in an epidemic model. J. Theor. Biol. **110**, 665–79 (1984). https://doi.org/10.1016/S0022-5193(84)80150-2
2. Anand, N., Sabarinath, A., Geetha, S., Somanath, S.: Predicting the spread of COVID-19 using SIR model augmented to incorporate quarantine and testing. Trans. Indian Natl. Acad. Eng. **5**, 141–148 (2020). https://doi.org/10.1007/s41403-020-00151-5
3. Ardabili, S.F., Mosavi, A., Ghamisi, P., Ferdinand, F., Varkonyi-Koczy, A.R., Reuter, U., Rabczuk, T., Atkinson, P.M.: COVID-19 Outbreak Prediction with Machine Learning. Preprints 2020040311. doi:10.20944/preprints202004.0311.v1 (2020)
4. Aron, J.L., Schwartz, I.B.: Seasonality and period-doubling bifurcations in an epidemic model J. Theor. Biol. **110**, 665–679. https://doi.org/10.1016/s0022-5193(84)80150-2
5. Babu, M., Marimuthu, S., Joy, M., Nadaraj, A., Asirvatham, E., Jeyaseelan, L.: Forecasting COVID-19 epidemic in India and high incidence states using SIR and logistic growth models. Clin. Epidemiol. Glob. Health (2020). https://doi.org/10.1016/j.cegh.2020.06.006
6. DelSole, T., Tippett, M.K.: Comparing forecast skill. Mon. Wea. Rev. **142**, 4658–4678 (2014). https://doi.org/10.1175/MWR-D-14-00045.1
7. Demšar, J.: Statistical comparisons of classifiers over multiple data sets. J Mach. Learn. Res. **7**, 1–30 (2006)
8. Diebold, F.X., Mariano, R.S.: Comparing predictive accuracy. J. Bus. Econ. Stat. **13**, 253–263 (1995). https://doi.org/10.1080/07350015.1995.10524599
9. Distante, C., Pereira, I., Gonçalves, L., Piscitelli, P., Miani, A.: Forecasting Covid-19 outbreak progression in Italian Regions: a model based on neural network training from Chinese data. MedRxiv (2020). https://doi.org/10.1101/2020.04.09.20059055
10. Eker, S.: Validity and usefulness of COVID-19 models. Hum. Soc. Sci. Com. (2020). https://doi.org/10.1057/s41599-020-00553-4
11. Flores, B.E.: The utilization of the Wilcoxon test to compare forecasting methods: A note. Int. J. Forecast. **5**, 529–535 (1989). https://doi.org/10.1016/0169-2070(89)90008-3
12. Guirao, A.: The Covid-19 outbreak in Spain. A simple dynamics model, some lessons, and a theoretical framework for control response. Infect. Dis. Model. https://doi.org/10.1016/j.idm.2020.08.010(2020)
13. Hanumanthu, S.R.: Role of intelligent computing in COVID-19 prognosis: a state-of-the-art review. Chaos Solit. Fract., 109947 (2020). doi:10.1016/j.chaos.2020.109947
14. Hassani, H., Silva, E.: A Kolmogorov-Smirnov based test for comparing the predictive accuracy of two sets of forecasts. Economics **3**(3), 590–609 (2015). https://doi.org/10.3390/econometrics3030590
15. He, J., Chena, G., Jiang, Y., Jin, R., Shortridge, R., Agusti, S., He, M., Wu, J., Duarte, C., Christakos, G.: Comparative infection modeling and control of COVID-19 transmission patterns in China, South Korea, Italy and Iran. Sci. Total Environ. **74**, 141447. https://doi.org/10.1016/j.scitotenv.2020.141447 (2020)
16. Hethcote, H.W.: The mathematics of infectious diseases. SIAM Rev. **42**(4), 599–653 (2000)
17. Hill, B.M.: Posterior distribution of percentiles: Bayes' theorem for sampling from a population. J. Am. Stat. Assoc. **63**, 677–691 (1968). https://doi.org/10.1080/01621459.1968.11009286
18. Hu, Z., Ge, Q., Li, S., Boerwincle, E., Jin, L., Xiong, M.: Forecasting and evaluating multiple interventions of Covid-19 worldwide. Front. Artif. Intell. **2020**, 00041 (2020). https://doi.org/10.3389/frai.2020.00041
19. Ibrahim, M.R., Haworth, J., Lipani, A., Aslam, A., Cheng, T., Christie, N.: Variational-LSTM Autoencoder to forecast the spread of coronavirus across the globe. MedRxiv (2020). https://doi.org/10.1101/2020.04.20.20070938
20. Ifguis, O., Ghozlani, M.E., Ammou, F., Moutcine, A., Abdellah, Z.: Simulation of the final size of the evolution curve of coronavirus epidemic in Morocco using the SIR Model. J. Environ. Pub. Health **2020**, Article ID 9769267. https://doi.org/10.1155/2020/9769267 (2020)
21. Jang, J.S.: ANFIS: adaptive-network-based fuzzy inference system. IEEE Trans. Syst. Man Cybern. **23**, 665–685 (1993). https://doi.org/10.1109/21.256541

22. Johnson, N., Kotz, S.: Some generalizations of Bernoulli and Polya-Eggenberger contagion models. Statist. Paper **32**, 1–17 (1991). https://doi.org/10.1007/BF02925473
23. Kermack, W.O., McKendrick, A.G.: A contribution to the mathematical theory of epidemics. Proc. R. Soc. Lond. A **115**, 700–721 (1927). https://doi.org/10.1098/rspa.1927.0118
24. Klyushin, D.A., Petunin, Y.I.: A nonparametric test for the equivalence of populations based on a measure of proximity of samples. Ukrainian Math J **55**(2), 181–198 (2003). https://doi.org/10.1023/A:1025495727612
25. Kolozsvári, L.R., Bérczes, T., Hajdu, A., Gesztelyi, R., Tiba, A., Varga, I., Szőllősi, G.J., Harsányi, S., Garbóczy, S., Zsuga, J.: Predicting the epidemic curve of the coronavirus (SARS-CoV-2) disease (COVID-19) using artificial intelligence. MedRxiv (2020). https://doi.org/10.1101/2020.04.17.20069666
26. Kumar, P., Singh, R., Nanda, C., Kalita, H., Sharma, S., Sharma, Y., Rani, M., Bhagavathula, A.: Forecasting COVID-19 impact in India using pandemic waves nonlinear growth models. MedRxiv (2020). https://doi.org/10.1101/2020.03.30.20047803
27. Li, R., Pei, S., Chen, B., Song, Y., Zhang, T., Yang, W., Bai, W., Lu, X., Zhang, W.: Substantial undocumented infection facilitates the rapid dissemination of novel coronavirus (sars-cov-2). Science **368**(6490), 489–493. https://doi.org/10.1111/jebm.12376
28. Magal, P., Webb, G.: Predicting the number of reported and unreported cases for the COVID-19 epidemic in South Korea, Italy, France and Germany (2019). SSRN: https://ssrn.com/abstract=3557360. doi.:https://doi.org/10.2139/ssrn.3557360
29. Matveichuk, S.A., Petunin, Y.I.: Generalization of Bernoulli schemes that arise in order statistics. I. Ukrainian Math. J. **42**(4), 459–466 (1990). https://doi.org/10.1007/BF01071335
30. Matveichuk, S.A., Petunin, Y.I.: Generalization of Bernoulli schemes that arise in order statistics. II. Ukrainian Math. J. **43**(6), 728–734 (1991). https://doi.org/10.1007/BF01058940
31. Mirjalili, S., Mirjalili, S.M., Lewis, A.: Grey wolf optimizer. Adv. Eng. Soft. **2014**(69), 46–61 (2014). https://doi.org/10.1016/j.advengsoft.2013.12.007
32. Nesteruk, I.: Statistics-based predictions of coronavirus epidemic spreading in mainland China. Innov. Biosyst. Bioeng. **4**(1), 13–8 (2020). https://doi.org/10.20535/ibb.2020.4.1.195074
33. Pires, A.: Interval estimators for a binomial proportion: comparison of twenty methods. REVSTAT Stat. J. **6**, 165–197 (2008). https://doi.org/10.1080/02664763.2012.713919
34. Rustam, F., et al.: COVID-19 future forecasting using supervised machine learning models. IEEE Access. **8**, 101489–101499 (2020). https://doi.org/10.1109/ACCESS.2020.2997311
35. Sujath, R., Chatterjee, J.M., Hassanien, A.E.: A machine learning forecasting model for COVID-19 pandemic in India. Stoch. Env. Res. Risk A **34**, 959–972 (2020). https://doi.org/10.1007/s00477-020-01827-8
36. Tuli, S., Tuli, S., Tuli, R., Gill, S.S.: Predicting the growth and trend of COVID-19 pandemic using machine learning and cloud computing. Internet Things **11**(100222) (2020). https://doi.org/10.1016/j.iot.2020.100222
37. Wang, N., Fu, Y., Zhang, H., Shi, H.: An evaluation of mathematical models for the outbreak of COVID-19. Precis. Clin. Med. **3**(2), 85–93 (2020). https://doi.org/10.1093/pcmedi/pbaa016
38. Wilcoxon, F.: Individual comparisons by ranking methods. Biometrika **1**, 80–83 (1945). https://doi.org/10.2307/3001968
39. Zhong, L., Mu, L., Li, J., Wang, J., Yin, Z., Liu, D.: Early prediction of the 2019 novel coronavirus outbreak in the mainland China based on simple mathematical model. IEEE Access. **8**, 51761–51769 (2020). https://doi.org/10.1109/ACCESS.2020.2979599

Artificial Intelligence and the Control of COVID-19: A Review of Machine and Deep Learning Approaches

Sakinat Oluwabukonla Folorunso, Emeka Ogbuju, and Francisca Oladipo

Abstract This study explores the prevalent Machine and Deep Learning approaches for the control of COVID-19. It reveals the impact of Artificial Intelligence in the case prediction, analysis, diagnosis, and treatment of the disease. Apart from discussing four (4) knowledge areas where Machine Learning and Deep Learning approaches were employed in the fight against the pandemic, we proposed a Generalized Artificial Intelligence Response Framework using those areas. We observed that most of the works seeking Artificial Intelligence scientific solutions to the pandemic were employing the use of chest X-ray images and chest computed tomography scans for prognosis and diagnosis while applying different Machine and Deep Learning approaches using available data dashboards. However, a production-ready landmark contribution towards the control of the disease through Artificial Intelligence is still at the moment a work in progress. Hence, the need for a response framework to give researchers and practitioners a working guide to finding solutions to the pandemic using computing techniques.

Keywords COVID-19 · AI response · Machine learning · Deep learning

S. O. Folorunso (✉)
Department of Mathematical Science, Olabisi Onabanjo University, Ago-Iwoye, Nigeria
e-mail: sakinat.folorunso@oouagoiwoye.edu.ng

E. Ogbuju · F. Oladipo
Department of Computer Science, Federal University, Lokoja, Nigeria
e-mail: emeka.ogbuju@fulokoja.edu.ng

F. Oladipo
e-mail: francisca.oladipo@kiu.ac.ug

F. Oladipo
Kampala International University, Kampala, Uganda

D. Oliva et al. (eds.), *Artificial Intelligence for COVID-19*, Studies in Systems, Decision and Control 358, https://doi.org/10.1007/978-3-030-69744-0_10

1 Introduction

The novel coronavirus originally called 2019-nCoV and then renamed COVID-19, is a leading cause of the closure of cities in China and other countries. The virus was first reported in China and led to the shutting down of markets, roads, and schools in the provinces of Hubei, Beijing, and Hong Kong [1]. The healthcare agencies of various nations and the World Health Organization (WHO) studied the virus by collecting data on its spread and prevalence to determine the precautionary measure to control it. However, the widespread human to human and objects to human transmission of the virus still led to both partial and total lockdowns of cities and towns across the world following its declaration as a global pandemic by the WHO.

The good news is that Artificial Intelligence (AI) and its new technologies like Machine Learning (ML), Deep Learning (DL), Big Data, and the Internet of Things (IoT) are crucial in predicting and fighting new diseases. AI is a powerful tool to fight against the current pandemic. Wang et al. (2020) [2] noted that while the World is facing the challenge of COVID-19, AI is being engaged in the fight against it with technological innovation and various sorts of ML and DL algorithms. Since the outbreak, research had concentrated on understanding how to use intelligence to fight against the disease. It is gradually becoming clear that AI is useful in determining the outbreak alerts and warnings, carrying out diagnoses and finding cures and treatments.

The technology however has not recorded successful breakthroughs against the pandemic due to the lack of adequate data or redundant data. Overcoming this constraint should take the form of creating a systemic balance between the interaction between AI and humans as well as the privacy of data and public health practice. Data may be available to fight the pandemic but needs adequate time to curate for training AI models [3]. The gathering of data on the diagnosis of individuals is critical in training AI models and saving lives with it. Notably, models based on data are useful in prediction, explanation, and pattern recognition. The model functionalities would help in diagnosing, recognizing, predicting, and treating infections of COVID-19 [3]. Some of the functionalities may be useful in managing the socio-economic impacts that result from the disease.

Apart from building ML and DL models, the other types of AI applications that can be useful against the COVID-19 pandemic include Computer Vision (CV) and Natural Language Processing (NLP). These applications can teach machines using Big Data on the prevalence of the disease condition. Since the outbreak of the virus, there has been an effort to deploy data analytic models and tools but the specific contribution of this study is the discussion of various applications of the AI technologies and the provision of four (4) coordinated knowledge areas where ML and DL approaches are applied in providing scientific solutions to the pandemic. We explore the potential and actual AI contributions in the fight against the pandemic and conclude that although the approaches are still in their infancy, the touch of a solution is not completely out of sight.

2 Knowledge Areas of AI in COVID-19 Control

There are four areas where AI can help fight against the current pandemic. These include the creation and collation of data dashboards, scientific prognosis, and diagnosis of the disease, provision of pharmaceutical cures and treatments, and enacting tracking and social control measures through an accurate ML prediction algorithm.

2.1 Prediction, Tracking and Social Control

AI can be used in managing the pandemic through the deployment of thermal imaging. The technology is useful in scanning public spaces for specific individuals who have the potential to be infected. It is then valuable to enforce lockdown and social distancing measures. Infrared cameras are used in train stations and airports across China to scan individuals for high temperatures. They were also deployed in facial-recognition to pinpoint individuals with high temperatures. Baidu is one of the producers of infrared cameras that use computer vision in scanning different individuals in the crowds [4]. The camera can scan 200 individuals every minute and recognize body temperature that exceeds 37 °C. However, thermal imaging has been inadequate in identifying a fever in individuals wearing glasses because the most reliable indication was the deployment of scanning of the inner tear duct. It was also hard to determine if a person's temperature was increased due to the COVID-19 pandemic or other sources. As noted earlier, AI is useful in predicting and diagnosing the pandemic but it is hampered due to the lack of historical data. However, robots and computer vision cannot be hindered by such limitations. This type of AI will be useful for social control. Related technologies like mobile phones with wearables and applications that have AI can help locate and control whole populations. In line with this, Barstugan et al. [5] did research to determine the effectiveness of social distancing in Europe which was conducted by the application of ML concept to determine the impact of social distancing on the spread of COVID-19. The very first and basic action that was taken against the coronavirus was social distancing so that the virus may not spread more rapidly or may be in order to control the virus. Although social distance measures may be awkward to normal social norms and some medic-patient interactions, it was still adopted because the condition is becoming a matter of life and death.

Apart from social control, AI can be useful for predicting and tracking individuals with COVID-19. The development follows a previous pandemic called the 2015 Zika virus, whereby AI helps in developing a dynamic neural network to understand the spread of the disease. Such models can be used with data from the COVID-19 pandemic, but they require re-training. The lack of unbiased and historical data to train AI models and the different characteristics of COVID-19 compared to previous epidemics, and panic behavior on social media may result in the lack of a model to predict and track COVID-19 [6]. The continued spread of the infection has resulted in the subsequent increase of traffic on social media, making it hard to determine the prevalence of the disease. One of the best ways to deal with the algorithm dynamics and the avalanche of big data is the deployment of content moderation on social media platforms. Most of the current models are not yet reliable and accurate, which means that several models to track and forecast COVID-19 do not deploy AI models [7]. Instead, the population uses susceptible infected and recovered models, such as an epidemic tracker, to predict the disease's spread. AI can be useful in reflecting success measures that can slow down or reduce the range of the COVID-19. They can further evaluate how scientists and governments are flattening the epidemiological curve of the disease.

So, authors in Metsky et al. (2020) [8] explained that various researches are being conducted on COVID-19 to identify their causes and effects. The death rate and the spread rate prediction of the disease could play a key role in finding a solution to the problem. There are various methods of machine learning that are helping in scanning and prediction of the rate of spread of COVID-19 in various countries. These estimations are important because they are playing a major part in enabling the government to pay attention to the issue and draft a proper solution for the issue. Practically, Apostolopoulos & Mpesiana (2020) [9] did research to predict the rate of COVID-19 infections and projections of deaths for the 50 states of the US. The research includes the overview of US state-by-state projections as well as the global projections of COVID-19 patients. According to the result of July, the number of cases reported in the US is five times less as compared to total cases.

In another similar development, Jiang et al. (2020) [10] developed a predictive model for Acute Respiratory Distress Syndrome (ARDS) among patients infected with COVID-19 based on the these symptoms: lymphocyte count, white blood count, temperature, cycle threshold, creatinine, hemoglobin, gender, CRP, age, fever, CK, LDH, Glu, ALT, AST, K+ , and N+ . The dataset consists of 53 hospitalized patients with COVID-19 in the dataset, all tested positive by throat swab with Real-Time Reverse Transcription Polymerase Chain Reaction (RT-PCR) assay from Wenzhou Central Hospital and Cangnan People's Hospital in Wenzhou, China. The three feature selection methods used were Information Gain, Gini index, and Chi-square statistics. The machine models used were Logistic Regression (LR), k-NN ($k = 5$), Decision Tree (DT) (based on Gain Ratio), DT (based on Gini Index), Random Forest (RF) and Support Vector Machine (SVM). SVM and k-NN performed best with 80% accuracy on the classification of COVID-19.

The essence of a predictive model is also to determine early warnings and alerts. For instance, BlueDot is a Canadian-based AI model that was funded for US$9 million. The model is better at sporting infectious disease outbreaks than humans. It predicted the outbreak of the infection by the end of 2019 and issued a warning to its customers at the end of the year before the world health organization's report on 9th January 2020. The researchers listed the top 20 destination cities where individuals from Wuhan would arrive after the outbreak. These would be at the forefront of the global spread of the COVID-19. HealthMap was also useful in giving an alarm at the end of 2019 to ensure that individuals understood that the virus could spread to various areas [11]. However, human input is optimal for AI applications because individuals can interpret and provide context to recognize the threat of the condition.

2.2 *Cures and Treatments*

ML algorithms are indeed helping in understanding how COVID-19 spreads and is speeding up research and discovering a proper treatment for COVID-19 [2]. AI was long used before they have COVID-19 pandemic to contribute to the discovery of new drugs. The number of research data centers and laboratories has increased to determine specific treatments and vaccines against the epidemic. The hope is that AI can be deployed in exhilarating the discovery of new drugs and repurposing existing ones. DeepMind from Google is an excellent example that has been used in predicting the structure of proteins in the formation of viruses [4]. Such information could be useful in developing new drugs. Exiting drugs can be explored also. For instance, Atazanavir is an existing drug that can be repurposed to treat COVID-19 using ML. Baricitinib is a drug that has been used to treat myelofibrosis and arthritis, and it has the potential to cure COVID-19 [4]. Alimadadi, et al. (2020) [12] showed that using ML algorithms, we can test multiple samples by simultaneously considering several potential antiviral agents by relying on DNA sequences, working on the protein structure, and potential drug binding sites of SARS-CoV-2. We can predict the proposed interactions between drugs and the virus and we could identify suitable medicine by understanding the best possible solution for COVID-19.

The vaccine is less likely to be available shortly, but much of the technology has been deployed in the current pandemic. Scientific checks and trades, as well as medical controls, are useful in ensuring that a drug can be helpful. It has to be approved after identification and screening, and this may take time. A vaccine may be ready after about one year despite the acceleration of AI. Some laboratories have reported that they will have the vaccine by September 2020 [13]. Still, such reports cannot be verified since it takes about two years to develop a fully functioning vaccine for a population.

In line with treatment, Yang et al. (2020) [14] described the latest research that is being conducted on ML algorithm and their application in reducing and alleviating the work stress of doctors that are treating patients who are suffering from COVID-19. The workload of medical staff was reduced because the effective application of ML algorithms helped in timely estimations and automated analyses to support clinicians. The example of this application is the fact that the chest Computed Tomology CT scans images are being used to detect COVID-19 lesions. These images are needed to be scanned by the trained radiologist but this need was eradicated by the application of ML tools. The research concluded that after the application of research tools on 400,000 Chests X-Rays (CXR), the use of images of the chest to diagnose COVID-19 is limited because of the fact that there are several factors that predict the chances of corona spread.

However, Brunese et al. (2020) [15] aimed at providing a fully automatic and faster diagnosis for COVID-19 using Deep Learning of VGG16 network with weights pre-trained on ImageNet on CXR images resized to 224 × 224 RGB image. They also provided explanations for their result to visualize class activation maps using Gradient-weighted Class Activation Mapping (Grad-CAM) algorithm. Their framework is first detecting the presence of pneumonia. The next phase then differentiates between COVID-19 and pneumonia. Then, the aim of the last phase is to localize the area of the COVID-19 incidence in the CXR. With a 6,523 CXR image dataset of different classes (COVID-19 (250), PB (2,753), and Healthy (3,520)) the average COVID-19 detection time is 2.5 s with 97% accuracy.

In the same vein, Li, et al. (2020) [16] proposed to build deep learning that detects COVID-19 and distinguish it from Community-Acquired Pneumonia (CAP) and other non-pneumonic lung disease using chest CT. They proposed, a deep learning model for COVID-19 detection using neural network (COVNet) to extract visual features from volumetric CT exams for the detection of COVID-19. CAP and other non-pneumonia CT exams were included to test the robustness of the model. The datasets were collected from 6 hospitals between August 2016 and February 2020. The dataset consists of 1296 instances for COVID-19, 1735 for CAP, and 1325 for non-pneumonia. Based on Area Under the Receiver Operating Characteristic Curve (AUC), sensitivity, and specificity metrics, the result of AUC of 0.96 was obtained for CT exams and AUC of 0.95 for CAP on CT exams. There is overlap in the chest CT imaging findings of all viral cases of pneumonia with other chest diseases which encourages a multidisciplinary approach to the final diagnosis used for patient treatment.

2.3 *Prognosis and Diagnosis*

Accurate and quick diagnosis of COVID-19 can be useful in generating data to train AI models. The information is also imperative and important in limiting the spread of the disease and saving lives. AI may provide valuable input in making a diagnosis based on images of chest radiography. AI can be as accurate as human beings in the diagnosis of various conditions such as COVID-19. It means that it can save the time that radiologists deploy in the prognosis of the disease. It also performs the diagnosis at a cheaper standard than a radiologist, and it is quicker than a human. Technologies like CT and CXR can be coupled with AI to ensure the detection of the disease. COVID-19 tests are currently expensive and in short supply, but all hospitals have CXR machines [17]. The technology can be used in smartphones to scan CT images. Many initiatives have been deployed to help understand the conditions, such as the deep Convolutional Neural Network (CNN) that uses CXR images to detect COVID-19.

For instance, Imran, et al. (2020) [3] developed and tested an AI-powered screening solution for COVID-19 infection that is deployable via a smartphone app. This app named AI4COVID-19 records and sends three 3-second cough sounds to an AI engine running in the cloud and returns a result within two minutes. Textual features were extracted from the cough sound with Mel-Frequency Cepstral Coefficients (MFCCs). The study approached this problem by investigating the distinctness of pathomorphological alterations in the respiratory system induced by COVID-19 infection when compared to other respiratory infections. The extracted features with 3 classes (COVID-19 likely, COVID-19 not likely, and Test inconclusive) were learned on 3 classifiers: Deep Transfer Learning-based Multi-Class classifier (DTL-MC), Classical Machine Learning based-Multi Class classifier (CML-MC) and Deep Transfer Learning-based Binary Class classifier (DTL-BC). Results obtained showed that DTL-MC outperforms with an accuracy of 92.64%, DTL-BC of 92.85%, and CML-MC (SVM) of 88.76%. AI4COVID-19 can distinguish among COVID-19 coughs and several types of non-COVID- 19 coughs. The accuracy is promising enough to encourage a large-scale collection of labeled cough data to gauge the generalization capability of AI4COVID-19.

Another initiative as from March 2020 that uses an AI model to diagnose COVID-19 deploys CXR images and has been used in the past to diagnose pulmonary Tuberculosis (TB). The potential has not yet been implemented in clinical practice settings, but several hospitals in China have used radiology technologies based on AI. Other radiologists have expressed concerns over the amount of data available to train AI models. Many hospitals in China are bound to suffer from selection bias because using CXR and CT scans can contaminate equipment and result in the increased spread of the disease [18]. The use of such scans in European hospitals reduced significantly after the pandemic broke to reflect the concern. Once an individual has been diagnosed with the condition, the fear intensifies and it may affect the patronage of the hospital. However, the point remains that ML algorithms can develop prognostic prediction models that predict mortality risks of infected individuals. They can provide more than 80% accuracy concerning an individual who has been infected and determine if he or she can develop acute respiratory distress syndrome.

For example, in the work of Yoo, et al. (2020) [19] who evaluated a deep learning-based decision-tree classifier for detecting COVID-19 from CXR images. The CXR images were grouped into four classes: normal, TB, non-TB, and COVID-19. They use four automated CXR imaging radiography systems (AXIRs). AXIR1 and AXIR2 are for the classification of images into abnormal/normal and TB/non-TB, respectively. If a good quality CXR is taken by AXIR1 and classified as an image of the normal state, no further action is taken. However, if the image is classified as abnormal, the next step (using AXIR2) is to determine whether it is TB or non- TB. AXIR3 and AXIR4 are used in the third step of the process, where the image is classified as COVID-19 or non-COVID-19, with or without TB. In each step, the prediction model is trained with a data group optimized for its intended purpose. The NIH ChestX-ray14 dataset was used in this study. The deep learning method is a 2-dimensional CNN with a PyTorch frame.

Similarly, in the work of Pereira et al. (2020) [20] where they proposed a multi-class and hierarchical classification schemas on their newly composed database named RYDLS-20, containing CXR images of pneumonia caused by different pathogens (COVID-19, MERS, SARS, Varicella, Streptococcus and Pneumocystis) as well as healthy lungs. These classes of pneumonia were unevenly distributed and overlapped so class imbalance treatment methods (ADASYN, SMOTE, SMOTE-B1/B2, AllKNN, ENN/RENN, TomekLinks, and SMOTE + TL) were applied as a data preprocessing method before classification. They applied some features extraction methods (LBP, EQP, LDN, LETRIST, BSIF, LPQ, oBIFs, and Inception-V3) on the CXR images. They also explored early and late fusion techniques in the schema in order to leverage the strength of multiple texture descriptors and base classifiers (k-NN, SVM, MLP, DT, and RF) at once. The proposed approach tested in RYDLS-20 achieved a F1-Score of 0.65 using a multi-class approach with MLP classifier using the LBP feature set and resampled with ENN. Furthermore, the proposed schema was also able to achieve an F1-Score of 0.89 for the COVID-19 identification in the hierarchical classification scenario using the early fusion combination of BSIF, EQP, and LPQ features resampled with SMOTE + TL.

Also, Hasan, et al. (2020) [21] proposed a feature extraction method based on the Q-Deformed Entropy (QDE) technique and Deep learning Features (QDE–DF) to classify COVID-19 coronavirus, pneumonia and healthy CT lung scans on 321 patients. They first applied a histogram threshold to segment the CT lung scan image. Then, CNN and QDE techniques are applied to extract features from the resultant image. Individual and combined features obtained were classified using four different ML models: Linear SVM, k-NN, Logistics Regression, and Long Short-Term Memory (LSTM) Neural Network. The combined feature set obtained the best accuracy of 99.68% with LSTM.

Likewise, Mei, et al. (2020) [22] proposed three AI models to classify CT scan images along with the clinical information of patients into COVID-19 (+), PTB, and SARS. The first model is based on a chest CT scan, the second model on clinical information, and the third on a combination of the two. CNN, MLP, SVM, RF models were deployed for the classification. The joint model using both clinical data and CT imaging achieved the highest values of 84.3% on sensitivity, 82.8% on specificity, and 0.92 on AUC.

Furthermore, Loey et al. (2020) [23] proposed a Generative Adversarial Network (GAN) with deep transfer learning for coronavirus detection in 307 CXR images with COVID-19, normal, pneumonia bacterial and pneumonia virus classes. They used GAN to generate more CXR images to increase their number. The three pre-trained models for transfer learning were Alexnet, Googlenet, and Restnet18. The GANed images were trained in three phases with the pre-trained model. Firstly, the Googlenet model was used on the images and achieving an accuracy of 80.6%. Secondly, Alexnet was trained and it achieved an accuracy of 85.2%. The last phase performed a classification with only 2 classes (COVID-19, and normal) with Googlenet achieving a 100% accuracy.

As well, Tartaglione et al. (2020) [24] presented a new COVID-19 dataset named CORDA with CXR images of 386 Patients with COVID negative and COVID positive classes from 4 different sources. They applied Histogram equalization to preprocess the images. U-Net was also applied to segment the lungs to create lung masks. ResNet-18, ResNet-50, and COVID-Net pre-training models were applied and compared on the CORDA dataset. Based on Accuracy, AUC, Sensitivity, Specificity, F-score, BA (balanced accuracy) and DOR (diagnostic odds ratio) measures with random shuffle split of 70: 30 train-test ratio, ResNet-50 with a certain CORDA + CXR combination performed best across all metrics.

Additionally, Abbas et al. (2020) [25] deployed Decompose, Transfer, and Compose (DeTraC) method for the classification of COVID-19, Normal, and SARS CXR images. For transfer learning, ImageNet and DeTraC pre-trained on ResNet 18. Principal Component Analysis (PCA) was applied to reduce the high-dimension of the feature space. The experimental results showed a high accuracy of 95.12%, a sensitivity value of 97.91%, and a specificity value of 91.87% obtained by the DeTraC method.

Also, authors in Sethy et al. (2020) [26] proposed the extraction of features from CXR lungs images with Deep features (ResNet50, AlexNet, VGG16, etc.). The different features extracted were then learned on the SVM model. The dataset [27–29] divided into three classes COVID-19, pneumonia, and normal was obtained from Kaggle and Github. ResNet + SVM obtained the best metric based on accuracy, sensitivity, False Positive Rate (FPR), and F1-score of 95.33%, 95.33%, 2.33%, and 95.34% respectively.

More so, Barstugan et al. (2020) [5] proposed the detection of COVID-19 with four different datasets formed by taking patches sized as 16 × 16, 32 × 32, 48 × 48, 64 × 64 from 150 CT images dataset [30] for two classes (coronavirus and non-coronavirus). The feature extraction process was applied to the patches to increase the classification performance. Grey Level Co-occurrence Matrix (GLCM), Local Directional Pattern (LDP), Grey Level Run Length Matrix (GLRLM), Grey-Level Size Zone Matrix (GLSZM), and Discrete Wavelet Transform (DWT) algorithms were used as feature extraction methods. SVM model applied with and without the extracted features. 2-fold, 5-fold, and 10-fold cross-validations were implemented during the classification process. Sensitivity, specificity, accuracy, precision, and F-score metrics were used to evaluate the classification performance. The best classification accuracy was obtained as 99.68% with 10-fold cross-validation and GLSZM feature extraction method.

2.4 Data Dashboards

Forecasting and tracking COVID-19 has caused the creation of an industry data dashboard to visualize the expected and actual spread. The best dashboards include HealthMap [31], the New York Times [31], the BBC [32], Thebaselab [33], John's Hopkins' CSSE [34], NextStrain [35] and UpCode [36]. Bing's COVID-19 tracker [36] is also a potential dashboard to help understand the spread of COVID-19 [37]. These dashboards give a global view and the increasing number of COVID-19 attacks. Emerging economies like South Africa have already established their dashboards for the COVID-19. Some use script in Python to illustrate how data can be extracted from the data set of the New York Times for COVID-19 and create a data visualization of infection progression. [38] in a comprehensive review provided a list of COVID-19 datasets and their descriptions as shown in Table 1.

3 Generalized AI Response to COVID-19

Following the knowledge areas explored in Sect. 2, we propose a generalized AI response framework to COVID-19 depicted in Fig. 1.

The framework shows possible application areas of AI to the pandemic and some of their various techniques. The application of AI in proffering solutions usually begins with a dataset hence the creation of various data dashboards is necessary to speed up the researches. While some computer scientists are engaging with the health practitioners in the creation of the dashboard, others are utilizing those resources to explore pharmaceutical cures and treatments, prediction, and social control measures as well as diagnoses to detect the virus.

In each of the areas, possible response activities are outlined. In the Prognosis and Diagnosis knowledge area, five (5) response activities may be employed recursively which includes data collection/collation, class labels identification, determination of the choice variables which is known as features engineering, creating of ML/DL models and detection of COVID using the models. The Fig. 1 shows that each of the response activities are techniques that may be applied iteratively in each of the areas and may overlap in another area. For example, both compartmental epidemic models and DL/ML models and simulations are possible under the prognosis and diagnosis response while contact tracing models, social distance models, and text-based NLP models are possible under the Prediction, Tracking and Social Control response. ML and DL approaches can predict the spread of the disease to help nations overcome the hazards of COVID-19, understand the virus in a better way, and map where it comes from so that policies could be made to contain the effects. In fact, even the prediction of the next pandemic is possible to enable the government plan ahead.

Machine Learning could help to save the lives of people and nations that are suffering from COVID-19 by helping in the identification of a person who is most at risk of COVID-19. It can make the diagnosis of patients and the development of drugs for patients of COVID-19 faster. It has the potentials to indicate existing drugs that can help patients of COVID-19 through the pharmaceutical responses with protein and DNA sequencing. DNA sequencing is a technological method that determines the order of bases in biological and medical researches. This and other response activities like working on the protein structure, and potential drug binding sites [12] are depicted in the Cures and Treatments knowledge area in the Fig. 1.

The essence of the response framework is to give both researchers and practitioners a working guide to what is possible in the quest to finding scientific solutions to the pandemic using the approach of the machine and deep learning techniques. We summarized in Tables 2, 3 and 4 the different approaches of ML and DL and their key findings in some existing researches discussed in this study.

Table 1 List of some COVID-19 datasets

Dataset name	Country/Region	Modality	Attributes
BSTI Imaging Database	United Kingdom	CT scans data	Patient CT scans
COVID CXR Dataset	Italy	CXR and reports	CXR Image, date, patient, demographics, findings, location and survival information
COVID-CT-Dataset	All Countries	Chest CT-scans	Scans with associated labels
COVID-19 CT segmentation dataset	Italy	Lungs CT scans	JPG image scans with segmentation and label report
COVID-19 Community Mobility Reports	131 Countries	Mobility statistics with textual Reports	Presence of people at grocery stores, pharmacies, recreational spots, parks, transit stations, workplaces, and residences
COVID-19 DATABASE	Italy	Radiology data	CXR and demographics
COVID-19 Open Research Challenge	All Countries	Research articles dataset	Published date, author list, journal name, full text
Coronavirus Source Data	All Countries	Case statistics	Time series of confirmed daily COVID-19 cases for countries around the world
Coronavirus COVID19 Tweets	All Countries	Public Tweets on COVID-19	UserID, location, hashtags, tweet text
COVID-19 Korea Dataset	Korea	Case statistics	Patient routes, age, gender, diagnosed date
CHIME	All Countries	Case statistics	Daily number of a susceptible, infected and recovered patient
Global research on COVID-19	All Countries	Database of research articles	Date, location, authors and journal
hCOV-19	All Countries	Genomic epidemiology	Genetic sequence and metadata
JHU CSSE COVID-19 Data	All Countries	Case statistics	Number of infections, number of cured patients, total mortality count, location

(continued)

Table 1 (continued)

Dataset name	Country/Region	Modality	Attributes
Kinsa Smart Thermometer Weather Map	USA	U.S. Health Weather Map	Temperature readings from internet-connected thermometers made by Kinsa Health.
LitCovid	All Countries	Dataset of research articles	Up-to-date research topics and geographic locations
nCoV2019 Dataset	China, Japan, South Korea, Hong Kong, Taiwan, Thailand, Singapore	Epidemiological data	Patient demographics, case reporting date, location, brief history
Novel Corona-virus 2019 dataset	All Countries	Case statistics	Patient demographics, case reporting date, location, brief History
New York Times dataset	USA	State-wise cumulative cases	Date, state name, number of cases, death count
Public Corona-virus Twitter Dataset	All Countries	Tweet IDs	Twitter ID with location
RCSB Protein Data Bank	All Countries	Clinical and pathology	Genomic sequences
RKI COVID19	Germany	Cases data	Number of infection cases

Source Latif et al. [38]

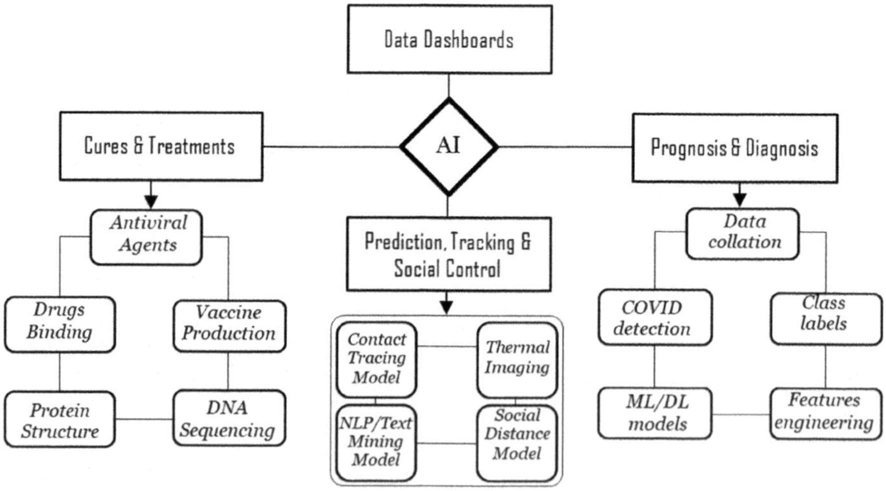

Fig. 1 AI response framework to COVID-19

Table 2 Summary of ML only approaches

S/N	Study	Dataset, classes	Classes	Feature extraction, selection	ML	Key findings
1	[10]	Text	ARDS, COVID-19	Information Gain, Gini Index, and Chi-square statistics	L R, *k*-NN (k = 5), DT, RF and SVM	SVM and k-NN performed best with 80% accuracy on the classification of COVID-19.
2	[26]	CT scan	COVID-19, pneumonia and normal	Deep features: ResNet50, AlexNet, VGG16, VGG19, etc., LBP, HOG, GLCM	SVM	ResNet + SVM obtained the best metric based on accuracy, sensitivity, FPR and F1-score of 95.33%, 95.33%, 2.33% and 95.34% respectively
3	[5]	CT scan	coronavirus /non-coronavirus	GLCM, LDP, GLRLM, GLSZM, and DWT	SVM	Accuracy of 99.68% with the GLSZM.
4	[20]	CXR	Normal, COVID-19, MERS, SARS, Varicella, Streptococcus and Pneumocystis	Sampling: ADASYN, SMOTE, SMOTE-B1/B2, AllKNN, ENN/RENN, TomekLinks, and SMOTE + TL Extraction methods: LBP, EQP, LDN, LETRIST, BSIF, LPQ, oBIFs, and Inception-V3	*k*-NN, SVM, MLP, DT, and RF	Multi-classification: F1-Score of 0.65 with MLP + LBP Hierarchical Classification: F1-Score of 0.89 with clustering + BSIF + EQP +LPQ + SMOTE + TL.

It may be noted that the prevalent ML technology is the SVM while the prevalent DL technology is the ResNet. Again, works that combine both ML and DL approaches, where feature extraction was done using the DL and modeling performed using the ML, used a combination of ResNet and SVM to achieve a highest a highest accuracy.

Table 3 Summary of DL only approaches

S/N	Study	Dataset	Classes	DL	Key findings
1	[24]	CXR	CORDA, CORDA&CXR, CORDA&RSNA, CORDA&COVID-CXR, COVID-CXR	ResNet-18, ResNet-50 and COVID-Net	Resnet 18 + COVID-19 + CXR obtained an accuracy of 100%
2	[15]	CXR	COVID-19, TB, Healthy	VGG-16 on ImageNet dataset	Average COVID-19 detection time was 2.5 s with 97% accuracy
3	[19]	CXR	normal, TB, non-TB, and COVID-19	ResNet 18 (29, 29) COVID-19 (9, 28)	An accuracy of 95%
4	[25]	CXR	COVID-19, normal and SARS	ImageNet and DeTraC on ResNet 18, PCA	DeTraC + ResNet18 achieved the highest Accuracy, Sensitivity and Specificity 95.12%, 97.91% and 91.87% respectively.
5	[16]	CT	COVID-19, CAP, and other non-pneumonia	COVNet	AUC of 0.96
6	[23]	CXR	COVID-19, normal, pneumonia bacterial and pneumonia virus	GAN GoogleNet, AlexNet, ResNet 18	Googlenet achieved an accuracy of 100%

4 Challenges

This section describes some of the challenges faced upon implementation of AI and ML models for the diagnosis and prognosis of COVID-19. The key objective of prediction and classification models is to build a good decision support system for domain experts.

Table 4 Summary of both ML & DL approaches

S/N	Study	Dataset	Classes	Feature extraction	DL	ML	Key findings
1	[21]	CT	COVID-19, pneumonia and healthy lungs	QDE, DF, QDE + DF, LBP, and LBP + DF	LSTM	Linear SVM, k-NN, LR	LSTM + QDE + DF achieved the best accuracy of 99.68%.
2	[22]	CT + Text	COVID-19+ PTB	CNN	CNN	MLP, SVM, RF	The joint model using both clinical data and CT imaging achieved an 84.3% sensitivity, an 82.8% specificity, and 0.92 AUC
3	[3]	Cough sound	COVID-19 likely, COVID-19 not likely and Test inconclusive.	MFCC, PCA	DTL-MC, DTL-BC	SVM	DTL-MC outperform with an accuracy of 92.64%

4.1 Small Data Sample Size

The major cause for the shortage of standard COVID-19 datasets is that the disease is relatively new and exclusion of data over different geographical regions. The deployment of deep learning and machine learning models to classification and prediction of COVID-19 needs vast volume of data. Also, the small sample available could be poorly biases. Consequently, developing models to analyze this small sample size is one of the main challenges in the classification and prediction of COVID-19. Some of solutions suggested is the use of textual descriptors to extract radiomic features from CXR and CTs. Also, obtaining more COVID-19 data will give precise prediction in the number of deaths and infections as most ML and DL models are highly accurate with vast amount of data [39].

4.2 Daily Case of Occurrences

The daily occurrences of COVID-19 incidences are modelled as time series problem. Modeling time series problem is one of the challenges of data mining models techniques [40]. The deployment of ML and DL methods such as LSTM and SVM can model the problem as a multiple time series problem simultaneously and also forecast as multi-step output. ML and DL methods models can forecast the daily occurrences as simultaneous joint model of multiple targets field (cases) simultaneously in order to capture dependencies between them.

4.3 Overlapping of Disease Symptoms

COVID-19 belongs to the family of pneumonia disease which is one of its main complications. The hierarchy of pneumonia infection by different organisms are viruses, bacteria or fungi [41] and COVID-19 cannot be regarded as a single disease or binary classification but rather as a group of different infections with different characteristics [20]. The challenge is that COVID-19 and pneumonia diseases have similar symptoms, hence, overlapping of disease symptoms. This is a class imbalance problem where one class have an extremely high number of sample size than the other class. The problem is compounded when allied with class overlap and disjucts. This problem will cause sub-optimal performance of models for classification [42]. This situation can be alienated using class imbalance schemes to form clear clusters for the classes, hence, improving classification.

4.4 Need for Robust and Effective for COVID-19

Most of the researches conducted were based on COVID-19 and other related pneumonia diseases. The results obtained from these researches may not be accurate as due to some other co morbidity factors such as like age, residency, gender, pulmonary, diabetes, hypotension, kidney and liver diseases. Hence, a symptom-based recognition model for COVID-19 should be developed to improve accuracy. Also, research should also be extended to other parts of the world with the COVID-19 epidemic as recent research is limited to top affected countries [39].

New opportunities can be maximized to facilitate domain expert and individuals in modeling and data analyses like WHO creating an anonymized platform for code and data sharing [43]. To take advantage these evolutions, international and interdisciplinary collaboration in terms of data collection, model building and validation is essential. Also, data registers are being created as more cases are being reported from many regions.

5 Conclusion

This study had discussed recent works that had applied AI towards the control of COVID-19. We found out that most of the works reviewed were done on image classification with CXR images and CTs for prognosis and diagnosis purposes. While the majority of the works used separate ML or DL approaches, a few used a combination of both approaches by extracting and selecting features with ML techniques and building the model with a DL technique. While most of the diagnostic approaches discussed are achieving good results, there is, however, no production-ready solution, and the scientific community is still working assiduously to improve the sensitivity of the AI models. A DL model can be useful in diagnosing COVID-19 from the CXR images or CT scans. The models show comparable performance with expert radiologists and can improve the efficiency of such individuals in clinical practice settings. It has the potential to relieve pressure from frontline radiologists and improve early isolation, diagnosis, and treatment. Therefore, the current level of the diagnostic efforts is already contributing to the control of the COVID-19 pandemic. While it is granted that AI has not yet played a critical role in fighting against COVID-19 from the viewpoints of pharmaceuticals, it is achieving some results in other areas while struggling to solve the constraint of a lack of historical data which may be overcome soon. Following the generalized response framework proposed in this study, researchers and practitioners may be guided on some of the things that are scientifically possible in exploiting AI approaches for the control of COVID-19.

References

1. Jamshidi, M., Lalbakhsh, A., Talla, J., Peroutka, Z., Hadjilooei, F., Lalbakhsh, P.,... Sabet, A.: Artificial intelligence and COVID-19: deep learning approaches for diagnosis and treatment. IEEE Access. **8**, 109581–109595 (2020)
2. Wang, S., Kang, B., Ma, J., Zeng, X., Xiao, M., Guo, J., Cai, M., Yang, J., Li, Y., Meng, X., Xu, B.: A deep learning algorithm using CT images to screen for Corona Virus Disease (COVID-19). MedRxiv (2020)
3. Imran, A., Posokhova, I., Qureshi, H.N., Masood, U., Riaz, S., Ali, K., John, C.N., Hussain, I., Nabeel, M.: AI4COVID-19: AI enabled preliminary diagnosis for COVID-19 from cough samples via an app. Inf. Med. Unlocked (2020)
4. Neri, E., Miele, V., Coppola, F., Grassi, R.: Use of CT and artificial intelligence in suspected or COVID-19 positive patients: statement of the Italian Society of Medical and Interventional Radiology. Radiol. Med. (Torino) **125**(5), 505–508 (2020)
5. Barstugan, M., Ozkaya, U., Ozturk, S.: Coronavirus (COVID-19) Classification using CT Images by Machine Learning Methods, p. 10 (2020)
6. Rodrigues, J.C.L., Hare, S.S., Edey, A., Devaraj, A., Jacob, J., Johnstone, A., ..., Robinson, G.: An update on COVID-19 for the radiologist-A British society of Thoracic Imaging statement. Clin. Radiol. **75**(5), 323–325 (2020)
7. Jin, C., Chen, W., Cao, Y., Xu, Z., Zhang, X., Deng, L., ..., Feng, J.: Development and evaluation of an AI system for COVID-19 Diagnosis. medRxiv (2020)

8. Metsky, H.C., Freije, C.A., Kosoko-Thoroddsen, T.S.F., Sabeti, P.C., Myhrvold, C.: CRISPR-based surveillance for COVID-19 using genomically-comprehensive machine learning design. BioRxiv 2020.02.26.967026 (2020)
9. Apostolopoulos, I.D., Mpesiana, T.A.: Covid-19: automatic detection from x-ray images utilizing transfer learning with convolutional neural networks. Phys. Eng. Sci. Med. **43**, 635–640 (2020)
10. Jiang, X., Coffee, M., Bari, A., Wang, J., Jiang, X., Huang, J., Shi, J., Jianyi, J., Cai, J., Zhang, T., Wu, Z., He, G., Huang, Y.: Towards an artificial intelligence framework for data-driven prediction of coronavirus clinical severity. Comput. Mater. Continua **63**(1), 537–551 (2020)
11. Rahmatizadeh, S., Valizadeh-Haghi, S., Dabbagh, A.: The role of artificial intelligence in management of critical COVID-19 patients. J. Cell. Mol. Anesthesia **1**, 16–22 (2020)
12. Alimadadi, A., Aryal, S., Manandhar, I., Munroe, P.B., Joe, B., Cheng, X.: Artificial intelligence and machine learning to fight COVID-19. Physiol. Genom. **52**(4), 200–202 (2020)
13. Jiang, Y., Wen, J.: Effects of COVID-19 on hotel marketing and management: a perspective article. Effects COVI Int. J. Contemp. Hosp. Manag. **32**(8), 2563–2573 (2020)
14. Yang, Z., Zeng, Z., Wang, K., Wong, S.S., Liang, W., Zanin, M., Liu, P., Cao, X., Gao, Z., Mai, Z., Liang, J.: Modified SEIR and AI prediction of the trend of the epidemic of COVID-19 in China under public health interventions. J. Thoracic Dis. **12**(3), 165 (2020)
15. Brunese, L., Mercaldo, F., Reginelli, A., Santone, A.: Explainable deep learning for pulmonary disease and coronavirus COVID-19 detection from X-rays. Comput. Methods Progr. Biomed. **196**(105608), 1–11 (2020)
16. Li, L., Qin, L., Xu, Z., Yin, Y., Wang, X., Kong, B., Bai, J., Lu, Y., Fang, Z., Song, Q., Cao, K., Daliang Liu, D., Wang, G., Xu, Q., Fang, X., Zhang, S., Xia, J., Xia, J.: Using artificial intelligence to detect COVID-19 and community-acquired pneumonia based on pulmonary CT: evaluation of the diagnostic accuracy. Radiology **296**(2), 65–72 (2020)
17. Zheng, N., Du, S., Wang, J., Zhang, H., Cui, W., Kang, Z., …, Ma, M.: Predicting COVID-19 in china using a hybrid AI model. IEEE Trans. Cybern. **50**(7), 2891–2904 (2020)
18. Alwashmi, M.F.: The use of digital health in the detection and management of COVID-19. Int. J. Environ. Res. Public Health **17**(8), 2906 (2020)
19. Yoo, S.H., Geng, H., Chiu, T.L., Yu, S.K., Cho, D.C., Heo, J., Choi, M.S., Choi, I.H., Van, C.C., Nhung, N.V., Min, B.J., Lee, H.: Deep learning-based decision-tree classifier for COVID-19 diagnosis from chest X-ray imaging. Front. Med. **7**(427), 1–8 (2020)
20. Pereira, R.M., Bertolini, D., Teixeira, L.O., Silla Jr., C.N., Costa, Y.M.G.: COVID-19 identification in chest X-ray images on flat and hierarchical classification scenarios. Comput. Methods Progr. Biomed. **194**, (2020)
21. Hasan, A.M., AL-Jawad, M.M., Jalab, H.A., Shaiba, H., Ibrahim, R.W., AL-Shamasneh, A.R.: Classification of Covid-19 coronavirus, pneumonia and healthy lungs in CT scans using Q-deformed entropy and deep learning features. Entropy, 517 (2020)
22. Mei, X., Lee, H., Diao, K., Huang, M., Lin, B., Liu, C., Xie, Z., Ma, Y., Robson, P.M., Chung, M., Bernheim, A., Mani, V., Calcagno, C., Li, K., Li, S., Shan, H., Lv, J., Zhao, T., Xia, J., Long, Q., Steinberger, S., Jacobi, A., Deyer, T., …, Yang, Y.: Artificial intelligence-enabled rapid diagnosis of patients with COVID-19. Nat. Med.: Lett. (2020)
23. Loey, M., Smarandache, F., Khalifa, N.E.M.: Within the lack of chest COVID-19 X-ray dataset: a novel detection model based on GAN and deep transfer learning. Symmetry **12**, 651 (2020)
24. Tartaglione, E., Barbano, C.A., Berzoviniy, C., Calandri, M., Grangetto, M.: Unveiling COVID-19 from Chest X-ray with deep learning: a hurdles race with small data. arXiv:2004.05405v1 [eess.IV] 11 Apr 2020 (2020)
25. Abbas, A., Abdelsamea, M.M., Gaber, M.M.: Classification of COVID-19 in chest X-ray images using DeTraC deep convolutional neural network. MedRxiv, pp. 1–14 (2020)
26. Sethy, P.K., Behera, S.K., Ratha, P.K., Biswas, P.: Detection of coronavirus disease (COVID-19) based on deep features and support vector machine and support vector machine. Int. J. Math. Eng. Manag. Sci. **5**(4), 643–651 (2020)
27. https://github.com/ieee8023/covid-chestxray-dataset [Online]
28. https://www.kaggle.com/andrewmvd/convid19-X-rays [Online]

29. Kermany, D.S., Goldbaum, M., Cai, W., Valentim, C.C., Liang, H., Baxter, S.L., Dong, J.: Identifying medical diagnoses and treatable diseases by image-based deep learning. Cell **172**(5), 1122–1131 (2018)
30. https://www.sirm.org/ [Online]
31. https://www.bbc.co.uk/news/resources/idt-4a11d568-2716-41cf-a15e-7d15079548bc [Online]
32. "https://www.bbc.co.uk/news/resources/idt-4a11d568-2716-41cf-a15e-7d15079548bc [Online]
33. https://coronavirus.thebaselab.com/ [Online]
34. https://coronavirus.jhu.edu/map.html [Online]
35. https://nextstrain.org/help/coronavirus/SARS-CoV-2 [Online]
36. https://co.vid19.sg/singapore/ [Online]
37. Ting, D.S.W., Carin, L., Dzau, V., Wong, T.Y.: Digital technology and COVID-19. Nat. Med. **26**(4), 459–461 (2020)
38. Latif, S., Usman, M., Manzoor, S., Iqbal, W., Qadir, J., Tyson, G., Castro, I., Razi, A., Boulos, M.N.K., Weller, A., Crowcroft, J.: Leveraging data science to combat COVID-19: A comprehensive review. Techrxiv (2020)
39. Swapnarekha, H., Behera, H.S., Nayak, J., Naik, B.: Role of intelligent computing in COVID-19 prognosis: A state-of-the-art review. Chaos, Solit. Fract. **138**, 109947 (2020)
40. Yang, Q., Wu, X.: Challenging Problems in Data mining. Int. J. Inf. Technol. Decis. Making **5**(4), 597–604 (2005)
41. Mackenzie, G.: The definition and classification of pneumonia. Pneumonia **8**(1), 14 (2016)
42. Fitkov-Norris, E., Folorunso, S.O.: Impact of sampling on neural network classification performance in the context of repeat movie viewing. In: Proceedings of Engineering Applications of Neural Networks (EANN 2013), Greece (2013)
43. W.H. Organization: Coronavirus disease (COVID-19) technical guidance: early investigations protocols. https://www.who.int/emergencies/diseases/ novel-coronavirus-2019/technical-guidance/early-investigations

Optimization of the International Trade Activities in the Period of COVID-19 by Proposing an Algorithm

Ouail El Imrani, Monsif Ben Messaoud Layti, Salmane Bourekkadi, Abdelhamid Boulaksili, and Issam Kabbassi

Abstract It is crucial to realize that maximizing transactions in international trade is necessary to allow people in a quarantine situation to establish an irregular pattern of behavior, particularly for international trade firms. This was par-ticularly the case when foreign trading activities were drastically reduced. In-stant tchnological access and management of knowledge eliminates distance miles, in an world where knowledge 's value and its regulation are which very intersting. However, in developing countries, especially in developing countries, these devices are not at the detriment of customers, but are often lacking in poli-cies. This article includes details on the position of the organization in the field of internal exchange in quarantine health (COVID19), and may con-tribute to develope knowledge and technologies.

Keywords Coronavirus · International trade · Intelligent system · Optimization

1 Introduction

The Covid-19 crisis will have a significant and lasting impact on international trade, of which we still have difficulty drawing the lines and the measurement if it is too early to assess the real impact of the various processes currently taking place, Knowing that researchers are trying to identify what could be the short and long term consequences of the pandemic on international trade. But the most important thing is that international trade is also one of the potential victims of the pandemic following the different scenarios of the future of commercial transactions around the world, we can highlight the reading grid that seems to be draw on the ground. To

O. El Imrani (✉) · M. Ben Messaoud Layti · A. Boulaksili
Abdelmalek Essaadi University, Tetouan, Morocco
e-mail: oelimrani@uae.ac.ma

S. Bourekkadi
Poitiers University, Poitiers, France

S. Bourekkadi · I. Kabbassi
Ibn Tofail University, Kenitra, Morocco

D. Oliva et al. (eds.), *Artificial Intelligence for COVID-19*, Studies in Systems, Decision and Control 358, https://doi.org/10.1007/978-3-030-69744-0_11

this end, we will attempt in this manuscript to propose an algorithm that will allow the optimization of trade transactions between countries in order to maximize wealth creation.

2 Application Model in International Exchange for the Proper Management of the COVID-19 Containment Period

Technically speaking, researchers and experts expect to see a global recession in 2020 that could take a severe form for some countries or regions. In this context, we should remember that JP Morgan Research forecasts a contraction in GDP over two quarters in the United States, ranging between -10% and -25%, and for the euro zone, between -15% and -22%. That means the world is expecting a huge drop in all economic indicators. Our goal of this article is to minimize the fallout from this crisis using a digital tool based on an algorithm.

The two connections that we research can be defined as follows:

- A core of services of foreign markets collects from the resources of the firms of the world of trading (upstream of the return chain) to deliver them downstream to the centers of the manufacturing industries. This foreign trades service center has to manage the gathered and sorted stocks, and the processing operations but with the lowest cost;
- A distribution hub for products from the core of retail services, breaks down such items into parts, and transfers them to the collaborator businesses of development, according to the expiration date. It handles inventories of materials and parts, as well as transport activities.

The characteristics of both connections are identical, which is why our issue can be examined with a single standardized prototype in linear programming.

Our study focusses on the implementation of a successful Covid-19 pandemic period management application in the international commercial sector, which in turn would involve a temporal multi-period model.

Generally speaking, while efforts are being made to minimize vagueness and the various risks, there is still some ambiguity. Thus, one of the major challenges of foreign exchange is the form of incoming goods.

3 Principle of Operation of the Optimization Model in International Trade

The theory of activity of our model of optimization within the foreign commercial market, which refers to the two links in the global chain of commerce, involves the phase from reception to distribution to the customers that can be described as a collection of activities that turn incoming products into outgoing goods. More broadly, the flows over a connection of the foreign chain come from the procurement of incoming products, by incoming storage, outgoing stockpiling, and transportation. Reason for which each production corporation would match offerings from all foreign trade service providers and cost-effective transport methods.

3.1 *Taking Quality into Account in Flows*

The selection of a broad range of goods is in International trade mainly depends on:

- Their nature: connections to various goods, such as in household appliances with washing machines, dish-washers, refrigerators of different brands;
- Their quality: the collected items come in various states, varying from fresh to unused.

Regarding the nature of the products, in a given sector, it is rather easy to relist the current sources. This will be in line with the notion of our modeling.

But it is difficult, if not impossible, to estimate the level of quality of the collected items. This is why there is confusion. We also defined a small number of possible attributes in our modelling. For every modeled connection, we identified 4 potential outgoing flows: return to the chain of direct trade foreign, continuation of that of reverse trade internationally, re-direction to a secondary market and evacuation to the removal hub. Of course, we then described four types of stages, alluded to before (A, B, C, and D).

It should be remembered that product quality assessment needs human intervention:

- For the international trade Benefits connection, the level of quality is calculated when sort by a specialist who assesses the condition of the product;
- For the transport link, the quality level of each part is determined immediately after the transport operation.

With respect to outgoing flow, preferably, of commodity of a given quality should be sent to the appropriate destination: for example, a level A product is usually intended for a connection of the foreign direct trade depending on the need of the providers. However, the distribution of goods does not generally lead to demands from these users. If the demand is too poor, it is therefore appropriate to store the outgoing items, due to getting the room sufficient to store them in good shape. If the de-making is too big, the relation doesn't have enough goods of the appropriate standard of consistency, it then seems stock breaks; these are also also repercussed by the corresponding costs for delay of delivery.

To promote the handling of outflows, multiple strategies are necessary to satisfy demands for goods or replacement parts or supplies. We also developed two alternative strategies, which are outlined in the following two pages.

3.2 Deterministic Model—Wait and See (WS)

In this section, we offer a description of the problems of foreign exchange and planning facilities optimization. It should be remembered that this is similar to the preparation of the two ties examined. We begin by adding indices, parameters and variables used in mathematical models in a standardized manner. This concept models are built in linear programming.

4 The Application's Algorithm for Optimizing the Operations of International Trade Companies

4.1 The Algorithm

The algorithm explains the Optimization mechanism between the outputs of foreign exchange of firms be it for the acquisition, production, delivery … etc. In the first position it is important to determine the need for products from the entry to the network one sees two buttons; first one is dedicated to the processing of the knowledge of internal business, second is destination.

The above algorithm clearly defines all options directly to companies with foreign trades; hence, after the identification with needs the customer can chose the products from a list of selects, then it moves to the entering of the sum desired then it moves to the check in the inventory of the entities that have this products. After this phase we go through filtering in order to get the best results in order to move to the stage of transport of the products. The optimum search outcome is shown at the browser in-sequence (depending upon the length or the expense of distribution of goods) (Fig. 1).

4.2 Discussion and Interpretation

In order to allow companies impacted by Covid-19 to establish a trend of irregular behavior, it could be conceivable that the optimization of foreign trade operations through an integrated framework is essential in order to improve their performance. Instant access and management of information via telecommunications reduce kilometers traveled in a world of increasing data power. New ICT innovations play an important role in socio-economic transitions across the world, from rich countries to less developing countries. Optimization of international trade activity through in-depth application encompasses all technologies used for sending and storing information, including computers, internet and telecommunications. The response from the ICT industry during COVID19 was good. Telecommunications companies around the world are working to promote the use of their networks. Much software can be

```
Si(stock==0)
  Ecrire ("Veuillez choisir votre  marchandise ") ;
  Ecrire ("Veuillez entrer votre quantité") ;
  Lire (quantité_marchandise)
    Pour i allant de 0 jusqu'à nombre_entreprises prestatires de
    l'international trade faire
       si(l'entreprise possède la marchandise)
         tab[i] = {id_entreprises prestatires polistique, nomn
         adresse,quantité disponibles}
       FinSis
    Finpour
      Pour i allant de 0 jusqu'à tab.sizeof faire
       Si (tab[i].demande = of_entreprises prestataires de
       l'international trade_D && credit=0)
         tab[k] = tab[i]
       sinon si (tab[i].demande > of_entreprises prestataires de
       l'international trade_D)
         tab[k] = tab[i] ;
         credit= tab[i].demande - of_entreprises prestataires de
         l'international trade _D
       FinSis

    Finpour
      Pour i allant de0 jusqu'à tab.sizezeof Faire
       Si (tab[i].delais > tab[i+1].delais
         tab[i]=tab_temps ;
         tab[i]= tab[i+1] ;
         tab[i+1]=tab_temps;
    Finpour
      Pour I allant de 0 jusqu'à tab.sizeof Faire
       Si(tab[i].Demande= OF_entreprises prestatires de l'international
       trade_D && dredit=0)
         tab[k]= tab[i] ;
       sinon si(tab[i].Demande > OF_entreprises prestataires de
       l'international trade_D)
         tab[k]= tab[i] ;
         credit= tab[i].Demande - OF_ entreprises prestataires de
         l'international trade_D)
       FinSis
    Finpour
       Choisir le meilleur choix des offres des entreprises prestatires
       de l'international trade
      Selon c=(choix) Faire
       Envoi de demande des marchandises à l'entreprises prestatire de
       l'international trade concernée
      Finselon
     FinSis
```

Fig. 1 Optimization algorithm for international trade companies distributed or modified for free, consumers can defer billing, defer charges for mobile small funds transactions, and increase or remove bandwidth limits.

5 Conclusion

To summarize and conclude this research work, we can say that in evaluating the output of international trading firms in the pandemic period, development of conditions must be as similar as practicable. We also recommend that the design should be implemented in development mode. For example, a production mode program will profit from optimizing processes in the development setting. Based on the needs of the firms in the foreign trading, this program helps to modulate optimum strategies in order to minimize manufacturing costs as well as to maximize the overall capital of the business. What is crucial is to consider what foreign trading companies can use as the basis for generating the highest benefit-added value with the least amount of capital. At least data from three foreign trading firms can be used to perform appropriate research.

References

1. Bourekkadi, S., E.L. Imrani, O., Kandili, M.E.L., Slimani, K., Khoulji, S., Babounia, A.: Intelligent solution based on information technologies - The correct value of the business in economic organization is intangible asset. In: Proceedings of the 33rd International Business Information Management Association Conference, IBIMA 2019: Education Excellence and Innovation Management through Vision 2020, pp. 6310–6317. Abd El-nasser Said, G.A., Mahmoud, A.M., El-horbaty, E.M. (no date) solving container terminals problems using computer-based modeling, Ain Shams University (2019)
2. Handiwibowo, G.A., Nasution, A.H., Kusuma Arumsari, Y., Puji Astuti, R.: Strategic fit implication of technological innovation capabilities for SMEs with new product development. Manag. Sci. Lett. **10**, 2875–2882 (2020). Growing Science
3. Elferjani, A.: Examination of port performance in a developing economy: a case study of Libyan ports. RMIT University (2015)
4. Akyeampong, E.K., Gates, H.l.: Dictionary of African Biography. Oxford University Press (2012)
5. Layti, M.B.M., El Imrani, O., Medouri, A., Rajaa, M.: logistics information systems and traceability of pharmaceutical products in public hospitals in Morocco: what solutions to improve the supply chain? In International Conference on Advanced Intelligent Systems for Sustainable Development (pp. 429–438). Springer, Cham (2019)
6. Alphaliner: Alphaliner - Top 100 : Operated fleets as per 12 October 2010, Alphaliner-TOP 100 (2017)
7. Ambrosino, D., Tànfani, E.: An integrated simulation and optimization approach for seaside terminal operations. In: Proceedings 26th European Conference on Modelling and Simulation (2012)
8. Caldeirinha, V., Felício, J.A., Dionísio, A.: Effect of the container terminal characteristics on performance, pp. 1–17. Évora University (UÉ) CEFAGE-UE, CEFAGE-UÉ (2013)

9. Anderson, R.E.: Implications of the information and knowledge society for education. In: dans Joke Voogt et Gerald Knezek (dir.) International Handbook of Information Technology in Primary and Secondary Education, vol. 20. Springer, Boston, MA, pp. 5–22 (2008)
10. Rajasekar, S., Philominathan, P., Chinnathambi, V.: Research Methodology. Methods, p. 23 (2006)
11. Rochon, J., Gondan, M., Kieser, M.: To test or not to test: preliminary assessment of normality when comparing two independent samples. BMC Med. Res. Methodol. **12**(1), 81 (2012)
12. Bourekkadi, S., Slimani, K., El Imrani, O., Ezzaki, M., Babounia, A., Fakhri, Y.: Toward increasing and investigating e-tourism data warehouse through a websites analysis strategy. J. Theoret. Appl. Inf. Technol. **98**(19), 3222–3232 (2020)

Internet of Things (IoT) and Real Time Applications

V. Nandalal and V. Anand Kumar

Abstract The IoT (Internet of Things) is the internet functioning of substantial machine, vehicles and other stuffs which consists of an embedded system with sensors, actuators and network connectivity that enable to collect and exchange data. Now all focus on body-centric communication technology, which integrates antennas and radio frequency (RF) systems (0.5–12 GHz) into clothes. These systems are developed with regard to size reduction, ease of integration and cost effectiveness as in COVID 19 situations. Body-centric applications are mainly focused in promoting personal communications, keeping track of body parameters like temperature, heart-beat, etc. and also to monitor people. Among several body-centric applications, monitoring people has become very popular wherein monitoring and protecting mentally challenged people has got a spot light. Our society is in need of monitoring mentally challenged especially the females and the children from becoming a victim of trafficking, as in these days trafficking has grown to a greater extent. At present COVID 19 situations without visiting the hospital, doctors can able to trace the medical record of the patients by connecting with wearable devices such as pulse oximeter which can be connected through IoT. At the point when issues with social significance are being tended to, the arrangements/frameworks produced for those issues must be moderate. Subsequently the need of great importance is to build up an IoT based streamlined body-driven wearable reception apparatus to screen and shield the simple-minded and ensure them if there should be an occurrence of crises like military dangerous tasks, woman trafficking and so forth, so as to encourage the continuous following of radio wire an IoT based wearable Antenna module has been fused.

Keywords IoT · RF · Body-centric wearable antenna · Wearable communication

---

V. Nandalal (✉)
Department of Electronics and Communication Engineering, Sri Krishna College of Engineering and Technology, Coimbatore, Tamilnadu, India
e-mail: nandalalskcet@gmail.com

V. Anand Kumar
Department of Electronics and Communication Engineering, Sri Eshwar College of Engineering and Technology, Coimbatore, Tamilnadu, India
e-mail: anand.kkr@gmail.com

D. Oliva et al. (eds.), *Artificial Intelligence for COVID-19*, Studies in Systems, Decision and Control 358, https://doi.org/10.1007/978-3-030-69744-0_12

1 Introduction and Key Discoveries

A recent trend in communication systems is to stay connected anywhere and at any time. The Internet of Things (IoT) enables new means of communication between people, things and the environment. The name Internet of Things that as of in recent time makes scorching individuals in business, scientists, designers and learners. The name that non-innovation related individuals consider as sort of enchantment and even threat to their security. The name that the EU set as one of the developing advancements and investigators gauge the overall market is relied upon to hit well more than 500 billion US dollars in 2022.

Let us roll back to 1970 s first. In 1973 the first Radio Frequency Identification (RFID) device was patented. This device, even if does not look nor reminds modern IoT devices, was the key enabling technology. The low power (actually here passive) solution with remote antenna large enough to collect energy from the electromagnetic field and power the device brought an idea of unique identifiable items. That somehow mimics well known EAN barcodes and their evolution we use nowadays like QR codes, but here every single thing has a different identity, while EAN barcodes present class of products, not an individual one. The possibility to identify a unique identity remotely became a fundamental of the IoT as we know today. Please note RFID is not the only technology standing behind IoT. In 1990's, rapid expansion of wireless networks, including broadband solutions like cellular-based transfers with its consequent generations brought the possibility to connect devices located in various, even distant geographical locations. Paralelly we encountered an exponential increment in the quantity of gadgets associated with the worldwide, Internet organize, including the Smartphone unrest that began around the mid of the main decade of the XXI century. On the equipment level, microchips and processors turned out to be truly littler and more vitality productive yet offering developing figuring capacities and memory size increment, alongside noteworthy value drops. Each one of those realities drove the presence of little, arranges situated, modest and vitality productive electronic gadgets.

Expression "IoT (Internet of Things)" has been utilized without precedent for 1999 by Kevin Ashton—a specialist on computerized advancement. Officially IoT was presented by the International Telecommunication Union (ITU) in the ITU Internet report in 2005 [14].

It speaks to an essential idea portraying the capacity of a few gadgets in a system to detect and gather information from various articles and afterward share the equivalent over the world through the web without human cooperation. The standard considering the web is including gadgets like PCs and mobiles that individuals are used for trading data among themselves. In any case, in real, web is not any more a human collaboration required stage. Today it has become a system where gadgets detect and speak with one another by gathering and communicating signals without human association. This is what is known as the "Internet of things". All such gadgets can't be straightforwardly called as the web of gadgets like the PC or the cell phones, henceforth the expression "Internet of Things" came.

Things in IoT are the devices that are part of the connected network. It may be a wearable health belt, an internet controlled door or an internet operated automatic train. The things in the internet of things gather data and then interpret it to make our live function better. But the actual things in IoT are present in the business sectors. These devices make the businesses run even smarter and more efficient. IoT offers tremendous potential for associations to change producing measures, business development and even the urban areas where individuals live. As the measure of information that associations approach increments, so too does the capacity to create experiences and see how to improve business productivity.

However, while IoT brings these and a lot more advantages, organizations should likewise know about the cyber security goals. Dangers can incorporate blackout of administrations, information misfortune administrative in compliance, reputational and direct money related misfortune. These give difficulties to organizations that may not yet have set up devoted IoT security arrangements, or battle with IT security financial plans. IoT security must be guaranteed at all levels: item advancement, client usage, and guideline. The advancement of secure IoT gadgets can be done based on secure activity frameworks and stages, and IoT-explicit security capacities ought to be actualized in the old style security answers for IT and telecom frameworks. There are as of now industry practices of creating IoT security proposals dependent on danger evaluations, and they should be upheld by the network and governments.

1. The utilization of IoT is now broad over a scope of business ventures: 61% of associations are presently utilizing IoT stages in their business.
2. IoT use is considerably higher in the IT and telecoms industry (71%) and fund (68%)
3. The developing pace of IoT expands the business requirement for information assurance and anticipation from digital occurrences.
4. Almost three-in-ten (28%) organizations utilizing IoT stages experienced occurrences including non figuring associated gadgets in the most recent year.
5. The unwavering quality of suppliers is no less significant, with in excess of a third (36%) of organizations giving outsiders admittance to their IoT stages.

The job of IoT in business has developed quickly as of late. Today, IoT frameworks can be utilized to acquaint cost decrease and reserve funds with organizations, just as open new income streams and make creation measures more straightforward.

As per a review, 61% of associations right now use IoT stages as business applications. Truth be told, there are really a few businesses where their utilization of IoT is much higher: 71% of those in the IT and telecoms industry use IoT, while 68% of those in the fund world go with the same pattern. Then, at utility and force of organizations (66%).

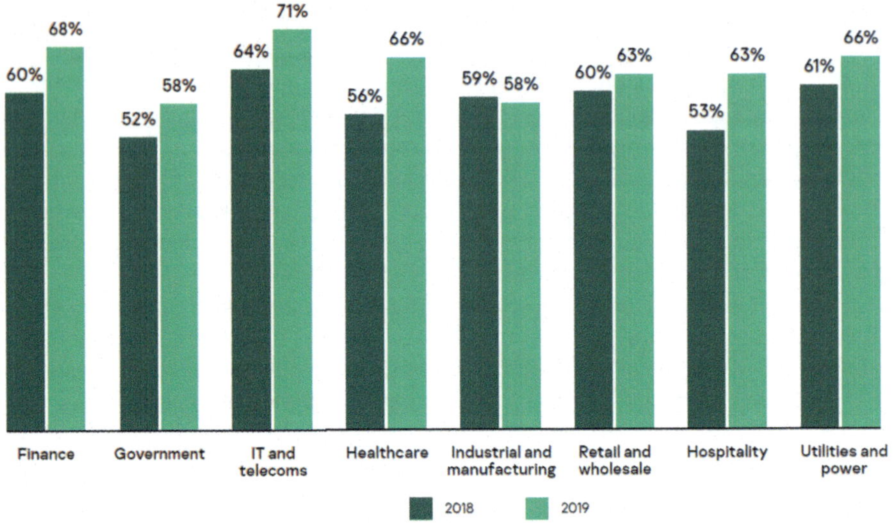

Fig. 1 What industries IoT platforms are used—year-on-year split [21]

1.1 *Year-on-Year Utilization of IoT Stages by Industry*

Prominently, all out IoT spending is set to reach \$1.1 trillion by 2025, bouncing by an enormous 567%, up from \$166 in 2016, as indicated by gauges from the GSMA and IDC. This noteworthy development is likely because of the more extensive degrees of utilization of IoT across business, industry and parts, for example, city arranging. Actually, we are as of now beginning to see IoT utilized for associated transportation, mechanical mechanization, the car business, the more extensive arrangement of smart city activities and initiatives (Fig. 1).

1.2 *IoT Safekeeping and Information Secrecy*

There are two ways to deal with the assurance of the idea of "data security":

1. **Data security**—the status of the wellbeing of data assets and the insurance of the authentic privileges of the character and society in the data circle.
2. **Data security** is a cycle of help for privacy, trustworthiness and openness of data.

Privacy: Ensuring admittance to data just to approved clients.

Trustworthiness: Support of unwavering quality and culmination of data and preparing techniques.

Availability: Ensuring admittance to data and related resources of approved clients as required.

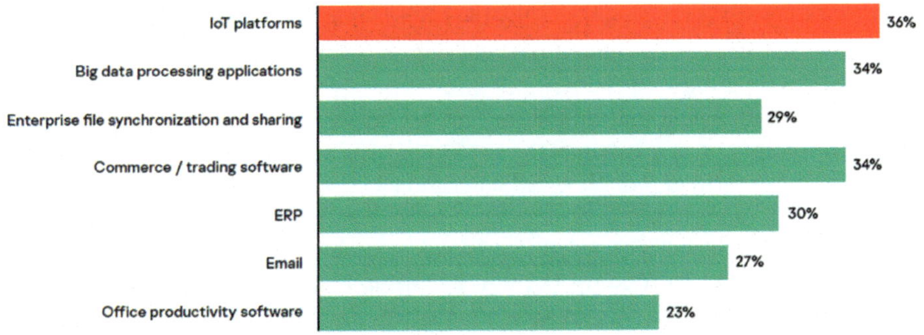

Fig. 2 What business applications are gotten to by outsiders [21]

As a result of their associated nature, IoT frameworks include numerous segments which sellers and outsiders may need to get to. For instance, in keen city ventures, frameworks, for example, traffic signals, CCTV and even utility supplies to residence, store a wide range of kinds of individual client information. Thusly, it's significant that the smart frame worked system is designed and secured to guarantee this information can't be unlawfully gotten to access.

As per an examination, 36% of organizations concede that outsiders approach their IoT stages. This is higher than for some different components of business framework, for example, office efficiency programming (23%), email (27%) or Enterprise Resource Planning (ERP; 30%) (Fig. 2).

Just as guaranteeing the dependability of outsiders who approach IoT frameworks, it is significant for associations to consider the security of these gadgets. This is featured by the 28% of organizations utilizing IoT stages who expressed that they encountered occurrences including noncompeting associated gadgets in the most recent year. This is higher than those influenced by crypto-mining assaults (26%), episodes including information sharing providers (27%) and framework occurrences including outsiders (27%). Given their associated nature, IoT stages join a wide range of gadgets on one system, every one of which can turn into a section point for an assault, causing the general assault surface to enlarge. Accordingly, it is significant for organizations and IT security experts to consider the difficulties and worries that may emerge with IoT execution, as spread out in the following area of this report.

The properties given above are central bases in the circle of insurance and security of data. Wellbeing of data—a status of the security of information on account of which their secrecy, openness and uprightness are given. Security of data is characterized by nonattendance of the unsatisfactory hazard associated with data spillage on specialized channels, unapproved and incidental effects on information or potentially on different assets of a mechanized data framework utilized in the automated system.

It is important to comprehend the estimation of three significant ideas plainly: hazard, danger and weakness.

The danger of data security—likelihood that this danger will have the option to utilize the weakness of a benefit or gathering of advantages and by that will make harm the association.

The danger is a potential or genuine threat of creation of any demonstration (activities or dormancy) guided against the subject to assurance (data assets) making harm the proprietor or client, which is indicated it is at risk for bending and misfortunes of data.

Weakness is an inadequacy; the mistake in usage which does conceivably the unanticipated effect on framework pulling in disappointments in framework activity is all the more regularly. Weaknesses are characterized by a lot of signs. One of the most significant signs—hurt which can be brought about by the framework, utilizing weakness. Regularly comprehend the particular misstep put forth in defense of plan or coding of the framework as a weakness.

In 2016 there was a column of occurrences which pulled in distinct fascination for the wellbeing of IoT. Among them, there were record DDoS-assaults against the French facilitating supplier OVH and Dyn DNS supplier of the USA. It is realized that these assaults are propelled utilizing the gigantic botnet comprising of switches, IP cameras, printers and different gadgets (Fig. 3).

"Significantly all the more upsetting is the way that among all IP addresses from which there were assaults there were some which put observing frameworks and additionally gadget administrations with corporate and defensive issues",—scientists state [15, 16].

Gadgets available to be purchased in outlets, cafés and corner stores have a place with analyzable; frameworks of advanced TV broadcasting; frameworks of physical security and observing of access; and gadgets of checking of the earth.

Analysts additionally discovered vindictive programming tainting a checking framework at the seismic station in Bangkok and furthermore mechanical programmable microcontrollers and the executive's frameworks a gracefully in different spots.

In lures, the assaults from China, Vietnam, Russia, Brazil and Turkey are found.

"The expanding number of the malevolent applications proposed for IoT gadgets and the related episodes of wellbeing shows genuine security of brilliant gadgets. 2016 I indicated that these dangers not exclusively are calculated yet in addition are genuine",—scientists state. "The current rivalry in the market of DDoS actuates cybercriminals to search for new assets for beginning of an ever increasing number of incredible assaults" (Fig. 4).

2 Malware Recognition Methods

For identification of the distorted conduct occurring in the current versatile condition (vindictive programming, an infection, a worm, and so forth.) were executed recognition based on marks, location based on conduct and discovery based on the

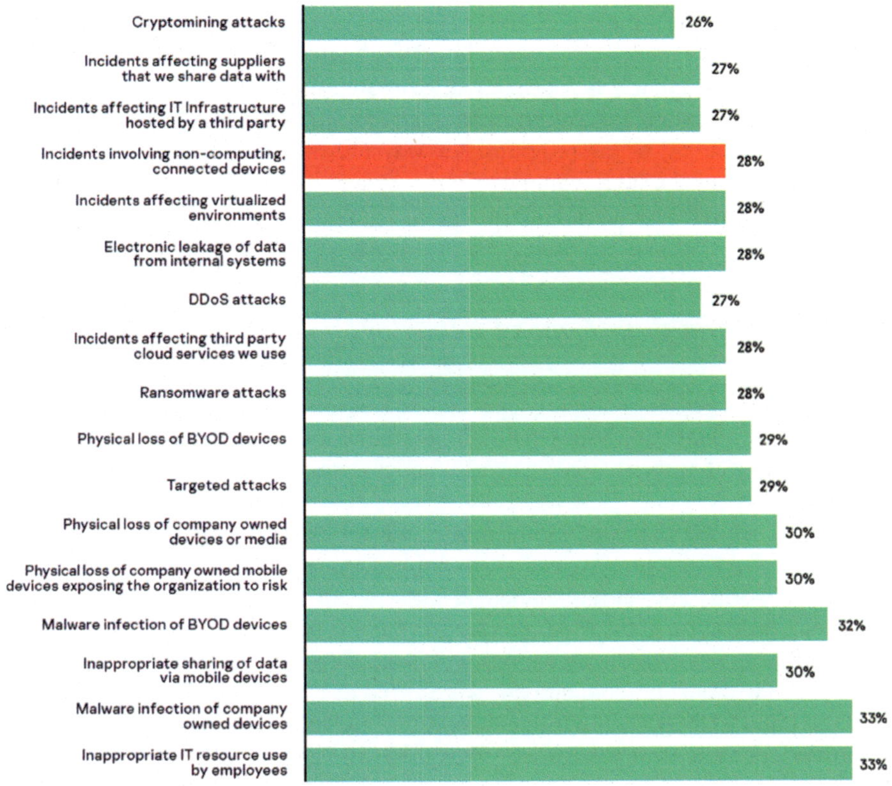

Fig. 3 What episodes are experienced by associations utilizing IoT stages [21]

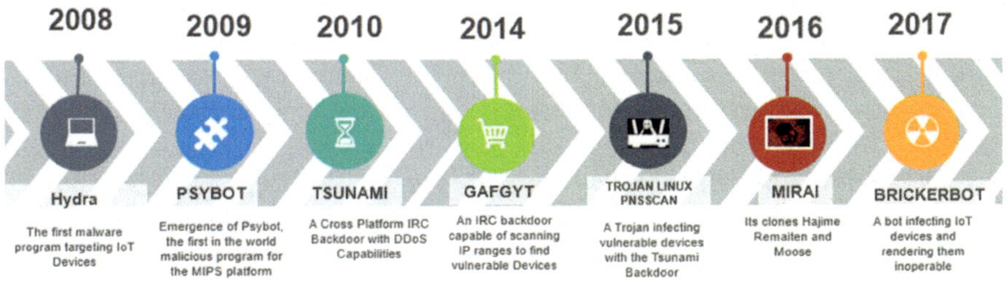

Fig. 4 Timeline of the most eminent malware for IoT

investigation. Inclinations of explores are summed up in the table underneath based on their techniques for recognition and gathered information.

Identification based on marks is the customary technique utilized for recognition of malevolent programming in the earth of the PC. For the assurance of the mark static and dynamic techniques are simultaneously utilized. Static examination is focused on a code of a source and an article and dissects codes without the real beginning of the program. It decompiles the source code of malevolent programming for identification of the weaknesses emerging in orders, directions, and so on (Table 1).

Dynamic investigation is a technique for search of specific layouts in memory release, a traffic stream and an information stream if there should be an occurrence of the real beginning of the program. Anyway use of this strategy to the portable condition requires the huge volume of memory and administration information on profitability is high for consistence of layouts [17].

2.1 IoT Precautions Code of Behaviors

As it was at that point consistently checked, IoT develops before the eyes, and along with it and the quantity of issues in the circle of security. For help of last, the complex of conventions of security is consistently fundamental for the help of due assurance of IoT gadgets.

The IoT conventions will assume a fundamental job in the total limited usage of innovation. They structure a reason for an information stream among sensors and the rest of the world. They are fundamental likewise for powerful framework activity and handy utilization of the MAC convention and the fitting steering convention. For various areas a few MAC conventions with access designs, accessible to the client, to TDMA (without the contentions) were offered, to CSMA (a low presentation of traffic) and FDMA (without the contentions, however requires extra outlines in hubs). Any of them isn't acknowledged as the norm, and with an enormous number of accessible gadgets search of a technique for uniform working of all gadgets will be increasingly more dangerous that obviously will request further investigates [18].

There are some undeniable things which can be made for joining of wellbeing into IoT: the most clear is backing of the web interface of the gadget. Basic things, for example, watch that names of clients and passwords were naturally changed during starting arrangement particularly help. What's more, changes will not permit employments of powerless passwords. Maybe, it is important to consider such measures as the lock of the bookkeeping passage after three-five unsuccessful endeavors of login. Consideration will be paid to passwords outside unique changes of settings. Check of system traffic to help on the way that codes of information don't go to clear content is a sensible advance, and it likewise has a place with any outlines of recuperation of the secret phrase. Plus, for touchy zones, for example, bookkeeping passages of the director; two-factor confirmation can be required [19].

2.2 Confidentiality in IoT

Control can be lost on the off chance that somebody hacks into the PDA or PC going about as a distant for different gadgets. On account of PCs and advanced mobile phones, this hacking should be possible distantly and frequently undetected.

Table 1 Malware recognition methods

Detection technique	Collected data	Description
Signature Based Technique	**Executable File Analysis**	Uses the readelf command to carry out static analysis on executable files using system calls
	Source Code Analysis	Uses the Android sandbox to carry out static/dynamic analysis on applications
	Packet Analysis	Uses functions such as packet-preprocessing and pattern matching to detect malware
	API Call History	Collects system events of upper layers and monitors their API calls to detect malware
Behavior Based Technique	**System Log Data**	Distinguishes inconsistencies as far as Linux pieces and screens traffic, part framework calls, and record framework log information by clients
	SMS, Bluetooth	Lightweight operators working in PDAs record administration exercises, for example, utilization of SMS or Bluetooth, contrasting the recorded outcomes and clients normal qualities to examine whether there is interruption or not
	Battery Consumption	Screens anomalous battery utilization of PDAs to identify interruption by recently made or as of now known assaults
	System Call	Screens framework calls of advanced cell portion to identify outside assaults through redistributing
	Process Information	Consistently screens logs and occasions and groups them into typical and irregular data
Dynamic Analysis Technique	**Information Marking**	Examines malware via completing static corrupt investigation for Java source code
	Information Marking	Adjusts stack casings to include corrupt labels into neighborhood factors and strategy contentions and follows the engendering cycle through labels to investigate malware

PDAs, much the same as PCs, convey a huge measure of individual data about their proprietors. They frequently connection to financial balances, email accounts, and at times family unit machines. Taken information can bring about major issues. Vehicles contain numerous PCs that control their capacity. At first, these PCs couldn't be hacked into. With the expanded network of the IoT, in any case, vehicles are currently in danger due to being associated with the Internet.

In another sense, control can be lost as an ever increasing number of organizations gather information about clients. This information frequently illustrates singular clients through the assortment of exercises on the web. All that you search, the entirety of your exercises on the web, is being followed by organizations that utilize that information.

There are numerous genuine issues with IoT protection and every one of them must be must be in point by point investigated, yet here are general ways IoT engineers can improve IoT security [20]:

Limit information obtaining: Software engineers should take a gander at the recurrence and the sort of information gathered with regards to the application and ought not to gather more information than the assignment requires. The stage should control which information an application gets.

Limit the quantity of information sources: Aggregation of information from various sources permits malevolent gatherings to distinguish touchy individual data of a person that could prompt protection infringement.

Limit crude information consumption: Raw information could prompt auxiliary utilization and security infringement. Thusly, IoT stages ought to consider changing over or changing crude information into auxiliary setting information.

Limit information disclosure: IoT applications ought to find just the information important to accomplish their essential goals. For instance, if the goal is to suggest food designs, the application ought not to endeavor to derive clients' wellbeing status without their unequivocal consent.

Limit information stockpiling: Raw information ought to be erased once an auxiliary setting is determined.

Limit the information maintenance period: More expanded maintenance periods give pernicious gatherings more opportunity to break and exfiltrate information.

Backing concealed information steering: To make it harder for web exercises to be followed back to the clients, this rule proposes that IoT applications should support and utilize an obscure directing system.

Anonymize information: Remove by and by recognizable data (PII) before the information gets utilized by IoT applications with the goal that the individuals portrayed by the information stay mysterious.

Scramble information interchanges: Typically, gadget to-gadget correspondences are encoded at the connection layer utilizing unique electronic equipment remembered for the radio modules.

Entryway to-cloud correspondence is commonly made sure about through HTTPS utilizing Secure Sockets Layer (SSL) or Transport Layer Security (TLS).

Encode information during handling: Sometimes the gathering preparing the information ought not have the option to peruse the information or the computational outcomes. Cycle information while they are in scrambled structure. For instance, homomorphic encryption is a type of encryption that permits calculations to be done on figure text, subsequently producing an encoded outcome that, when unscrambled, matches the aftereffect of activities performed on the plaintext.

Scramble information away: Encrypted information stockpiling lessens any security infringement because of noxious assaults and unapproved access.

Decrease information granularity: IoT applications should demand the base degree of granularity that is needed to play out their essential errands. A more elevated level of granularity could prompt auxiliary information utilization and inevitably security infringement. For instance, area can be coarse, in view of cell tower area or fine, in light of the location.

Question replying: Raw information can prompt distinguishing proof and protection infringement because of optional use. Rather than giving a numeric reaction to an inquiry a relative scale, Eq. 1–5 ought to be utilized.

Square rehashed questions: Query reactions should obstruct different inquiries that malignantly could find information that abuses client security, for example, breaking down convergences of various outcomes.

Circulate information handling: Distributed information preparing keeps away from incorporated enormous scope information get-together and exfiltration.

Circulate information stockpiling: Distributed information stockpiling lessens any protection infringement because of malevolent assaults and unapproved access. It additionally decreases protection chances due to unconsented auxiliary information disclosure.

3 Real Time Application of IoT

IoT (Internet of Things), a framework that overcomes any barrier between day by day questions and the web, is quickly changing the manner in which we play out our everyday errands. From design and retail to security and car, the effect of IoT is reverberating in pretty much every vertical today. The innovation has picked up such a great amount of energy throughout the long term that it isn't viewed as a promotion any longer. Essentially any physical gadget these days can be changed over into an IoT gadget. IoT lessens the endeavors in everyday life and helps a machine or gadget to deal with things that ordinarily require human endeavors easily. It is an innovation that is the consequence of humankind's exertion and eagerness to have a helpful existence.

3.1 A Real Time IoT-Based Wearable Communication Enabled Jacket to Monitor and Analyze the COVID-19

Recent trend in communication systems is to stay connected anywhere and at any time. Persuaded by the idea of a body-centric communication technology, many research projects have been initiated to integrate antennas and radio frequency (RF) systems (0.5 GHz to 12 GHz) into clothes. These systems have to be developed also with regard to size reduction, ease of integration and cost effectiveness as in COVID 19 situations. Body-centric applications are mainly focused in promoting personal communications, keeping track of body parameters like temperature, heartbeat, etc. and also to monitor people. Among several body-centric applications, monitoring people has become very popular wherein monitoring and protecting mentally challenged people has got a spot light. Our society is in need of monitoring mentally challenged especially the females and the children from becoming a victim of trafficking, as in these days trafficking has grown to a greater extent Without visiting the hospital doctors can able to trace the medical record of the patients by connecting with wearable devices which is connected through IoT. They have to be protected from traffickers and ought to be rescued when being trafficked. When problems with social importance are being addressed, the solutions/systems developed for those issues have to be affordable. Hence the need of the hour is to develop an IoT based economized body-centric wearable antenna to monitor and safeguard the mentally challenged and protect them in case of emergencies. The Internet of Things (IoT) enables new means of communication between people, things and the environment. By using this technology differently abled people can improve their life style as normal people do. In order to facilitate the real time tracking of antenna an IoT based wearable Antenna module has been incorporated.

Microstrip antennas are advantageous due to their simple design, easy construction and the presence of a large ground plane there is a significant reduction in radiated energy into the body. Advancements in microstrip antenna technology had led to the development of wearable microstrip antennas which play a vital role in body area communication, health monitoring and military applications. Research in wearable antennas has been paving way for excellent performances with respect to various applications. Recently, wearable antennas with circular polarization are being developed for navigation applications. A compact circularly polarized antenna for bio telemetric devices at ISM 2.4 GHz was proposed with an integrated band pass filter to reduce interferences and cross talks [1]. An Integrated radiator cum filter module with compact design, circular polarization and good frequency selectivity was developed for wearable devices with low SAR. The antenna has an impedance bandwidth of 12.2% [2]. Ink jet technique was used to make the antenna thin, lightweight and flexible. A wearable magneto-electric dipole textile antenna with combined effect of electric and magnetic resonances to improve the bandwidth and reduce the back radiations was proposed [3]. The antenna had a meager reduction in performance due to bending and a low SAR level of about 2 W/kg. A flexible embroidered textile antenna was proposed with multiband operation operating at GSM, PCS and WLAN bands

[4]. The antenna was made using a metal coated polymer fiber thus providing excellent mechanical flexibility and low losses. A body worn antenna integrated within an inflammable live jacket was published to use for Copas-Sarsat personal locator beacons (PLBs) [5]. The frequencies of operation are 121.5 and 406 MHz. A wearable textile antenna with wideband circular polarization property at ISM 2.4 GHz for low power transmission was presented [6]. The antenna was tested and the results were interpreted which shows a maximum gain of 4.9 dBi with an impedance and axial ratio bandwidths of 44% and 23% respectively. A rectangular circularly polarized dual band patch antenna for Iridium and GPS bands were proposed and comparative studies with different textile materials were also discussed [7]. Middle East respiratory syndrome corona virus (MERS-CoV) causes severe acute respiratory infection with as yet unclear epidemiology. MERS-CoV counteracts parts of the innate immune response in human bronchiolar cells. Here we analyzed respiratory functions using respiratory sensor to accessory proteins 3, 4a, 4b, and 5 for their abilities to inhibit the type I interferon response. Accessory protein 4a was found to block interferon induction at the level of melanoma differentiation-associated protein 5(MDA5) activation presumably by direct interaction with double-stranded RNA [8].

The advancements in wearable antenna in our country have grown to a greater extent. Scientists have been combining many novel techniques with the wearable antennas to improve their performances and to integrate them with wide range of wireless systems. An analysis on wearable antenna was done wherein the design issues of wearable antennas with respect to the various effects like human body, environment, conformability and testing were discussed [9]. An inset feed wearable textile antenna on flexible substrate for ISM 2.4–2.4835 GHz was developed [10]. The antenna uses EBG structures for enhanced gain, bandwidth and return loss performances. The antenna also has low SAR. A comparative study of performances of rectangular microstrip patch antenna on various textile materials for wearable applications was presented [11]. The textile material used was cotton with different dielectric constants ranging between 2.2 and 12. A novel microstrip antenna design with low front to back ratio was developed for telemedicine application [12]. The objective of this antenna is to monitor the health condition of target individuals [13]. The Endoplasmic Reticulum Stress Sensor IRE1α Protects Cells from Apoptosis Induced by the Corona virus Infectious Bronchitis Virus.

Applying the knowledge of technology for social issues like COVID 19 is the first and foremost duty of every graduated citizen. Hence we step forward to contribute ourselves through the development of an economized wearable navigation antenna to monitor and safeguard the mentally challenged individuals from traffickers, who use them for illegal activities. The proposal aims at the design and development of a wearable conformal antenna which is circularly polarized. The proposed antenna will operate in the L5 band of IRNSS as the main band and L2 band of GPS as auxiliary band. The L5 IRNSS band is chosen, as the proposal mainly focuses in addressing a serious issue in our country where our indigenous navigation system, IRNSS was deployed recently. The antenna will be made using low cost flexible substrates or even using the textile materials as substrates so that the target individual can afford it thus making it an economized one. The Internet of Things (IoT) enables new

Table 2 Design specifications

Specifications	Nominal range
Frequency	1176.42 and 1227.60 MHz
Input impedance	50 Ω
VSWR	<2:1
Peak Gain	3 dBi (min)
3 dB Beam width	60 degrees
Polarization	Circular (RHCP)
Axial ratio	<3 dB
Dimensions	70 mm X 70 mm (max)

means of communication between people, things and the environment. By using this technology differently abled people can improve their life style as normal people do. In order to facilitate the real time tracking of antenna an IoT module has been incorporated.

Global Positioning System (GPS) is a satellite based navigation system that provides location and time information. The use of this system is tremendous that it can locate one's absolute position, relative movement and time transfer anywhere at any time. GPS systems use circular polarization for better signal alignment irrespective of the orientation of the receiver antenna. Initially GPS was developed for defense purposes and later had got extended to civilian too. Among those frequency bands used for GPS, L5 (1176.45 MHz) is now being used in India for IRNSS (Indian Regional Navigation Satellite System) programme. Hence to meet our objective of monitoring and rescuing mentally challenged individuals, this frequency band can also be used in addition to an auxiliary GPS band, L2 (1227.60 MHz) (Table 2).

3.2 Microstrip Patch Antennas

Microstrip patch antennas are planar and can be fabricated easily. These antennas are now being made on flexible substrates so that they can be used for conformal applications. Microstrip patch antennas are being used widely for wearable applications due to their low profile nature. They have a large ground plane which results in high directivity, gain. They also have reduced back lobe emissions and hence have a little effect on human tissues when used for wearable applications.

Microstrip patch antenna can support circular polarization and is being widely used for navigation applications. In spite of all these advantages, they also have few disadvantages like low bandwidth and less efficiency but several approaches have been developed to improve the bandwidth of patch antenna. The antenna can be fed in many ways wherein coaxial feed has an impact on quality factor by creating a shunt inductance thereby reducing it. This leads to bandwidth improvement of patch antenna (Figs. 5 and 6).

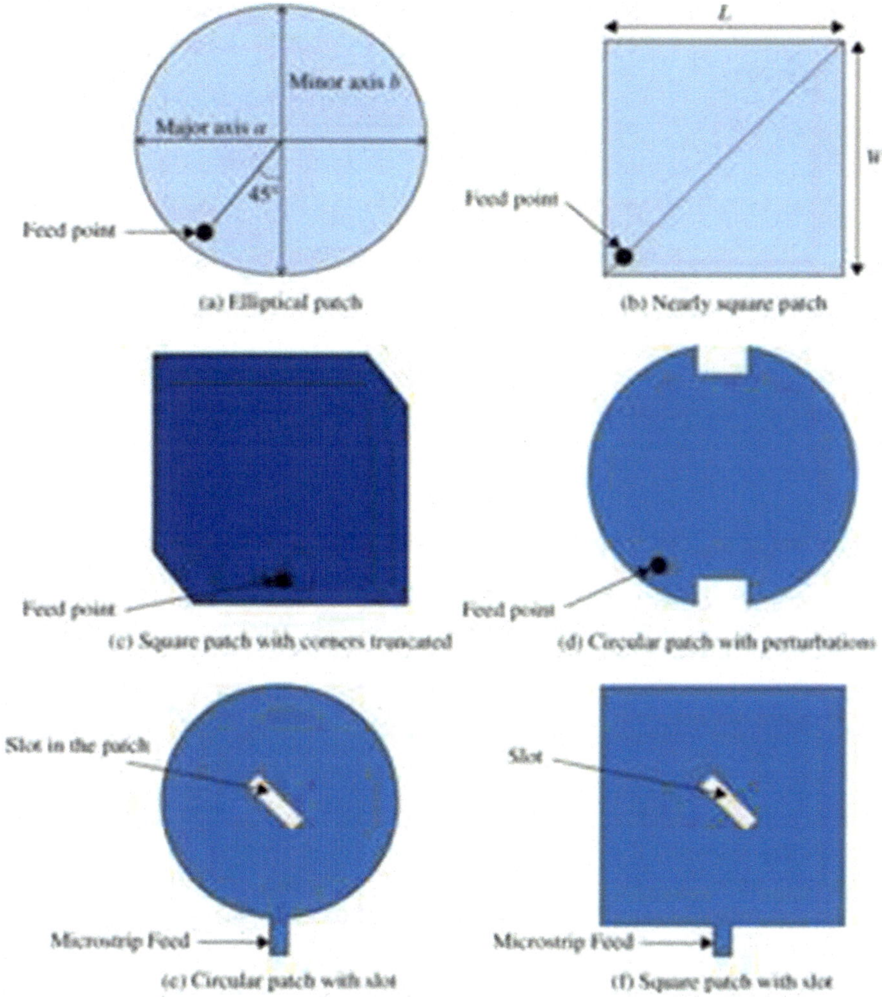

Fig. 5 Several topologies of circularly polarized Microstrip patch antenna

3.3 Block Diagram of Navigation System

100% woven polyester Nickel-copper-Nickel plated conductive (Rip-stop type)) laid on the lower woven polyester layer. It acts as the ground plane for the same fabrics laid on the upper non-woven polyester layer. The size of woven, nonwoven polyester and electro-textile made ground plane for the simulation and fabrication are taken as $0.54 \times 0.54\lambda 02$. The single capacitive probe feed is used to improve the return loss. It is connected to the upper electro-textile layer through an annular gap which acts as capacitor to nullify the effect of probe inductance, while the lower electro-textile

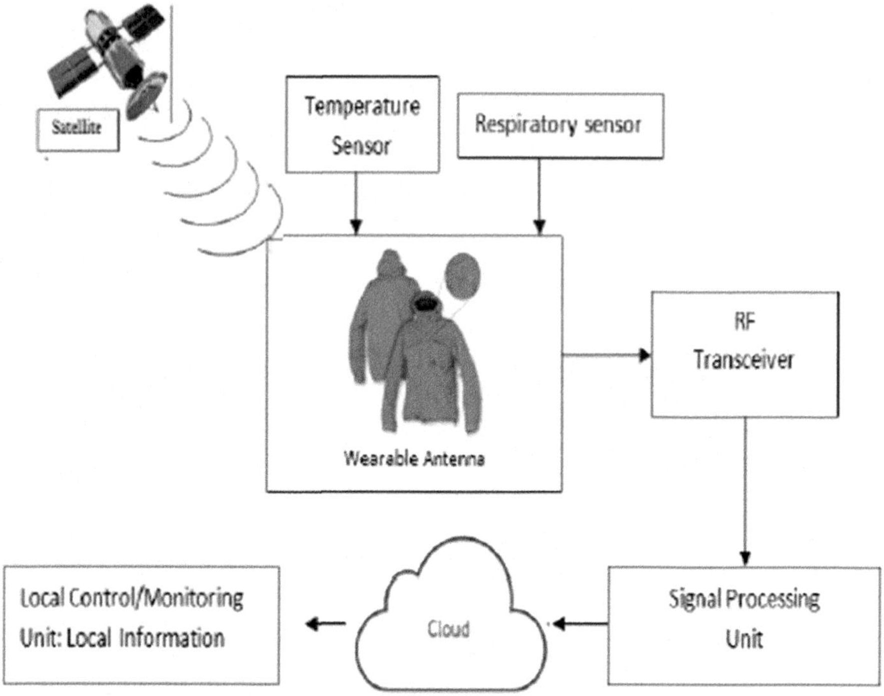

Fig. 6 Diagram of navigation system

layer is fed with an indirect contact by a small clearance hole between the probe and the patch as shown in Fig. 7.

Several navigation systems are being used by different countries. GPS is owned by the US. It has 24 satellites. The Indian indigenous navigation system IRNSS has 7 satellites to cover our nation. The USSR navigation system GLONASS has 24 satellites. GALELIO, the European Union's navigation system has 30 satellites and it is under development. The China's COMPASS navigation system which is also being developed is said to have 35 satellites. Out of these varied navigation systems, the GPS and GLONASS are being used predominantly across the globe. Since the project focuses in developing a solution for a social issue in our nation, we have proposed to develop wearable antennas that work in IRNSS frequency bands with GPS as auxiliary frequency band of operation.

The satellite navigation system can pin point one's location. A typical Satellite Navigation system's block diagram is shown in Fig. 6. The navigation satellites deployed in space are revolving around the earth continuously. These satellites are transmitting signals all day. As and when a navigation receiver with a navigation antenna picks up the signal, the RF front end of the receiver does the RF filtering and the down conversion process where the down converted signal is processed by

Fig. 7 Circularly polarized textile antennas

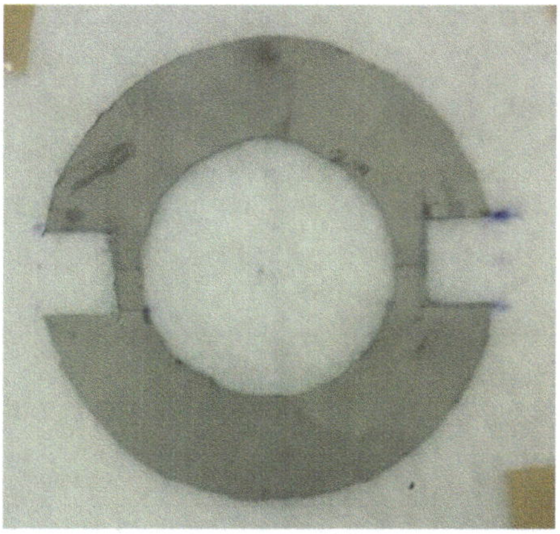

(a) Top View

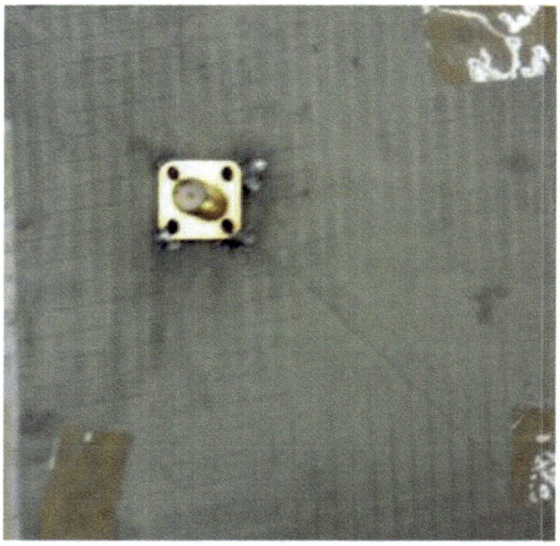

(b) Bottom View

the signal processing unit and the location information is transmitted to the local monitoring centre.

With the exact location information of an individual, it becomes easy for us to track and monitor them. The navigation system thus by providing the exact location information of a person along with its temperature range and respiratory (inhale and exhale duration and its cycles) if there is any deviations from the reference value it will be intimated to the doctors. The Internet of Things (IoT) enables new means of communication between people, things and the environment. By using this technology differently abled people can improve their life style as normal people do. In order to facilitate the real time tracking of antenna an IoT module has been incorporated.

The social issue addressed here is to ensure the safety of mentally challenged individuals and children who are being abducted and used illegally by anti-social people. Thus there is a requirement for a system that continuously monitors and alerts the location and movement of the preferred individuals. Satellite Navigation was conscripted to serve our purpose and the objective has been framed to design and develop a low profile wearable antenna that can be embedded in the clothes of mentally challenged individuals and children to monitor and rescue them.

The antenna has to be a low profile, conformal one and should to be embedded in the clothes to make them wearable. Hence a thorough literature survey will be done and based on that, the topology of the antenna will be selected. After gathering all the requisites, the antenna simulation will be carried out. The results will be verified with the specifications. If the specifications are not met, further tuning can be done to match the specifications. Once the specifications are met, the fabrication process will follow that and as the fabrication gets over, the return loss of the antenna will be measured using a Vector Network Analyzer. The radiation pattern of the antenna will also be measured in a shielded anechoic chamber. If there are any mismatches with the simulated and the measured results, tuning can be made accordingly. A prototype will be developed later and real time testing can be done by deploying the embedded antenna prototypes in an open area or in a practical scenario. The Internet of Things (IoT) enables new means of communication between people, things and the environment. By using this technology differently abled people can improve their life style as normal people do.

4 Conclusion

The IoT can possibly drastically expand the accessibility of data, and is probably going to change organizations and associations in for all intents and purposes each industry around the globe. Thusly, discovering approaches to use the intensity of the IoT is relied upon to factor into the vital goals of most innovation organizations, paying little mind to their industry center. The quantity of various innovations needed to help the sending and further development of the IoT places a premium on interoperability, and has brought about boundless endeavors to create norms and specialized determinations that help consistent correspondence between IoT gadgets and segments. Cooperation between different principles advancement gatherings and solidification of some current endeavors will in the long run bring about more noteworthy lucidity for IoT innovation organizations. From home and brilliant (Smart Cities) urban areas to cultivating and retail, the employments of IoT are numerous and the innovation keeps on growing its viewpoint. In spite of the fact that there are as yet eminent accomplishments left to be found in the use of IoT for self-propelled vehicles, early signs foresee a decent picture ahead. At present COVID 19 situations without visiting the hospital, doctors can able to trace the medical record of the patients by connecting with wearable devices such as pulse oximeter which can be connected through IoT. When problems with social importance are being addressed, the solutions/systems developed for those issues have to be affordable. Hence the need of the hour was developed an IoT based economized body-centric wearable antenna to monitor and safeguard the mentally challenged and protect them in case of emergencies like military risky operations, woman trafficking etc.,. In order to facilitate the real time tracking of antenna an IoT based wearable Antenna module has been incorporated.

References

1. Jiang, Z.H., Gregory, M.D., Werner, D.H.: Design and experimental investigation of a compact circularly polarized integrated filtering antenna for wearable biotelemetric devices. IEEE Trans. Biomed. Circuits Syst. **10**(2) (2016)
2. Jiang, Z.H., Gregory, M.D., Werner, D.H.: A Compact, wideband circularly polarized co-designed filtering antenna and its application for wearable devices with low SAR. IEEE Trans. Antennas Propag. **63**(9) (2015)
3. Yan, S., Soh, P.J., Vandenbosch, G.A.E.: Wearable Dual-band magneto-electric dipole antenna for WBAN/WLAN applications. IEEE Trans. Antennas Propag. **63**(9) (2015)
4. Wang, Z., Lee, L.Z., Psychoudakis, D., Volakis, J.L.: Embroidered multiband body-worn antenna for GSM/PCS/WLAN communications. IEEE Trans. Antennas Propag. **62**(6) (2014)
5. Lilja, J., Pynttäri, V., Kaija, T., Mäkinen, R., Halonen, E., Sillanpää, H., Heikkinen, J., Mäntysalo, M., Salonen, P., de Maagt, P.: Body-worn antennas making a splash: lifejacket-integrated antennas for global search and rescue satellite system. IEEE Antennas Propag. Mag. **55**(2) (2013)
6. Lui, K.W., Murphy, O.H., Toumazou, C.: A wearable wideband circularly polarized textile antenna for effective power transmission on a wirelessly powered sensor platform. IEEE Antennas Propag. Mag. **61**(7) (2013)
7. Kaivanto, E.K., Berg, M., Salonen, E., de Maagt, P.: Wearable circularly polarized antenna for personal satellite communication and navigation. IEEE Trans. Antennas Propag. **59**(12) (2011)
8. Niemeyer, D., Zillinger, T.: Middle East respiratory syndrome coronavirus accessory protein 4a Is a Type I interferon antagonist. J. Virol. (2013)
9. Patel, T., Sahoo, M.: design issues of wearable antennas. Int. J. Sci. Res. (IJSR) **5**(5) (2016)
10. Rajya Lakshmi, V., Manikanth, M.: Design of wearable textile antenna for ISM band with low SAR. Indian J. Modern Eng. Res. (IJMER) **5**(12) (2015)
11. Murali1, D., Narada Maha Muni1, B., Dilip Varma1, Y., Chaitanya, S.V.S.K.: Development of wearable antennas with different cotton textiles. Int. J. Eng. Res. Appl. (IJERA) **4**(7) (2014)
12. Survase, S.C., Deshmukh, V.V.: Design of wearable antenna for telemedicine application. Int. J. Eng. Sci. Innov. Technol. (IJESIT) **2**(2) (2013)
13. Fung, S., Liao, T.: The endoplasmic reticulum stress sensor IRE1α protects cells from apoptosis induced by the coronavirus infectious bronchitis virus. J. Virol. (2014)
14. ITU Internet Reports 2005: The Internet of Things. http://www.itu.int/osg/spu/publications/internetofthings/
15. https://www.helpnetsecurity.com/2018/01/16/internet-of-things-securityissues-2018/
16. https://securelist.com/honeypots-and-the-internet-of-things/78751/
17. Khan, R., Khan, S.U., Zaheer, R., Khan, S.: Future Internet: The Internet of Things architecture possible applications and key challenges. In: Proceedings of the 10th International Conference FIT, pp. 257–260 (2012)
18. Oh, S.R., Kim, Y.G.: Security requirements analysis for the IoT. 2017 International Conference on Platform Technology and Service (PlatCon), pp. 1–6 (2017)
19. Reza Ghorbani, H., Hossein Ahmadzadegan, M.: Security challenges in the internet of things: survey. In: 2017 IEEE Conference on Wireless Sensors (ICWiSe), pp. 1–6 (2017)

20. https://www.networkworld.com/article/3221474/internet-of-things/30-ways-toimprove-iot-privacy.html
21. https://media.kasperskydaily.com/wpcontent/uploads/sites/92/2020/02/27074211/2020_Kaspersky_IoT_report.pdf

Optimum Scheduling of the Disinfection Process for COVID-19 in Public Places with a Case Study from Egypt, a Novel Discrete Binary Gaining-Sharing Knowledge-Based Metaheuristic Algorithm

Said Ali Hassan, Prachi Agrawal, Talari Ganesh, and Ali Wagdy Mohamed

Abstract The aim of this paper is to introduce an improved strategy for controlling COVID-19 and other pandemic episodes as an environmental disinfection culture for public places. The scheduling aims at achieving the best utilization of the available working day-time hours, which is calculated as the total consumed disinfection times minus the total loosed transportation times. The proposed problem in network optimization identifies a disinfection group who is likely to select a route to reach a subset of predetermined public places to be regularly disinfected with the most utilization of the available day-working hours. A Nonlinear Binary Model is introduced with a detailed real application case study involving improving the scheduling of Coronavirus disinfection process for some Educational Institutions as an example of crowded public places in Cairo, Egypt. The case study mathematical model is solved using a novel Discrete Binary Gaining-Sharing knowledge-based optimization algorithm (DBGSK). The results of this study show that the novel optimization algorithm can efficiently solve the proposed Problem.

S. A. Hassan
Department of Operations Research and Decision Support, Faculty of Computers and Artificial Intelligence, Cairo University, Cairo, Egypt
e-mail: saidalihassan@yahoo.com

P. Agrawal · T. Ganesh
Department of Mathematics and Scientific Computing, National Institute of Technology Hamirpur, Hamirpur 177005, Himachal Pradesh, India
e-mail: prachiagrawal202@gmail.com

T. Ganesh
e-mail: ganimsc2007@gmail.com

A. W. Mohamed (✉)
Operations Research Department, Faculty of Graduate Studies for Statistical Research, Cairo University, Giza 12613, Egypt
e-mail: aliwagdy@gmail.com

Wireless Intelligent Networks Center (WINC), School of Engineering and Applied Sciences, Nile University, Giza, Egypt

D. Oliva et al. (eds.), *Artificial Intelligence for COVID-19*, Studies in Systems, Decision and Control 358, https://doi.org/10.1007/978-3-030-69744-0_13

Keywords Disinfection process scheduling · COVID-19 · Public places · Nonlinear binary constrained optimization · Gaining sharing Knowledge-Based optimization algorithm

1 Introduction

Nowadays, the new Coronavirus (COVID-19) put humans in all countries in front of the huge danger. The entire world is suffering from a global epidemic of COVID-19 that has infected thousands of people in almost all countries [1]. In December last year, Wuhan in China, was the origin of a pneumonia of unknown cause. By Jan in this year, assured cases were detected outside Wuhan [2]. The Centers for Decease Control and Prevention (CDC) declares the major signs of COVID-19 so that any individual can discover whether or not he has such symptoms [3, 4].

The risk in these diseases is that there is no vaccine for treatment yet; the matter is further complicated by the fact that the incubation period of the virus is up to 14 days; therefore, officials of the examination in screening places will not be able to discover all the possible patients carrying the disease [5].

The continuous disinfection process for public places should be performed regularly to control COVID-19 or similar epidemic or pandemic episodes currently and in the future. Surfaces and objects in Public Places that are frequently touched may include: doors and door handles; keyboards and desks; seating areas; sinks and sink handles; handrails; drinking fountains; touch screens; all bathroom surfaces; refrigerators copiers and printers; food service areas; desks; tables; counters, halls, workshops, labs, stands, doors, computer keyboard, practical training tools, phones and other objects, [6]. Figure 1 shows a scheme representing the continuous disinfection process for public places. The responsible groups start performing the disinfection of public buildings contaminated with the virus, but sooner, the virus appears again as

Fig. 1 Contamination and disinfection cycle of the public places

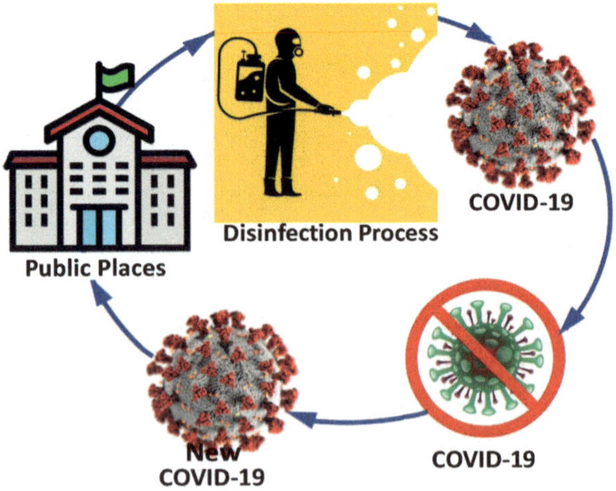

a result of the infected people. Thus, the public places are contaminated again where they need to be cleaned once more, and this process is continuously repeatedly.

A proposed problem for an environmental Disinfection Culture for Public Places (DCPP) in network optimization is defined for a disinfection group that want to settle on the foremost effective route for disinfection of several candidate places. The group begins from a predetermined position and next go to each chosen place exactly once within the day working hours.

The target of the scheduling is to determine the optimum scheduling route for the disinfection group to maximize the utilization of daily available time measured as the total active disinfection time minus the total wasted travelling time in the chosen route. In order to solve the complicated mathematical model for the DCPP, a novel binary version of recently developed Gaining-Sharing knowledge-based optimization algorithm (GSK) to solve binary optimization problems is proposed [7].

The structure of the paper is as follows: This section is for the introduction. The second section introduces the new Disinfection Culture for Public Places (DCPP). As educational institutions are considered one of the important public places crowded with people, several faculties will be chosen as a real application case study.

The mathematical model of the Disinfection Culture for Public Places (DCPP) Problem is designed in Sect. 3 including all needed formulations. The steps of the solution procedure are also explained. A real application case study is presented in Sect. 4; its complete mathematical model is formulated.

In Sect. 5, a novel Discrete Binary version of a recently developed gaining-sharing knowledge-based optimization technique (GSK) is introduced for solving the DCPP. GSK cannot solve the problem with discrete binary space; therefore, Discrete Binary-GSK optimization algorithm (DBGSK) is proposed with two new discrete binary junior and senior stages to inspect the problem search space efficiently. The experimental results of the case study obtained by DBGSK is also presented. Section 6 summarizes the conclusions and the suggested points for future researches

2 Disinfection Scheduling Strategies for Public Places

All countries suffer from the virus attack and taking into consideration that this is a vast evolving case, new situation changes may not be represented at once [8]. The updated worldwide total cases and deaths of coronavirus are recorded daily [9]. The greatest risk also lies in travelling from one country to another, the risks of travel recently include all countries of the world [10].

The rate of the virus spreading affirmed by its reproductive number is estimated in the early stages of the disease to be 2.2 [11]. Updated information about COVID-19 indicate clearly that the current and the near future situations are not quite right in such a way that foreshadows a catastrophe for most of the countries of the world.

Strict measures should be taken at the level of governments and peoples, including disinfection of places where large crowds of people gather. Disinfection process according to the strict procedures announced by the Centers of Disease Control and

Prevention (CDC) website [12] should be taken into consideration wherever the cases of coronavirus infection appear, such a protocol involves particular steps to be performed [13].

The standards of cleaning and disinfection protocols include the thorough cleaning process to remove dirt and impurities. The cleaning process is followed by disinfection using appropriate chemicals to kill the virus on surfaces that have been exposed to infected people.

The disinfection teams consist of specialists who are well versed in cleaning and disinfection services [14]. The group' specialists maintain the World Health Organization (WHO) instructions [15].

To optimize the scheduling of the disinfection problem, a new defined problem which we will call Coronavirus Travelling-Disinfection Problem (TDP) in network optimization is proposed for a disinfection group member who want to choose the most effective route for approaching several candidate places located in different predetermined positions. The group begins in a starting point, and next wants to transport to some chosen subset of places each one exactly once within the day working time. The aim of the TDP is to choose precisely a route to maximizes the actual working hours in the places and minimizing the total transportation times between different institutions.

The new proposed Problem is designated over a graph G with a set of n nodes V representing the places and an additional node denotes the location where the disinfection group starts the job, and a set of arcs representing the travelling times between two distinct places [16]. While the disinfection group should start the route from a chosen position, they end the route at the last visited workplace, while the driver will return with the vehicle and equipment.

3 Mathematical Model Formulation for the Disinfection Scheduling Strategies

The Disinfection Culture for Public Places (DCPP) Problem is then defined as:

- Each workplace is visited only once by the disinfection group,
- The tour starts at a predetermined position and terminates at the latest visited public place,
- The overall goal of the problem to be achieved is the best utilization of the available working day hours, calculated as the total active disinfection time minus the total wasted travelling time in the chosen route.

3.1 Mathematical Model

3.1.1 Decision Variables

Let:

1, if place i is approached by the Disinfection on position m of his route, i
$x_i^m =$ and $m = 1, 2, \ldots, n$.
0, otherwise.

Constraints:

(1) **Positions Constraints:**

Each position m in the Disinfection route has at most one place:

$$\sum_{i=1}^{n} x_i^m \leq 1, m = 1, 2, \ldots, n \quad (1)$$

(2) **Places Constraints**:

Each place i can be in one position of the Disinfection route or not visited:

$$\sum_{m=1}^{n} x_i^m \leq 1, i = 1, 2, \ldots, n. \quad (2)$$

(3) **Consecutive Positions Constraints:**

A position (m + 1) cannot exist in the Disinfection tour unless the preceding position m exists, this is achieved by the following set of constraints:

$$\sum_{i=1}^{n} x_i^{m+1} \leq \sum_{i=1}^{n} x_i^m, m = 1, 2, \ldots, n - 1 \quad (3)$$

If $\sum_{i=1}^{n} x_i^{m+1} = 1$, then $\sum_{i=1}^{n} x_i^m = 1$, $m = 1, 2, \ldots, n - 1$,

If $\sum_{i=1}^{n} x_i^{m+1} = 0$, then there is no restriction on the value of $\sum_{i=1}^{n} x_i^m$, $m = 1, 2, \ldots, n - 1$.

(4) **Working hours/Day Constraints:**

The total time spent by the Disinfection in travelling and site inspection should be within the maximum working hours/day $= T = 8$ h.

$$\sum_{i=1}^{n} t_{0i}x_i^1 + \sum_{m=1}^{n}\sum_{i=1}^{n}(t_i x_i^m) + \sum_{i=1}^{n}\sum_{\substack{j=1 \\ j\neq i}}^{n} t_{ij}.(\sum_{m=1}^{n-1} x_i^m.x_j^{m+1}) \leq T. \tag{4}$$

where:

t_{0i} = Transportation time between the headquarter and workplace i, $i = 1, 2, \ldots, n$,

t_{ij} = Transportation time between the two adjacent places i and j, $i, j = 1, 2, \ldots, n$,

t_i = Inspection time for workplace i, $i = 1, 2, \ldots, n$.

This is a quadratic inequality in two variables, the first part is for travelling from the headquarter to the first position in the route, the second part is the inspection times at places and the third part is the travelling time between different positions in the route.

(5) **Binary Constraints**:

All the decision variables are 0–1.

$$x_i^m = 0 \text{ or } 1, i, m = 1, 2, \ldots, n \tag{5}$$

(6) **The Objective Function**

The Total Disinfection Time (TDT) is considered as gain and the Total Travelling Time (TTT) is considered as losses. So, the objective functions are formulated as:

$$\text{Maximize Z} = \text{(TDT)}-\text{(TTT)} =$$

$$= [\sum_{m=1}^{n}\sum_{i=1}^{n}(t_i x_i^m)]-[\sum_{i=1}^{n} t_{0i}x_i^1 + \sum_{i=1}^{n}\sum_{\substack{j=1 \\ j\neq i}}^{n} t_{ij}\cdot(\sum_{m=1}^{n-1} x_i^m\cdot x_j^{m+1})] \tag{6}$$

Finally, we have a suggested a model that contains (n^2) binary variables and ($3n$) constraints.

Any finally obtained optimal solution will produce two distinct situations:

(1) If $\sum_{m=1}^{n} x_i^m = 1, i = 1, 2, \ldots, n$, then all the n-places are visited by the disinfection-group in one working day and the problem is completed.

(2) If $\sum_{m=1}^{n} x_i^m = 0$ for any i, then the corresponding place i is not visited by the disinfection-group in the first working day. In this case, it is needed to eliminate the visited places, subjoin other candidate places to be disinfected, add one more day and then repeat the procedure for another working day. The solution procedure is presented in Fig. 2.

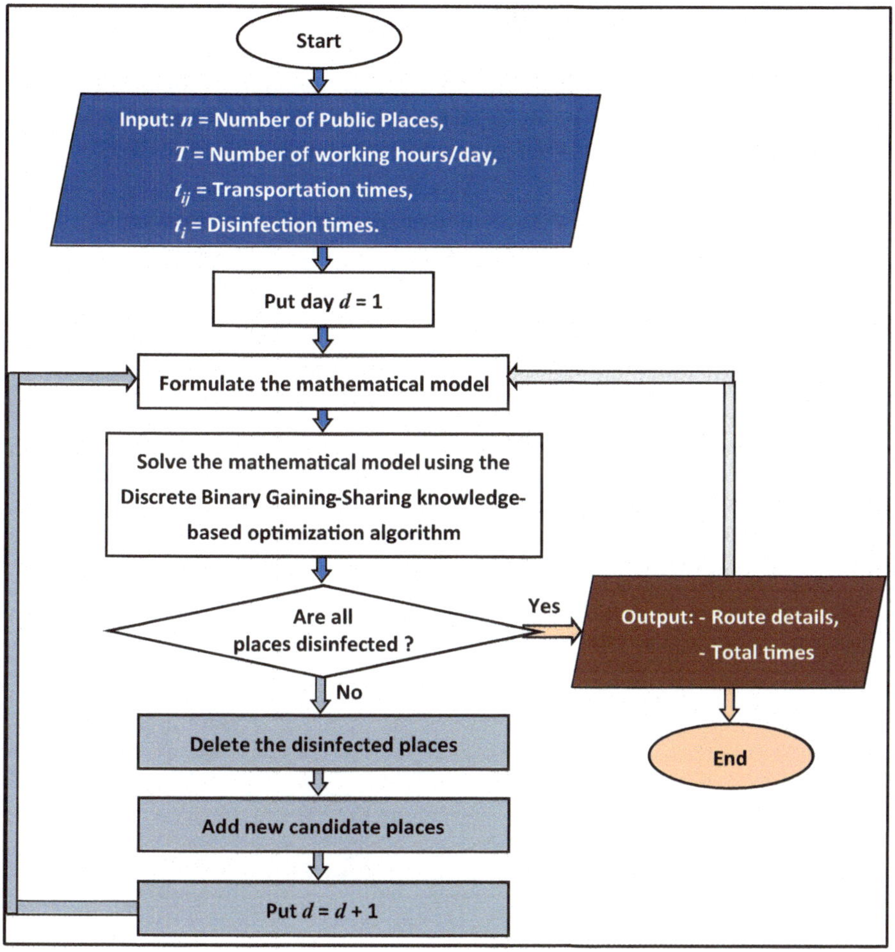

Fig. 2 Steps of the solution procedure of the TDP

4 A Real Application Case Study: Educational Institutions, Cairo, Egypt

The chosen real application case study addresses some very important educational institutes where people (staff, students, and employees) are crowded like other public places. Ain Shams University management and the main two campuses are located in the area of Abbasia, Cairo. It comprises two high institutes and fifteen faculties, it has 7 campuses located in Great Cairo. It has 3 adjacent campuses, at Abassia and 5 faculties each on an independent campus in Ramsis street, El Sarayat St., Al Maqrizi Street, Asmaa Fahmy Street and Shoubra El-Kheima, [17].

A disinfection group of 10-persons working as one team is applied to these 5 separated faculties. Table 1 and Fig. 3 show the names, address and locations of each of them. Based on many recorded travels and expert's opinions, Table 2 demonstrates the estimated average travelling and needed disinfection times, where numbers inside the cells (i, j) represent the travelling times t_{ij} for the problem.

The mathematical formulation for the given case is worked out by substituting in the previously described model.

Table 1 The five separate-faculty' campuses for the case study

#	Faculty	Address
MH	Ministry of Health and Population	Parliament of Egypt street, Al Munirah, El-Sayeda Zainab, Cairo
1	Faculty of Specific Education	Ramsis street, Abassia
2	Faculty of Engineering	1 El Sarayat St., Abassia, Al Waili, Cairo
3	Faculty of Education	Al Maqrizi Street, Mansheya El-Bakry, Heliopolis, Roxy, Cairo
4	Faculty of Women	Asmaa Fahmy Street, Nabil El Waqqad Street, from Ahmed Tayseer Street, Cairo
5	Faculty of Agriculture	Shubra Al Kheimah, Al Qalyubia Governorate

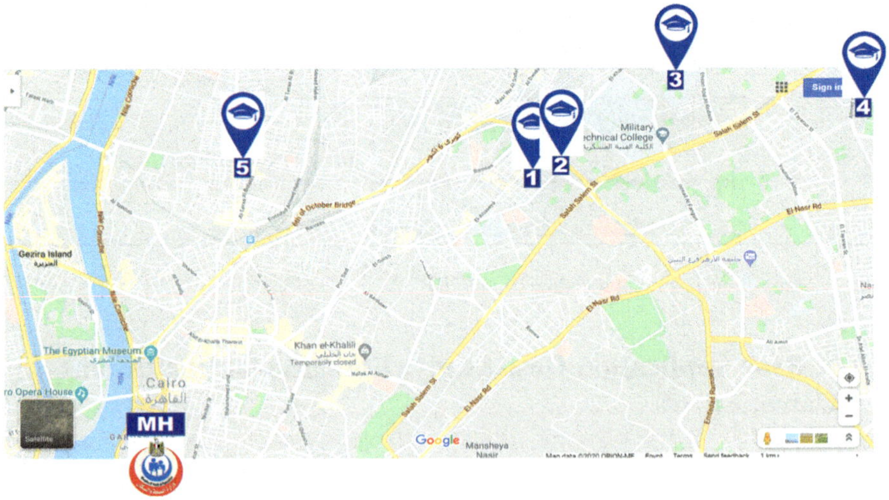

Fig. 3 Locations of the five separate-faculty' campuses for the case study

Table 2 Travelling and disinfection times for the problem

	i/j	0	1	2	3	4	5
t_i	**0**		0.50	0.75	1.00	1.25	1.25
2.50	**1**			0.25	0.25	0.50	1.25
2.00	**2**					0 .50	1.00
3.00	**3**					0.25	1.25
1.50	**4**						1.50
2.25	**5**						

5 The Proposed Methodology

Metaheuristic approaches are developed for the complex optimization problems with continuous variables [18–24]. Mohamed et al. [7] recently proposed a novel Gaining Sharing Knowledge-based optimization algorithm (GSK), setup on acquiring knowledge and share it with others throughout their lifetime. The original GSK solves optimization problems over continuous space, but it can't solve the problem with binary space as the case in this study. So, a new variant of GSK is introduced to solve the proposed prolem. A novel Discrete Binary Gaining Sharing knowledge-based optimization algorithms (DBGSK) is proposed over discrete binary space with new binary junior and senior gaining and sharing stages [25, 26]. On the other hand, there are many constraint handling techniques in the literature [27]. In their work, the augmented Lagrangian method is used in which an unconstrained optimization problem is obtained from a constrained optimization one, [28, 29]. The proposed methodology is described below.

5.1 Gaining Sharing Knowledge-Based Optimization Algorithm (GSK)

The human-based algorithm GSK is of two-stages: junior and senior gaining and sharing stage. All persons acquire knowledge and share their views with others. The people from early-stage gain knowledge from their small networks such as family members, relatives, neighbours, etc. and want to share their opinions with the others who might not be from their networks, due to curiosity of exploring others. These may not have the experience to categorize the people. In the same way, the people from the middle or later age enhance their knowledge by interacting with friends, colleagues, social media friends, etc. and share their views with the most suitable person, so that they can improve their knowledge. These people have the experience to judge other people and can categorize them (good or bad). The process human-based thinking mentioned above can be formulated mathematically in the following steps:

Step 1: To get a starting point of the optimization problem, the initial population must be created randomly within the boundary constraints.

Step 2: The dimensions of junior and senior stages are computed

Step 3: Junior gaining sharing knowledge stage: In this stage, the early aged people gain knowledge from their small networks and share their views with the other people who may or may not belong to their group. With the same principle, individuals are updated.

Step 4: Senior gaining sharing knowledge stage: This stage comprises the impact and effect of other people (good or bad) on the individual. The updated individual can be determined as follows:

The individuals are classified into three categories (best, middle and worst) after sorting individuals into ascending order (based on the objective function values).

For every individual x_t, choose the top and bottom $100p\%$ individuals for gaining part and the third one (middle individual) is chosen for the sharing part so that the new individual is updated.

5.2 Discrete Binary Gaining Sharing Knowledge-Based Optimization Algorithm (DBGSK)

For solving problems in discrete binary space, a novel Discrete Binary Gaining Sharing knowledge-based optimization algorithm (DBGSK) is suggested. In DBGSK, the new initialization and the working mechanism of both stages (junior and senior gaining sharing stages) are introduced over discrete binary space, and the remaining algorithms remain the same as the previous one. The working mechanism of DBGSK are presented in the following subsections

Discrete Binary Initialization:

The initial population is obtained in GSK and updated using an equation for binary population, where the round operator is used to convert the decimal number into the nearest binary number.

Discrete Binary Junior gaining and sharing stage:

The discrete binary junior gaining and sharing stage is based on the original GSK where the individuals are updated using a special procedure.

Discrete Binary Senior gaining and sharing stage:

The individuals are updated in the original senior gaining sharing stage that contains two cases. The two cases further modified for binary senior gaining sharing stage.

6 Experimental Results

The problem is handled by using the proposed novel DBGSK algorithm with appropriate parameters. DBGSK runs over personal computer Intel ® CoreTM i5-7200U CPU @ 2.50 GHz and 4 GB RAM and coded on MATLAB R2015a. To get the optimal solutions, 30 independent runs are complete, and the obtained statistics are provided in Table 3, including the best, median, average, worst solutions and the DBGSK standard deviations. Moreover, Fig. 4 shows the convergence graph of the solutions using DBGSK. From the figure, it can be observed that after the 24th iteration, it converges to the global optimal solution (6.00), which shows the robustness of the DBGSK.

The route provided by the optimum solution can be seen in Fig. 5. The route begins in the Ministry of Health (MH) and then is composed of 3 faculties numbers 1, 3 and 4 which are: Faculty of Specific Education, Faculty of Education and Faculty of Women respectively. The corresponding route length is 8 h, which means that all the available working daytime is utilized completely without any slack. The total disinfection time is 7 h and the total traveling time is only 1 h.

The remaining two faculties numbers 2 and 5 are added to the new list of places to be disinfected and the process of continuous disinfection will be repeated for another day.

Table 3 Statistical results using DBGSK

Algorithm	Best (Maximum)	Median	Average	Worst (Minimum)	Standard Deviation
DBGSK	6.00	6.00	6.00	6.00	0.00

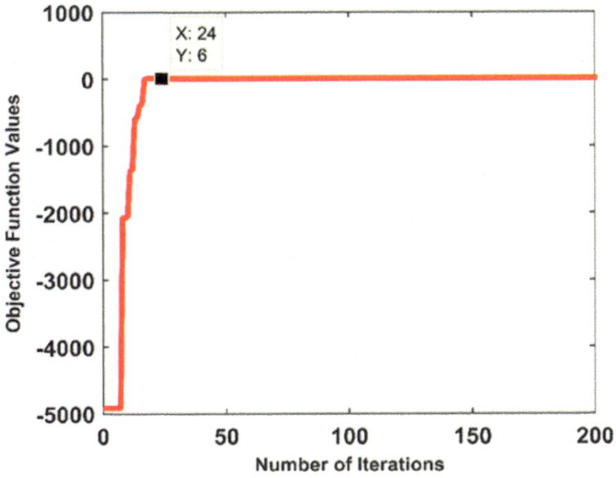

Fig. 4 Convergence graph of DBGSK

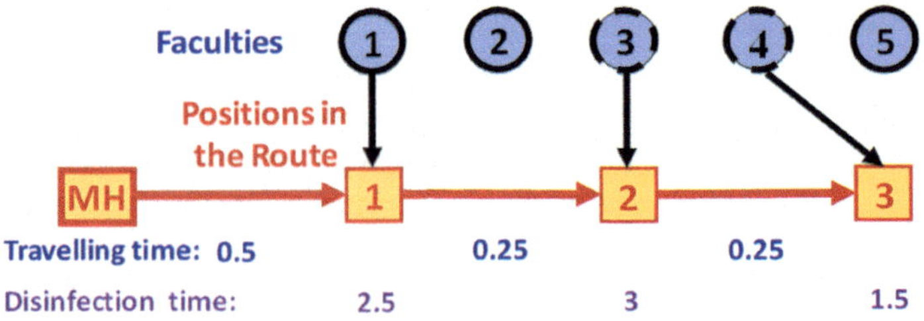

Fig. 5 Optimum solution for the case study example

7 Conclusions and Points for Future Researches

The main conclusions for this paper can be summarized as follows:

1. An improved scheduling a continuous disinfection process of the new Coronavirus (COVID-19) and similar epidemic or pandemic episodes is introduced. The scheduling is aiming at achieving the best utilization of the available day time in the disinfection process.
2. A nonlinear binary constrained mathematical model is formulated for the given problem. The binary decision variables represent the allocation of chosen public places in the positions of the chosen route of the disinfection process.
3. The nonlinear binary mathematical model and the solution method are used to solve a real application case study for disinfecting Educational Institutions in Ain Shams University, Cairo, Egypt. The detailed mathematical model and the solution procedure are exhaustively explained.
4. The proposed problem is solved by a novel Discrete Binary Gaining Sharing Knowledge based Optimization algorithm (DBGSK). It proves the ability of finding the solution of the problem, and the obtained results demonstrates the robustness and convergence towards the optimal solutions.

The points for future researches can be stated in the following points:

1. To propose other mathematical models' formulation for the same problem comprising the designing the objective function, the decision variables and the constraints and then comparing the effectiveness of computations for each model.
2. To extend the problem to cover extended variations like: Time windows, multiple disinfection groups, Stochastic Problem, Multi-objective Problem and other variations.
3. To check the performance of the DBGSK approach in solving different complex optimization problems, and further works can be investigated by the extension of DBGSK with different kinds of constraint handling methods.

References

1. Cleemput, S., Dumon, W., Fonseca, V., Abdool Karim, W., Giovanetti, M., Alcantara, L.C., Deforche, K., de Oliveira, T.: Genome Detective Coronavirus Typing Tool for rapid identification and characterization of novel coronavirus genomes, Bioinformatics, btaa145, 28 February 2020 (2020). https://doi.org/10.1093/bioinformatics/btaa145
2. THE LANCET website: A novel coronavirus outbreak of global health concern, retrieved on March 30, 2020 (2020). https://www.thelancet.com/journals/lancet/article/PIIS0140–6736(20)30185-9/fulltext
3. World Health Organization (WHO) website (2020a) Novel Coronavirus (2019-nCoV) Situation Report – 7, Data as reported by 27 January 2020
4. Guan, W., Ni, Z., Hu, Y., Liang, W., Ou, C., He, J., Liu, L., Shan, H., Lei, C., Hui, D.S.C., Du, B., Li, L.: Clinical Characteristics of Coronavirus Disease 2019 in China. The New England Journal of Medicine, February 28, 2020. https://doi.org/10.1056/nejmoa2002032 https://www.nejm.org/doi/full/10.1056/NEJMoa200203
5. Bai, Y., Yao, L., Wei, T., Tian, F., Jin, D.Y., Chen, L., Wang, M.: Presumed asymptomatic carrier transmission of COVID-19. JAMA **323**(14), 1406–1407 (2020)
6. Environmental Consultants Inc. APEX: General guidance for building managers regarding novel coronavirus (2020). https://www.smrecover.com/wp-content/uploads/2020/03/COVID-19-General-Guideline-for-Building-Managers-Final.pdf
7. Mohamed, A.W., Hadi, A.A., Mohamed, A.K.: Gaining-sharing knowledge-based algorithm for solving optimization problems: a novel nature-inspired algorithm. Int. J. Mach. Learn. Cybern. **11**, 1501–1529 (2020)
8. Wikimedia Commons website (2020). Accessed 3 April 2020. https://commons.wikimedia.org/wiki/File:COVID-19_Outbreak_World_Map.svg
9. Worldometer website (2020a) COVID-19 Coronavirus pandemic. Accessed 3 April 2020. https://www.worldometers.info/coronavirus/#ref-13
10. Centers for Decease Control and Prevention (CDC) website (2020a) COVID-19 Travel Recommendations by Country. Accessed 3 April 2020. https://www.cdc.gov/coronavirus/2019-ncov/travelers/map-and-travel-notices.html
11. Li, Q., Guan, X., Wu, P., Wang, X., Zhou,L., Tong, Y., Ren, R., Leung, K.S.M., Lau, E.H.Y., Wong, J.Y., Xing, X., Xiang, N., et al.: Early transmission dynamics in Wuhan, China, of Novel Coronavirus–Infected Pneumonia. New England J. Med. (2020)
12. Centers of Disease Control and Prevention (CDC) website (2020b). Coronavirus disease 2019, retrieved on April 11, 2020. https://www.cdc.gov/
13. ServiceMaster DSI website (2020) Preventive cleaning & decontamination, COVID-19 Coronavirus Disinfection. Accessed 30 Mar 2020. https://servicemasterdsi.com/coronavirus-decontamination/
14. Sentrex website (2020) UK Coronavirus Infection Control & Fogging. Accessed 28 Mar 2020. https://sentrex.co.uk/service/coronavirus-infection-control/
15. World Health Organization (WHO) website (2020b), Guidance for health workers. Accessed 29 Mar 2020. https://www.who.int/emergencies/diseases/novel-coronavirus-2019/technical-guidance/health-workers
16. Pinter, C.C.: A Book of Set Theory, Dover Publications Inc. ISBN10 0486497089, ISBN13 9780486497082 (2014)
17. Ain Shams University official web site (2020) History, retrieved at: http://www.asu.edu.eg/
18. El-Qulity, S.A., Mohamed, A.W., Bafail, A.O., Abdelaal, R.M.S.: A multistage procedure for optimal distribution of preparatory-year students to faculties and departments: A mixed integer nonlinear goal programming model with enhanced differential evolution algorithm. J. Comput. Nonlinear Dyn. **13**(11), 7847–7863 (2016)
19. Ali Khater, M, Ali Wagdy, M.: Control Parameters in differential evolution (DE): A short review. Robot Autom Eng J. **3**(2), 555607 (2018)

20. Khater, M., Wagdy, A., Elfeky E.Z. Saleh. M.: Solving constrained non-linear integer and mixed integer global optimization problems using enhanced directed differential evolution algorithm. In Machine Learning Paradigms: Theory and Application, Cham, Switzerland: Springer, (2019)
21. Mohamed, A.W.: Solving stochastic programming problems using new approach to differential evolution algorithm. Egyptian Informatics J. **18**(2), 75–86, (2017)
22. Hadi, A.A., Mohamed, A.W., Jambi, K.M.: LSHADE-SPA memetic framework for solving large-scale optimization problems. Complex & Intell. Syst. **5**(1), 25–40 (2019)
23. Song, Y., Wu, D., Wagdy Mohamed, A., Zhou, X., Zhang, B., Deng, W.: Enhanced success history adaptive DE for parameter optimization of photovoltaic models. Complex. **2021**, Article ID 6660115, pp. 22 (2021)
24. Mohamed, A.W., Mohamed, A.K., Elfeky, E.Z. Saleh, M.: Enhanced directed differential evolution algorithm for solving constrained engineering optimization problems. Int. J. Appl. Metaheuristic Comput. **10**(1) 1–28 (2019)
25. Agrawal, P., Ganesh, T., Mohamed, A.W.: Solving knapsack problems using a binary gaining sharing knowledge-based optimization algorithm. Complex Intell. Syst. (2021)
26. Agrawal, P., Ganesh, T. Mohamed, A.W.: A novel binary gaining–sharing knowledge-based optimization algorithm for feature selection. Neural Comput & Applic. (2020)
27. Muangkote, N., Photong, L., Sukprasert, A.: Effectiveness of constrained handling techniques of improved constrained differential evolution algorithm applied to constrained optimization problems in mechanical engineering (2019)
28. Long, W., Liang, X., Huang, Y., Chen, Y.: A hybrid differential evolution augmented Lagrangian method for constrained numerical and engineering optimization. Comput.-Aided Design **45**(12), 1562–1574 (2013)
29. Bahreininejad, A.: Improving the performance of water cycle algorithm using augmented Lagrangian method. Adv. Eng. Softw. **132**, 55–64 (2019)
30. Deb, K.: An efficient constraint handling method for genetic algorithms. Comput. Methods Appl. Mech. Eng. **186**(2–4), 311–338 (2000)
31. Coello, C.A.C.: Theoretical and numerical constraint-handling techniques used with evolutionary algorithms: a survey of the state of the art. Comput. Methods Appl. Mech. Eng. **191**(11–12), 1245–1287 (2002)

Predicating COVID19 Epidemic in Nepal Using the SIR Model

Pawan Thapa

Abstract **Background:** The propagation of infectious diseases through a population is a natural spatial and temporal process of great importance for modern society. Thus, the SIR model of COVID 19 proposed a greater understanding of the disease's spatial diffusion and prediction. It develops a model that simulates the spread of illness. **Methods:** The study creates a simulating SIR model in a worst-case scenario COVID-19. It estimates the models' parameters by minimizing the negative log-likelihood function using the Nelder- Mead method. According to this model, the pandemic height reached by the mid of August, the end of October. About 1 million people of age group 10–19 and 20–29 with a probability of 30% infected by then, which translates to about 552 severe cases, about 175 cases in need of intensive care (there are about 1595 *ICU beds*, and 840 ventilators are available in 194 hospitals in Nepal, WHO, 2020) and up to 30 deaths per day. **Conclusion:** This simulation type can help improve comprehension of disease spread dynamics and provide control measures for an epidemic outbreak. The suggestion that authorities need to implement a strict containment strategy over a long period to control disease spreading on the community and humans.

Keywords Susceptible · Infectious · Recovered · SIR model · COVID 19 · Predication

1 Introduction

COVID-19 has spread in 213 countries, infecting more than two hundred million confirmed cases worldwide (as on August 21, 2020) [1]. The outbreak was announced by the World Health Organization (WHO) as a pandemic on March 11, 2020, like Italy, Iran, South Korea, and Japan reported surging numbers of cases [2]. The number of cases outside China quickly increased [3, 4]. A report on January 24 recommends using personal protective equipment and intense testing require [5–7]. Several other

P. Thapa (✉)
Department of Geomatics Engineering, Kathmandu University, Dhulikhel, Nepal
e-mail: pawan.thapa@ku.edu.np

D. Oliva et al. (eds.), *Artificial Intelligence for COVID-19*, Studies in Systems, Decision and Control 358, https://doi.org/10.1007/978-3-030-69744-0_14

studies have estimated that numbers of infections in many countries are likely to be considerably more significant than the reported cases [8, 9].

Nepal confirmed the first case on January 23, 2020, when a 31-year-old student returned to Kathmandu from Wuhan on January 9, tested positive for the disease [10]. The first case of local transmission confirms on April 4 in Kailali District. The first death that occurred on May 14 in Nepal was that of a 29-year-old postnatal woman from Sindhupalchok [11]. A country-wide lockdown came into effect on March 24, 2020, and ended on July 21, 2020 [12]. As of August 17, 2020, the Ministry of Health and Population (MoHP) has confirmed 27,241 cases, 17,495 recoveries, and 107 deaths in the country [13]. In the meantime, 529,427 PCR tests in 40 laboratories across the country [14]. Nepal, on January 23, bordering districts of India, were reported to be in high alert, and medical personnel puts various entry points along the Indo-Nepal border [11, 12, 14].

Many studies have been recently reported by researchers to understand the dynamics of this pandemic [15, 16]. In Nepal, the forecast for COVID-19 has few studies to understand the COVID-19 epidemic spread [17, 18]. This paper study of the epidemiological Susceptible-Infected-Recovered (SIR) model for the spread of COVID-19 of Nepal and analysis the correlation with its neighbors China and India [4, 19]. It will forecast 90 days, which will be the guideline to address this pandemic and plan the economic, social activities. This model result depends on the quality of data available, and the progress of the spread of the virus's spread may also affect the predictions [20–22].

2 Materials and Methods

2.1 *Study Area*

The study area is Nepal and its neighboring countries China and India. Nepal faces tremendous increase of confirmed case after end of lockdown and allowing economic activities due to government unable to increase test rate, ventilator, ICUs, and designated hospitals during that period [23–25]. Another is migrant worker coming back here, through numerous ways which risk its own family and community [26] (Fig. 1).

2.2 *Data Collection*

The study used datasets acquired from different sources are shown in Table 1.

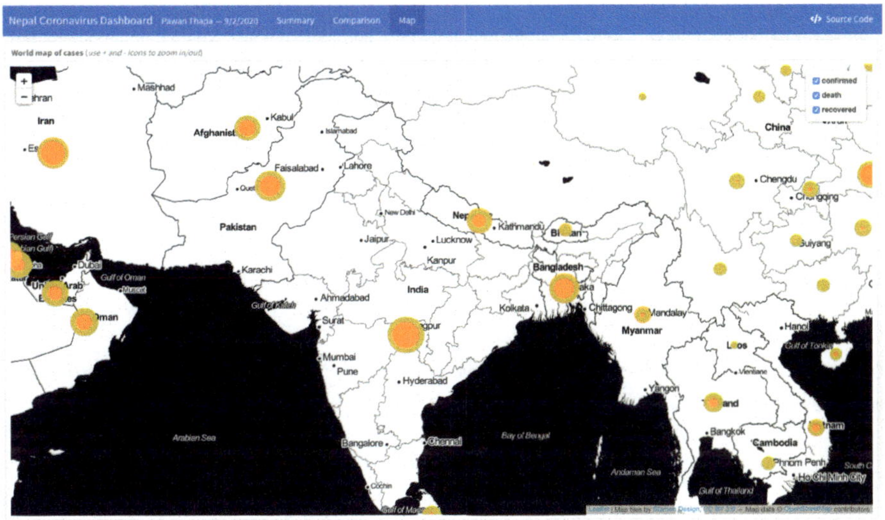

Fig. 1 Study area used for predicating COVID 19 [29]

Table 1 The datasets used for the SIR modelling

Datasets	Data source
	From Wikipedia, the free encyclopedia
COVID 19	https://en.wikipedia.org/wiki/COVID-19_pandemic_in_Nepal Ministry of Health and Population, Government of Nepalhttps://www.mohp.gov.np/eng/
Population	World Population Prospects 2019
	https://population.un.org/wpp/

2.3 Methods

The SIR is one of the simplest compartmental models consists of Susceptible (S), Infectious (I), and Removed (R) [27]. S means the people who have less immune to the disease, I represent those who are contacted and confirmed of disease, and R are those who have recovered from the disease. The population data consider during this outbreak do not include new births, death, and migration (Fig. 2).

N = S + I + R = Constant.

The SIR model of ordinary differential equations [24]:

$$\frac{dS}{dt} = -\frac{\beta IS}{N} \tag{1}$$

$$\frac{dI}{dt} = -\frac{\beta IS}{N} - \gamma I \tag{2}$$

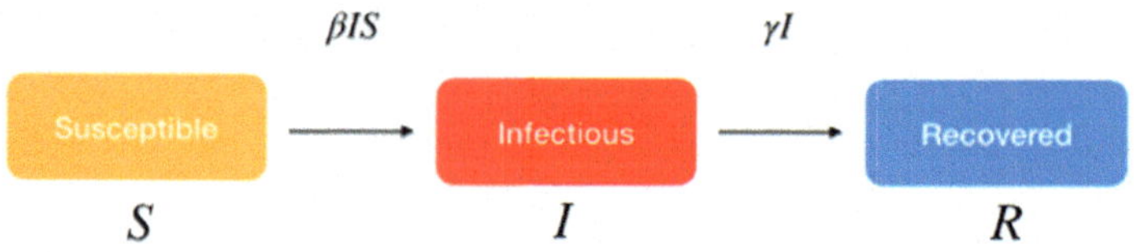

Fig. 2 The methodological framework for SIR model (Kai Sasaki)

$$\frac{dI}{dt} = -\gamma I \tag{3}$$

where, S(t) is the number of susceptible persons at time t, I = I(t) is the number of infected persons at time t, R(t) is the number of recovered persons in time t, β is the contact rate, and 1/γ is the average infectious period. In particular, the model with three equations can reduce to one function about the total infection count (C = I + R) [28]. The epidemiological data collected from the Ministry of Health and Population, Government of Nepal (https://www.mohp.gov.np/eng/) till 30 August 2020 from the date of the first case detected, and other states in (Table 1). The simulations of the SIR model perform on the Rstudio [4, 18, 29].

3 Results

The results showed that India's new confirmed cases plummeted. However, Nepal and China have increases in gradual phase (Fig. 3a); the two types: confirmed and death (Fig. 3b), where India confirmed cases reach more than 3.5 million, where

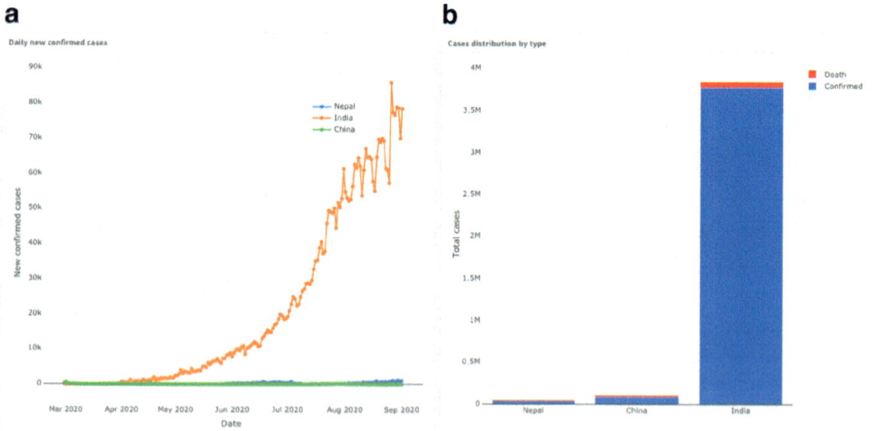

Fig. 3 Line graph of daily confirmed cases Coronavirus of Nepal, China and India (**a**) Bar graph of death and confirmed cases of Nepal, China, and India (**b**)

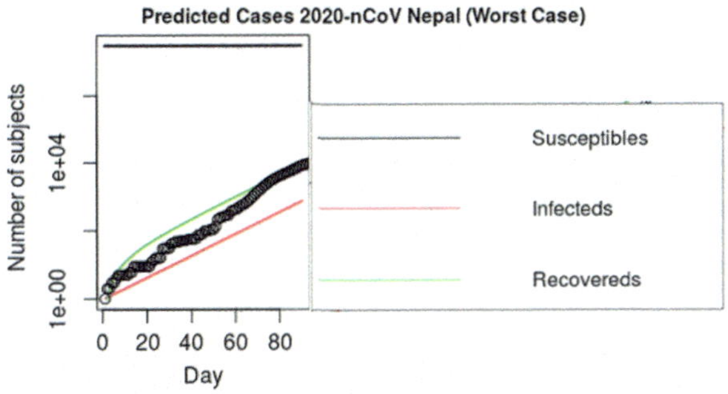

Fig. 4 SIR model predicating the cases of COVID 19 for 90 days

Nepal and China are increasing in gradual phase. Nepal cases will increase as PCR testing has significantly available throughout the nation.

The SIR model was used to determine the coronavirus cases for 90 days (Fig. 4) of Nepal. The predication shows the suspect of new cases in black, the infected cases in red, and recovered in green. There is sharp growth of three cases: susceptible, infected, recovered starting from 20 days up to 90 days.

The potential age group line graph of Nepal generates in Rstudio by using Nepal's population data through the united nations world population prospects (Fig. 4). It's a category into ten age groups of males and females. The age group 0–9 has around 9% population, and more than 10% are age group 10–19, and 20–29, starting from 30–39 the line graph sharply decline around 1% of 80–89 of the total population. This study shows that two age groups, 10–19 and 20–29, are susceptible to coronavirus with a probability of 30% [24, 30, 31]. Therefore, the government, health workers, hospitals, and other stakeholders should take an intensive measure of tracing, tracking, and testing to reduce this pandemic's risk (Fig. 5).

4 Discussion

A simple S-I-R model refers to this as one of the baseline models [32]. The study shows the cumulative number of confirmed cases plummeted from mid-August in Nepal and India. One of the main reasons is increasing the test sample from all over Nepal hospitals, other through the incoming of people from different people. According to the ministry, COVID-19 confirmed cases highest on the age group 20–29, 10–19, and 30–39. The confirmed cases among people aged between 20 and 29 years stand at 1,792, representing nearly 39% of total infections. Likewise, according to the Health Ministry, 1,195 cases in the age group from 10 to 19 years and 975 cases confirmed in 30–39 years. Nepal was considered one of the highest risk areas for the pandemic and one of the least prepared [21, 33, 34]. However, WHO later re-classified Nepal to "Very Vulnerable." [35]. It sees a significant influx of people return from India [36]. The first COVID-19 case confirmed returned from China on 9 January [4, 37].

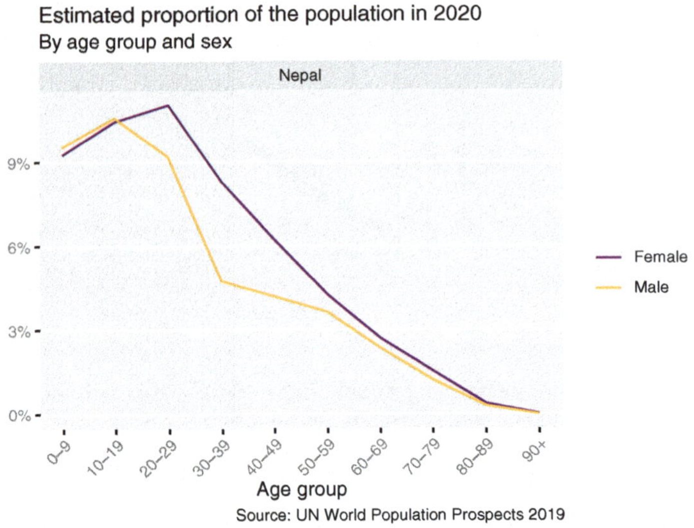

Fig. 5 Nepal Population Male and Female categorized in different age-groups

By 4 April, six additional cases had confirmed in abroad return people; and patients that day, the first local transmission case was confirmed [38]. The figures nearly doubled on a single day on 17 April, when 12 Indian nationals from Delhi, quarantined in a mosque in Bhulke of Udayapur, tested positive for the disease [39]. Increased testing in the Bhulke area discovered 16 new cases within a week [40, 41]. The four new patients found in Bhulke in the following weeks; the first case outside Bhulke confirms on 14 May in a journalist from Gaighat Bazaar who had reported from Bhulke and attended other coronavirus-related events, bringing the total in Udayapur to 33 [41, 42]. The comparison also plays a significant role as India and china cases increased, Nepal also increases as these neighboring countries are similar to culture and religion. People of the north are their relationship with neighboring China, and the south side has a close relationship with India. Therefore, this will provide an understanding of the situation and make decisions to open borders and even apply compulsory PCR tests for crossing borders. Due to several confirmed cases where patients do not know from whom they get it, it significantly proves the community transmission denied by the health ministry [15, 43, 44]. The last few months' significant rises in the number of cases and no signs of abating show this pandemic transmitted on the community.

5 Conclusions

The SIR model determines the behavior of a pandemic and prediction. It minimizes the negative log-likelihood function using the Nelder-Mead method. The result shows the pandemic height reached by the mid of August, the end of October. About 1 million people of age group 10–19 and 20–29 with a probability of 30% infected by then, which translates to about 552 severe cases, about 175 cases in need of intensive care (there are about 1595 *ICU beds*, and 840 ventilators are available in 194 hospitals in Nepal, WHO, 2020 [45]) and up to 30 deaths per day. This simulation can help improve comprehension of disease spread dynamics and provide control measures for an epidemic outbreak. The suggestion is that authorities need to implement a strict containment strategy over a long period to control the pandemic situation successfully. Underdeveloped countries are always a high risk of health pandemic. They should learn lessons to strengthen their health system through continuous updating, maintenance, and up-gradation.

References

1. 20200512-covid-19-sitrep-113.pdf. Accessed 3 Sept 2020. [Online]. https://www.who.int/docs/default-source/coronaviruse/situation-reports/20200512-covid-19-sitrep-113.pdf?sfvrsn=feac3b6d_2
2. Statement on the second meeting of the International Health Regulations (2005) Emergency Committee regarding the outbreak of novel coronavirus (2019-nCoV). https://www.who.int/news-room/detail/30-01-2020-statement-on-the-second-meeting-of-the-international-health-regulations-(2005)-emergency-committee-regarding-the-outbreak-of-novel-coronavirus-(2019-ncov. Accessed 3 Sept 2020
3. WHO Director-General's opening remarks at the media briefing on COVID-19 - 11 March 2020. https://www.who.int/dg/speeches/detail/who-director-general-s-opening-remarks-at-the-media-briefing-on-covid-19—11-March-2020. Accessed 3 Sept 2020
4. COVID-19 pandemic in Nepal, Wikipedia. 2 Sept 2020, Accessed: Sep. 03, 2020. [Online]. https://en.wikipedia.org/w/index.php?title=COVID-19_pandemic_in_Nepal&oldid=976372442
5. Blog—Science and Revolution. http://scienceandrevolution.org/blog. Accessed 3 Sept 2020
6. Clinical features of patients infected with 2019 novel coronavirus in Wuhan, China - The Lancet. https://www.thelancet.com/journals/lancet/article/PIIS0140-6736(20)30183-5/fulltext. Accessed 3 Sept 2020
7. Timeline of the COVID-19 pandemic in January 2020. Wikipedia. Aug. 29, 2020. [Online]. https://en.wikipedia.org/w/index.php?title=Timeline_of_the_COVID-19_pandemic_in_January_2020&oldid=975553379. Accessed 3 Sept 2020
8. Flaxman, S. et al.: Estimating the effects of non-pharmaceutical interventions on COVID-19 in Europe. Nature **584**(7820), Art. no. 7820 (2020)). https://doi.org/10.1038/s41586-020-2405-7
9. Lau, H., et al.: The association between international and domestic air traffic and the coronavirus (COVID-19) outbreak. J. Microbiol. Immunol. Infect. **53**(3), 467–472 (2020). https://doi.org/10.1016/j.jmii.2020.03.026
10. Shrestha, R., Shrestha, S., Khanal, P., Kc, B.: Nepal's first case of COVID-19 and public health response. J. Travel Med. **27**(3) (2020). https://doi.org/10.1093/jtm/taaa024
11. https://kathmandupost.com/sitemap/news/66/columns/2020/03/30/covid-19-weakest-links/national/2020/03/08/icymi-top-stories-from-sunday-march-8. Accessed 3 Sept 2020

12. DoHS-Annual-Report-FY-2074-75-date-22-Ashad-2076-for-web-1.pdf. [Online]. https://dohs.gov.np/wp-content/uploads/2019/07/DoHS-Annual-Report-FY-2074-75-date-22-Ashad-2076-for-web-1.pdf. Accessed 3 Sept 2020
13. crisis solution_current. https://nepalresearch.com/crisis_solution/index.html. Accessed 3 Sept 2020
14. Ghimire, S.S.: 206 Nepalis die of coronavirus across the globe as of Saturday evening. My Republica. http://myrepublica.nagariknetwork.com/news/96983/. Accessed 3 Sept 2020
15. Government decides to lift the four-month-long coronavirus lockdown, but with conditions. https://kathmandupost.com/national/2020/07/21/government-decides-to-lift-the-four-month-long-coronavirus-lockdown-but-with-conditions. Accessed 3 Sept 2020
16. Report 13 - Estimating the number of infections and the impact of non-pharmaceutical interventions on COVID-19 in 11 European countries. Imperial College London. http://www.imperial.ac.uk/medicine/departments/school-public-health/infectious-disease-epidemiology/mrc-global-infectious-disease-analysis/covid-19/report-13-europe-npi-impact/. Accessed 3 Sept 2020
17. A Comprehensive Public Health Evaluation of Lockdown as a Non-pharmaceutical Intervention on COVID-19 Spread in India: National Trends Masking State Level Variations. https://www.ncbi.nlm.nih.gov/pmc/articles/PMC7310653/. Accessed 3 Sept 2020
18. Europe PMC. https://europepmc.org/articles/pmc7310653/bin/85905-2020.05.25.20113043-1.docx. Accessed 3 Sept 2020
19. PDF) COVID-19 in India: State-wise Analysis and Prediction. ResearchGate. https://www.researchgate.net/publication/341037704_COVID-19_in_India_State-wise_Analysis_and_Prediction. Accessed 3 Sept 2020
20. PDF) A Short Communication on Agent-based modeling approach applied to the spread of cholera. ResearchGate. https://www.researchgate.net/publication/342513642_A_Short_Communication_on_Agent-based_modeling_approach_applied_to_the_spread_of_cholera. Accessed 3 Sept 2020
21. Salam Kathryn, R.A.: Is South Asia Prepared for the Wuhan Virus? Foreign Policy. https://foreignpolicy.com/2020/01/28/south-asia-prepared-wuhan-virus-china-nepal-india-health/. Accessed 3 Sept 2020
22. D. Guerrero, "Spread of Covid-19: a Study Case of Honduras, Forecasting with Logistic Model and SIR Model," p. 13
23. "Cabinet decides to ease lockdown in phases. https://kathmandupost.com/national/2020/06/10/cabinet-to-discuss-ways-to-ease-lockdown. Accessed 3 Sept 2020
24. Health Sector Response to Novel Coronavirus (2019-nCoV) English.pdf. [Online]. https://www.mohp.gov.np/attachments/article/543/Health%20Sector%20Response%20to%20Novel%20Coronavirus%20(2019-nCoV)%20English.pdf. Accessed 3 Sept 2020
25. Nepal relaxes COVID-19 lockdown for most economic activities - Xinhual English.news.cn. http://www.xinhuanet.com/english/2020-06/12/c_139132345.htm. Accessed 3 Sept 2020
26. Gill, P.: COVID-19: Nepal in Crisis. https://thediplomat.com/2020/06/covid-19-nepal-in-crisis/. Accessed 3 Sept 2020
27. Hethcote, H.W.: The mathematics of infectious diseases. SIAM Rev. **42**(4), 599–653 (2000). https://doi.org/10.1137/S0036144500371907
28. Estimation of the final size of the COVID-19 epidemicl medRxiv. https://www.medrxiv.org/content/10.1101/2020.02.16.20023606v5. Accessed 3 Sept 2020
29. COVID-19 in Belgium. Stats and R. https://www.statsandr.com/blog/covid-19-in-belgium/. Accessed 3 Sept 2020
30. World Population Prospects - Population Division - United Nations. https://population.un.org/wpp/. Accessed 3 Sept 2020
31. Nepal Population (2020) - Worldometer. https://www.worldometers.info/world-population/nepal-population/. Accessed 3 Sept 2020
32. PDF) SIR Model, ResearchGate. https://www.researchgate.net/publication/341001056_SIR_Model. Accessed 3 Sept 2020

33. Nepal ill-prepared for coronavirus outbreak. https://thehimalayantimes.com/nepal/nepal-ill-prepared-for-coronavirus-outbreak/. Accessed 3 Sept 2020
34. Nepal ranks 111th in health security index. The Himalayan Times, Feb. 08, 2020. https://thehimalayantimes.com/nepal/nepal-ranks-111th-in-health-security-index/. Accessed 3 Sept 2020
35. N. Times, Nepal lockdown to be extended. https://www.nepalitimes.com/latest/nepal-lockdown-to-be-extended/. Accessed 3 Sept 2020
36. Amid Covid-19 threat, Banbasa border sees a sudden influx of people returning home from India. https://kathmandupost.com/sudurpaschim-province/2020/03/18/amid-covid-19-threat-banbasa-border-sees-a-sudden-influx-of-people-returning-home-from-india. Accessed 3 Sept 2020
37. Nepal confirms first case of deadly coronavirus - The Economic Times. https://economictimes.indiatimes.com/news/international/world-news/nepal-confirms-first-case-of-deadly-coronavirus/articleshow/73590302.cms. Accessed 3 Sept 2020
38. P.| Apr 4, 2020, and 15:48 Ist, Nepal confirms 3 new coronavirus cases - Times of India. The Times of India. https://timesofindia.indiatimes.com/world/south-asia/nepal-confirms-3-new-coronavirus-cases/articleshow/74981586.cms. Accessed 3 Sept 2020
39. Republica, COVID-19 cases jump to 16 in Nepal as two more patients tested positive (with video). My Republica. http://myrepublica.nagariknetwork.com/news/92625/. Accessed 3 Sept 2020
40. B. ANUPAM/RSS, State-1 sees three COVID-19 cases today; taking number of patients to 27. My Republica. http://myrepublica.nagariknetwork.com/news/93027/. Accessed 3 Sept 2020
41. Two new persons detected with COVID-19 taking infection count to 47. The Himalayan Times, Apr. 23, 2020. https://thehimalayantimes.com/nepal/two-new-persons-detected-with-covid-19-taking-infection-count-to-47/. Accessed 3 Sept 2020
42. First Covid-19 case outside Bhulke found in Udayapur. https://kathmandupost.com/province-no-1/2020/05/17/first-covid-19-case-outside-bhulke-found-in-udayapur. Accessed 3 Sept 2020
43. Government to close down border with India and China for a week. https://kathmandupost.com/national/2020/03/22/government-to-close-down-border-with-india-and-china-for-a-week. Accessed 3 Sept 2020
44. Hyolmo, K.: Nepal is untouched by coronavirus so far, say govt authorities. My Republica. http://myrepublica.nagariknetwork.com/news/85487/. Accessed 3 Sept 2020
45. Situation report, p. 12

Feature Extraction of Coronavirus X-Ray Images by RNN, Correlational Networks, and PNN

V. Kakulapati and Appiah Prince

Abstract Today, the entire world is suffering and fear with the epidemic of coronavirus. The statistics of coronavirus as on current data, 213 countries affected by this pandemic, more than 1.1 cr people, suffering from this killer virus, and about 6L fatality are recording. This virus is spreading speedily, and the patients are mainly suffering from breathing. The patient having previous health issues will get more possibility of this disease. In this work, try to evaluate the COVID 19 patient x-ray images by using DL (deep learning) techniques developed on the grouping of a recurrent neural network (RNN) and a correlational network to identify COVID-19 automatically is used in the prediction of high-risk outbreaks to learn on the prognostic code sequences of patients. By use of RNNs helps the model to assess difference in patient status in terms of time and thereby improve predictive precision. A correlational neural network is to identify the salient features for CORONAVIRUS, and these features are feed into a Probabilistic neural network (PNN) for better corona diagnosis. The experimental result gives improved accuracy for analyzing coronavirus disease.

Keywords PNN · Correlation · Neural · Recurrent · Diagnosis · Corona · Accuracy

1 Introduction

Coronavirus is detected in the Wuhan province of china, raising the risk to human health, commerce, and the financial system. The infection displays substantially similar characteristics to some of the other bacterial infections. Consequently, the condition is challenging to handle, owing to the increasing spread rate of the virus.

V. Kakulapati (✉)
Sreenidhi Institute of Science and Technology, Yamnampet, Ghatkesar, Hyderabad 501301, Telangana, India
e-mail: vldms@yahoo.com

A. Prince
ITMO University, St. Petersburg, Russia
e-mail: princeappiah35@gmail.com

D. Oliva et al. (eds.), *Artificial Intelligence for COVID-19*, Studies in Systems, Decision and Control 358, https://doi.org/10.1007/978-3-030-69744-0_15

As the COVID-19 global epidemic continues to evolve, analysts attempt to improve, recognize, reduce, and prevent its progression. Primary research fields include researching the spread of COVID-19, promoting its diagnosis, designing potential vaccination and therapies, and considering the disease outbreak's socio-economic impacts.

If the epidemic continues and the number of actual cases and sufferers with severe renal distress and respiratory diseases rises, there could be legitimate reasons to be highly worried about the effects of this infectious disease outbreak [1]. Significant focus has been paid to defining effective ways of seeking effective solutions relevant to COVID-19. But the growing volume of information, massive volumes of data that targets themselves used during the battle against the epidemic, remains a significant challenge for investigators and decision-makers to address.

A chest radiology assessment is quite prevalent and is an economically viable methodology for digital diagnostics. The doctor's manifestations of chest or x-ray can also be very demanding. Nevertheless, CT (computed tomography) imaging of lungs may even be more problematic than chest diagnosis. The intelligent public datasets are scarce. It is indeed challenging to diagnose and identify with assistive devices significant therapeutic at various medical facilities employing pulmonary X-rays. The lack of characteristics to interpret an image is noticeable, especially to massive x-ray images datasets.

Although medical imaging assessments can be performed faster and are much more accessible provided the proliferation of chest radiology imaging systems [2] in sophisticated healthcare providers, a need for more specialized radiologists to characterize the x-ray images poses a limitation according to the specific visual markers observed in the images.

Because of its infectiousness and acceleration, the COVID-19 epidemic can be seen as severe [3]. The medicare sector's effect is also essential based on the number of patients who need ICU admission and long-term automatic ventilators [4]. Early diagnostics are imperative to accurately control healthcare, possibly to relieve stress. AI strategy for COVID-19 and some pneumonic forms can provide an inexpensive and accurate assessment in this scenario.

Though a wide range of deep learning AI systems have a significant improvement for predicting the potential of COVID-19 by using x-ray analysis, most of them are restricted sources and aren't really open to the scientific community and stimulation of this kind of applications.

The treatment strategy to COVID-19, depending on digital diagnostics, has been the priority in many medical applications, with more research researching diagnostic detection technologies. Recently discovered an investigation of papers in the domains of AI in response to this, which utilize patient's health information to predict disease severity and existing non-invasive assessments to monitor diagnoses from Computer Tomography (CT) and X-Ray scans.

Recent years have seen significant development of machine learning (ML) and AI. Machine learning and Artificial intelligence methods have played a key role in healthcare applications such as healthcare image analysis, computerized diagnoses, image recognition, image synthesis, image classification, segmentation techniques, picture-led care, image recovery, and analysis ML object detection method from photographic images are a powerful and efficient representation of information. The ML and AI help doctors to detect and forecast the likelihood of illness correctly and more effectively and to avoid it in time. This increases physicians'and analysts' ability to consider how the generic variants leading to infection can be studied. In studying the disease, many investigators use deep learning algorithms, such as CNN, RNN (Recurrent Neural Network), Correlation Network, etc. In this chapter, apart from CNN, RNN, and applied Correlational neural network, probability neural network in the analysis of covid 9 lung images.

This chapter should be arranged: The Sect. 1 outlines the presentation of the theme. Section 2 discusses several works related to the classification of the lung X-ray images or lung nodule. Section 3 gives an explanation for this analysis. Section 4 provides a thorough overview of the methods used. Section 5 addresses the findings of the study of disease methods. The related topic is discussed in the Sect. 6 topic. Section 7 outlines the study while Sect. 8 presents future directions for study.

2 Related Work

Diagnosis of COVID-19, chest X-Ray images, especially thoracic x-rays, may also be used. During areas with restricted access to appropriate healthcare facilities like CT scanners, the usability and accessibility of imaging tools required may be an option. As seen in [5–7], it is possible to choose Deep Learning (DL) techniques in X-Ray imaging utilizing specific frameworks that are used for CT scans, for example, ResNet [8] and CNN [9].

A coronavirus detection system [10] is focused on a deep architecture using X-ray images. The x-ray images in data set are 76 images of coronavirus instances, pneumonia cases images are 4290, and normal patient images are 1583 images. For coronavirus cases, the procedure has reached 98.3% precision. A Transfer Learning Technique with CNN [11] is suggested to efficiently detect coronavirus instances by withdrawing critical characteristics from the chest x-rays.

ML and AI approaches are the basis of Automatic or CAD (Computer Assisted Diagnostic System) applications. The DL technology for identifying coronavirus (COVID-Net) [12] has describable precision in standard, pneumonia, and COVID-19, which obtained a ranking of 92.4%. Identified with DL models [13] in X-ray images, COVID-19 recommended the COVIDX-Net variant of 7 CNN architecture models. SVM classification was utilized [14] to group features from multiple neural networks altering models in X-ray images and achieved the highest precision of the ResNet50 model. A DL model has been developed in [15], utilizing 224 images of COVID-19 and attained an accuracy of 98.75% and 93%. Precision 98% attained for the identification of chest CT images using ResNet 50 [16].

CT and CXR imaging techniques are essential for diagnosing COVID-19. Many researchers are utilized in developing diagnosis models ranging from predictive models to feature learning have extensively analyzed the historical conception of image diagnostic systems.

In coronavirus, diagnostics from x-ray becomes one of the most common and successful methods. Newly updated developments to coronavirus identification have carried out many investigations [17–19]. For instance, CNN [20] has been utilized to detect Coronavirus in CT dependent on the formation network. CT images were categorized into three groups in the fully - connected layer: stable coronavirus and contagious pneumonia. In [14], CXR a specific ImageNet model has been pre-processed to extract high-level functionality These functions have been integrated into SVM to predict COVID-19 cases as an ML classifier. A transmission-based CNN-based architecture [21], known as COVID-Net, was utilized to identify images into four classes: standard, infectious, non-coronavirus, and Virus infections.

Inaccurately identifying bacterial pneumonia, ML techniques are utilized, specifically for radiography and x-ray images, growth prognosis, and cryptoscopic image study [22]. In the chest X-ray and CT images, infectious pathogenic variations comprise a variety of features [23]. The anomalous division and shading in the image are seen by coronavirus [24] by utilizing CNN-based techniques on X-ray and CT studies [25]. In research undertaken before using the CNN process, analysis with other attribute extraction techniques are usually used.

To develop DL models for detection of the coronavirus transfer learning (TL) approach [26]. Three DL models were chosen and modified to accurately detect and analyze coronavirus utilizing x-ray, inception ResNet V2, InceptionNetV3, and NASNetLarge and used a dataset containing 850 coronaviruses confirmed cases, 500 non-coronavirus cases, and 915 regular X-ray images. Among these, InceptionNetV3 produced the maximum results with 98.6% and 99% precision, respectively, data intensification in model training.

Developed a deep ensemble model [27] that incorporates deep pneumonia-class performances from all transfer methodologies using a DL concept. Several around 5200 X-rays were classified into 1300 standard X-ray images, 3900 irregular X-rays [28]. A 3.6% classification error was noticed in the model, with 99.6% accuracy in test results from the dataset. In a deep TL model, a CS (Compressed Sensing) [29] was developed to achieve physicians by automatic classification of pneumonia in X-ray. Simulation-based findings revealed that the suggested solution can diagnose the 2.66% mal-classification classification of pneumonia (abnormal/standard).

Considering that neural activity inputs can only pass in that dimension from source to destination at feed-forward networks. Utilizing RNN as it enables transmissions to both routes to the future that permit internal links among secret units [22]. The RNN integrates sequence feeds, unlike an RNN, through a persistent hidden state, wherein initiation depends on the preceding it one step; hence the network can exhibit dynamic temporal conduct [23].

Amenities for identifying COVID-19 from CXR images using a profoundly learned decision-tree classification (32) described that classifier includes three dual Decision Trees (DTs), individually proficient in a DL technique with a CNN developed on a PyTorch frame. During the first statistical model, CXR images are categorized as standard and pathological. The second tree detects irregular images containing infectious diseases, and the third detects inconsistent images bearing contagious diseases. Both first and second DTs are 98 and 80%, respectively, while the third tree's overall precision is 95%. By pre-screening of patients, using DL based decision-tree cataloging is visible for case management and rapid-track decisions.

3 About Coronavirus X-Ray Images

Pneumonia is major complications associated with coronavirus. The bacteria epidemic, which can be affected by environmental pathogens like viruses, bacteria, or parasites, the alveoli, alveolar ducts and pulmonary bronchioles become part of the lung responsible. Infections should not be categorized as anonymity and cluster of various kinds of diseases [31].

Till today, no appropriate therapies publicly available for this epidemic. To assess infectious disease or align the assessment, which aims to improve the broader understanding of its modes of transmission, the spread of lung parenchyma, and related patterns [32] and promote the development of a curative treatment. AI, chest X-Ray, and CT (computed tomography) radionics are suitable tools for diagnosing the disease and screening. As described in [33] in the peripheral and posterior CT images, recognizable abnormalities of ground grass opacity predict coronavirus pneumonia. Consequently, in the exact diagnosis of Covid-19 CT could play a significant role.as advanced images when data from chest x-rays show a coronavirus. AI technologies and Chest X-ray radiology characteristics are of substantial assistance in acquaintance with extensive screenings for each country with access to Devices or diagnostic services for coronavirus [34].

AI and DL strategies used some of their main significant achievements in the characterization of image features. It would even detect signs of the coronavirus in X-ray images and CT scans if that could pick precise details through high-resolution pictures.

An RT-PCR examination of mouth saliva samples and swabs is the primary medical diagnosis for SARS-CoV-2 contaminating [35]. Consequently, as a time of incubation of approximately 14 days is possible [36], the risk for the RT-PCR's negative results should be considered in the preliminary stage. CT will validate cases fixed and making the prognostics of complicated cases significantly more comfortable in the first few days following the onset of indications [37]. The CT captures breathing variations at an elevated in persistent with coronavirus.

Lung x-ray scientific results consider that lung colouring associated with COVID-19 is less sensitive [38]. Also, it should be 90% capable of accurately detecting the infection, which is precision. The small group may have led to responsiveness disparities. The duration between the acute indications and the CT scan may be an essential component in the accuracy of X-ray observations. Whereas during the first three days following the onset of cough and temperature, no infection symptoms were still apparent in the X-rays. Within a week, they were more evident [39].

This risk involved seems to be demonstrated by an Italian experiment of 72 diagnosable patients released in April 2020 [38]. All patients were under isolation at residence before the scanning technique was performed and were hospitalized as everyone's symptoms worsened. The chest X-ray's significance was 69% [40].

Consistent with a FSC (Fleischer Society consensus) statement available on Apr. 7, 2020 [41]:

- Screening of confirmed COVID-19 and conservative patient features of patients is not anticipated because they are a threat to the disease's progression.
- Patients with COVID-19 and deteriorating breathing conditions are seen in the image.
- The severe clinical care of enduring with confirmed coronavirus, which exhibit relatively high-serious medical aspects and increased risk of infection, an x-ray is demonstrated in an information-controlled setting.

Potential consequences are correlated with the regular performance of CT for diverse patients [42]:

- Middle range services, in specific the PPE, due to inappropriate use.
- The severity of spreading to employees, enduring, and carers increased since coronavirus effected individuals are analogous to Radiology's direct and indirect institutions.
- More susceptibility to ionizing radiation

The fundamental impacts on CT were mentioned in adulthood as [43–46]:

- GGOs (ground-glass opacities): longitudinal, micro-pleural, cerebral
- Septal thickening inter/intra-lobular
- Consolidation of airspace
- Vascular bronchial lesion thickening
- Bronchiectasis traction.

3.1 A Common Finding of CT Images

Only in a limited minority of patients should such observations intensify worries about viral infections and other extremely-added diagnoses.

- Lymphadenopathy of the mediastinal process
- Bronchial epidemics: will arise as a COVID-19 complication.
- Slight respiratory nodules
- Blood tree.
- Airborne Thorax.
- cavity.

3.2 *Changes in Chronological CT*

Four CT aspects were characterized:

- Initial stage: regular CT 0–4 days
- Two days after initial infection, approximately 50% of patients have regular CT scans
- Incremental phase (five to eight days): enhanced GGO visibility and outrageous paving
- Peak phase (9 to 13 days):
- Fascination phase (>14 days): "starchy patterns" develop and abnormalities resolve in a month or more after an improvement about infection.

4 Methodology

4.1. CNN: It is one of the most robust profound learning networks with multiple hidden layers. These occult layers are very efficient in transforming and, ultimately, sampling to obtain low-to-high levels of data input characteristics [47]. Thus, for such a data set, the success of CNN is evaluated first. A specific type of multi-layer vision is a CNN, but unlike profound learning architecture, a rudimentary neural network can't recognize complex features. The basic principle underlying CNN [48] is that it should get distinctive features from high-school inputs and convert them to lower-schools for much more unique properties. CNN provides coevolutionary (FC) layers, which are pooled and fully connected.

4.2. Feature selection: Two aspects depend on the success of the forecast. These are the separation characteristics and classification performance. Image segmentation in different classifiers plays a significant role. There are several characteristics of the datasets used to distinguish. Most of them are unrelated to the grouping either in part or entirely. The list of functions is then used to pick various essential features to achieve a reasonable consistency of classification compared with all elements.

With the current growing impact of processing power, DL methods have been used to generate various complicated neural systems like CNNs [49] or RNNs (recurrent neural networks) [50]. Such an approach enables natural language processing, image recognition, speech recognition, and various areas to expand. RNN methods are based on handling estimation problems of time series and include input layer, hidden layers, and one output layer. In the present layer input and output of the previous layer, the hidden layer's result is determined. The use of this method allows an RNN to document process information. Data from the last layer are separated into the following sequence via the exchange between the hidden layers, which builds the relationship in time sequences.

RNNs provide a hidden layer that is transmitted by time, and much-transmitted data can be preserved. Most widely used in prediction applications is that they can handle sequential data of varying lengths.

The set of features can be described as a pre-processing step utilized in computer education to remove outliers, eliminate irrelevant data, optimize learning accuracy, and improve performance perception. A filtration algorithm is used for the correlation-based probabilistic testing procedure, such as the Correlation-based Feature Selection. CFS consists of two critical phases; the first step tests matrix associations between function and function. A further step is to analyze the function space, which is intended to achieve the possible subset. The elevated number of features is extortionate to search all possible subsets to recognize the best. There are several evolutionary computing methods, like the strongest one to define functional space in a properly inferred manner.

The core analysis is using "Probabilistic Neural Network (PNN), and it does better training. In the adaptive classification model in which mathematical modeling variants have been ineffective, PNN incorporates quantitative concepts with machine learning. The PNN explains microbial contamination without growing conditions and the possibility. Transformation in working conditions [51] is caused by mutation. It's a form of the network on a radial basis and refers to the Bayesian decision rule and the probability density function estimators. PNN also involves the identification properties of statistic pattern, which involves nonlinear mappings and grouping. A neural feed-forward network is a supervised PNN algorithm for one-pass learning, also consists of three layers. PNN has training potential to gather data in the scarce form.

5 Implementation

Proposed COVID-19 detection involves many stages, as display in Fig. 1. The steps are briefly explaining here.

1. Collecting X-ray images of patients of COVID-19 as well as healthy patients.
2. Generate 1500 chest X-ray images
3. Provide feature selection on images applying machine learning algorithms (Neural Network).
4. Divide dataset into two groups, training group, and validation group
5. Evaluate the performance of the algorithm on the validation dataset.

5.1 Dataset

The dataset used for this project was obtained from a Kaggle database, which contains an X-ray test on COVID-19 patients. These data set were used for evaluation involving a patient with and without COVID-19. The description of the data is given in Table 1. Only the X-ray images of both persons were employed. The total images for the study 160 image. The imbalance was controlled using the data augmentation method and improving convergence to contribute a better outcome.

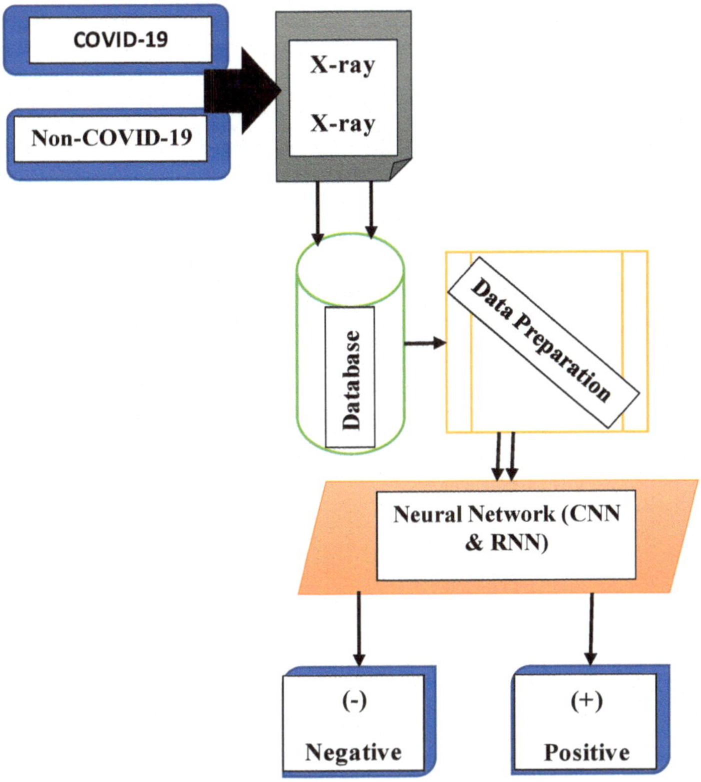

Fig. 1 Propose machine learning diagnose system architecture

Table 1 Dataset

X-ray images	**Frequency**
COVID-19	60
Healthy	100
Total	**160**

Pre-processing x-ray images: The images are pre-processing of data and resize the image as an input for the algorithm. Pre-processed some image Techniques for optimizing machine efficiency and training time acceleration.

5.2 Evaluation Metrics

Metrics like precision, accuracy, recall, and Area under curve graph were used to access the reliability of the two proposed machine learning algorithms. These metrics are computed based on the true-positive, true-negative, false-negative and false-positive.

$$Accuracy = \frac{(TP + TN)}{(TP + TN + FN + FP)}$$

$$Precision = \frac{TP}{(TP + FP)}$$

The accuracy metric measures the percentage of correctly identify cases relative to the provided dataset. Most machine learning performing better if the accuracy is higher.

Precision measures the exactness, which is computed as the percentage of optimistic prediction, which was true positive divided by the number of predicted positives.

The recall is the completeness, which is computed as the percentage of positive that were correctly identified as true positive divided by the number of real positives.

$$Recall = \frac{TP}{TP + FN}$$

F-measure is calculated, combining precision and recall, which is significant for a test dataset involving an imbalance class.

$$F - measure = 2\frac{Precision * Recall}{(Precision + Recall)}$$

The X-ray images were load for pre-processing, preparation, and cleaning to avoid data trawling. The Orange application widget was used for the training of the data as well as its validation. Sample of the data used (X-ray) images are shown in Figs. 2 and 3. The X-ray images had 1024 × 1024 pixels when the model train was pretrained using 224 × 224 pixel images.

The model design for diagnosing COVID-19 was based on CNN, RNN, and PNN. The model was designed to perceive COVID-19 using lung X-ray images. The orange application comes with an image analyzer, which is very powerful and can code to suit the kind of patterns need within the image provided for training.

The detector for COVID-19 was trained and tested on the collected dataset, 70% for training, and 30% as a remainder for testing. To reduce the imbalance of data, the class weight technique was applied. Probably more accurately adjust the weight in the input data to class frequencies. Each model was able to distinguish between the dataset for higher classification accuracy.

The result of the study was very encouraging in the field of diagnosing method in COVID-19. Multiple epochs were applied to train the VGG16 based model of CNN, RNN, and PNN. The use of the machine learning technique was effective. The prediction model for CNN achieved a higher accuracy of 97.2% and an F-measure of

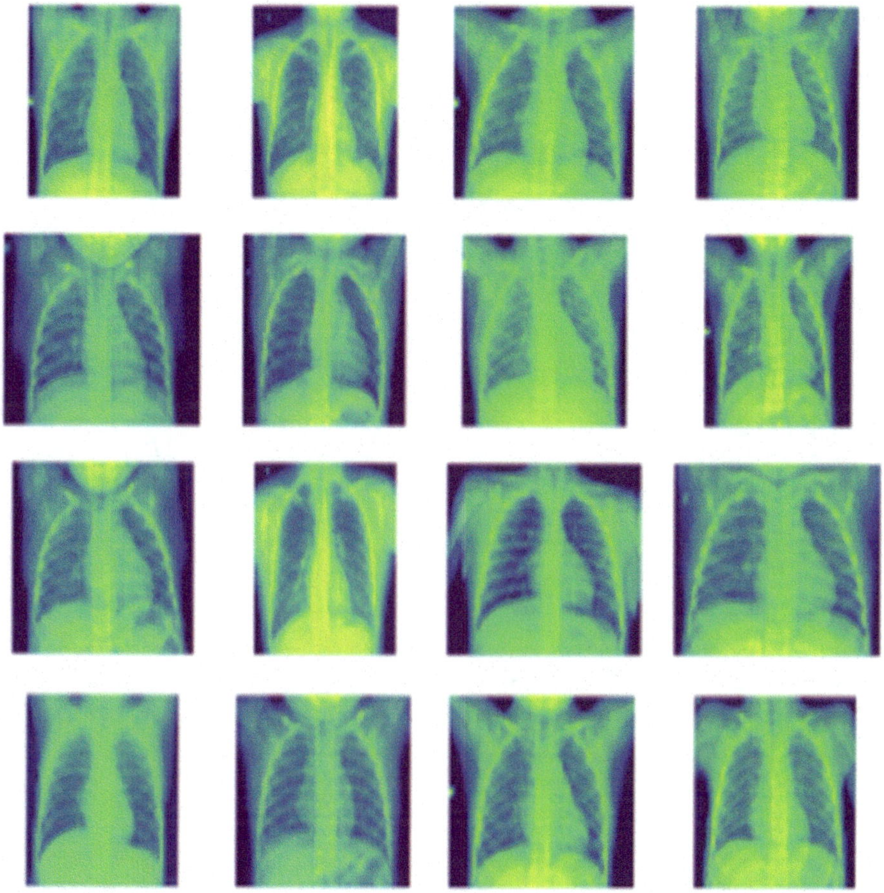

Fig. 2 Normal X-ray images

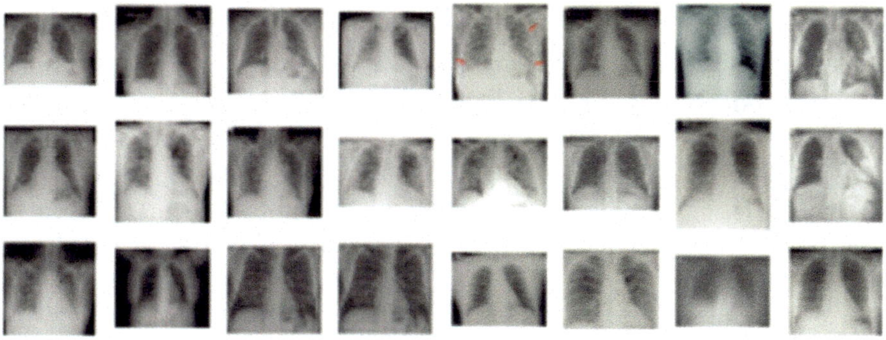

Fig. 3 Abnormal X-ray images

Fig. 4 CNN training and validating accuracy

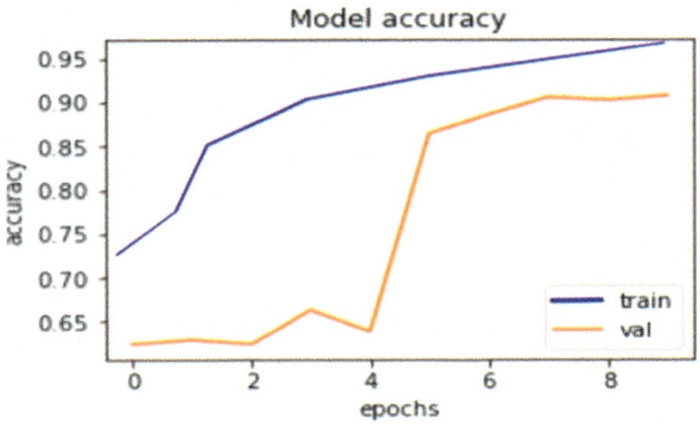

Fig. 5 RNN training and validating accuracy

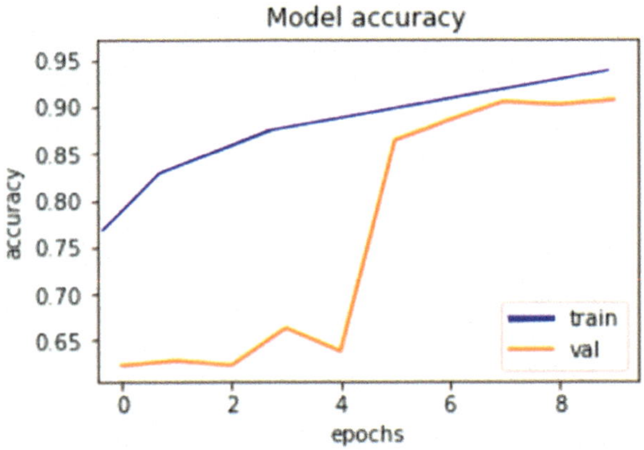

94%. The PNN attained an accuracy of 93.4%, F-measure of 92%, the RNN model for achieving an accuracy of 86.32%, and F-measure of 87%. Figures 4, 5, 6, 7, 8 and 9 shows the performance of both the neural network model to classification accuracy.

6 Discussion

In this chapter, A deep transfer learning of the CNN and RNN Models was developed and tested to identify and recognize X-ray chest images of COVID-19. Each proposed model obtains a better result. Comparing our model accuracy and precision with other models, the CNN, COVID-19 prediction is best. Receiving 97.7% for accuracy and 96.4% for precision. The best training process was gained as the difference between the training and validation became closer. A robust COVID-19 detector was built as the F-measure improved to 0.97. The metrics of AUC was impressive as the model achieved 0.9. Figure 6 shows the result of the metric AUC. Thus, the COVID-19 diagnosis model trained on the x-ray data provides superior performance. metrics.

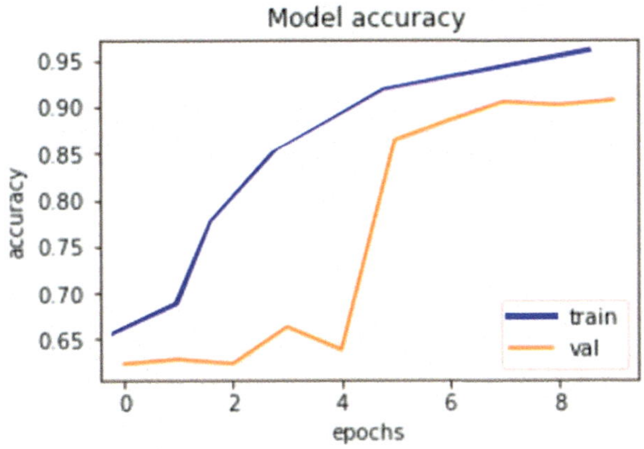

Fig. 6 PNN training and validating accuracy

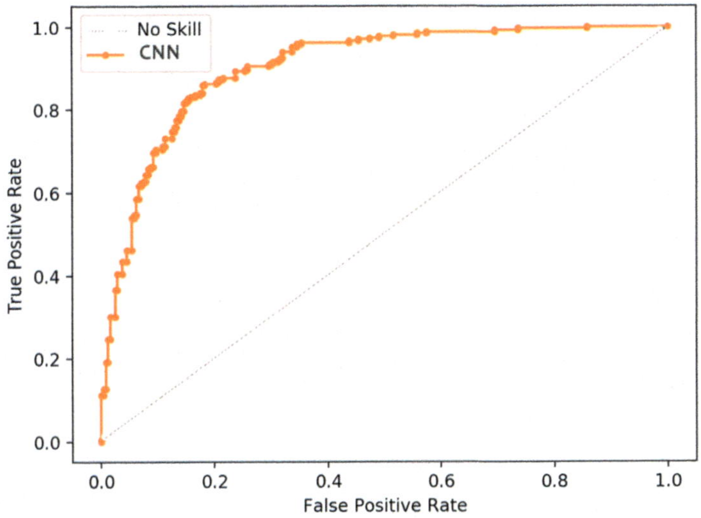

Fig. 7 Area under the curve of CNN

Using CNN is highly sensitive, as it can be seen from Fig. 6, we recommend scientists working on COVID-19 to depend on systems with models built using CNN.

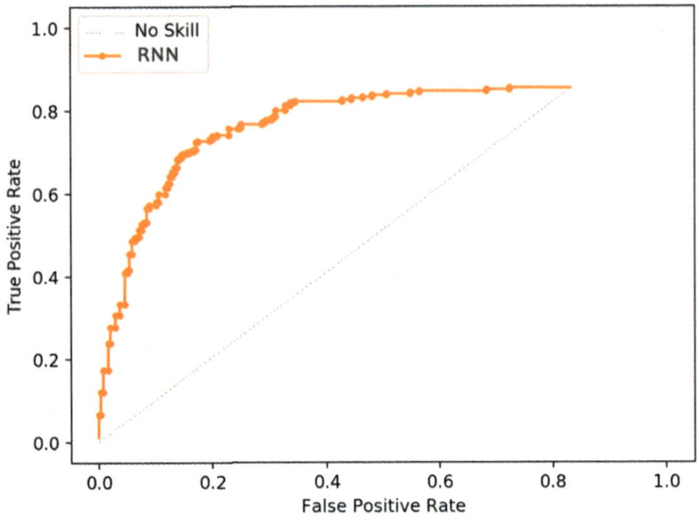

Fig. 8 Area under the curve of RNN

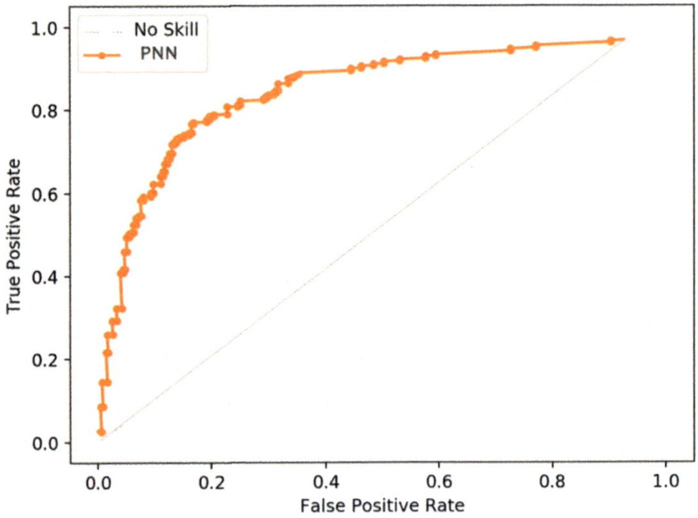

Fig. 9 Area under the curve of PNN

7 Conclusion

The exponential increase of COVID-19 across the globe and an increasing number of deaths need urgent actions from all departments. Future forecasting of potential infections will enable authorities to battle the consequences effectively. In this chapter, the machine learning algorithm was used to analyze COVID-19. COVID-19 with chest X-ray images was detected in the process of modeling utilizing CNN, PNN, and RNN.

8 Future Enhancement

In the future, consider diagnosing COVID-19 in RT-PCR using the VGG-16 version and compare their performance using a high volume of the dataset. Risk modeling is also taken out by using inferential statistics, compartmentalized modeling methods to explain and forecast the health consequences of communicable diseases. The automation of coronavirus prevention uses an extensive data set and develops similarity measures of pandemic symptoms. Utilize the clustering techniques based on location wise and transmission of the spread of the coronavirus. Providing recommendations to prevent the disease which can be built using deep learning techniques. Develop new strategies to enhance classification accuracy and efficiency of corona patient privacy and provide a personalized recommendation to the patient for better diagnosis by applying nature-inspired optimization techniques.

References

1. Guo, T., et al.: Cardiovascular implications of fatal outcomes of patients with coronavirus disease 2019 (COVID-19). JAMA Cardiol. early access, Mar 27, 2020. https://doi.org/10.1001/jamacardio.2020.1017
2. https://www.vision-systems.com/non-factory/life-sciences/article/14173262/covid-19-chest-radiography-deep-learning-virus-detection
3. Tolksdorf, K., et al.: Influenza-associated pneumonia as reference to assess seriousness of coronavirus disease (COVID-19), Euro surveillance 25 (11) (2020)
4. Grasselli, G., et al.: Critical care utilization for the COVID-19 outbreak in lombardy, Italy: early experience and forecast during an emergency response, JAMA (2020)
5. Abbas, A., et al.: Classification of COVID-19 in chest X-ray images using DeTraC deep convolutional neural network. arXiv preprint arXiv:200313815 (2020)
6. Bukhari, S.U.K., et al.: The diagnostic evaluation of Convolutional Neural Network (CNN) for the assessment of chest X-ray of patients infected with COVID-19. medRxiv (2020)
7. Hammoudi, K., et al.: Deep Learning on Chest X-ray Images to Detect and Evaluate Pneumonia Cases at the Era of COVID-19. arXiv preprint arXiv:200403399 (2020)
8. He, K., et al.: Deep residual learning for image recognition. In: Proceedings of the IEEE Conference on Computer Vision and Pattern Recognition, 2016, pp. 770–778
9. LeCun, Y., et.al.: Deep learning. Nature **521**(7553), 436–444 (2015)
10. Ucar, F., et al.: COVIDiagnosis-Net: deep Bayes-SqueezeNet based diagnosis of the coronavirus disease 2019 (COVID-19) from X-ray images. Med. Hypotheses **140**, (2020). https://doi.org/10.1016/j.mehy.2020.109761
11. Apostolopoulos, I.D., et al.: Covid-19: automatic detection from X-ray images utilizing transfer learning with convolutional neural networks. Phys. Eng. Sci. Med., 1–8 (2020). https://doi.org/10.1007/s13246-020-00865-4
12. Wang, L., et al.: COVID-Net: A tailored deep convolutional neural network design for detection of COVID-19 cases from chest radiography images. arXiv preprint arXiv:2003.09871 ((2020))

13. Hemdan, E., et al.: COVIDX-Net: A framework of deep learning classifiers to diagnose COVID-19 in x-ray images. arXiv preprint arXiv:2003.11055 (2020)
14. Sethy, P.K., et al.: Detection of coronavirus Disease (COVID-19) based on Deep Features (2020)
15. Ioannis, D., et al.: COVID-19: Automatic detection from X-ray images utilizing Transfer Learning with Convolutional Neural Networks, arXiv:2003.11617 (2020)
16. Narin, A., et al.: automatic detection of coronavirus disease (COVID-19) Using X-ray images and deep convolutional neural networks. arXiv preprint arXiv:2003.10849 (2020)
17. Dong, D., et al.: The role of imaging in the detection and management of covid-19: a review. IEEE Rev Biomed Eng. (2020)
18. Li, L., et al.: Artificial intelligence distinguishes covid-19 from community acquired pneumonia on chest ct. Radiology p 200905 (2020)
19. Shi, F., et al.: Review of artificial intelligence techniques in imaging data acquisition, segmentation and diagnosis for covid-19 IEEE Reviews in Biomedical Engineering (2020)
20. Wang, S., et al.: A deep learning algorithm using CT images to screen for corona virus disease (covid-19) medRxiv (2020)
21. Wang, L., et al.: Covid-net: A tailored deep convolutional neural network design for detection of covid-19 cases from chest radiography images (2020)
22. Negassi, M., et al.: Application of artificial neural networks for automated analysis of cystoscopic images: a review of the current status and future prospects. World J. Urol. (2020)
23. Koo, H.J., et al.: Radiographic and CT features of viral pneumonia. Radiographics **38**(3), 719–739 (2018)
24. Wang, D., et al.: Clinical characteristics of 138 hospitalized patients with 2019 novel coronavirus-infected pneumonia in Wuhan, China. JAMA **323**(11), 1061–1069 (2020)
25. Murala, S., Wu, Q.J.: Local ternary co-occurrence patterns: a new feature descriptor for MRI and CT image retrieval. Neurocomputing **119**, 399–412 (2013)
26. Albahli, S., et al.: Detection of coronavirus disease from X-ray images using deep learning and transfer learning algorithms. J. X-ray Sci. Technol. **28**(5), 841–850 (2020)
27. Chouhan, V., et al.: A novel transfer learning based approach for pneumonia detection in Chest X-ray images. Appl. Sci. **10**, 559 (2020)
28. Kermany, et al.: Identifying medical diagnoses and treatable diseases by image-based deep learning. Cell **172**, 1122–1131 (2018)
29. Islam, et al.: Automatic detection of pneumonia on compressed sensing images using deep learning. In: Proceedings of the 2019 IEEE Canadian Conference of Electrical and Computer Engineering (CCECE), Edmonton, AB, Canada, 5–8 May 2019, pp. 1–4
30. Yoo, S.H., et al.: Deep learning-based decision-tree classifier for COVID-19 diagnosis from chest X-ray imaging. Front. Med. **7,** 427 (2020). ISSN = 2296-858X
31. Mackenzie, G.: The definition and classification of pneumonia. Pneumonia **8**(1), 14 (2016)
32. https://quibim.com/tag/chest-x-ray
33. https://pubs.rsna.org/doi/10.1148/radiol.2020200274
34. .https://www.auntminnie.com/index.aspx?sec=sup&sub=xra&pag=dis&ItemID=127983
35. Deutsche Röntgengesellschaft, AG Thoraxdiagnositik. https://www.drg.de/de-DE/5995/covid-19/
36. Robert Koch-Institut. https://www.rki.de/SharedDocs/FAQ/NCOV2019/FAQ_Liste.html#FAQId13818896
37. Xie, X., et al.: Radiology 2020. https://doi.org/10.1148/radiol.2020200343
38. Choi, H., et al.: Radiology: Cardiothoracic Imaging 2020. https://doi.org/10.1148/ryct.2020200107
39. Wong, H.Y., et al.: Radiology 2020. https://doi.org/10.1148/radiol.2020201160
40. Lee, E.Y.P., et al.: COVID-19 pneumonia: what has CT taught us? [online] thelancet.com. Published: February 24, 2020 (2020)
41. Rubin Geoffrey, D., et al.: The role of chest imaging in patient management during the COVID-19 pandemic: a multinational consensus statement from the Fleischner Society. Radiology, p. 201365

42. Constantine, A., et.al.: Chest CT and coronavirus disease (COVID-19): a critical review of the literature to date. Am. J. Roentgenol. (2020)
43. Wang. D., et.al.: Clinical characteristics of 138 hospitalized patients with 2019 novel coronavirus-infected Pneumonia in Wuhan, China. JAMA (2020)
44. Pan, F., et.al.: Time course of lung changes on chest CT during recovery from 2019 novel coronavirus (COVID-19) pneumonia. Radiology (2020)
45. Shi, H., et.al.: Radiological findings from 81 patients with COVID-19 pneumonia in Wuhan, China: a descriptive study. [online] thelancet.com 24 February 2020 (2020)
46. Wei, Z., et.al.: Relation between chest CT findings and clinical conditions of coronavirus disease (COVID-19) pneumonia: a multicentre study. Am. J. Roentgenol. (2020)
47. Li, J., et al.: Deep convolutional neural network for latent fingerprint enhancement. Signal. Process. Image Commun. **60**, 52–63 (2018)
48. Gers, F.A., et.al.: Recurrent nets that time and count. Proc. IEEE-INNS-ENNS Int. Joint Conf. Neural Netw. (IJCNN) **3**, 189–194 (2000)
49. Galvez, R.L., et.al.: Object detection using convolutional neural networks. In: IEEE Reg. 10 Annu. Int. Conf. Proceedings/TENCON. Institute of Electrical and Electronics Engineers Inc.; 2019. pp. 2023–2027
50. Chung, J., et.al.: Empirical evaluation of gated recurrent neural networks on sequence modeling (2014)
51. Fekrazad, F.: A best approach in intrusion detection for computer network PNN/GRNN/RBF. Int. J. Comput. Sci. Issues **11**, 182 (2014)
52. Jeatrakul, P., et.al.: Comparing the performance of different neural networks for binary classification problems. In: 2009 Eighth International Symposium on Natural Language Processing. IEEE, Bangkok pp. 111–115 (2009)

Text Mining for Covid-19 Analysis in Latin America

Josimar Chire Saire and Anabel Pineda-Briseño

Abstract The oubtreak of coronavirus, name coined by World Health Organization (WHO) and declared pandemic in March 2020, has enormously impacted differents sectors of countries such as health, economy, education, politics, society, etc. Currently, scientists groups are working to develop a vaccine to strengthen immunological system against Covid-19. During the pandemic, governments promote partial, total lockdowns to prevent Covid-19 proliferation. Then, people was forced to stay at home, ration expenses, lost their job and some companies closed because of the low demand of their services/products. Therefore, academical people can study the pandemic and its effects from economic, health, social fields. The aim of this chapter is collect what was studied from January to July, discuss and contribute with extra analysis in Latin American region. Besides, motivate/promote the community to get involved on this main topic: Covid-19 impact in Latin America.

1 Introduction

In this section, the topic of Covid-19 is introduced. First, a general overview in the world is presented, starting from the first cases of Covid-19 in China and Latin America. Next, a review of text mining applications in health, specifically in an epidemiology context. Finally, an outline of research work related to Covid-19 in Latin America.

J. Chire Saire (✉)
Institute of Mathematics and Computer Science (ICMC), University of São Paulo (USP), São Carlos, SP, Brazil
e-mail: jecs89@usp.br

A. Pineda-Briseño
Tecnológico Nacional de México campus Matamoros, H. Matamoros, Tamaulipas, Mexico
e-mail: anabel.pb@matamoros.tecnm.mx

D. Oliva et al. (eds.), *Artificial Intelligence for COVID-19*, Studies in Systems, Decision and Control 358, https://doi.org/10.1007/978-3-030-69744-0_16

1.1 Covid-19 Outbreak in the World

At the end of 2019 it originated in China Wuhan District a novel infectious disease named Covid-19 (coronavirus). This disease caused an outbreak of viral pneumonia with high level of contagion and rapid spread across the world, which caused that WHO declared this pandemic an international concern of public health emergency in March of this year [1–3]. To date this disease has infected millions of people, and has killed thousands of them. In addition to generating a negative impact in other areas such as economy, education, politics, tourism, etc. By August 31, 2020, the WHO confirmed globally 25,144,524 positive cases and 844,410 deaths by Covid-19 [4]. The Table 1 shows the top 10 countries in the world with the most confirmed cases until August 31. Unlike the previous Table 1, the Table 2 shows the top 10 countries with cumulative cases total and cumulative deaths total until July 31, without considering the countries of Latin America, since this work focused on the analysis of information collected within the period from January to July. According to the data displayed in the Table 1, of the top 10, the countries Brazil, Peru, Colombia, Mexico and Chile belong to Latin America, which represent 50% of the list. It can also be observed in both tables that the United States of America was the country with the most confirmed cases to date and was the country that reported the first case of Covid-19 in the American continent on January 20. It is important to clarify that this list is without considering the amount of the total population of the countries and is in order to contextualize the general situation of Covid-19 in the world.

Table 1 Top 10 countries of coronavirus disease (Covid-19)

#	Country	Cases—cumulative total (Aug 31)	Deaths—cumulative total (Aug 31)
1	United States of America	5,899,504	181,689
2	Brazil	3,846,153	119,504
3	India	3,621,245	64,469
4	Russian Federation	995,319	17,176
5	Peru	639,435	28,607
6	South Africa	625,056	14,028
7	Colombia	599,914	19,064
8	Mexico	591,712	63,819
9	Spain	464,306	29,119
10	Chile	409,974	11,244

Table 2 Top 10 countries of coronavirus disease (Covid-19) excluding Latin American countries

#	Country	Cases—cumulative total (Jul 31)	Deaths—cumulative total (Jul 31)	First case date
1	United States of America	4,388,566	150,054	Jan 20
2	India	1,638,870	36,511	Jan 30
3	Russian Federation	839,981	13,963	Jan 31
4	South Africa	482,169	7,812	Mar 5
5	Spain	288,281	28,510	Feb 2
6	Iran	301,530	16,569	Feb 19
7	The United Kingdom	302,305	41,169	Feb 1
8	Saudi Arabia	274,219	2,869	Mar 2
9	Bangladesh	232,194	3,083	Mar 8
10	Pakistan	278,305	5,951	Feb 26

1.2 Covid-19 in Latin America

This subsection introduces the context of Latin America, from February to July. The Table 3 presents a summary of total cases in Latin American region and the Fig. 1 displays a Latin America map to shows the cumulative cases total, employing a logarithmic scale.

1.3 Text Mining Applications

There are diverse text mining applications around the world in the context of health. However, in this subsection we will only highlight some proposals presented in recent years, focused on epidemiology topic. A search has been made in the main databases such as IEEE Xplorer, Springer, ACM, Scopus, ArXiv and MedrXiv using the keywords "text mining", "data mining", "epidemic", "pandemic", "epidemiology", "twitter", "social networks", "covid-19" and "coronavirus". The Table 4 summarizes the general search parameters using as examples the advanced search query strings employed in IEEE Xplore database. All the proposals presented in this section exclude those developed in Latin America and include some relevant works that have been published as a preprint.

The Tables 5 and 6 present the selected from the different databases consulted from 2010 to date. The Table 5 presents a list of proposals without considering those with a Covid-19 approach. Of the selected articles, the proposals [21–25] that represent a 71.42%, focus their application on monitoring and prediction of infectious disease such as zika, dengue, cholera, H1N1 and hay fever. In most of the works the combination of text mining and machine learning is proposed. For its part, the paper

Table 3 Information about Latin American countries, population (thousands)

Country	Population	Cases (cumulative total)	Deaths (cumulative total)	First case
Argentina	45,479	185,373	3,466	Mar 03 [4]
Bolivia	11,640	75,234	2,894	Mar 10 [5]
Brasil	211,716	2,625,612	91,607	Feb 25 [6]
Chile	18,187	353,536	9,457	Mar 03 [7]
Colombia	49,085	286,020	9,810	Mar 06 [8]
Ecuador	16,905	84,370	5,657	Feb29 [9]
Peru	31,915	407,492	19,021	Mar 06 [10]
Paraguay	7,192	5,207	47	Mar 07 [11]
Uruguay	3,388	1,243	41	Mar 13 [12]
Venezuela	2020	17,859	158	Mar 13 [13]
Costa Rica	5,098	17,290	140	Mar 06 [14]
El Salvador	6,481	16,632	448	Mar 18 [15]
Honduras	9,235	41,426	1,312	Mar 10 [16]
Nicaragua	6,203	3,672	116	Mar 18 [17]
Guatemala	17,153	48,826	1,867	Mar 13 [18]
Panama	3,894	64,191	1,397	Mar 09 [19]
Mexico	134,829	416,179	46,000	Feb 28 [20]

[26] that represents 14.23%, provides a review containing the main techniques of data mining, a field of science that is included within data mining. The paper [27], that represents the remaining 14.23%, addresses the importance of social networks such as Twitter, Facebook and Instagram in outbreaks and epidemiological surveillance.

On the other hand, Table 6 shows a selected list of proposals with a Covid-19 approach. The papers [28, 29], the 28.32%, focus their work to infoveillance for surveillance proposals based on the combination of text mining and natural language processing (NLP). Other 28.32% of the articles ([30, 31]) propose the combination of text mining and machine learning for the detection and diagnosis of fake news and patients with symptoms of Covid-19 respectively. Regarding the papers [32, 33] (28.32%), these are based on machine learning to predict Covid-19 contagion risks. Finally, the article [31] that represents 14.23%, employs machine learning techniques and text mining for text analytics and visualization. Although the objective of this subsection is not to present an exhaustive study, it can be clearly seen that the negative impact of Covid-19 highlighted the need to put in operation algorithms, platforms, techniques and models in real world scenarios. The aforementioned to mitigate the staggered crisis that the pandemic has caused, not only in the public health sector (both physical and mental) but also in other areas such as the economy, education, tourism, etc.

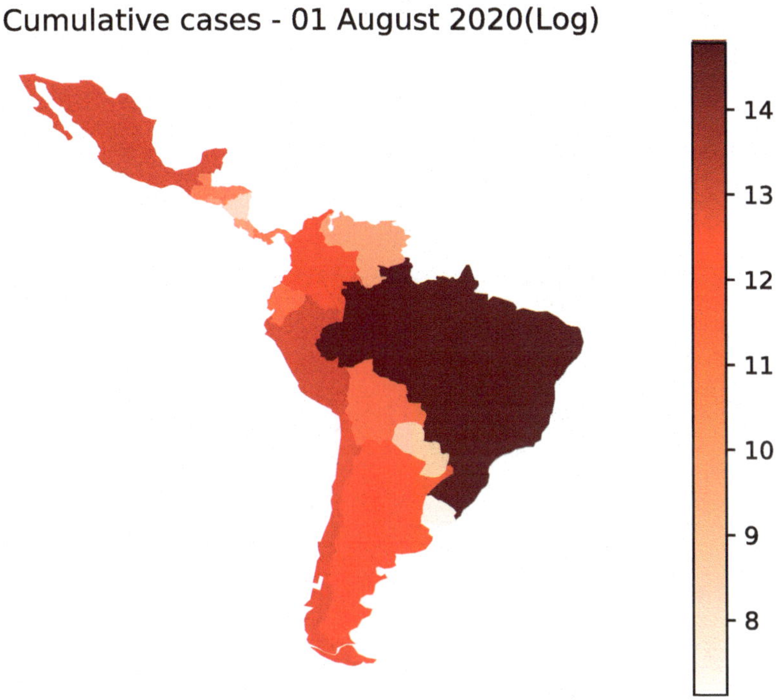

Fig. 1 Map of Latin America

Table 4 Advanced search in database

Query	Advanced search query string
Query 1	(text mining OR data mining) AND (epidemic OR pandemic OR epidemiology) AND (twitter OR social networks OR digital media) NOT (covid-19 OR coronavirus)
Query 2	(text mining OR data mining) AND (epidemic OR pandemic OR epidemiology) AND(twitter OR social networks OR digital media) AND (covid-19 OR coronavirus)

1.4 Research in Latin America

The focus of the chapter is around Covid-19 applications/research in Latin America. A search in the main repositories related to computer science and health was carried out and the data range considered for this search was from January to July.

Table 5 Selected literature—Query 1

Author	Title	Scope	Keywords	Date
Saire [21]	Building Intelligent Indicators to Detect Dengue Epidemics in Brazil using Social Networks	Brazil	Text Mining; Machine Learning; Applied Science; Dengue	Aug 1, 2019
Bates [22]	Tracking Disease: Digital Epidemiology Offers New Promise in Predicting Outbreaks	Not applicable	Diseases; Cholera; Internet; Public healthcare; Real-time systems; Twitter; Patient monitoring; Medical services	Jan 24, 2017
Subramani et al. [23]	Text Mining and Real-Time Analytics of Twitter Data: A Case Study of Australian Hay Fever Prediction	Australian	Twitter; Machine learning; Text mining Information retrieval Knowledge discovery	Sep 22, 2018
de Araujo et al. [27]	Social Networks Applied to Zika and H1N1 Epidemics: A Systematic Review	Not applicable	Social media; Collaboration in health; Health surveillance; Zika; H1N1; Twitter; Facebook; Instagram	Aug 5, 2018
Tekieh and Raahemi [26]	Importance of Data Mining in Healthcare: A Survey	Not applicable	Data mining; Health data analysis; Data quality; Predictive modelling; Health big data; Data mining applications	Aug 25, 2015
Edo-Osagie et al. [24]	A scoping review of the use of Twitter for public health research	Not applicable	Disease tracking; Event forecasting; Pharmacovigilance; Public health; Syndromic surveillance	May 16, 2020
Lwin et al. [25]	Temporal and textual analysis of social media on collective discourses during the Zika virus pandemic	Not applicable	Facebook; Health communication; Public health; Social media; Twitter; Zika	May 29, 2020

Table 6 Selected literature—Query 2

Author	Title	Scope	Keywords	Date
De Santis et al. [28]	An Infoveillance System for Detecting and Tracking Relevant Topics From Italian Tweets During the COVID-19 Event	Italy	Natural language processing; topic tracking; topic detection; social network analysis; text mining; COVID-19; infodemiology; infoveillance	Jul 17, 2020
Albahri et al. [30]	Role of biological Data Mining and Machine Learning Techniques in Detecting and Diagnosing the Novel Coronavirus (COVID-19): A Systematic Review	Not applicable	Coronaviruses; MERS-CoV; SARS-CoV-2; COVID-19; Artificial Intelligence; Biological Data Mining; Machine Learning	May 25, 2020
Elhadad et al. [31]	COVID-19-FAKES: A Twitter (Arabic/English) Dataset for Detecting Misleading Information on COVID-19	Not applicable	Not applicable	Aug 21, 2020
Fu et al. [32]	Be Aware of the Hot Zone: A Warning System of Hazard Area Prediction to Intervene Novel Coronavirus COVID-19 Outbreak	Not applicable	Hazard area prediction; epidemic feature engineering; classification with reinforcement	Jul 25, 2020
Abd-Alrazaq et al. [29]	Top concerns of tweeters during the COVID-19 pandemic: A surveillance	Not applicable	2019-ncov; Coronavirus; covid-19; Disease surveillance; Health informatics; Infodemiology; Infoveillance; Public health; Sars-cov-2; Social media; Twitter	Apr 4, 2020
Muthusami et al. [34]	Covid-19 outbreak: Tweet based analysis and visualization towards the influence of coronavirus in the world	Not applicable	COVID-19; Machine learning algorithms; Sentiment analysis; Text mining; Tweets	Jun 30, 2020
Kim et al. [33]	Hi-COVIDNet: Deep Learning Approach to Predict Inbound COVID-19 Patients and Case Study in South Korea	South Korea	Coronavirus; Deep learning; Neural networks; Covid-19; inflow infection prevention; pandemic	Jul 06, 2020

1.4.1 IEEE Xplorer

This repository has available the use of logical operators to do a specific search. The search is considering: books, conferences, courses, journal & magazines, standards, authors, citations.

- Query 1: ("All Metadata":covid-19 OR "All Metadata":coronavirus) AND ("All Metadata":text mining OR "All Metadata":data mining), results: 1
- Query 2: ("All Metadata":covid-19 OR "All Metadata":coronavirus) AND ("All Metadata":text mining OR "All Metadata":data mining) AND ("All Metadata":america), results: 0.

Query 1 is performed to know how many papers are related to the general area. And, Query 2 for specific context of Latin America. It is remarkable to find only one result, in spite of [35] presents an infoveillance system to track topics using posts of Twitter (social network) from Italy.

1.4.2 Springer

This repository has a diversity of areas, one of them is computer science, public health and more. Then, a search can cover more areas and let us know how is the production around Covid-19.

- Query 1: 'covid-19, coronavirus and text mining, data mining', results: 0
- Query 2: 'covid-19, coronavirus and text mining, data mining and america', results: 0

Queries show there is any indexed work in this repository now.

1.4.3 ArXiv

This repository is popular to present pre-print to the community and get feedback to strengthen the work.

- Query 1: order: -announced_date_first; size: 50; date_range: from 2020-01-01 to 2020-07-31; include_cross_list: True; terms: AND all = coronavirus; AND all = text mining, results: 7, see Table 7.
- Query 2: order: -announced_date_first; size: 50; date_range: from 2020-01-01 to 2020-07-31; include_cross_list: True; terms: AND all = covid-19; AND all = text mining. The results of this query is presented in Table 8 and include results of Table 7.
- Query 3: order: -announced_date_first; size: 50; date_range: from 2020-01-01 to 2020-07-31; include_cross_list: True; terms: AND all = covid-19; AND all = text mining; AND title=america, results: 0.

Table 7 ArXiv results, Query one

Author	Title	Scope	Keywords	Date
Nguyen [36]	Artificial Intelligence in the Battle against Coronavirus (COVID-19): A Survey and Future Research Directions	Not applicable	Artificial intelligence; AI; machine learning; coronavirus; COVID-19; SARS-CoV-2; pandemic; epidemic; outbreak; survey; review; overview; future research directions	30 July
Chen et al. [37]	Coronavirus Knowledge Graph: A Case Study	Not applicable	Applied computing, Health informatics; Biological networks; Computing methodologies, Information extraction; Knowledge representation and reasoning; Information systems	4 July
Lee et al. [38]	Answering Questions on COVID-19 in Real-Time	Not applicable	Not applicable	29 June
Wang et al. [39]	CORD-19: The COVID-19 Open Research Dataset	Not applicable	Not applicable	10 July
Gao et al. [40]	NAIST COVID: Multilingual COVID-19 Twitter and Weibo Dataset	Not applicable	Not applicable	17 April
Fister et al. [41]	Discovering Associations in Covid-19 Related Research Papers	Not applicable	COVID-19, data science, metro maps, optimization	6 April
Saire and Navarro [42]	What is the people posting about symptoms related to Coronavirus in Bogota, Colombia	Colombia	Natural Language Processing, Text Mining, Symptomatology, Coronavirus, Covid-19	25 Mar

Table 8 ArXiv results, Query two

Author	Title	Scope	Keywords	Date
Tekumalla and Banda [43]	Characterization of Potential Drug Treatments for COVID-19 using Social Media Data and Machine Learning	Not applicable	Not applicable	20 July
Soni and Roberts [44]	An Evaluation of Two Commercial Deep Learning Based Information Retrieval Systems for COVID-19 Literature	Not applicable	Not applicable	27 July
Peng et al. [45]	COVID-19-CT-CXR: a freely accessible and weakly labeled chest X-ray and CT image collection on COVID-19 from biomedical literature	Not applicable	Not applicable	11 June
Georgiou [46]	A Study of Knowledge Sharing related to Covid-19 Pandemic in Stack Overflow	Not applicable	Covid-19; Stack Overflow; Data Analytics	18 April
Zavarrone [47]	CO.ME.T.A. covid-19 media textual analysis. A dashboard for media monitoring	Not applicable	Not applicable	16 April
Lopez et al. [48]	Understanding the perception of COVID-19 policies by mining a multilanguage Twitter dataset	Not applicable	Not applicable	23 Mar

1.4.4 MedrXiv

- Query 1: for full text or abstract or title "(covid19 or coronavirus) and (text mining or data mining)" (match whole all) and posted between "01 Jan, 2020 and 31 Jul, 2020", results: 208. The next table, Table 9, presents the first 10 results.
- Query 2: for term "(covid19 or coronavirus) and (text mining or data mining) and (america)" and posted between "01 Jan, 2020 and 31 Jul, 2020", results: 16. Table 10, presents the first 10 results.

1.5 PubMed

PubMed is a popular repository of life sciences and biomedical topics, maintained by National Library of Medicine of USA.

- Query 1: (covid19 or coronavirus) and (text mining or data mining) and (america), results: 1.

The unique results was: Li [68] et al. conducts a spatio temporal study to analyze the correlation of Covid-19 impact on mental health using social data mining on the United States of America.

In summary, considering the results of the queries in the previous repositories IEEE Xplorer, Springer, ArXiv, MedrXiv, PubMed only the next countries of Latin America are studied: Colombia, Peru, Mexico, Brazil, and South America as region. Therefore, Covid-19 analysis is still opened to conduct studies from different fields, considering each country has an own context about economy, health, education, culture. Finally, the closure of this section is to motivate/encourage Latin American people to start national/international collaboration projects to analyze how the pandemic impacted on your territory. Besides, the analysis of the top users show they are related to mass media: television, radio, magazines, newspapers.

2 NLP Applied to South America

The first case in Latin America was reported in Brazil, this country is located in South American region and the official language is Portuguese, see Table 3. In this section will cover the conducted studies with the aim of understanding South American region. South America has the next countries: Argentina, Bolivia, Brazil, Chile, Colombia, Ecuador, Peru, Paraguay, Uruguay, Venezuela.

Figure 2 presents the maps to summarize information presented in Table 3 related to South American countries. Left side presents the numbers of cumulative cases per country using logarithmic scale, this graphic is good to compare number of total infections of Covid-19. But, it is not fair because each country has different size of

Table 9 Ten first results of Query 1—MedrXiv

Author	Title	Scope	Keywords	Date
Chire Saire and Oblitas [49]	Covid19 Surveillance in Peru on April using Text Mining	Peru	Natural Language Processing, Text Mining, People behaviour, Coronavirus, Covid-19	25 May
Xie and Li [50]	Health and Demographic Impact on COVID-19 Infection and Mortality in US Counties	USA	Not applicable	11 May
Zou et al. [51]	Public Reactions towards the COVID-19 Pandemic on Twitter in the United Kingdom and the United States	UK, Usa	Coronavirus, COVID-19, Twitter, Soci al media, Public health, Pandemic	28 July
Wang et al. [52]	Public Opinions towards COVID-19 in California and New York on Twitter	USA	COVID-19; coronavirus; social media	14 July
Azarafza et al. [53]	Clustering method for spread pattern analysis of corona-virus (COVID-19) infection in Iran	Iran	COVID-19, Data mining, Machine learning, Clustering method, Spatio temporal distribution, Iran	28 May
Tran et al. [54]	Studies of Novel Coronavirus Disease 19 (COVID-19) Pandemic: A Global Analysis of Literature	Not applicable	Scientometrics; content analysis; text mining, COVID-19	08 May
Shuja et al. [55]	COVID-19 Open Source Data Sets: A Comprehensive Survey	Not applicable	COVID-19, coronavirus, pandemic, machine learning, artificial intelligence, open source, data set	23 Mar
Chandu [56]	Identification of spatial variations in COVID-19 epidemiological data using K-Means clustering algorithm: a global perspective	Not applicable	Not applicable	05 June
Aznab [57]	Evaluation of COVID 19 infection in 279 cancer patients treated during a 90-day period in 2020 pandemic	Iran	COVID-19, Cancer, Treatment, Solid Tumor, Hematology Malignancy	01 June
Kumar et al. [58]	Accurate Prediction of COVID-19 using Chest X-Ray Images through Deep Feature Learning model with SMOTE and Machine Learning Classifiers	Not applicable	COVID-19, X-ray, Feature Extraction, Deep Learning, Machine Learning	17 April

Table 10 Results of Query 2 -MedrXiv

Author	Title	Scope	Keywords	Date
Chire Saire and Oblitas [49]	Covid19 Surveillance in Peru on April using Text Mining	Peru	Natural Language Processing, Text Mining, People behaviour, Coronavirus, Covid-19	25 May
Chire Saire and Pineda-Briseno [59]	Text Mining Approach to Analyze Coronavirus Impact: Mexico City as Case of Study	Mexico	Natural Language Processing, Text Mining, People behaviour, Coronavirus, Covid-19	12 May
Drias and Drias [60]	Mining Twitter Data on COVID-19 for Sentiment analysis and frequent patterns Discovery	Not applicable	tweets Analytics, COVID-19, sentiment analysis, frequent patterns, association rules mining	18 May
Chire Saire [61]	How was the Mental Health of Colombian people on March during Pandemics Covid19?	Colombia	Not applicable	04 July
Chire Saire [62]	Infoveillance based on Social Sensors to Analyze the impact of Covid19 in South American Population	South America	COVID-19, coronavirus, pandemic, machine learning, artificial intelligence, open source, data set	11 April
Souza et al. [63]	Predicting the disease outcome in COVID-19 positive patients through Machine Learning: a retrospective cohort study with Brazilian data	Brazil	COVID-19, prediction model, disease outcome, machine learning, Brazil	28 June
Samuel et al. [64]	Feeling Positive About Reopening? New Normal Scenarios from COVID-19 Reopen Sentiment Analytics	Usa	Not applicable	02 June
Stamm et al. [65]	Clinical practice guidelines and recommendations in the context of the COVID-19 pandemic: systematic review and critical appraisal	Not applicable	Coronavirus, COVID-19, SARS CoV-2, Recommendations, Guidelines, Clinical practice guidelines	20 June
Strohbehn et al. [66]	COVIDOSE: Low-dose tocilizumab in the treatment of Covid-19	Not applicable	Not applicable	26 July
Teheran et al. [67]	Epidemiological characterization of asymptomatic carriers of COVID-19 in Colombia	Colombia	COVID-19; Asymptomatic; Carrier States; Risk factors, Novel Coronavirus	20 June

population, from Brazil with more than 210,000 thousands and Uruguay with less of 3,500. The map of the center is showing the rate between cumulative cases and population. And right side, is presenting the proportion of cumulative cases and total deaths.

The analysis of the previous graphics show the high number of infections in Brazil, but Chile has a bigger ratio of infections/population. In spite of the disaster generated by Covid-19 in Ecuador during the first months and decreasing pattern during the next weeks, Ecuador still has the biggest rate of mortality, and the second is Peru.

The existent papers for this subsection, with the aim of presenting papers related to South American countries are presented in graphic Fig. 3. From March to July, there is a total of 6 papers, analyzing Colombia, South America, Peru, Brazil and the most frequent country is Colombia.

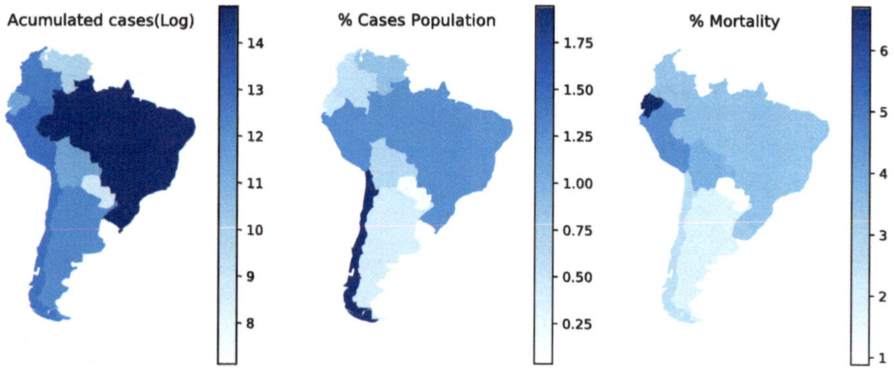

Fig. 2 Maps of South America

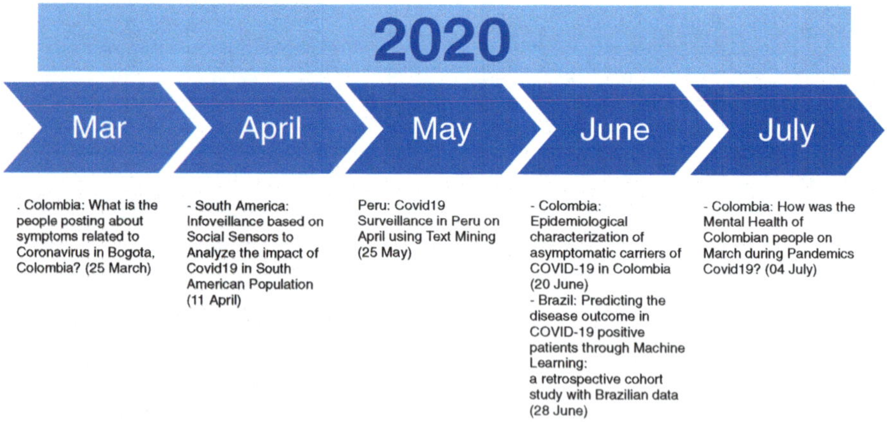

Fig. 3 Timelime of papers with focus in South America

2.1 March

The first reported case in Colombia was on March 06 [42], it conducts study using Twitter as source data. The collected data was from 08-03-2020 to 14-03-2020, the aim of the paper is detect evidence of symptoms in users from Bogota, Colombia. An example of the terms are: 'fiebre'(fever), 'tos'(cough), 'gripe'(flu), 'estornudar'(sneeze), 'contagio'(contagioun). Graphics presented in Fig. 4, left side shows the increasing number of teets/posts from March 08 until March 18 in Bogota, right side the number of total cases in Colombia, then with more cases in Colombia more people starts to talk about Covid-19 symptoms. Besides the possibility of trusting or not about the posts from Colombian users arise, one proposal strategy is to check user creation date.

Finally, the illustration Fig. 5 presents the cloud of words per day, with higher font are the most frequent words and dolor(pain), fiebre (fever), contagio (contagion) are frequent during the week. Authors conclude Twitter is a useful source to get data and text mining supports the analysis of the collected text to understand the topic related symptoms and Covid-19 in Bogota, Colombia.

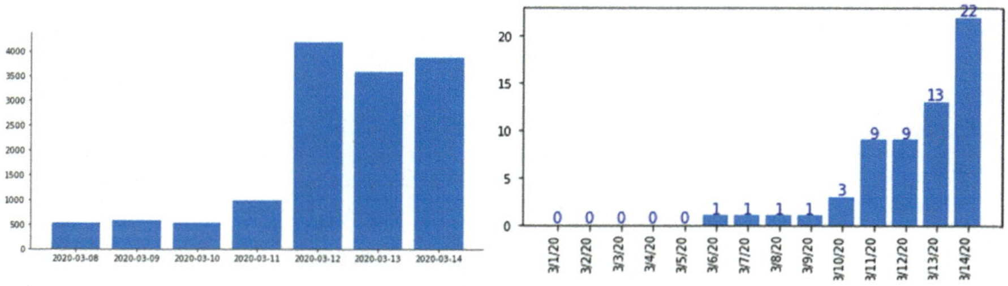

Fig. 4 Number of publications, number of cases in Colombia [42]

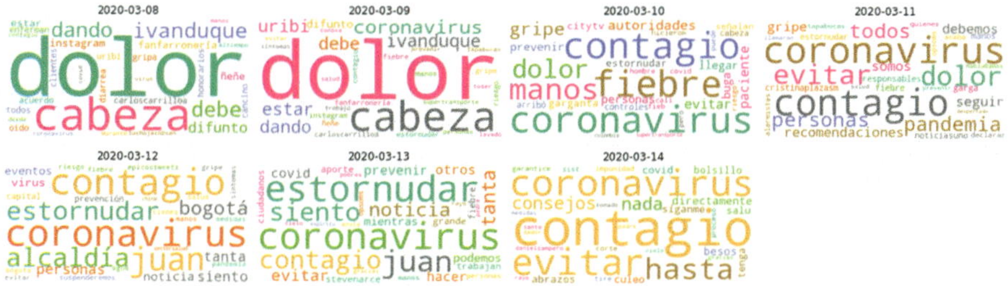

Fig. 5 Cloud of words per day, Bogota [42]

2.2 *April*

South American region is composed of Argentina, Bolivia, Brazil, Chile, Colombia, Ecuador, Peru, Paraguay, Uruguay and Venezuela. Almost all the countries has Spanish as official language, except Brazil has Portuguese. The conducted work presented in paper [62], has the objective of analyzing South American countries with Spanish speakers from 08-03-2020 to 21-03-2020. Considering the access to Internet, the scope of the study includes capitals, where the access to technology is affordable and existent, see Table 11.

The possibility of finding noise in the data is mentioned, a strategy of filtering the one hundred users with more number of posts, thinking they can be trustful. Figure 6 presents the number before (left side) and after of filtering (right side). The distribution is very similar, but Venezuela has a decreasing number of posts. Bolivia is not the smallest country in terms of territory, population but it has the lowest number of total posts. In contrast, Colombia is the most populated country but it has the third position, Argentina is the country with more number of total tweets. These results can show two main things: Argentina could have more active users or the density of Buenos Aires, Argentina is concentrated around the center of the capital.

Besides, the analysis of the top users show they are related to mass media: television, radio, magazines, newspapers. For details, see Table 12.

Table 11 South America cartography information [62]

Name	Capital	Territory (km^2)
Argentina	Buenos Aires	2.792.600
Bolivia	La Paz	1.098.581
Chile	Santiago	756.102
Colombia	Bogotá	1.141.748
Ecuador	Quito	283.561
Paraguay	Asunción	406.752
Peru	Lima	1.285.216
Uruguay	Montevideo	176.215
Venezuela	Caracas	916.445

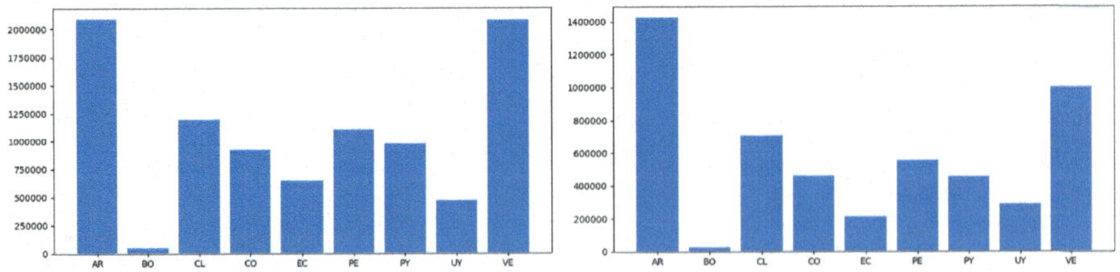

Fig. 6 Number of publications, number of cases in Colombia [62]

Table 12 Eleven nicknames from the top 100 users [62]

Name	Nicknames
Argentina	Portal Diario, Clarin, Radio DoGo, Camila, El Intransigente, Agustina, Pablo, #FrenteDeTodos,
	Ale, Lucas, Diario Cronica
Bolivia	Pagina Siete, La Razon Digital, Radio SPLENDID, RTP Bolivia, FmBolivia, Radio Lider 97 FM,
	Bolivia Social, El Alto Se Respeta, Javierdeltoro, Red Bolivision, Bolivia.com
Chile	Cooperativa, Fabian Parraguez, Fernando Luis, #YoApruebo, Publimetro, Felipe, 24 Horas,
	Cristian, Rodrigo,#RenunciaPi era, Pablo
Colombia	El Espectador, EL TIEMPO, Radio Nacional CO, Juan, La FM, Diario La Republica,
	Erika Fontalvo, RCN Mundo, Roberto Salazar, La vida es bella, Canal Citytv,
Ecuador	Teleamazonas, Primicias, Pichincha Comunicaciones, Marieta Ocampo, Roque Rivas Zambrano,
	Ricardo Paredes Egas, Edicion Medica Ec, Patricio eguez, Alfonso Parraga, Cristian Mosquera
Paraguay	ARTexpress, Victor Araujo, Marcos Ozuna, Radio anduti, ABC Cardinal 730 AM,
	Leli Ramirez Lugo, CPeraltaSocialMedia, Fernando Nu ez, ultima Hora,
	Graciela Jacqueline Ricciardi Paredes, Zoraida Palacios
Peru	Agencia Andina, Diario La Republica, Luis VF, El Comercio, Diario Trome,
	Diario Correo, Diario Gestion, Jose, Luis, Libero, Gizlaine
Uruguay	Agence France-Presse, El Observador, Telemundo, Luis, Carlos, Rita Montelongo,
	Pablo, Adriana, Teledoce #QuedateEnCasa, Alfredo Badolati (Badoleitor 5.0), dianarocio17
Venezuela	CaraotaDigital, DolarToday, El Nacional, Maduradas.com, El Cooperante,
	AlbertoNews, TalCual, Efecto Cocuyo, teleSUR TV, ultimas Noticias, Runrunes

Finally, the author presented a summary of top terms using cloud of words (see Fig. 7). It is important to consider/remember that health authorities promoted different health policies in the countries, on diverse dates.

The most frequent terms are: caso (case), covid, nuevo (new), medida (action) and the name of the country respectively. By consequence, it is possible to conclude that the users are talking about the first cases in their countries and health policies from the governments.

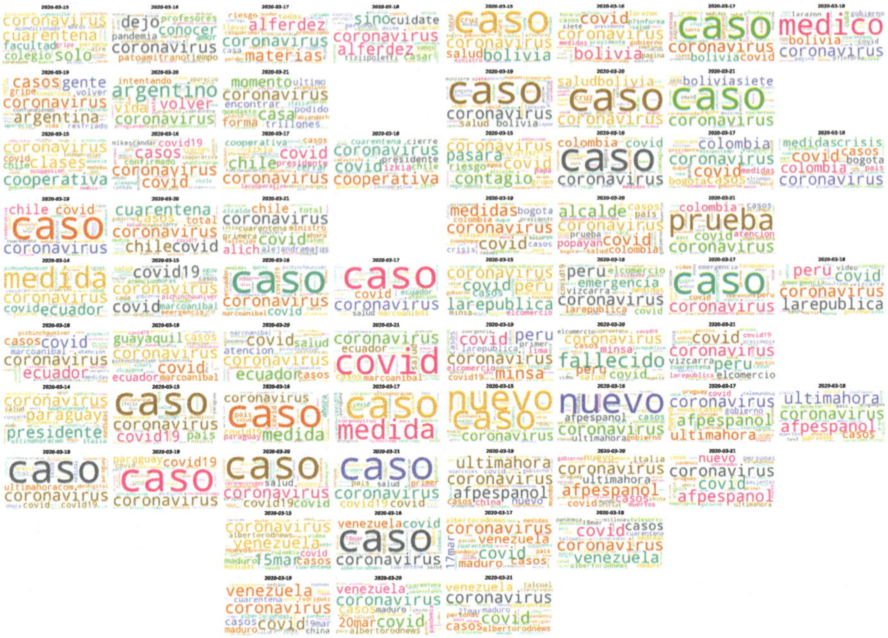

Fig. 7 Countries: Argentina, Bolivia, Chile, Ecuador, Peru, Paraguay, Uruguay, Venezuela [62]

2.3 May

Authors [49] conducted a study to analyze the incidence of Covid-19 in Peru country, from 01-04-2020 to 31-04-2020. It is important to consider that each South American country has a different name geopolitical names to explain geographical distribution or borders. For example, Peru has regions, province, city and district. Besides, Peru has 24 regions and one province with the title of region, Table 13 presents a summary of this data.

Regions of Iquitos, Ucayali, Madre de Dios, Puno, Cusco are the 5 largest but the density of population is not present there. Lima, Piura, La Libertad, Arequipa, Cajamarca have more population. It is important to remark this area because this context can represent an extra information about access to technology and high concentration of power in the capital of Peru. Besides, the Fig. 8 represents the geolocalization of the capital of each region, this places were selected to collect data from Twitter. Also, the number of tweets coming from each city are represented in the Fig. 9.

Considering previous affirmation, the number of tweets are related to the size of population, even other factors can influence access to technology, age distribution, etc. Lima has the biggest number of Tweets.

Then focus the analysis in Lima for the number of posts, a cloud of bigrams is created, see Fig. 10, considering first 15 days. Terms frequent are: ser querido

Table 13 Geopolitical Data—Peru

Region	Capital	Territory (km^2)	Population
Amazonas	Chachapoyas	39 249.13	379 384
Áncash	Huaraz	35 914.81	1 083 519
Apurímac	Abancay	20 895.79	405 759
Arequipa	Arequipa	63 345.39	1 382 730
Ayacucho	Ayacucho	43 814.80	616 176
Cajamarca	Cajamarca	33 317.54	1 341 012
Callao	Callao	146.98	994 494
Cusco	Cusco	71 986.50	1 205 527
Huancavelica	Huancavelica	22 131.47	347 639
Huánuco	Huánuco	36 848.85	721 047
Ica	Ica	21 327.83	850 765
Junín	Huancayo	44 197.23	1 246 038
La Libertad	Trujillo	25 499.9	1 778 080
Lambayeque	Chiclayo	14 231.3	1 197 260
Lima	Lima	34 801.59	9 485 405
Loreto	Iquitos	368 851.95	883 510
Madre de Dios	Puerto Maldonado	85 300.54	141 070
Moquegua	Moquegua	15 733.97	174 863
Pasco	Cerro de Pasco	25 319.59	254 065
Piura	Piura	35 892.49	1 856 809
Puno	Puno	71 999.00	1 172 697
San Martín	Moyobamba	51 253.31	813 381
Tacna	Tacna	16 075.89	329 332
Tumbes	Tumbes	4669.2	224 863
Ucayali	Pucallpa	102 410.55	496 459

(beloved familiar), quedate casa (stay home), recien comienza (it just starts), covid19 and coronavirus. Therefore, users are worried for the pandemic and the infection of their families.

A manual analysis is performed to identify topics in each city: economy, fun, national situation, regional situation, transport, internation situation, covid-19, politics, corruption, religious. The Fig. 11 summarizes the incidence of topic in each city. A remarkable topic is religious in Cajamarca, Cuzco and Huanuco, a possible reason of finding this related terms: there are religious traditional activities.

Besides, analyzing the general context through the Fig. 12, the terms/posts related to regional situation are scarcely. Predominantly, international situation of Covid-19 is the popular topic.

In short, Peruvian citizens are worried about Covid-19, international situation and economy, politics from Peru and a minor worrying about religion and transport.

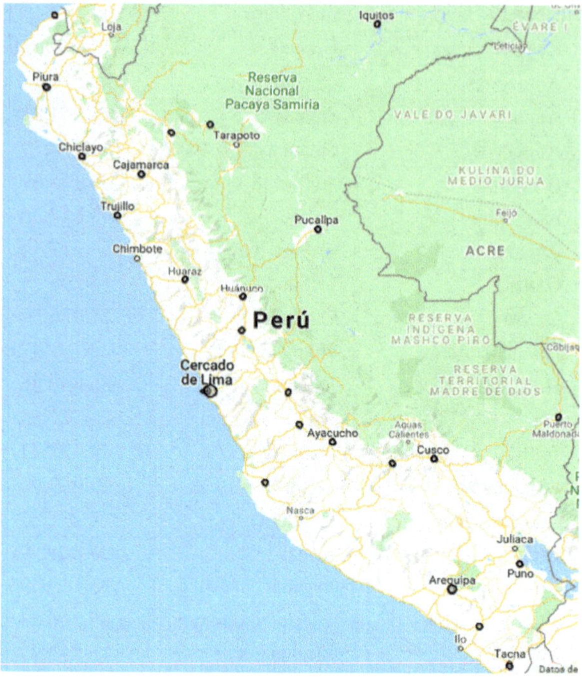

Fig. 8 Geolocalization of regions of Peru [49]

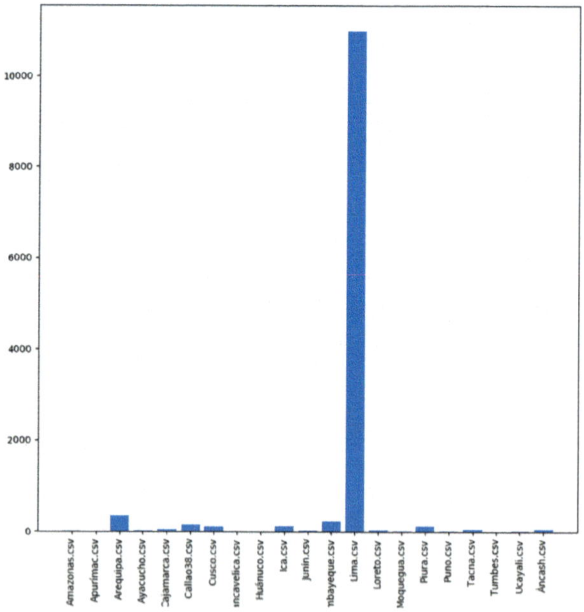

Fig. 9 Number of tweets—cities [49]

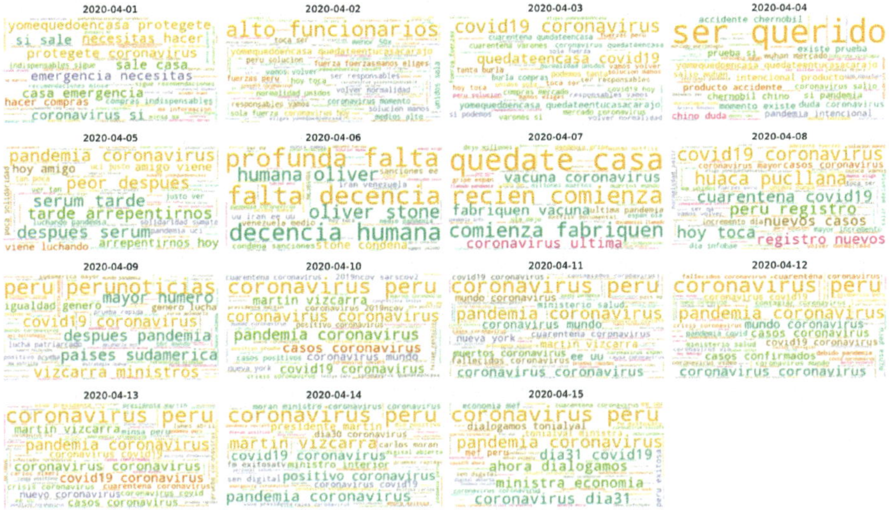

Fig. 10 Cloud of words: Lima [49]

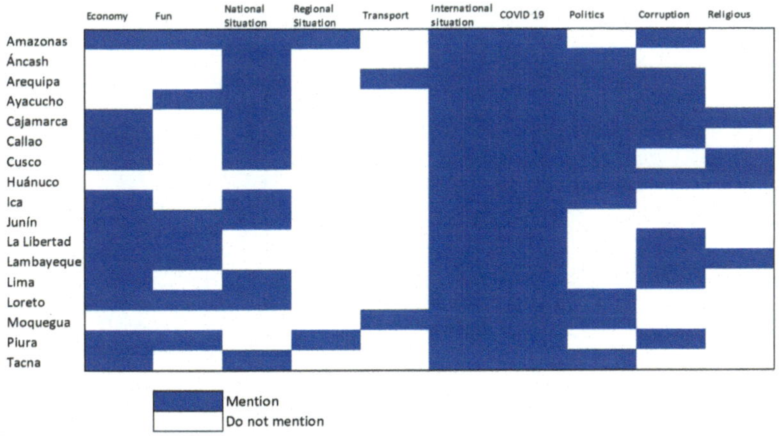

Fig. 11 Words by region [49]

2.4 June

Teheran et al. [67] started a study to describe the asymptomatic people in Colombia because this group can infect other and increase Covid-19 propagation. This citizens can be a silent carrier in public places then it is important describe to identify them early, besides there is bias identifying asymptomatic and pre-symptomatic people [69–71]. The study uses a dataset produced by National Institute of Health (INS) from Colombia, updated until May 23, 2020. Records with no health status information (symptomatic, asymptomatic) were discarded. The available variables/attributes are:

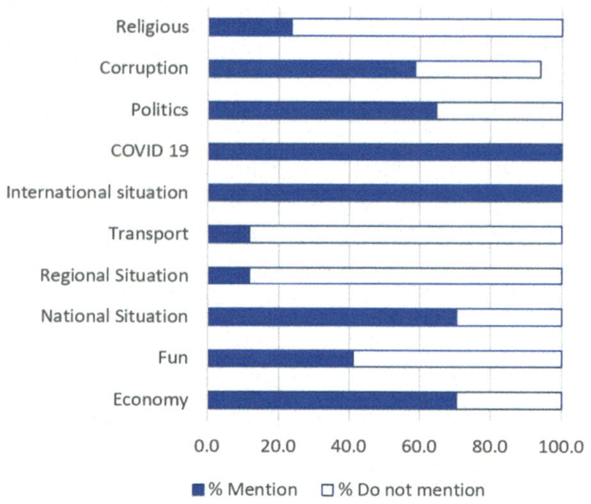

Fig. 12 Mentioned words [49]

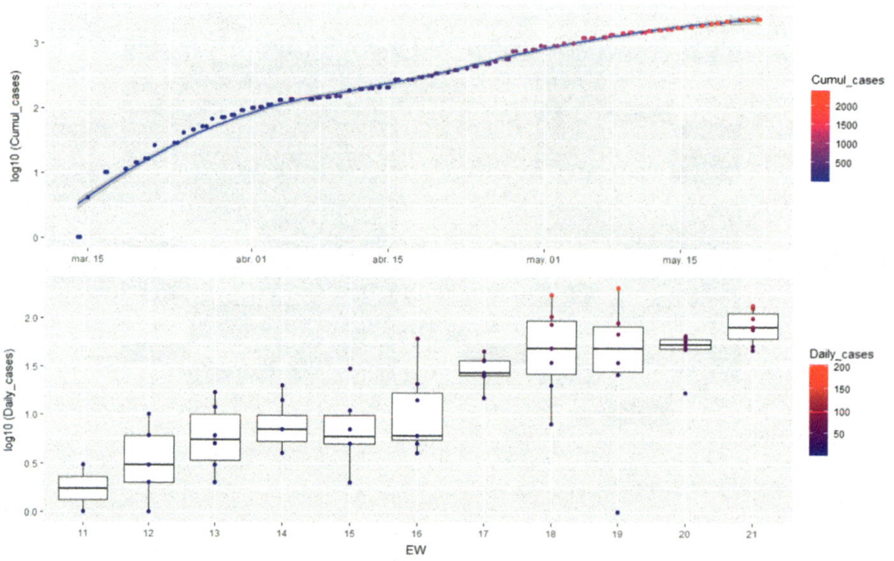

Fig. 13 Colombia covid-19 reported cases daily, weekly [67]

age, care setting (home, nursing home, hospital, intensive care unit), case type, country of origin diagnosis, outcome (recovered, convalescent, deceased), sex. Figure 13 summarizes the daily cases and cases weekly from week 11–21.

Besides, a heatmap graphic was generated to analyze the number of symptomatic, asymptomatic in every department until May 23, see Fig. 14.

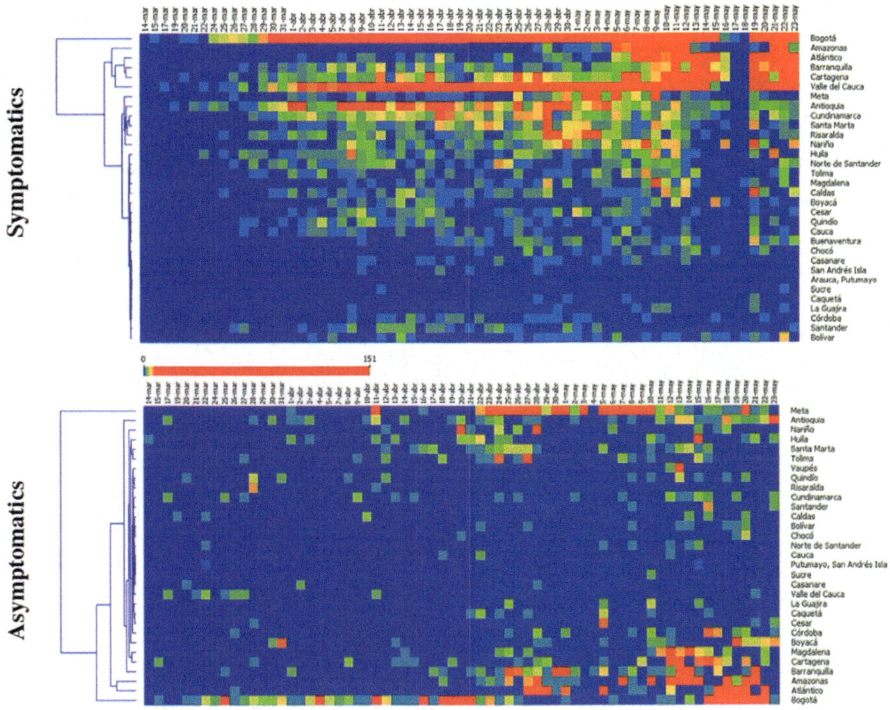

Fig. 14 Heatmap symptomatic, asymptomatic [67]

The main finding are: the identification of 2388 Asymptomatic cases more, 11.83% more than the reported cases in the national dataset. The countries of origin, mainly from Spain, Europe and the next ones, North and South America. The Colombians arriving from Spain, USA were detected with high frequency in Bogota, Valle del Cauca. Department of Amazonas only received imported cases from South American countries. Almost the half of this cases were located in Meta and Bogota. Finally, house was the common place of care 85.7% and 13.9% recovered. A limitation commented by authors was the lack of mass screening for Covid-19 in Colombia.

According the abstract, Souza et al. [63] performs experiments to classify poor diagnosis in patients with covid-19 (positives) using machine learning algorithms. But, after a careful reading of introduction, the work is oriented to make prognosis or early identification of patients, using a dataset of Espirito Santo State from Brazil. The available dataset [72] includes data related to patients, i.e. age, sex, gender, besides symptoms: cough, sore throat, headache and some comorbities: obesity, smoking, and the outcome, i.e. cure, death. Data cleaning and selection of attributes of the experiments are explained in the second section. A comparison between Logistic Regression (LR), Linear Discriminant Analysis (LDA), Naive Bayes (NB), K-Nearest Neighbors (KNN), Decision Trees (DT), XGBoost (eXtreme Gradient Boosting) and Support Vector Machine (SVM) was made. The experiments

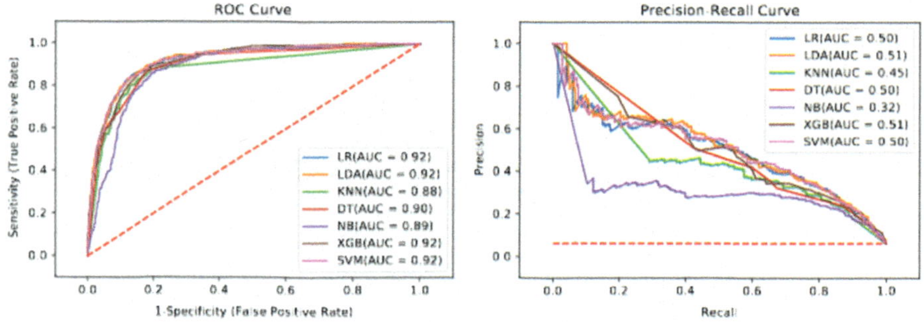

(a) ROC AUC (b) PR AUC

Fig. 15 ROC, AUC curves

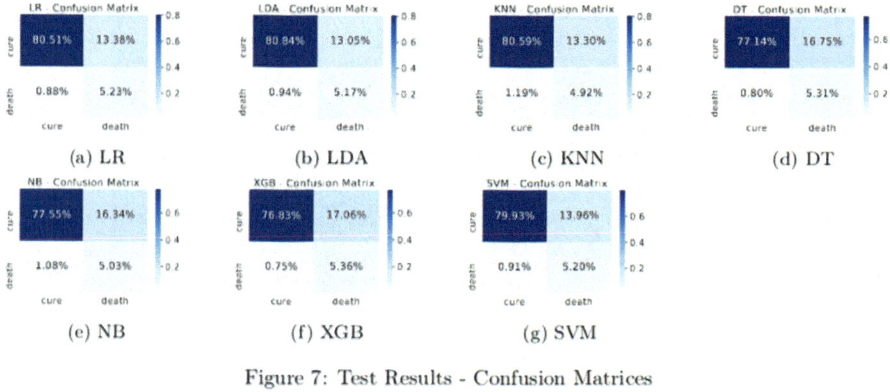

Fig. 16 Confusion matrix of algorithms

performed used: dataset 1 from February 29 to May 23 and dataset 2 from May 24 to May 30. First experiment compared results of the algorithms with the first dataset, later second experiment used the first dataset for training and second for testing.

Results summarizing Area Under Curve (AUC) and ROC (Receiver Operating Characteristic) graphics, which are presented in the Fig. 15, besides a confusion matrix that is presented in the Fig. 16.

LR and LDA got the best results, besides of the influence of features is performed, and hypertension history, coronary heart disease has discriminatory variables.

2.5 July

An analysis about mental health during pandemic in Bogota, Colombia [61] is conducted, many South American countries established an strict lockdown. Then, people staying at home for long periods can affect emotional, mental health. The study is

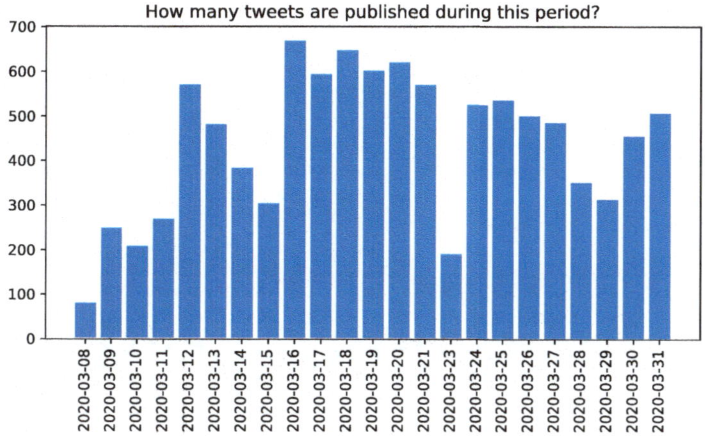

Fig. 17 Frequency of post per day [61]

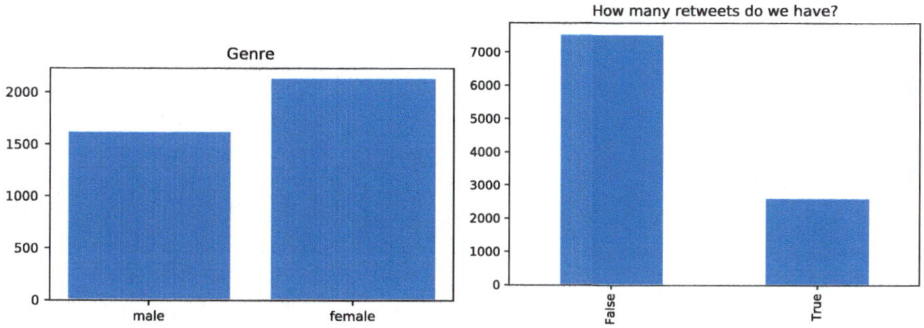

Fig. 18 Genre distribution, number of retweets [61]

considering Twitter as source data, date range from 08-03-2020 to 31-03-2020. Selected words, i.e. miedo (fear), morir (die), familiar (family member), sobrevivir (survive), etc. Frequency of posts (Fig. 17) with the presence of this terms evidence, an initial state with no high impact or interest at the beginning of March, but there is a peak between March 16 to 21.

Although it is not possible to recover genre data from users in Twitter, considering Spanish language, a proposal is presented in Fig. 18 (left side), usually male names finish with 'o' letter and female ends with 'a'. Therefore, an estimation of the genre distribution is possible, female users are posting more than male. Besides, the users can write, post or share whatever they want but some people prefers share, post ideas, content from other users, then this behaviour can be captured or represented by the retweet option. By consequence, right side of Fig. 18 suggests people is preferring share post from someone else and this can be a signal of mental health issue.

Specifically, use of Internet can be represented getting the hour of the posts, see Fig. 19.

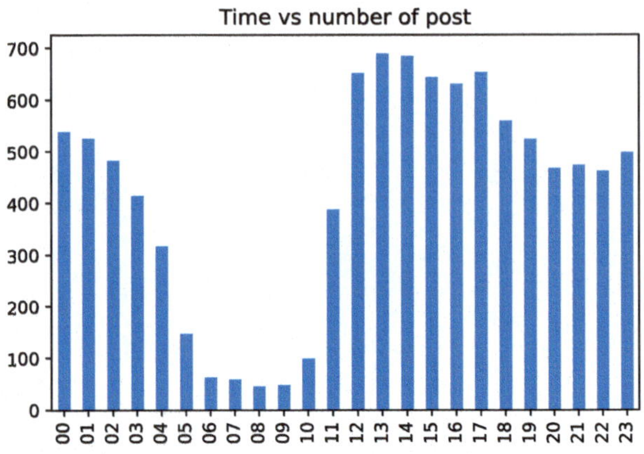

Fig. 19 Post distribution hourly [61]

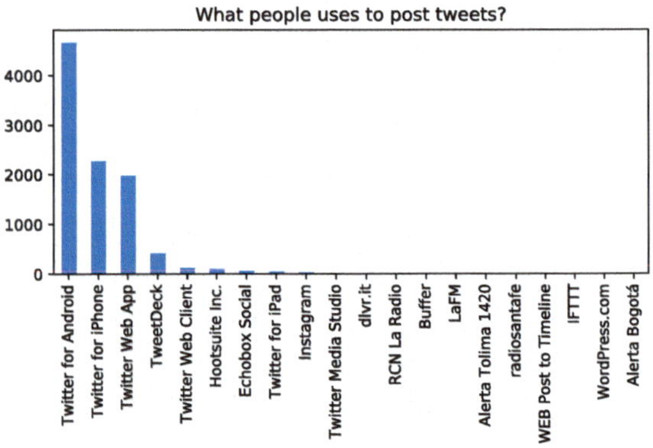

Fig. 20 Source of posting tweets [61]

Currently, it is not possible to get some social, economical information from the users but the device used to share posts can represent a clue about this feature from users. Figure 20 plots the frequency of the devices, i.e. Android, IPhones, etc.

Finally, cloud of words representation are showed in Fig. 21, left side is introducing the terms of size one and right side, the bi-grams (two terms). Terms of size one, i.e. familia—family (March 21, 24, 27 and 29), bigrams: puedo sobrevivir—can survive (10), voy morir—go to die (12), esperanza william—hope william (15), atrapados miedo—trapped fear (19), salir casa—leave home (24) can evidence a constant warning about health, Covid-19, family and some negativism presents a initial concern related to mental health.

3 NLP Applied to Central America

The Fig. 22 presents the maps that summarize the information presented in the Table 3 about of Central American countries. Central America is divided in the next countries: Costa Rica, El Salvador, Guatemala, Honduras, Nicaragua, and Panama. From

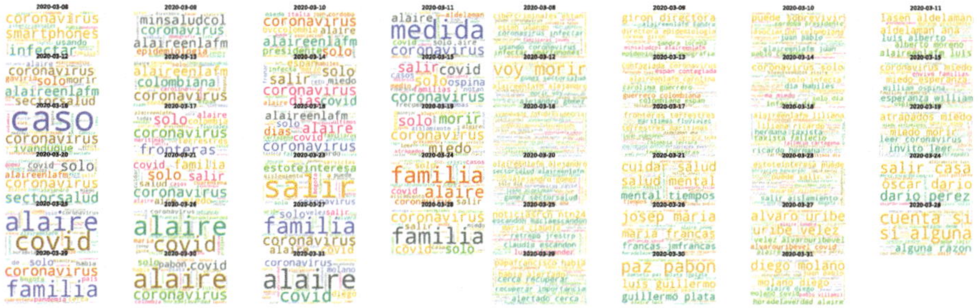

Fig. 21 Cloud of words [61]

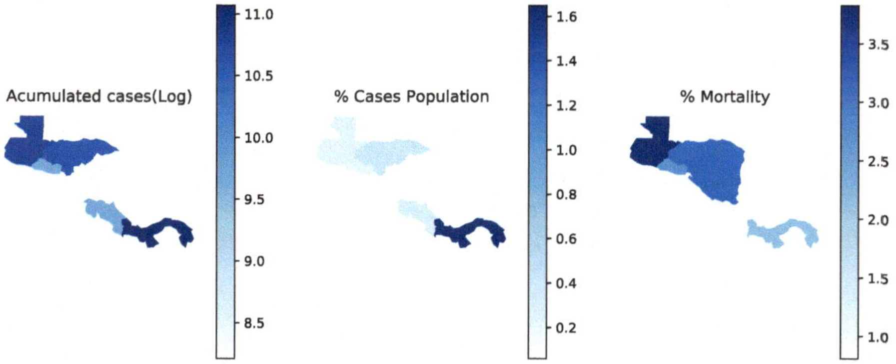

Fig. 22 Maps of central America

left to right are presented the maps to show the cumulative cases total employing logarithmic scale; the rate between cumulative cases total and population; and the proportion of cumulative cases total and cumulative deaths total for each country. After carrying out a general analysis of what is shown in the graphs, the countries Panama, Guatemala and Honduras present a high rate of infections by Covid-19. Of these countries, Panama leads the Central American countries with the highest proportion of infections in relation to its population, while Honduras has the highest mortality rate.

After conducting a general search of the research work related to the use of natural language processing (NLP) combined with social networks, in order to use the latter as information sensors that allow relevant public health information during the development of Covid-19, it was possible to verify the little work carried out so far in this region of Latin America. As proof of the above, the only work that was identified and that will be addressed in this subsection is a scientific article that precedes the formal peer review and publication.

Basically, the authors in the work [73] illustrate how data generated through Twitter can be used to help the implementation of strategies to address pandemic emergence in Central America countries. This study considered only Spanish native language and the capital cities of each country.

Summarizing this article, the authors conducted some experiments focused on analyzing the posts of Twitter users during the period between April 4 and 11. Specifically, they analyzed three aspects for each capital city: the number of publications, the Twitter users with the highest number of publications, and the terms most used in user publications in relation to Covid-19. The main findings were:

- Costa Rica was the country with the highest number of posts while Honduras and Nicaragua were the countries with the lowest numbers. This information can be verified in Fig. 23.

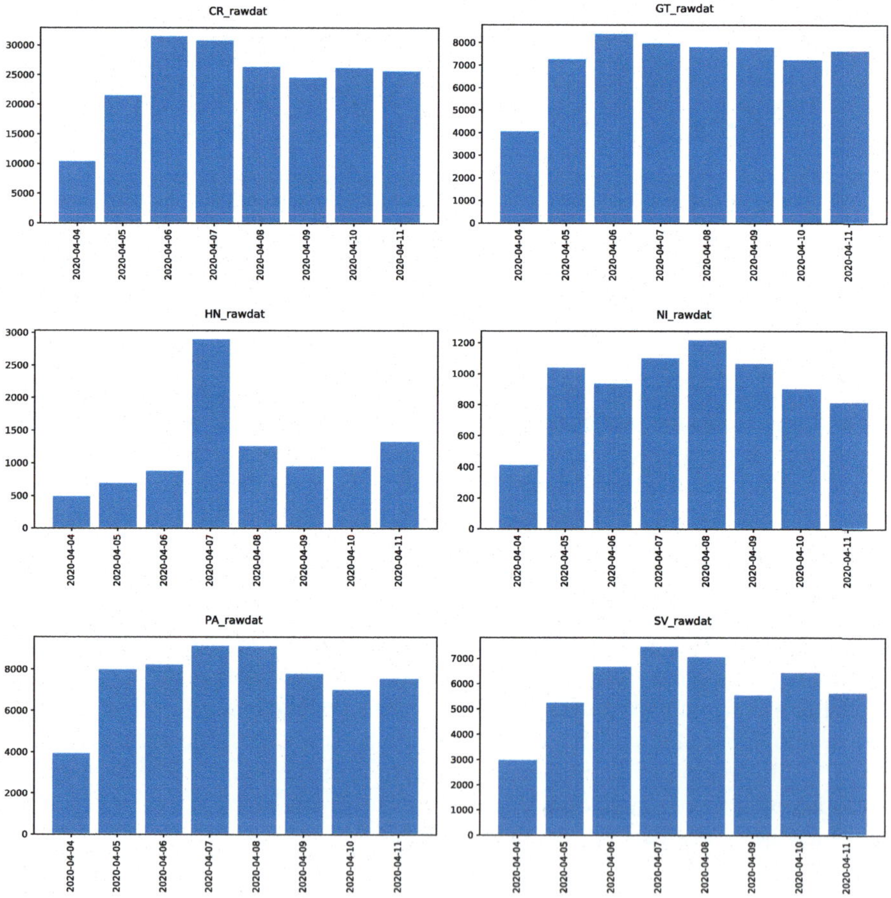

Fig. 23 Number of posts per day in Costa Rica, Guatemala, Honduras, Nicaragua, Panama and El Salvador [73]

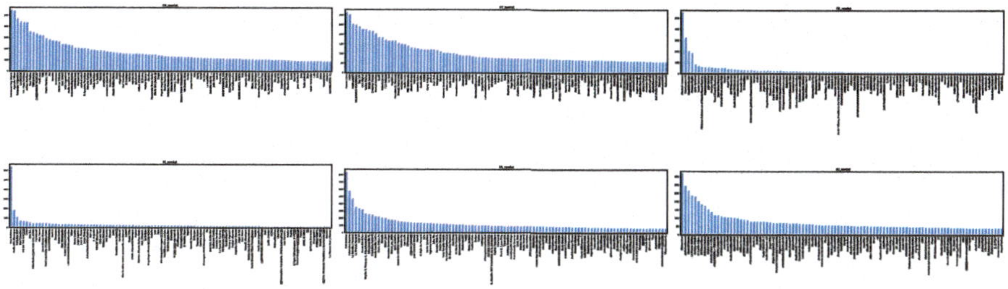

Fig. 24 Top 100 Twitter users in Costa Rica, Guatemala, Honduras, Nicaragua, Panama and El Salvador [73]

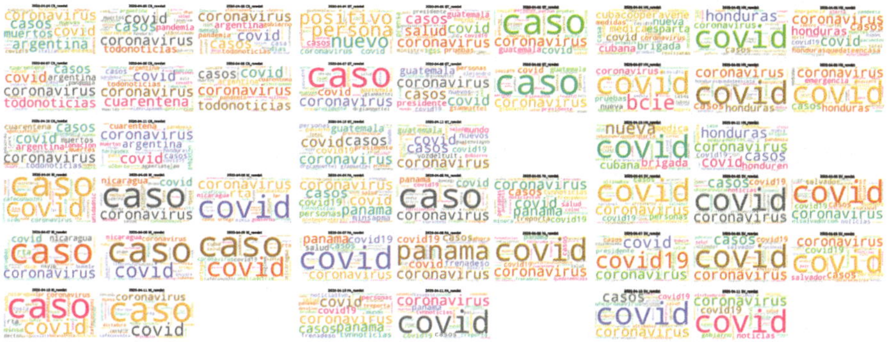

Fig. 25 Cloud of words of Costa Rica, Guatemala, Honduras, Nicaragua, Panama, and El Salvador [73]

- The Top 5 Twitter users for Costa Rica, Nicaragua, Panama and El Salvador were media accounts while for Guatemala and Costa Rica their Top 5 were a combination of media and personal accounts. A histogram with the top 100 Twitter users of each country can be seen in Fig. 24.
- Regarding the most published words, all countries published about Covid-19 or coronavirus, and on their national cases. This information can be seen through the clouds of unigrams and bigrams shown in Figs. 25 and 26.
- The most published bigrams by country are summarized in Table 14.

In short, the paper concludes that the surveillance tool is useful both for detection and prevention of infectious diseases such as pandemic Covid-19 which is affecting whole world currently.

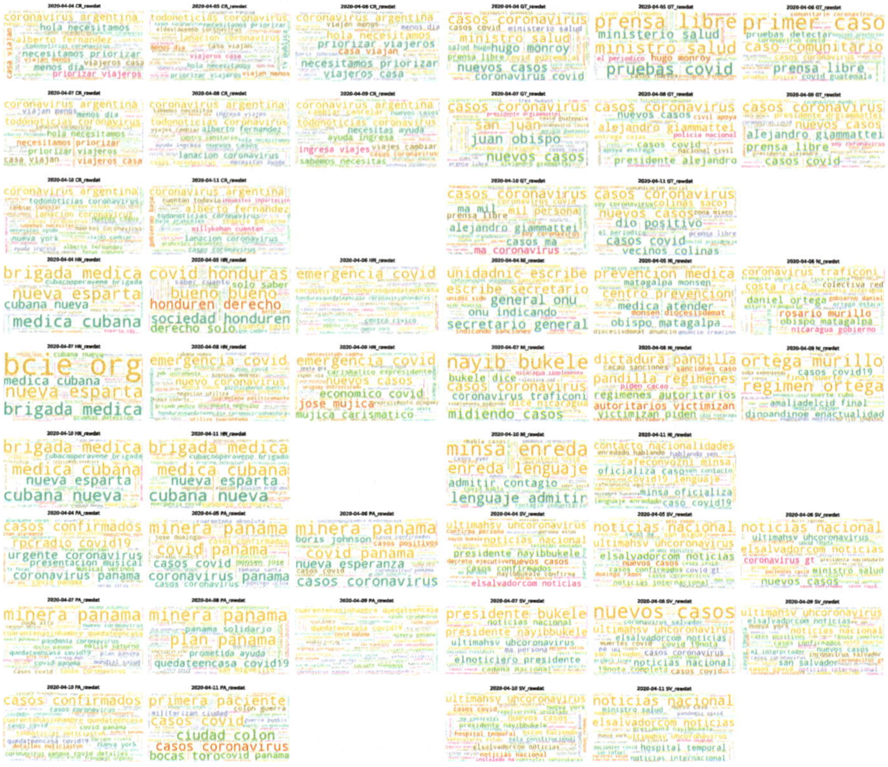

Fig. 26 Cloud of wordbis of Costa Rica, Guatemala, Honduras, Nicaragua, Panama and El Salvador [73]

Table 14 The most published bigrams by country in Central America

Country	Most published words
Costa Rica	'viajeros casa', 'priorizar pasajeros' and 'ingresa viajes'
Nicaragua	'prevencion medica'
Panama	'casos covid', 'casos coronavirus' and 'casos confirmados'
Honduras	'emergencia covid' and 'brigada medica'
Guatemaala	'primer caso'
El Salvador	'casos nuevos' and 'nuevos casos'

4 NLP Applied to North America

North America is made up of the countries Bermuda, Canada, United States, Greenland and Mexico. The latter is the only country in North America that in turn is part of Latin America because it has Spanish as its official language. For that reason, in this subsection we will only explore text mining studies on population data from this country.

Similar to Central America, for North America only one relevant work was found that aligns with the objectives of this article. In the paper [59] the authors present a study with the purpose to identify the principal concerns of the population during of outbreak stage of Covid-19 in Mexico City.

Summarizing this article, the authors conducted some experiments focused on analyzing the posts of Twitter users during the period between March 3 to 20. Specifically, they analyzed three aspects: the number of publications during the period, the Twitter users with the highest number of publications, and the terms most used in user publications in relation to Covid-19. The main findings were:

- The number of post or tweets per day during the period explored was increasing according was increasing the number of positive Covid-19 cases confirmed by the Ministry of Health of the Government of Mexico. This information can be confirmed in the Fig. 27.
- The most published words were "coronavirus" and "covid", which suggest as principal theme of concern the preventive and health security measures to prevent the spread of Covid-19 implemented by the Government of Mexico (see Fig. 28).
- The Twitter user with the highest number of publications was "La Silla Rota", a Mexican digital newspaper. This media posted 50% more than the next best publisher, which was "Noticieros Televisa". This information can be corroborated through the Fig. 29.
- After categorizing and remove media (written press, radio and television) tweets, the most published words were "coronavirus" and "covid" for non-media users accounts (seeFig. 30). These results were similar to the results of the experiment

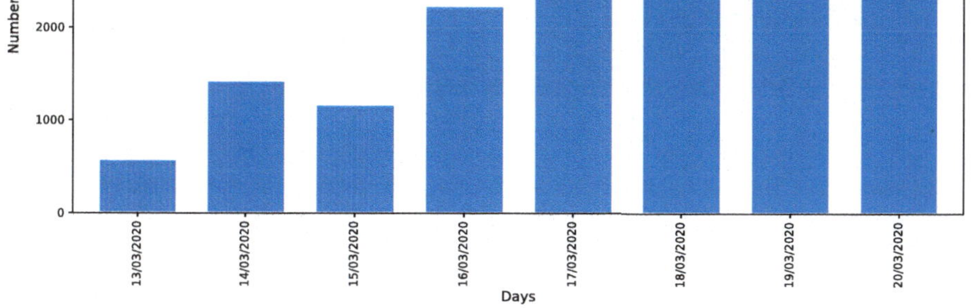

Fig. 27 Number of tweets by per day in Mexico City [59]

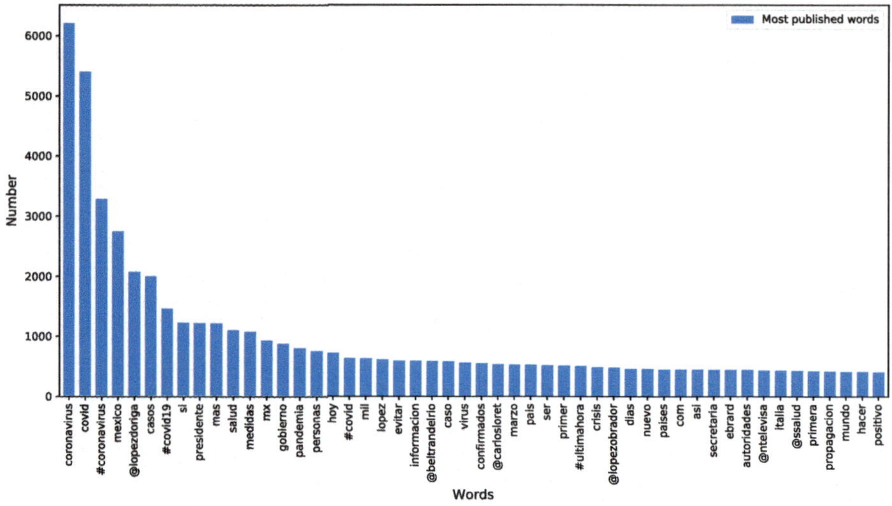

Fig. 28 Top 50 of the most posted words in Mexico City [59]

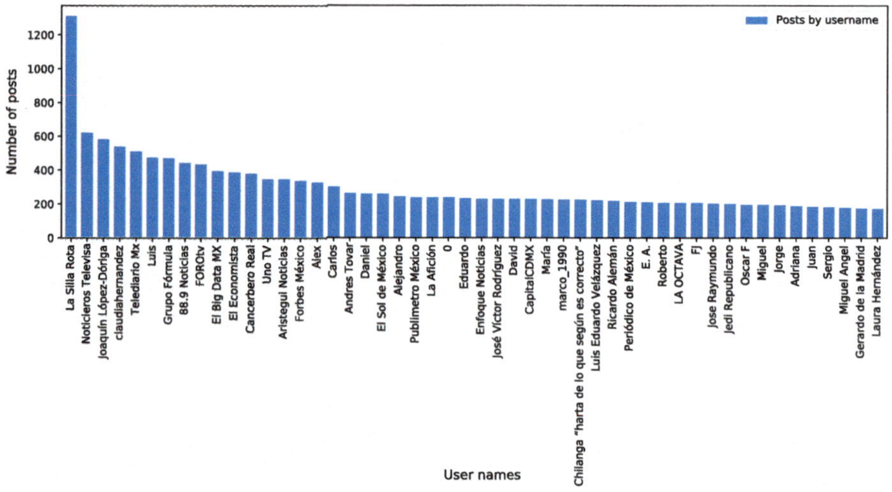

Fig. 29 Top 50 Twitter users with most posts in Mexico City [59]

in which all Twitter user accounts are considered. This suggests that there is no influence of the media on the population, at least in this study that considers Mexico City.

The authors identify after a general exploratory that the preventive and health security measures implemented by the Government of Mexico were the central concerns of citizens during the Covid-19 outbreak phase in Mexico City.

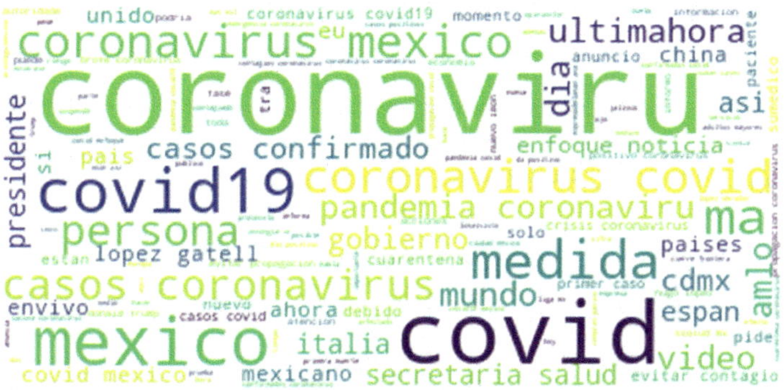

Fig. 30 Cloud of words published by the non-media in Mexico City [59]

5 Conclusions

In this chapter was presented an overview of Covid-19 research work published this year in Latin America. It was of particular interest for this work only consider for the analyses those proposals that employ text mining techniques and social networks, the latter as information sensors. Articles published and in preprint from January to July were considered. The main databases that include the topics of computer science and health were consulted, such as: IEEE Xplorer, Springer, ACM, Scopus, ArXiv, MedrXiv and PubMed. This work started with an overview of Covid-19 outbreak in the world and Latin America. However, order to analyze the information according to the context of each Latin America region, the results were grouped in South America, Central America and North America, The scientific community showed greater interest in using this field of Artificial Intelligence to monitor the development of the Covid-19 pandemic in South America than in Central and North America. However, even so, the results obtained reveal the scarce scientific work in this field of knowledge and the range of opportunities and challenges that it imposes. For example, it is clear that the negative impact of Covid-19 highlighted the need to put algorithms, platforms, techniques and models to work in real world scenarios.

As a final reflection, it is believed that this research work can become a reference for future proposals that involve text mining as the central axis. Likewise, to also be a motivator and promoter of collaboration in order to contribute to the solution of the problems derived from the Covid-19 outbreak in Latin America, not only in public health but in other areas such as economy, education, politics, tourism, religion, etc., where Artificial Intelligence can provide high-impact solutions.

6 Future Work

Considering the actual progress related to global Covid-19 research, the future work will extend the actual review to the complete year of 2020. Because, the collected papers were considering situation previous to July month. And, it is very possible more works related to Covid-19 and Text Mining were done and released. Therefore, all the papers related to Text Mining, Covid-19 will be condensed in a survey of 2020 papers to facilitate the work of research groups, industry tasks of Latin American community and the other regions.

Acknowledgements Authors wants to thank to Research4tech, an Artificial Intelligence (AI) community of Latin American Researcher with the aim of promoting AI, build science communities to catapult and enforce development of Latin American countries supported on science and technology, integrating academic community, technology groups/communities, government and society.

References

1. WHO: Who statement regarding cluster of pneumonia cases in Wuhan, China. WHO, Beijing, vol. 9 (2020)
2. Wang, C., Horby, P.W., Hayden, F.G., Gao, G.F.: A novel coronavirus outbreak of global health concern. The Lancet **395**(10223), 470–473 (2020)
3. Sohrabi, C., Alsafi, Z., O'Neill, N., Khan, M., Kerwan, A., Al-Jabir, A., Iosifidis, C., Agha, R.: World health organization declares global emergency: a review of the 2019 novel coronavirus (covid-19). Int. J. Surg. (2020)
4. Clarín (2020). https://www.clarin.com/sociedad/coronavirus-confirmaron-primer-caso-argentina-espera-conferencia-gobierno_0_awnywhZX.html. Accessed 21 Aug 2020
5. Los-Tiempos (2020). https://www.lostiempos.com/actualidad/pais/20200310/confirman-dos-primeros-casos-coronavirus-bolivia. Accessed 21 Aug 2020
6. de Saúde, M. (2020). https://www.saude.gov.br/noticias/agencia-saude/46435-brasil-confirma-primeiro-caso-de-novo-coronavirus. Accessed 21 Aug 2020
7. Reuters (2020). https://www.reuters.com/article/us-health-coronavirus-chile/chile-records-first-confirmed-case-of-coronavirus-health-ministry-idUSKBN20Q2UU. Accessed 21 Aug 2020
8. MinSaludCol (2020). https://mobile.twitter.com/MinSaludCol/status/1236020009127890951. Accessed 21 Aug 2020
9. Comercio, E. (2020). https://mobile.twitter.com/elcomerciocom/status/1233773816825946113. Accessed 21 Aug 2020
10. Reuters (2020). https://www.reuters.com/article/us-health-coronavirus-peru/peru-records-first-confirmed-case-of-coronavirus-president-vizcarra-says-idUSKBN20T1S9. Accessed 21 Aug 2020
11. Herald, D. (2020). https://www.deccanherald.com/international/paraguay-reports-first-coronavirus-case-811730.html. Accessed 21 Aug 2020
12. Observador, E. (2020). https://www.elobservador.com.uy/nota/un-desafio-inedito-202031321363. Accessed 21 Aug 2020
13. NTN24 (2020). https://www.ntn24.com/america-latina/venezuela/regimen-de-maduro-confirma-dos-primeros-casos-de-coronavirus-120128. Accessed 21 Aug 2020
14. AméricaEconomia (2020). https://www.americaeconomia.com/politica-sociedad/mundo/costa-rica-reporta-primer-caso-de-coronavirus-en-centroamerica-en-una. Accessed 21 Aug 2020

15. Gráfica, P. (2020). https://www.laprensagrafica.com/elsalvador/Primer-caso-de-COVID-19-en-El-Salvador-pudo-haber-entrado-por-punto-ciego-en-Metapan-se-ha-activado-cerco-sanitario-por-48-horas-en-ese-municipio-20200318-0064.html. Accessed 21 Aug 2020
16. de Salud, S. (2020). https://covid19honduras.org/?q=primeros-casos-confirmados. Accessed 21 Aug 2020
17. Reuters (2020). https://www.reuters.com/article/us-health-coronavirus-nicaragua-idUSKBN21608Q. Accessed 21 Aug 2020
18. Libre, P. (2020). https://www.prensalibre.com/guatemala/comunitario/coronavirus-alejandro-giammattei-confirma-el-primer-caso-de-covid-19-en-Guatemala/. Accessed 21 Aug 2020
19. Garda (2020). https://www.garda.com/crisis24/news-alerts/321101/panama-first-covid-19-case-confirmed-march-9-update-1. Accessed 21 Aug 2020
20. Angeles, C.L. (2020). https://losangeles.cbslocal.com/2020/02/28/mexico-confirms-its-first-2-coronavirus-cases/. Accessed 21 Aug 2020
21. Saire, J.E.C.: Building intelligent indicators to detect dengue epidemics in brazil using social networks. In: 2019 IEEE Colombian Conference on Applications in Computational Intelligence (ColCACI), pp. 1–5. IEEE (2019)
22. Bates, M.: Tracking disease: digital epidemiology offers new promise in predicting outbreaks. IEEE Pulse **8**(1), 18–22 (2017)
23. Subramani, S., Michalska, S., Wang, H., Whittaker, F., Heyward, B.: Text mining and real-time analytics of twitter data: a case study of Australian hay fever prediction. In: International Conference on Health Information Science, pp. 134–145. Springer (2018)
24. Edo-Osagie, O., De La Iglesia, B., Lake, I., Edeghere, O.: A scoping review of the use of twitter for public health research. Comput. Biol. Med. 103770 (2020)
25. Lwin, M.O., Lu, J., Sheldenkar, A., Cayabyab, Y.M., Yee, A.Z.H., Smith, H.E.: Temporal and textual analysis of social media on collective discourses during the Zika virus pandemic. BMC Public Heal. **20**, 1–9 (2020)
26. Tekieh, M.H., Raahemi, B.: Importance of data mining in healthcare: a survey. In: Proceedings of the 2015 IEEE/ACM International Conference on Advances in Social Networks Analysis and Mining 2015, pp. 1057–1062 (2015)
27. de Araujo, D.H.M., de Carvalho, E.A., da Motta, C.L.R., da Silva Borges, M.R., Gomes, J.O., de Carvalho, P.V.R.: Social networks applied to zika and h1n1 epidemics: a systematic review. In: Congress of the International Ergonomics Association, pp. 679–692. Springer (2018)
28. De Santis, E., Martino, A., Rizzi, A.: An infoveillance system for detecting and tracking relevant topics from italian tweets during the covid-19 event. IEEE Access **8**, 132527–132538 (2020)
29. Abd-Alrazaq, A., Alhuwail, D., Househ, M., Hamdi, M., Shah, Z.: Top concerns of tweeters during the covid-19 pandemic: infoveillance study. J. Med. Internet Res. **22**(4), e19016 (2020)
30. Albahri, A., Hamid, R.A., et al.: Role of biological data mining and machine learning techniques in detecting and diagnosing the novel coronavirus (covid-19): a systematic review. J. Med. Syst. **44**(7), (2020)
31. Elhadad, M.K., Li, K.F., Gebali, F.: Covid-19-fakes: a twitter (arabic/english) dataset for detecting misleading information on covid-19. In: International Conference on Intelligent Networking and Collaborative Systems, pp. 256–268. Springer (2020)
32. Fu, Z., Wu, Y., Zhang, H., Hu, Y., Zhao, D., Yan, R.: Be aware of the hot zone: a warning system of hazard area prediction to intervene novel coronavirus covid-19 outbreak. In: Proceedings of the 43rd International ACM SIGIR Conference on Research and Development in Information Retrieval, pp. 2241–2250 (2020)
33. Kim, M., Kang, J., Kim, D., Song, H., Min, H., Nam, Y., Park, D., Lee, J.G.: Hi-covidnet: Deep learning approach to predict inbound covid-19 patients and case study in south korea. In: Proceedings of the 26th ACM SIGKDD International Conference on Knowledge Discovery & Data Mining, pp. 3466–3473 (2020)
34. Muthusami, R., Bharathi, A., Saritha, K.: Covid-19 outbreak: tweet based analysis and visualization towards the influence of coronavirus in the world. Gedrag en Organisatie **33**(2) (2020)
35. De Santis, E., Martino, A., Rizzi, A.: An infoveillance system for detecting and tracking relevant topics from italian tweets during the covid-19 event. IEEE Access **8**, 132527–132538 (2020)

36. Nguyen, T.T.: Artificial intelligence in the battle against coronavirus (covid-19): a survey and future research directions (2020). http://dx.doi.org/10.36227/techrxiv.12743933.v1
37. Chen, C., Ebeid, I.A., Bu, Y., Ding, Y.: Coronavirus knowledge graph: a case study (2020)
38. Lee, J., Yi, S.S., Jeong, M., Sung, M., Yoon, W., Choi, Y., Ko, M., Kang, J.: Answering questions on covid-19 in real-time (2020)
39. Wang, L.L., Lo, K., Chandrasekhar, Y., Reas, R., Yang, J., Burdick, D., Eide, D., Funk, K., Katsis, Y., Kinney, R., Li, Y., Liu, Z., Merrill, W., Mooney, P., Murdick, D., Rishi, D., Sheehan, J., Shen, Z., Stilson, B., Wade, A., Wang, K., Wang, N.X.R., Wilhelm, C., Xie, B., Raymond, D., Weld, D.S., Etzioni, O., Kohlmeier, S.: Cord-19: the covid-19 open research dataset (2020)
40. Gao, Z., Yada, S., Wakamiya, S., Aramaki, E.: Naist covid: multilingual covid-19 twitter and weibo dataset (2020)
41. Fister Jr. I., Fister, K., Fister, I.: Discovering associations in covid-19 related research papers (2020)
42. Saire, J.E.C., Navarro, R.C.: What is the people posting about symptoms related to coronavirus in Bogota, Colombia? (2020)
43. Tekumalla, R., Banda, J.M.: Characterization of potential drug treatments for covid-19 using social media data and machine learning (2020)
44. Soni, S., Roberts, K.: An evaluation of two commercial deep learning-based information retrieval systems for covid-19 literature (2020)
45. Peng, Y., Tang, Y.X., Lee, S., Zhu, Y., Summers, R.M., Lu, Z.: Covid-19-ct-cxr: a freely accessible and weakly labeled chest x-ray and ct image collection on covid-19 from biomedical literature (2020)
46. Georgiou, K., Mittas, N., Angelis, L., Chatzigeorgiou, A.: A study of knowledge sharing related to covid-19 pandemic in stack overflow (2020)
47. Zavarrone, E., Grassia, M.G., Marino, M., Cataldo, R., Mazza, R., Canestrari, N.: CO. ME. TA.–covid-19 media textual analysis. a dashboard for media monitoring (2020)
48. Lopez, C.E., Vasu, M., Gallemore, C.: Understanding the perception of covid-19 policies by mining a multilanguage twitter dataset (2020)
49. Chire Saire, J.E., Oblitas, J.: Covid19 surveillance in Peru on April using text mining. medRxiv (2020). https://doi.org/10.1101/2020.05.24.20112193. https://www.medrxiv.org/content/early/2020/05/25/2020.05.24.20112193
50. Xie, Z., Li, D.: Health and demographic impact on covid-19 infection and mortality in us counties. medRxiv (2020). https://doi.org/10.1101/2020.05.06.20093195. https://www.medrxiv.org/content/early/2020/05/11/2020.05.06.20093195
51. Zou, C., Wang, X., Xie, Z., Li, D.: Public reactions towards the covid-19 pandemic on twitter in the united kingdom and the united states. medRxiv (2020). https://doi.org/10.1101/2020.07.25.20162024. https://www.medrxiv.org/content/early/2020/07/28/2020.07.25.20162024
52. Wang, X., Zou, C., Xie, Z., Li, D.: Public opinions towards covid-19 in California and Newyork on twitter. medRxiv (2020). https://doi.org/10.1101/2020.07.12.20151936. https://www.medrxiv.org/content/early/2020/07/14/2020.07.12.20151936
53. Azarafza, M., Azarafza, M., Akgun, H.: Clustering method for spread pattern analysis of corona-virus (covid-19) infection in iran. medRxiv (2020). https://doi.org/10.1101/2020.05.22.20109942. https://www.medrxiv.org/content/early/2020/05/28/2020.05.22.20109942
54. Tran, B.X., Ha, G.H., Nguyen, L.H., Vu, G.T., Phan, H.T., Le, H.T., Latkin, C.A., Ho, C.S., Ho, R.C.: Studies of novel coronavirus disease 19 (covid-19) pandemic: a global analysis of literature. medRxiv (2020). https://doi.org/10.1101/2020.05.05.20092635. https://www.medrxiv.org/content/early/2020/05/08/2020.05.05.20092635
55. Shuja, J., Alanazi, E., Alasmary, W., Alashaikh, A.: Covid-19 open source data sets: a comprehensive survey. medRxiv (2020). https://doi.org/10.1101/2020.05.19.20107532. https://www.medrxiv.org/content/early/2020/07/13/2020.05.19.20107532
56. Chandu, V.: Identification of spatial variations in covid-19 epidemiological data using k-means clustering algorithm: a global perspective. medRxiv (2020). https://doi.org/10.1101/2020.06.03.20121194. https://www.medrxiv.org/content/early/2020/06/05/2020.06.03.20121194

57. Aznab, M.: Evaluation of covid 19 infection in 279 cancer patients treated during a 90-day period in 2020 pandemic. medRxiv (2020). https://doi.org/10.1101/2020.05.26.20102889. https://www.medrxiv.org/content/early/2020/06/01/2020.05.26.20102889
58. Kumar, R., Arora, R., Bansal, V., Sahayasheela, V.J., Buckchash, H., Imran, J., Narayanan, N., Pandian, G.N., Raman, B.: Accurate prediction of covid-19 using chest x-ray images through deep feature learning model with smote and machine learning classifiers. medRxiv (2020). https://doi.org/10.1101/2020.04.13.20063461. https://www.medrxiv.org/content/early/2020/04/17/2020.04.13.20063461
59. Chire Saire, J.E., Pineda-Briseno, A.: Text mining approach to analyze coronavirus impact: Mexico city as case of study. medRxiv (2020). https://doi.org/10.1101/2020.05.07.20094466. https://www.medrxiv.org/content/early/2020/05/12/2020.05.07.20094466
60. Drias, H.H., Drias, Y.: Mining twitter data on covid-19 for sentiment analysis and frequent patterns discovery. medRxiv (2020). https://doi.org/10.1101/2020.05.08.20090464. https://www.medrxiv.org/content/early/2020/05/18/2020.05.08.20090464
61. Chire Saire, J.E.: How was the mental health of Colombian people on march during pandemics covid19? medRxiv (2020). https://doi.org/10.1101/2020.07.02.20145425. https://www.medrxiv.org/content/early/2020/07/04/2020.07.02.20145425
62. Chire Saire, J.E.: Infoveillance based on social sensors to analyze the impact of covid19 in South American population. medRxiv (2020). https://doi.org/10.1101/2020.04.06.20055749. https://www.medrxiv.org/content/early/2020/04/11/2020.04.06.20055749
63. Souza, F.S.H., Hojo-Souza, N.S., Santos, E.B., Silva, C.M., Guidoni, D.L.: Predicting the disease outcome in covid-19 positive patients through machine learning: a retrospective cohort study with brazilian data. medRxiv (2020). https://doi.org/10.1101/2020.06.26.20140764. https://www.medrxiv.org/content/early/2020/06/28/2020.06.26.20140764
64. Samuel, J., Rahman, M.M., Ali, G.G.M.N., Samuel, Y., Pelaez, A., Chong, P.H., Yakubov, M.: Feeling positive about reopening? New normal scenarios from covid-19 reopen sentiment analytics. medRxiv (2020). https://doi.org/10.1101/2020.06.01.20119362. https://www.medrxiv.org/content/early/2020/06/02/2020.06.01.20119362
65. Stamm, T.A., Andrews, M.R., Mosor, E., Ritschl, V., Li, L.C., Ma, J.K., Campo Arias, A., Baker, S., Burton, N.W., Eghbali, M., Fernandez, N., Ferreira, R., Gaebler, G., Makri, S., Mintz, S., Moe, R., Morasso, E., Murphy, S.L., Ntuli, S., Omara, M., Simancas Pallares, M., Horonieff, J., Gartlehner, G.: Clinical practice guidelines and recommendations in the context of the covid-19 pandemic: systematic review and critical appraisal. medRxiv (2020). https://doi.org/10.1101/2020.06.19.20134767. https://www.medrxiv.org/content/early/2020/06/20/2020.06.19.20134767
66. Strohbehn, G.W., Heiss, B.L., Rouhani, S.J., Trujillo, J.A., Yu, J., Kacew, A.J., Higgs, E.F., Bloodworth, J.C., Cabanov, A., Wright, R.C., Koziol, A., Weiss, A., Danahey, K., Karrison, T.G., Edens, C.C., Ventura, I.B., Pettit, N.N., Patel, B., Pisano, J., Strek, M.E., Gajewski, T.F., Ratain, M.J., Reid, P.D.: Covidose: low-dose tocilizumab in the treatment of covid-19. medRxiv (2020). https://doi.org/10.1101/2020.07.20.20157503. https://www.medrxiv.org/content/early/2020/07/26/2020.07.20.20157503
67. Teheran, A.A., Camero, G., Prado de la Guardia, R., Hernandez, C., Herrera, G., Pombo, L.M., Avila, A., Florez, C., Barros, E.C., Perez Garcia, L., Paniz Mondolfi, A., Ramirez, J.D.: Epidemiological characterization of asymptomatic carriers of covid-19 in Colombia. medRxiv (2020). https://doi.org/10.1101/2020.06.18.20134734. https://www.medrxiv.org/content/early/2020/06/20/2020.06.18.20134734
68. Li, D., Chaudhary, H., Zhang, Z.: Modeling spatiotemporal pattern of depressive symptoms caused by COVID-19 using social media data mining. Int. J. Environ. Res. Public Heal. **17**(14) (2020)
69. Zhang, W.: Estimating the presymptomatic transmission of covid19 using incubation period and serial interval data. medRxiv (2020). https://doi.org/10.1101/2020.04.02.20051318. https://www.medrxiv.org/content/early/2020/04/06/2020.04.02.20051318

70. Tindale, L., Coombe, M., Stockdale, J.E., Garlock, E., Lau, W.Y.V., Saraswat, M., Lee, Y.H.B., Zhang, L., Chen, D., Wallinga, J., Colijn, C.: Transmission interval estimates suggest pre-symptomatic spread of covid-19. medRxiv (2020). https://doi.org/10.1101/2020.03.03.20029983. https://www.medrxiv.org/content/early/2020/03/06/2020.03.03.20029983
71. Lavezzo, E., Franchin, E., Ciavarella, C., Cuomo-Dannenburg, G., Barzon, L., Del Vecchio, C., Rossi, L., Manganelli, R., Loregian, A., Navarin, N., Abate, D., Sciro, M., Merigliano, S., Decanale, E., Vanuzzo, M.C., Saluzzo, F., Onelia, F., Pacenti, M., Parisi, S., Carretta, G., Donato, D., Flor, L., Cocchio, S., Masi, G., Sperduti, A., Cattarino, L., Salvador, R., Gaythorpe, K.A., , Brazzale, A.R., Toppo, S., Trevisan, M., Baldo, V., Donnelly, C.A., Ferguson, N.M., Dorigatti, I., Crisanti, A.: Suppression of covid-19 outbreak in the municipality of vo, Italy. medRxiv (2020). https://doi.org/10.1101/2020.04.17.20053157. https://www.medrxiv.org/content/early/2020/04/18/2020.04.17.20053157
72. do Estado do Esp ırito Sant, G. (2020) https://coronavirus.es.gov.br/painel-covid-19-es. Accessed 02 Sept 2020
73. Saire, J.E.C., Lemus-Martin, R.: Infoveillance to analyze covid19 impact on central america population. medRxiv (2020)

Spread of COVID-19 in Odisha (India) Due to Influx of Migrants and Stability Analysis Using Mathematical Modeling

Aswin Kumar Rauta, Yerra Shankar Rao, and Jangyadatta Behera

Abstract **Aim/Objectives:** To ascertain the effect of migrant workers on the spread of COVID-19 in Odisha, India and to examine both local and global stability. **Study Design:** Out-migrants are diagnosed at compartment (A), those who were confirmed positive, they were sent to the infected compartment (I) for treatment and the remaining healthy individuals are sent to quarantine compartment (Q) for a period of twenty one days under surveillance or observation. Then basing on the principle of mathematical epidemiology, the set of ordinary (nonlinear) differential equations is formulated. **Methodology/Approach:** Jacobian Matrices are employed to find eigen values of the system for stability behaviour. Routh-Hurwitz Criterion and Poincare-Bendixson theorem are used for stability analysis. The set of ordinary (nonlinear) differential equations are solved using Runge-Kutta fourth order method. The simulation of numerical data is performed using MATLAB. **Results**: The study shows that the prevalence of COVID-19 would remain nearly 250 to 300 days in Odisha since the inception of entry of infected migrants to the state till the disease is stable. Further the study proves that it persists to endemic equilibrium for global stability when basic reproduction number greater than unity. The numerical and analytical results of the study establish that the disease free equilibrium is locally stable when basic reproduction number is less than unity and unstable when it is more than unity. **Conclusions:** As there is no specific treatment, vaccine or medicine available for the disease till the date, so the only intervention procedure called quarantine process is devised in this model to check the stability behaviour of the disease. Due to intervention of quarantine, lock-down, shutdown and other social distancing rules, the study shows that the system is stable after a certain period of time. This mathematical

A. K. Rauta (✉) · J. Behera
Department of Mathematics, S.K.C.G. (Autonomous) College, Paralakhemundi 761200, Odisha, India
e-mail: aswinmath2003@gmail.com

J. Behera
e-mail: jangyabhr09@gmail.com

Y. S. Rao
Department of Mathematics, GIET Ghangapatana, Bhubaneswar 752054, Orissa, India
e-mail: sankar.math1@gmail.com

D. Oliva et al. (eds.), *Artificial Intelligence for COVID-19*, Studies in Systems, Decision and Control 358, https://doi.org/10.1007/978-3-030-69744-0_17

modelling embedded with important risk factor like migration could be adopted for each state that will be helpful for better prediction of the entire country and world.

Keywords Global and local stability · Modeling · Migration · Equilibrium · Quarantine · Virus

Nomenclature

S	Susceptible compartment
I	Infected compartment
Q	Quarantine compartment
R	Recovered compartment
A	Diagnosed compartment
β	Rate of contact
γ	Rate at which the infected population is quarantined
ε	Rate at which quarantine population is recovered
T	Rate of newborn
δ_1	Death rate other than COVID-19
δ_2	Death rate due to COVID-19
Λ	Migrant population
P	Proportion of migrants detected COVID-19

1 Introduction

Being the second most populous country in the world, it is an urgent need to investigate the spread and control of disease in India. However, due to diversity of vast population, uncertainty of infection, varying rate of recovery, state wise different COVID-19 induced death rate and non-uniform quarantine policy of the states, it is strenuous to predict the spread and control of disease accurately in the country. Therefore, we have considered one of the states in India is Odisha having population nearly equal to the population of Spain because the entry of huge migrants to the state suddenly enhanced the number of COVID-19 patients from below two hundred to more than eight hundred within one week even after forty days of lockdown period.

An unknown and unexpected disease having symptoms of fever, cough, cold, fatigue, headache, and shortness of breath leads to severe pneumonia that causes death was first detected in Wuhan city of China in December 2019. The disease is confirmed as due to a phylogenetically SARS-CoV-2 clade novel corona virus that is called COVID-19 disease. In India, the first COVID-19 case was detected from the state of Kerala on 30th January 2020. The patient was a student from Wuhan returnee. Gradually, many cases have been reporting from different states of the country everyday [1–7]. In Odisha the first COVID-19 patient [8–13] was a 31 year young man detected from Bhubaneswar (state capital) on 16th March 2020 who was returned from Italy and second case was a 77 year old man from U.K. returnee was detected on 20th March 2020. Then on 21th March 2020 the state government declared lockdown in five districts and supported by the Janata curfew on 22nd March 2020 appealed by the prime minister of India. Then the government of India declared complete lockdown in the entire country from 24th March 2020 midnight to 15th April 2020 to break the chain of transmission of COVID-19. The first death case due to COVID-19 in the state was reported on 6th April 2020. The deceased was a 72 year old man from Bhubaneswar who was also suffering from pre-existing diseases. Odisha is the first state in India that had extended the 2nd lockdown up to 30th April 2020. By the time, the government of India implemented second, third and fourth lockdowns from 16th April 2020 to 3rd May 2020, 4th May 2020 to 17th May 2020 and 18th May 2020 to 31th May 2020 respectively with relaxations in some services. The number of cases enhanced in the state after the government of India allowed the migration of workers across the country. Odisha was a least concerned state regarding COVID-19 till 6th may 2020 with only below 200 members of cases reported but suddenly the number raised after the entry of huge numbers of migrants during the third lockdown period from different hotspot areas like Surat(Gujarat), Mumbai(Maharashtra), Chennai(Tamilnadu), Kerala, West Bengal, New Delhi and other parts of the country. Especially the migrants of Surat (India) returnee were detected more positive cases in the state that enhanced the number of positive cases from 200 (during first and second lockdown period) to more than 800 within one week. It is seen that the districts where more number of migrants entered from different hotspot areas of the country were reported more positive cases than the districts where less number of migrants were entered. These hotspot districts were Ganjam, Jajpur, Balasore, Bhadrak, Khurda, Kendrapara, Puri, Sundargarh, Cuttack, Anugul, Mayurbhanj. But the disease had been spread twenty three districts out of thirty districts of the state. Ganjam district was free from COVID-19 till 6th may 2020 but became the hotspot area of the state after the entry of at least fifty thousand Surat returnees to the district. More than four lakh workers [14] of Ganjam district had been working in Surat town only. Nearly six lakh migrants from different parts of the country have registered for return to the state. Around one lakh fifty thousand migrants from different districts of state had reached to the state till 18th May 2020. So it is a great concern to predict or forecast the spread of disease and its control if all the migrant people would enter to the state. The government of Odisha has made temporary health centers in the villages and urban areas to provide quarantine facilities to all migrant people coming to the state to control the disease.

The mathematical models are developed on COVID-19 for India are very few and perhaps no model has been developed on Odisha regarding COVID-19 so for our knowledge. Chayu Yang et al. [15] have investigated the spread of COVID-19 in Wuhan, China using SEIR mathematical model emphasizing on the concentration of corona virus in the environmental reservoir and its role in the spread of disease. Their study included birth rate but lack of influx of immigrants and migrants.

Shilei Zao et al. [16] have developed the SUQC mathematical model to study the dynamics of COVID-19 in China and interpreted the role of quarantine effects on the control of disease. Rajesh Singh et al. [17] have used age structured SIR model to study the spread of COVID-19 in India. They have suggested the social distancing as the most effective means of mitigation. They have found three week's lockdown in India was insufficient to check the resurgence of the disease. Their forecast of stability in India is about the periodic lockdown with relaxation of 67 days or completely lockdown of 49 days. P.V Khrapov et al. [18] have considered the simple SIR model but modified the equations based on the difference of time period between the onsets of the disease, its diagnosis, recovered or death to study the development of COVID-19 in China. They simply computed the numerical simulations without undergoing the analysis of stability. Manav. R. Bhatanagra [19] has proposed a mathematical model on community spread of COVID-19 using the data of USA, Italy and India and forecasted the increasing numbers of COVID-19 and preventing measures. Kaustuv Chatterjee et al. [20] have developed SEIR model on COVID-19 in India and predicted that the peak of infection will be during the month of July2020 and spread will be overwhelmed by the end of May. They have suggested proper health care with ICU facilities to reduce the death rate. Palash Ghosh et al. [21] have analyzed state wise contact rate of COVID-19 in India. They have studied exponential, logistic and SIS model jointly for each state and observed some states are showing decreasing trend in contact rate where as some states are showing increasing trend in contact rate. So they have suggested for lockdown policy to minimize the contact rate. Kaushalendra Kumar et al. [22] have developed SIR model to study the COVID-19 case in India and forecasted that 3 million people of India would be infected by October 2020. Further, their study reveals that the pandemic will persist from two months to more than six months.

Though many mathematical models have been implemented by many researchers on the investigation regarding COVID-19 in India but they have lack of important parameters and risk factors of the disease. So detailed investigation of the disease by considering the responsible factors like immigration is an emerging necessity in the study of COVID-19 to provide better understanding of the disease control, make decision, implement public health policy and explore the research dynamics in the interdisciplinary subjects. Thus, we have developed a mathematical model in which new compartment called diagnosed compartment (A) is used where the migrants were tested whether they were infected or not. Then, they were sent to susceptible and infected compartment for further investigation as per the principle of dynamical system. Entry of migrants characterized by death due to COVID-19, non COVID-19 death and new born have been addressed in this article for the stability behavior of the disease in Odisha (India). Therefore, the investigation done in this paper is an original, innovative and authentic work. This work may be extended for investigation of whole India as well as the world.

2 Mathematical Modeling and Basic Assumptions

The total population is distributed into five compartments as shown in Fig. 1. Diagnosed population (A) for migrants who are screened at the check post (Railway Station, State Border and Quarantine centre),Susceptible population (S) for healthy individuals, Infected population (I) for attacked individuals, Quarantine population (Q) for isolated individual and Recovered population (R) for cured individuals or those have reported negative in quarantine class. The whole population is N = S+I + Q+A + R. The susceptible population enhanced by the new born (T) but decreased due to contact of infected population at the rate β and diminished by the death due to other reason at the rate δ_1. The infected population size increases with change of time but then reduced due to recovery and death. Quarantine population also increases initially then decreases due to recovery as well as death but recovered population always increase by huge susceptible and migrant individuals after they get out of quarantine class though there is small death rate δ_1. On the basis of this criteria, the flow of the model is shown in the following diagram.

The following set of ordinary differential equations is generated as per the principle of Epidemic models;

$$\begin{aligned}
\frac{dS}{dt} &= T - \beta SI - \delta_1 S \\
\frac{dA}{dt} &= \Lambda - PA - (1-P)A - \delta_1 A \\
\frac{dI}{dt} &= \beta SI + PA - (\gamma + \delta_1 + \delta_2)I \\
\frac{dQ}{dt} &= (1-P)A + \gamma I - (\epsilon + \delta_1 + \delta_2)Q \\
\frac{dR}{dt} &= \epsilon Q - \delta_1 R
\end{aligned} \tag{1}$$

Subject to the initial conditions S(0), I(0), Q(0), R(0) and A(0) all are positive.

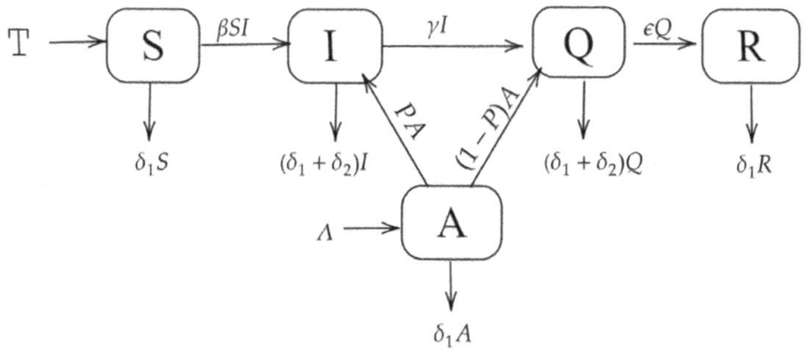

Fig. 1 Diagrammatic representation of the model

2.1 Basic Assumptions

i. COVID-19 spreads due to direct or indirect contact between susceptible and infected individuals.
ii. The latent period is ignored i.e. instantly the disease spreads.
iii. It is assumed that the population is homogeneous i.e. the rate of contact is independent of population size.
iv. Out—migrants who have registered in the government portal to return to the state are taken into consideration.
v. Birth and death rates are considered as constant.

Since the above set of equations is not in closed form, so, it could not be solved using any standard form of Ordinary Differential Equations. Hence, Runge-Kutta fourth order numerical method is employed to find the solutions with the help of MATLAB software.

2.2 Existence of Boundedness and Positive Invariant of the Solutions

Here, total population size,

$$N = S + A + I + Q + R$$
$$\Rightarrow \frac{dN}{dt} = \frac{dS}{dt} + \frac{dA}{dt} + \frac{dI}{dt} + \frac{dQ}{dt} + \frac{dR}{dt}$$
$$\Rightarrow \frac{dN}{dt} = T + \Lambda - \delta_1 N - \delta_2(I + Q)$$

In the absence of any diseases, $\frac{dN}{dt} = T + \Lambda - \delta_1$

Then, total population carries $N \to \frac{T+\Lambda}{\delta_1}$ as $q \to \infty q \to \infty$

Thus, it follows the solution of (1) exists in the region defined by $\Gamma = \left\{(S, A, I, Q, R) \in R_+^5 : S + A + I + Q + R \leq \frac{T+\Lambda}{\delta_1}\right\}$.

2.3 Basic Reproduction Number and Existence of Equilibrium

Basic reproduction number of the system (1) will be obtained as;

$$R_0 = \frac{\beta S_0}{(\gamma + \delta_1 + \delta_2)}$$

Two equilibrium points are

i. Diseases free equilibrium $\Gamma_{DFE}\left(S_0 = \frac{T}{\delta_1}, A = 0, I = 0, Q = 0, R = 0\right)$
ii. Endemic Equilibrium $\Gamma_{EE}(S = S^*, A = A^*, I = I^*, Q = Q^*, R = R^*)$
For the steady-state conditions, the endemic equilibrium $\Gamma_{EE}^*(S^*, A^*, I^*, Q^*, R^*)$ of the system (1) is determined by the equations

$$\begin{aligned}
&T - \beta SI - \delta_1 S = 0\\
&\Lambda - PA - (1-P)A - \delta_1 A = 0\\
&\beta SI + PA - (\gamma + \delta_1 + \delta_2)I = 0\\
&(1-P)A + \gamma I - (\varepsilon + \delta_1 + \delta_2)Q = 0\\
&\varepsilon O - \delta_1 R = 0
\end{aligned} \tag{2}$$

Solving the above equations simultaneously; we get

$$\begin{aligned}
S^* &= \frac{T}{\beta I^* + \delta_1}\\
A^* &= \frac{\Lambda}{\delta_1 + 1}\\
Q^* &= \frac{\Lambda(1-P) + \gamma I^*(\delta_1+1)}{(\delta_1+1)(\delta_1+\delta_2+\epsilon)}\\
R^* &= \frac{\epsilon\Lambda(1-P) + \gamma I^*(\delta_1+1)}{\delta_1(\delta_1+1)(\delta_1+\delta_2+\epsilon)}
\end{aligned}$$

2.4 Local Stability Analysis

The local stability analysis of system (1) is performed using the Jacobian matrix at the equilibrium points.

Theorem 1 *If $R_0 < 1$, the disease-free equilibrium $\Gamma_0\left(\frac{T}{\delta_1}, 0, 0, 0\right)$ of the system (1) is locally asymptotically stable in the region. If $R_0 > 1$ then Γ_0 is unstable and it continues to be endemic equilibrium.*

Proof At the diseases free equilibrium point $\Gamma_0\left(\frac{T}{\delta_1}, 0, 0, 0\right)$, the Jacobian matrix is

$$J_{DFE} = \begin{pmatrix}
-\delta_1 & 0 & -\beta\frac{T}{\delta_1} & 0\\
0 & -(\delta_1+1) & 0 & 0\\
0 & P & \left(\beta\frac{T}{\delta_1} - (\gamma+\delta_1+\delta_2)\right) & 0\\
0 & (1-P) & \gamma & -(\delta_1+\delta_2+\varepsilon)
\end{pmatrix}$$

Clearly, the eigen values are

$$\begin{aligned}
\lambda_1 &= -\delta_1\\
\lambda_2 &= -(\delta_1+1)\\
\lambda_3 &= -(\delta_1+\delta_2+\varepsilon)
\end{aligned}$$

For, $\lambda_4 = \beta\frac{T}{\delta_1} - (\gamma + \delta_1 + \delta_2)\frac{\beta T}{\delta_1(\gamma+\delta_1+\delta_2)} < 1 \Rightarrow R_0 < 1.$ □

Thus, all the Eigen values have negative real parts. Therefore, by Routh-Hurwitz criterion of stability, the system (1) is locally asymptotically stable at the Diseases free equilibrium points.

Theorem 2 *The endemic equilibrium* $\Gamma^*(S^*, A^*, I^*, Q^*, R^*)$ *is locally asymptotically stable when* $R_0 > 1$.

Proof At the endemic equilibrium $\Gamma^*(S^*, A^*, I^*, Q^*, R^*)$, the Jacobian matrix is

$$J_{EE} = \begin{pmatrix} -\beta I^* - \delta_1 & 0 & -\beta S^* & 0 & 0 \\ 0 & -(1+\delta_1) & 0 & 0 & 0 \\ \beta I^* & P & \beta S^* - (\delta_1 + \delta_2 + \gamma) & 0 & 0 \\ 0 & (1-P) & \gamma & -(\delta_1 + \delta_2 + \varepsilon) & 0 \\ 0 & 0 & 0 & \varepsilon & -\delta_1 \end{pmatrix}$$

After calculation, the eigen values are

$$\lambda_1 = -\delta_1$$
$$\lambda_2 = -(\delta_1 + \delta_2 + \varepsilon)$$
$$\lambda_3 = -(1 + \delta_1)$$

Other two eigen values are obtained from the Quadratic equation of the form $\lambda^2 + a_1\lambda + a_2 = 0$

where

$$a_1 = \beta I^* + 2\delta_1 + \delta_2 + \gamma - \beta S^* > 0$$
$$a_2 = (\beta I^* + \delta_1)(\delta_1 + \delta_2 + \gamma - \beta S^*) + \beta^2 I^* S^* > 0$$

If $R_0 > 1$, then $a_1 a_2 > 0$. Again by the Routh-Hurwitz Criterion, the system is locally asymptotically stable. □

2.5 Global Stability for the Endemic Equilibrium

Theorem 3 *If* $R_0 > 1$, *then the endemic equilibrium* $\Gamma^*(S^*, A^*, I^*, Q^*, R^*)$ *is globally stable in the given region.*

Proof Since the first and third equation of the system (1) are independent of Quarantine and Recovered class, so we can apply the Dulac's criteria with multiplier $D = 1/I$. □

Let's consider equations
$$M_1 = T - \beta SI - \delta_1 S$$
$$M_2 = \beta SI - (\delta_1 + \delta_2 + \gamma) + PA$$

Then, $DM_1 = \frac{T}{I} - \beta S - \frac{\delta_1 S}{I}$
$DM_2 = [\beta S - (\delta_1 + \delta_2 + r)] + \frac{PA}{I}$

So we have, $\frac{\partial(DM_1)}{\partial S} + \frac{\partial(DM_2)}{\partial I} = -\left(\beta + \frac{\delta_1}{I} + \frac{PA}{I^2}\right) < 0$

Hence, by the Poincare-Bendixson theorem, all the solutions starting in the positive quadrant of SI plane with $I > 0$ and $S + I \leq \frac{T}{\delta_1}$ approaches (S_*, I_*) as $t \to \infty$. In this case, the limiting forms for other three equations of the system (1) shows $A \to A^*, Q \to Q^*, R \to R^*$. Thus, the endemic equilibrium $\Gamma^*(S^*, A^*, I^*, Q^*, R^*)$ is globally stable in the region Γ for the system (1).

3 Interpretation of the Numerical Results

Odisha is the only state in India that was adopted quarantine period for over 28 days (21 days government quarantine and 7 days home quarantine) instead of 14 days quarantine when the infection spread in the state due to entry of migrants after the end of second lockdown in the country. Presently, the total population of the state is around 4.5 crore [13, 23]. The total number of migrants registered to return to the state [8, 9] under government's custody is more than five lakhs but some people had returned to the state by the means of cycle, walking, rail and vehicles. We have fixed the initial conditions for all compartments as per the data [8–13] available up to 18th May 2020. Hence, the initial condition for diagnosed compartment of migrant individuals is set as A (0) = 600000 and the initial condition for other compartments are assumed as S(0) = 45000000, I(0) = 695, R(0) = 220 and Q(0) = 600052. This study was carried out from 23rd March 2020 to 18th May 2020 (approximately 55 days). For the sake of convenience to plot the graphs, the initial values are scaled to unity as S(0) = 1, I(0) = 0.00013, Q(0) = 0.013333, R(0) = 0.00061555 and A(0) = 0.013333. The parametric values are taken per unit time i.e. per day. The contact rate of Odisha was in between 0.01 to 0.13, so $\beta = 0.01$ to 0.13. The quarantine period at the government level was 21 days. Therefore, $\gamma = 1/21 = 0.047$, $\varepsilon = 1/21 = 0.047$. Since the crude birth and death rates are 20 and 8.3 per one thousand in the state, so per unit time T = (20/1000)/365 = 0.000054 and $\delta_1 = (8.3/1000)/365 = 0.00022$. Again it has been reported that there are 4 deaths due to COVID-19 out of 876 confirmed infected cases in the period of 55 days, hence the death rate of this disease per day is $\delta_2 = (4/876)/55 = 0.000083$, The total number of migrants are assumed as $\Lambda = 1000000$ and rate of the proportion of infected migrants is calculated as P = 0.0034.

Figure 2 is plotted for basic reproduction number $R_0 = 0.943$ in support of Theorem 1, that shows the system is stable when $R_0 < 1$ i.e. no new infections occurs. The susceptible population remains at the same level with a slight increase due to entry of new-born and as long as no new infection occurs with progress of time or infection is reduced due to adoption of quarantine. It means that the disease will die out and susceptible class will be stable without any impact on the share of other compartments that are at zero level except the recovered class which is just above

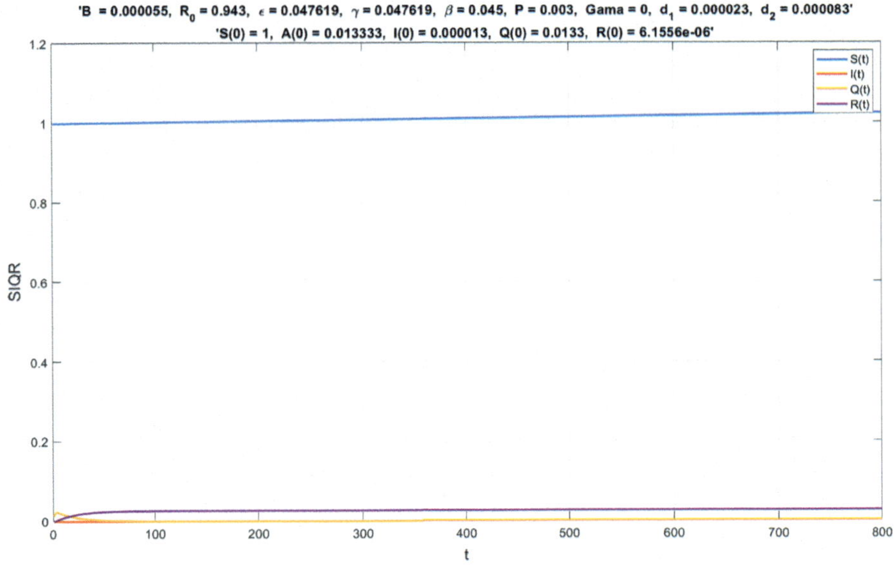

Fig. 2 S,I,Q,R versus time graph for basic reproduction number less than unity

the zero level because of the recovery of infected individuals. Also Theorem 1 states that the system is unstable when $R_0 > 1$ i.e. the disease leads towards the endemic for some periods of time which is verified in Figs. 3, 4 and 5.

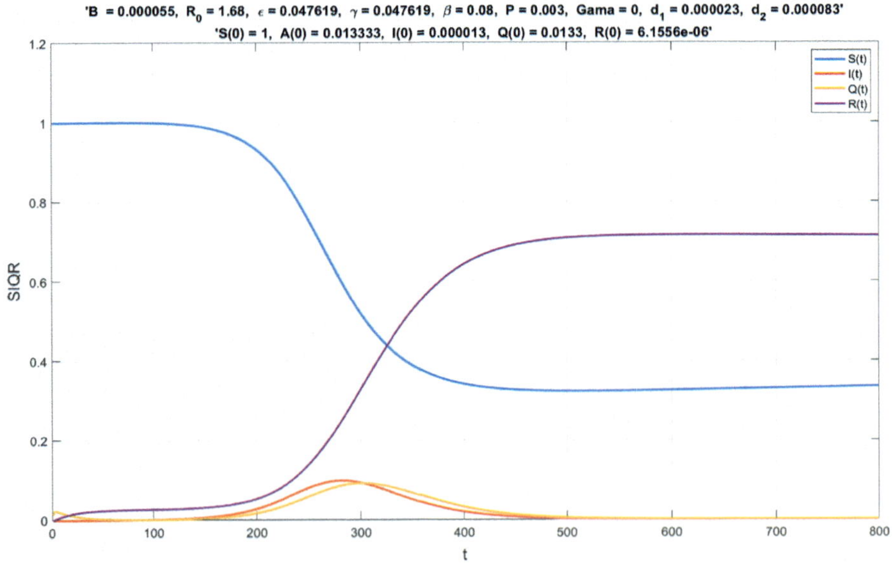

Fig. 3 S,I,Q,R versus time graph for basic reproduction number greater than unity

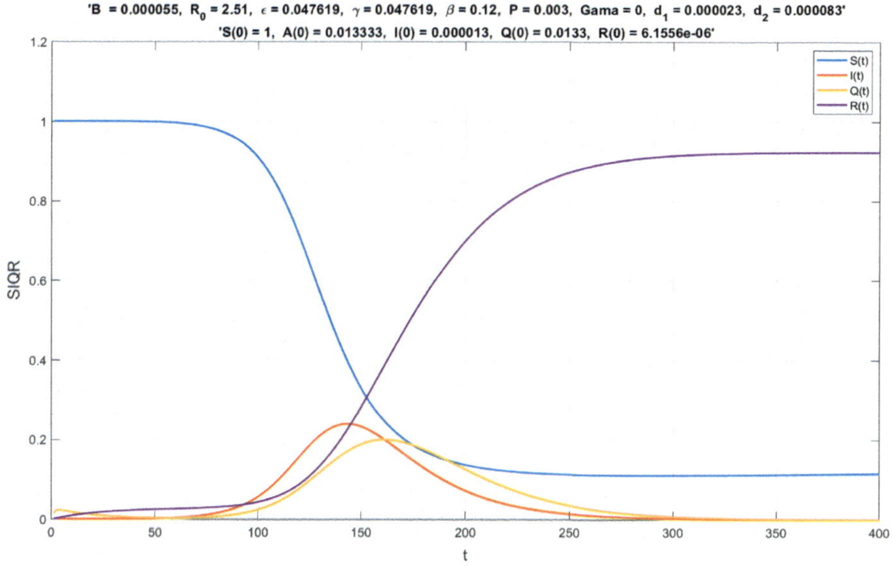

Fig. 4 S,I,Q,R versus time graph for basic reproduction number greater than unity

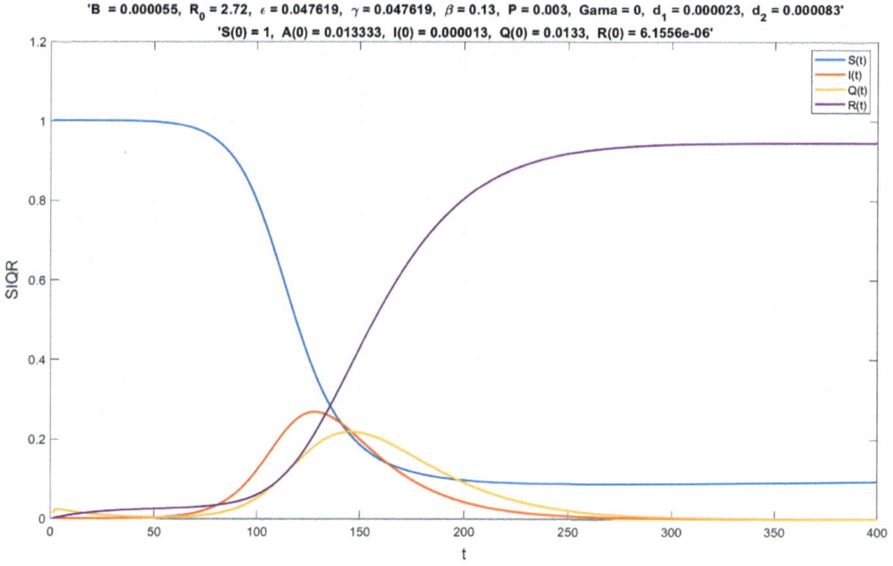

Fig. 5 S,I,Q,R versus time graph for basic reproduction number greater than unity

Figures 3, 4 and 5 are drawn for $R_0 = 1.68$, $R_0 = 2.51$ and $R_0 = 2.72$ respectively to validate Theorem 2 and Theorem 3. Theorem 2 states that the endemic equilibrium is stable when $R_0 > 1$. The simultaneous study of S, I, Q, R in Figs. 3, 4 and 5 illustrates that the susceptible class decreases for a certain time period due to infection of susceptible class then becomes stable as the infection is declined by the quarantine process and a large number of individuals are recovered in the long run. The infected population increases for a particular period then diminished due to recovery and quarantine of large number of individuals. The recovered line shows the enhanced pattern due to the low death rate and high recovery rate of infected and migrant individuals. Size of R increases over the long run and then asymptotically converges towards stability. This exhibits the global stability of the system that is analytically proved in Theorem 3. The recovered class is not approaching to zero level indicates that the disease has disappeared before the infection spread over the whole susceptible population (S).

Figure 6 shows the graph of infected versus time in the presence of migrants. It shows that the curves are rising with a peak as the basic reproduction number increases due to influx of migrants in the early phase of the epidemic, but due to effective quarantine policy and recovery of huge population with a low death rate, the curves become flatter with higher slopes that in turn indicates that the infected cases are reducing and finally the system is getting stable. It is observed that the prevalence of COVID-19 is likely to be continued for long term approximately 300 days.

Figure 7 shows the infected versus quarantine graph. It infers that the number of fresh infection is reduced due to an increase in number of quarantine individuals but do not approach to zero level due to persisting nature of the epidemic outbreak. The

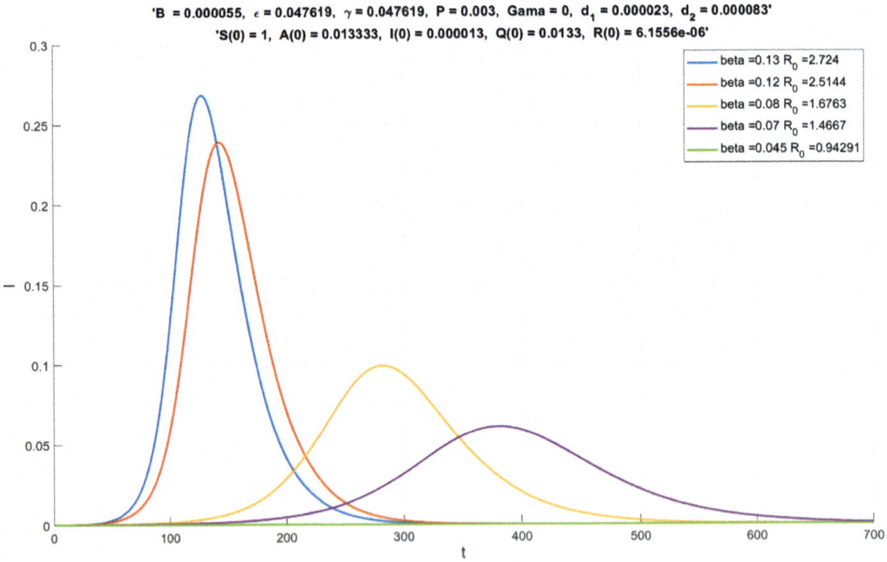

Fig. 6 Infected versus time

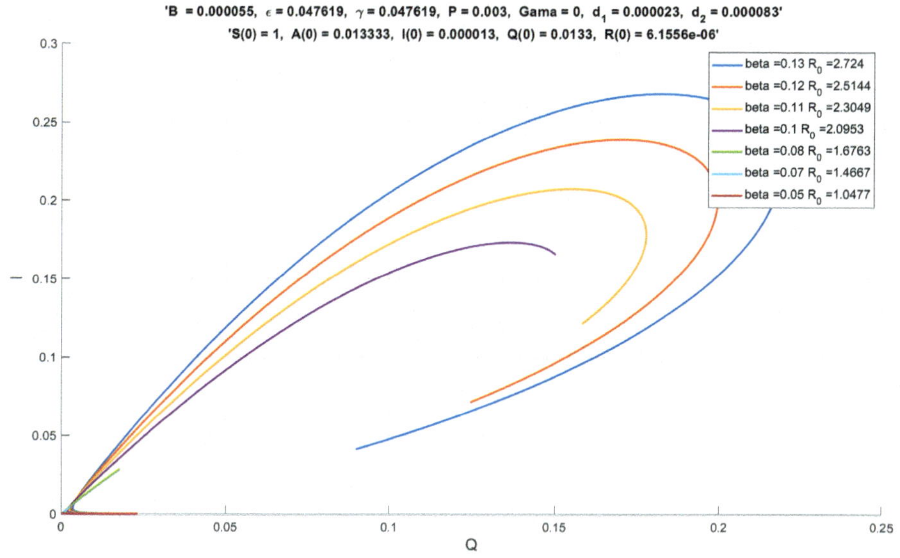

Fig. 7 Infected versus quarantine graph

quarantined individuals do not infect other people and do not transmit the disease after getting out of quarantine compartment. So the infection is reduced on the time evolution.

The phase portrait graph of S versus I is shown in Fig. 8. It interprets that the infection is raised due to entry of infected migrants and other infected individuals decreases after the progress of time due to huge recovery and low death rate upon the lockdown and quarantine rules.

4 Conclusion

The model developed in this article is suited to the present scenario of COVID-19 in Odisha (India). The analytical and numerical interpretations of results are both in good agreements. The stability behavior of the disease is analyzed using different theorems that are supported by numerical simulation and graphs. It is found that the stability is characterized by effective quarantine policy of the state. The absence of quarantine leads the system to be unstable. Both endemic and diseases free equilibriums are derived from the equations. The study shows that the system is stable at disease free equilibrium point when basic reproduction number (R_0) is less than one and is unstable for R_0 greater than one which persist to endemic or pandemic. Routh-Hurwitz condition is used for showing the stability of the differential equations at disease free and endemic equilibrium points. The endemic of disease is felt for certain period of time but global stability is achieved in long terms as per Dulac's

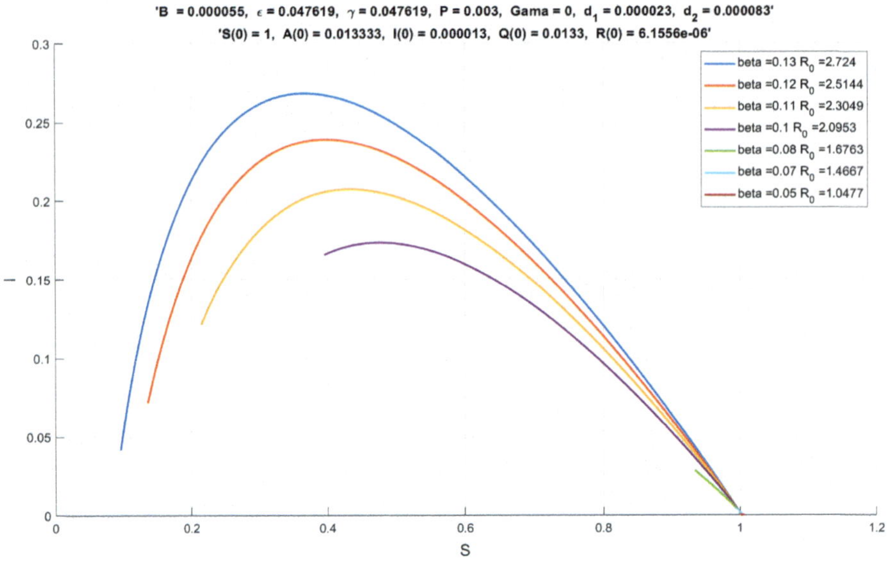

Fig. 8 Phase portrait graph of S versus I

criteria. The investigation done in this paper shows that the prevalence of COVID-19 will remain nearly 250 to 300 days in Odisha as for as the infected migrants would have been entering to the state as per the current trends. So, in order to reduce the spread of the disease, it is suggested that the proper screening of immigrants, more testing of susceptible as well as contact tracing of invectives is required in addition to the controlling technique quarantine policy. Other studies as well as our investigation have forecasted the long term persistence of COVID-19 globally. So, it is suggested to survive with empowering the socio-economy activities in addition to management of disease using all precautionary measures like social distancing, use of mask, lockdown/shutdown/containment rules, hand washing, sanitization, cleanliness with the existing health care facilities.

There are also some limitations in our study. The investigation does not include parameters like saturated incidence, age structured, severe and mild cases, vertical transmission, preexisting diseases and many more risk factors. Our study is limited to only one state in India but could be extended to other states of India as well as to world. In the future scope of study, other relevant parameters may be considered. Also, this study may include exposed compartment and double quarantine classes. Any other approaches for stability behaviors may be employed and other epidemic model is encouraged to adopt for study of this problem.

References

1. https://mygov.in
2. https://india.mohfw.gov.in
3. https://www.who.int
4. https://www.worldmeters.info
5. https://www.pharmaceutical_technology.com
6. https://www.statista.com
7. https:// www.covid19 india.org
8. https://health.odisha.gov.in
9. https:// covid19.odisha.gov.in
10. https://osdma.org
11. https://ndma.org
12. https://nrhmorissa.gov.in
13. www.google.com
14. https://ganjam.nic.in
15. Yang, C., Wang, J.: A mathematical model for the novel corona virus epidemic in Wuhan, China: Math. Biosci. Eng. **17**(3), 2708–2724 (2020).https://doi.org/10.3934/mbe.2020148
16. Zhao, S., Chen, H.: Modelling the epidemic dynamics and control of COVID-19 outbreak in China: Quantitive Biology, Higher Education Press and Springer, GmbH Germany (2020). doi:10.1007/S40484-020-0199-0
17. Singh, R., Adhikari, R.: Age structured impact of social distancing on COVID-19 epidemic in India: arxiv: 2003.12055 V1 [q-bio.PE] 26 Mar. 2020 (2020)
18. Khrapov, P.V., Loginova, A.A.: Mathematical Modelling of the dynamics of the COVID-19 epidemic development in China. Int. J. Open Inf. Technol. **8**(4), 13–16 (2020). ISSN 2307-8162
19. Bhatanagar, M.R.: COVID-19: Mathematical Modelling and Predictions, www.reserachgate.net/piblication/340375647, https://doi.org/10.13140/rg.2.2.29541.96488 (2020)
20. Chatterjee, K., Kumar, A., Shankar, S.: Healthcare Impact of COVID-19 Epidemic in India: a Stochastic Mathematical Model. Med. J. Armed Forces India (2020). https://doi.org/10.1016/j.mjafi.2020.03.022
21. Ghosh, P., Ghosh, R., Chakraborty, B.: COVID-19 in India: State wise Analysis and Prediction: MedRxiv (2020). doi:https//doi.org//https://doi.org/10.1101/2020.04.24.20077792
22. Kumar, K., Meiteei, W.B., Sing, A.: Projecting the future trajectory of COVID-19 Infection in India using susceptible-infected-recovered(SIR) model: An Analytical Paper for Policymakers (2020). https://www.iipsindia.ac.in/content/COVID19-information
23. https://censusindia.gov.in

COVID-19 Epidemic Analysis and Prediction in Virudhunagar District Using Machine Learning

M. Shanmuga Eswari, N. Indumathi, and R. Ramalakshmi

Abstract In this era, the universe is facing the new pandemic situation. Every person feared about this new situation and new virus. That virus is named as COVID-19. This Corona virus is impinge on respiratory and leads to fatal. But this virus is connected to the same family of corona viruses such as Severe Acute Respiratory Syndrome (SARS) and Middle East Respiratory Syndrome (MARS). The mortal rate is sky-scraping when compared to previous SARS-COV with fatal rate of 10% and MARS-COV with rate of 30% of world population. The proposed covid-19 study gives the impression of being up rural place of Tamil nadu's Virudhunagar district in India. This analysis has been taken between the pandemic lockdown period of March 13 and July 26 of 2020. This study has shown the infectious growth rate in Virudhunagar and Sivakasi during the above mentioned outbreak time of 0.01754, 0.036643 respectively in the overall population. In Sivakasi, the Covid-19 spreading rate is high of 22.47% and death rate of 32.55% compared to other taluk in Virudhunagar. The morality age was an average of 61.5. This learning is implemented simple k-nearest neighbor and optimizable k-nearest neighbor classifier for predicting the pandemic situation in Virudhunagar district. Acquired an accuracy of 94.09% and 98.06% and the performance metric of Area Under Curve of Receiver Operating Characteristic according to 0.88,0.94 and respectively. This has been shown the corona virus affected the old age and pre medical conditioned existing people. This study is providing assistance to welfare department for taking safety measures as well as, public to get motivation to keep them safe.

Keywords Knn · Optimizable knn · Covid-19 · Machine learning

M. Shanmuga Eswari · N. Indumathi
Department of Computer Applications, Kalasalingam Academy of Research and Education, Krishnankoil 626126, Tamil Nadu, India
e-mail: mse.skc@gmail.com

N. Indumathi
e-mail: induarivu27@gmail.com

R. Ramalakshmi (✉)
Department of Computer Science and Engineering, Kalasalingam Academy of Research and Education, Krishnankoil 626126, Tamil Nadu, India
e-mail: rama@klu.ac.in

D. Oliva et al. (eds.), *Artificial Intelligence for COVID-19*, Studies in Systems, Decision and Control 358, https://doi.org/10.1007/978-3-030-69744-0_18

1 Introduction

The epidemic of COVID-19 has brought a critical, complicated and unexpected scenario to the entire world. It is a global health crisis that has brought the world to a stalemate with unprecedented and unexpected impacts on everyone's lives, our financial systems, our social structures and our livelihood opportunities.

The emergence and extend of the novel coronavirus (SARSCoV-2) in 2019 has caused a dramatic increase in the prevalence and deaths since the very first discovery in Wuhan, China, in December 2019. The infection can cause illnesses varying from cold or flu to acute respiratory ailments and mortality [1].

Actually, the main epidemiological risk factor for novel corona virus disease in 2019 involves near direct contact with an infected persons with an incubation period of 2–14 days. The very first case outside China was identified in Thailand on 13 January 2020. Since, this ongoing epidemic has extended to more than 50 other countries in the world [2].

Symptoms of the disease include fever, cough, shortness of breath, and vomiting and diarrhea. In much more extreme cases, COVID-19 may lead to pneumonia and sometimes even mortality [3]. WHO announced Coronavirus Disease 2019 (COVID-19) an universal epidemic on 11 March 2020 (Figs. 1 and 2). The virus has spread to 210 countries and regions around the world, with a total of over two million reported cases [4].

This figure represents the corona virus around the world. Note the spike proteins for corona virus visualization. On the surface of the avian infectious bronchitis virus (left in the

insect collage). They produce an effect close to the solar corona (visible during the total eclipse) and give its name to the Coronaviridae family. Corona viruses are encompassed with the positive sense of RNA virus. It's varying from 60 nm to 140 nm in diameter with spike like projections on its surface giving it a crown like appearance under the microscope of the electrons [5].

India confirmed its first COVID-19 case in Kerala on 30 January which by 3 February, rose to three cases; all were students who had returned from Wuhan,

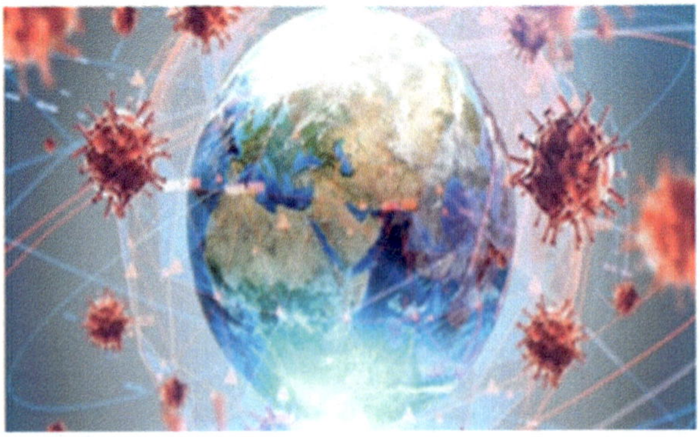

Fig. 1 Corona virus spread around the world (*Source* https://www.pharmaceutical-technology.com/)

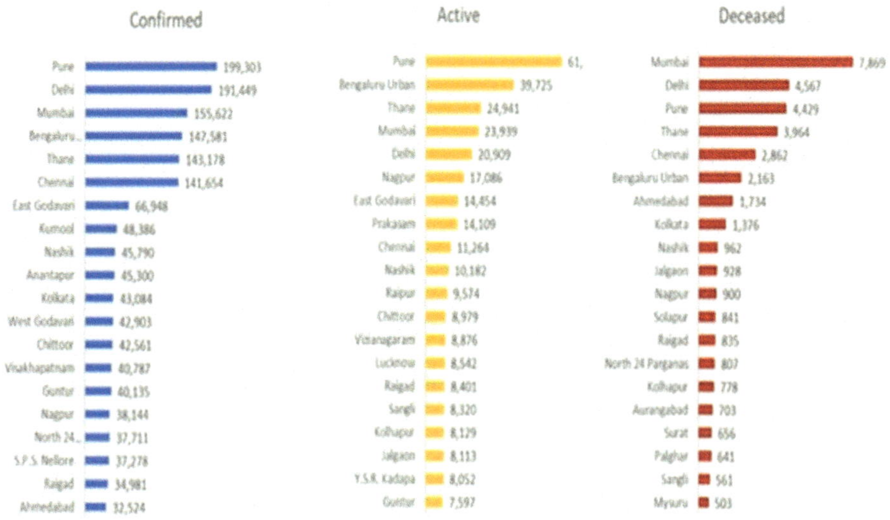

Fig. 2 In India corona case status as of September 7 (*Source* MOH)

China. The Ministry of Health, and Family welfare reported 4,846,427 cases in all, 3,780,107 recoveries and 79,722 deaths in India up to September 14 [6].

The corona virus is spreading the following criteria [7].

1. A country/region is experiencing imported infected cases with travel history from the countries hit by viruses during this time.
2. During this process, a country/region gets new infections from people who have not had travel history but have come into contact with people identified in stage 1.
3. This is group transmission infection. In this time, a person who has not been in contact with an infected person or someone with a travel history of virus-hit countries is experiencing new infection.
4. The spread of the virus is virtually uncontrollable at this point, and the country may have several large clusters of infection.

1.1 Preventive Measures

The Government Measures Dataset of COVID19 collects all the steps taken by governments around the world to respond to the Corona virus pandemic. The processing of data is requiring secondary data for the analysis. The accessible researched knowledge falls under five categories [8]. Those are all listed below,

- Social distance
- Restrictions on travel

- Actions on public health
- Social and Economic Behavior
- Curfew (Lockdown).

1.1.1 Social Distance

Social distancing, also known as "physical distancing," involves maintaining a secure space between yourself and others who are not in your family. To practice social or physical distance, keep at least 6 feet (about 2 arms in length) away from other people who are not in your home, both indoor & outdoor [9].

1.1.2 Restriction of Travel

Travel increases the chances of COVID-19 spreading level. Staying at home is the safest way to defend the peoples from COVID-19, and others. So the government restricts the travelling to other countries and states. Do steps to protect yourself and others from COVID- 19 during your trip [10]. That constraints are,

- When in outdoor areas, wear a mask to keep the nose and mouth covered.
- Avoid physical contact with someone who is not from your household by remaining at least 6 feet apart (about 2 arms' length).
- Using hand sanitizer (with at least 60% alcohol) or wash your hands regularly.
- Evite touch with someone is ill.

1.1.3 Quarantine

A person who have affected any deceases, stay in a ventilated room, if possible with an attached or separate restroom. If some other member who wants to stay in the same room, they are advised to keep maintain the distance of at least of 1 m between of the persons [11]. Quarantines can be used in following ways

- Outbreaks: A sudden spike in an area of illness cases.
- Epidemics: Disease outbreak across a wider region, or across a country.
- Pandemics: A common illness that threatens the whole globe and affects many people worldwide.

1.1.4 Isolation

To isolate people who are sick from everyone else so as not to transmit the disease.

1.1.5 Curfew

The shutdown had prevented people from leaving their homes. All transport systems of airways, road, and rail were discontinued, with exemptions for the transport of an important goods, fire service, police, and emergency needs. Educational institutions, industrial establishments, and hospitality services were also suspended [12].

2 Coronavirus Pandemic in Virudhunagar District, Tamilnadu Literature

2.1 History of Virudhunagar

The district of Virudhunagar was created through the separation of Old Ramanathapuram district from 1985. The district lies in the southern part of the state of Tamil Nadu (Fig. 3). The Virudhunagar district is the India's biggest player in match unit, fireworks industry and printing, concentrated mostly in and around Sivakasi. Virudhunagar is the largest oil, chicory, coffee bean, dried chillies, and pulses market. In the District there are two commercial centre's one in Virudhunagar and another one in Rajapalayam [13].

Virudhunagar having the highest number of cases in the south zone. The district recorded the highest proportion of new cases after Chennai. Virudhunagar has total number of cases as of now 13,683, recovered 13045, and death 202. A 60 year old man, first case of covid-19 found in the month of April from the area of Rajapalayam.

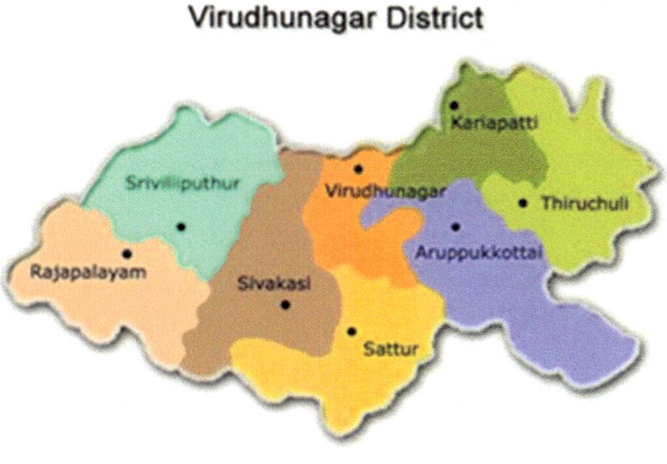

Fig. 3 Map of Virudhunagar district, Tamilnadu (*Source* http://dcmsme.gov.in/)

In this district have large number of different industries and giving the employment is high. Here the people

are working large group and survived always crowd. So they are not known the awareness of Covid-19. That is the main reason for spreading level. In this article, analyzed inhabitants understanding of the symptoms of COVID-19, perceived risk of coronavirus contraction, and anxiety related to the COVID-19 pandemic, infection rate and their relationship to changes in behaviour and stress from lockdown.

2.2 Significance of the Study

When the novel corona virus transformed into an epidemic within the next few months, the effects to the human race is on a wide scale. The spread of the novel corona virus has caused terrible human distress and a significant impact on global health and the economy. The only way to get out of such a emergency situation is to take preventive and precautionary steps to monitor the spread of this virus. People should known much more about COVID-19 communicable diseases, and they should also be aware of preventive steps to fight this coronary virus disease. In this district, virus spreading level gradually increased to attain the peak of positive cases. The main reasons for this situation are lack of awareness about the pandemic, not possible to follow the curfew and social distancing due to financial situation. This study intends to identify the infection ratio, death prediction and comparative study among the Virudhunagar district and Sivakasi area.

The key objectives of this study have been,

1. To know the level of coronavirus cases in Virudhunagar district during the proposed period.
2. To compare the case history of covid19, between Virudhunagar and Sivakasi.
3. To analysis of the infection ratio of covid19.
4. Finding death rate accuracy among genders
5. An implication based on the findings of the study

The above listed factors are achieved through machine learning implementation and visualization techniques.

2.3 Review of Literature

As a result of its rapid spread, COVID-19 is becoming a global pandemic. It is very difficult to diagnose infected individuals since they do not necessarily show signs of the disease. It is therefore important to find a way of estimating the number of potentially infected persons on a regular basis in order to follow the necessary intervention.

Artificial Intelligence (AI) and Machine Learning (ML) technologies has been used to enhance the accuracy of predictions for both pathogenic and nonpathogenic disinfect [14]. MYCIN was developed to apply 450 rules obtained from a health professional to treat viral infection by recommending drugs to patients. Such an advisory system acts as strategic decision-making support for physicians and medical experts [15]. Latest research on the potential of ML and AI technologies for different pandemic outbreaks help health experts in different infectious and non-infectious diseases (SARS, EBOLA, HIV, COVID 19) outbreak [16]. ML can be used to treat massive data and intelligently forecast the disease transmission. AI has started to emerge as scientific breakthrough of the twenty-first century and has identified multiple applications in the area of climate modeling, astronomical investigation, and emerging technologies [17].

AI can be used to test an individual for COVID-19 as an alternative to conventional time- consuming and costly methods. While several studies have been performed research on the use of AI in forecasting cases and, patients diagnosed with corona infection by chest X-ray images [18]. In ML, models are constructed using historical data, and these models are being used to predict new outcomes. Regression, classification, clustering, and deep learning are some of the machine learning approaches that have been widely used in a number of fields, such as image processing, speech recognition, health knowledge, and etc. [19].

Many uses of machine learning techniques for Covid-19 have been suggested, such as prediction and diagnosis, clinical performance prediction, disease monitoring and forecasting, drug creation, vaccine discovery, and false news prediction [20].

Viral epidemics are a major threat. corona isn't the first, and it's not the last. Machine learning is encouraging us do that [21].

- Identify which are most at risk
- Diagnostic patients
- Develop drugs more quickly
- Discover successful medications that can benefit you
- Predict the spread of the disease
- better grasp the viruses
- Trace where the viruses originate, and
- Predict for the next disease outbreak

Machine learning has proved to be useful in forecasting risks in many fields. Explicitly with health risks, it is potentially important in three main ways of infection risk, severity risk and outcome based risk.

3 Materials and Methods

3.1 Data Collection

Real time Data were used for this analysis. Data were collected from various resources related to newspapers, local organizations and web scraping. For this data were taken the range between March 13,2020 and July 26,2020 of infectious places of Virudhunagar district includes taluks like Sivakasi, Virudhunagar, Srivilliputhur, Rajapalayam, Thiruchuli, Aruppukottai and Karriapatti. This dataset ranges from March 13, 2020 and July 26, 2020, total days of 137. which holds the details of day wise details of Confirmed active cases, discharged and number of deaths along with gender and premedical conditions of each infected peoples in above listed virdhunagar taluks. From this, valid data sheet was made for further processing which holds the information about talukname, date, total, confirmed, death, active, patient's pre medical conditions and gender. Along with the statistical visualization used for Sivakasi's infectious conditions, and the machine learning model was used to predict virdhunagar's infectious rate.

3.2 Data Preprocessing

First step, created a valid data sheet based on availability of data. Then removed missing values and unwanted data from the existing list. Then Principle Component Analysis was employed for features selection. The following Selected parameters attributes namely confirmed, active cases, death and total were given as input to the model training. Pre processed data set was segmented into two sets namely training set and testing set with 70 and 30% of data.

3.3 Machine Learning Classifiers

Main purpose of this analysis to predict the Sivakasi's infection rate based on containment region, moderate or safe region. This phase includes data preprocessing, model building, training the model and validating the model (Figs. 4 and 5).

Machine learning optimizable knn applied using training dataset and testing dataset facilitated in accuracy computation. An entire flow depicted in the Figs. 6 and 7.

K nearest neighbor

KNN is used for both classification and regression predictive problems with optimization. This is non parametric and lazy learning algorithm.

Algorithm steps

Input: virdhucovid -19 dataset march13,2020- july26,2020 Steps

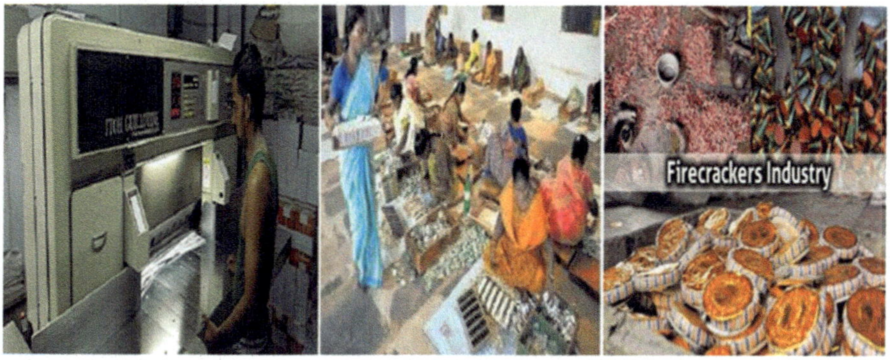

Fig. 4 Industrial platform of virudhunagar (*Source* https://www.sivakasionline.com/)

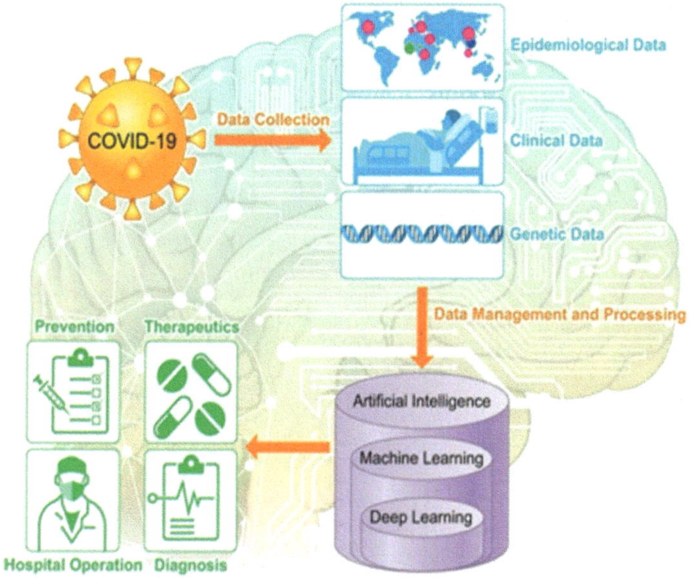

Fig. 5 Machine learning and artificial intelligence on covid19 (*Source* https://www.researchgate.net)

1. Load Virudhunagar district covid-19 dataset
2. Choose the nearest value of k
3. Do the following in test data

   - distance calculation be on Euclidean, hamming, city block and etc. and choose
   - sorting value in ascending based on available distance
   - write max label value from k

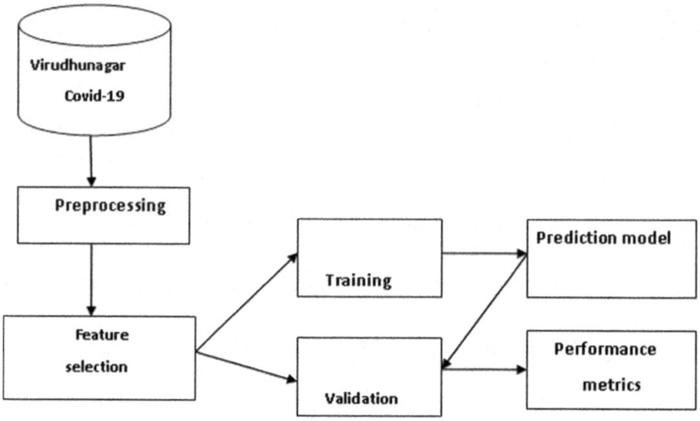

Fig. 6 Implementation of Machine learning for Virudunagar Covid-19 data

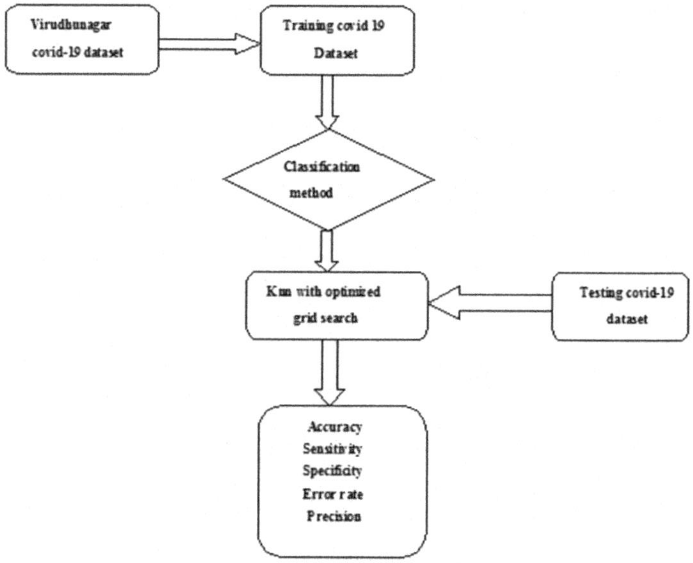

Fig. 7 Methodology used in proposed Knn with grid search optimization

- calculate average k reference points
- repeat the steps 3.1 to 3.4

4. Fit the model and predict
5. Do performance measure
6. Tune the hyper parameter
7. Optimized the result using grid search
8. Validate the test set

Table 1 Testing performances formulae

Metrics	Formulae
Acc(Accuracy)	$\frac{Number of correctly classified data}{Total number of data}$
Error Rate	$\frac{Number of misclassification data}{Total number of data}$
Pre(Precision)	$\frac{Number of true positives}{Number of true positives + Number of false positives}$
Sen (Sensitivity)	$\frac{Number of true positives}{Number of true positives + number of false negatives}$
Spc (Specificity)	$\frac{Number of negatives}{Number of negatives + Number of false positives}$

Output: Infectious prediction rate in S, V region of safe, containment, moderate

After training of classification algorithms, the models require to validate by using many methods like accuracy prediction, error rate, precision, specificity and sensitivity. The formulas for testing performances were embodying in the Table 1.

4 Results and Discussions

The work is carried out by a Matlab2020a, which is a flexible one since it supports many packages and functions. Classification prediction model is created and classified the zone classes as containment, moderate and safe during the period March 2020–July 2020. Optimizable knn algorithm was work proficiently according to its entity competence. Prediction model fitness was assessed based training, testing and validation

In optimizable knn the advanced options were set to optimizing the error rate, precision, true values and false negative values. In this hyper parameter values distances were set as different parameter namely city block, chebyshev, correlation, cosine, Euclidean, hamming, jaccard, mahalanobis and cubic. Distance weight set as default equal, then check with inverse and squared inverse to optimized the covid viruthunagar data. For tuning the parameter based on number of neighbors as 3.

Next optimizer was chosen as grid search with the following parameters with ten grid divisions, and training limit set as 300 s. Grid search used for finding the optimal tuning of parameters of a model to predict the results in a superior accuracy. After the training the error rate was minimized. Based on this, the model was fit for the prediction of covid-19 ratio in Sivakasi and Virudhunagar district. After an evaluation the performance metric was listed in the Table 2.

The oknn model got an Area Under Curve of ROC 0.94. it was depicted on Fig. 8. If the curve lied on top most left side, shows that the model was good to fit.

Table 2 Performance of knn and optimizable knn model for virudhunagar COVID-19 data

Classifiers	Accuracy Rate (%)	Error Rate (%)	Precision (%)	Sensitivity (%)	Specificity (%)
Knn	94.09	5.91	97.78	96.04	97.01
Optimizable knn (Oknn)	98.06	1.94	98.3	98.04	98.6

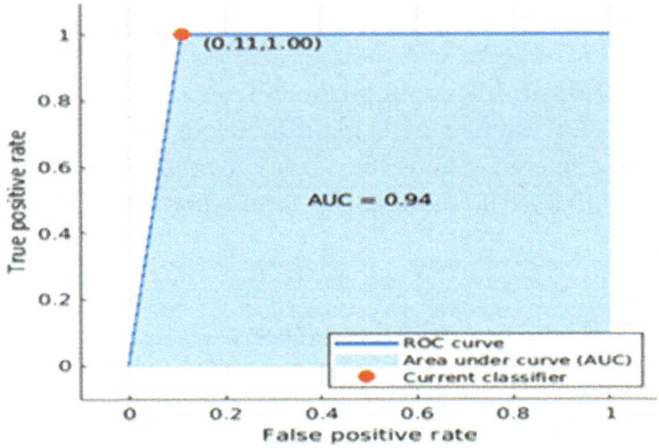

Fig. 8 AUC of ROC in Oknn

4.1 *Data Visualization of Sivakasi and Virudhunagar*

Data visualization, after finding the statistical arithmetic mean of fatal persons age and infection rate of virthunagar district taluks.

Tableau and excel were used for visualizing the data to make a presentable one. It helped a people to understand the present situation swift. From this the people can recognize their importance in the society (Fig. 9).

Data were collected from news paper and various sources. During the period of first lockdown to fourth lockdown period as per the data of 26 July 2020. The total population of viruthunagar district is about 2052365 (Table 1) and Sivakasi is about 234700 (Table 2).

4.2 *Infection Rate Growth Phase*

For this visualization, following parmeters were based on the number of infectious cases in number of days (Table 3). First hundred cases were reached after 58 days from the first case of corona case assessment. But Second hundred cases were found rapid within 27 days of first 100 cases. Next 300 cases were addressed within 10 days (Fig. 10).

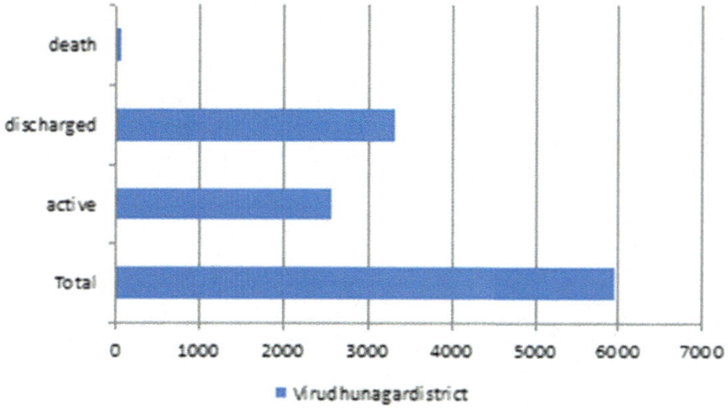

Fig. 9 Covid-19 status of Virudhunagar district as per 26 July 2020

Table 3 Infection Rate growth

No. of cases	No. of days
0–100	58
100–200	27
200–500	10
500–750	3
750–1000	3
1000–1500	2
1500–2000	3
2000–2500	3
2500–3000	3
3000–3500	3

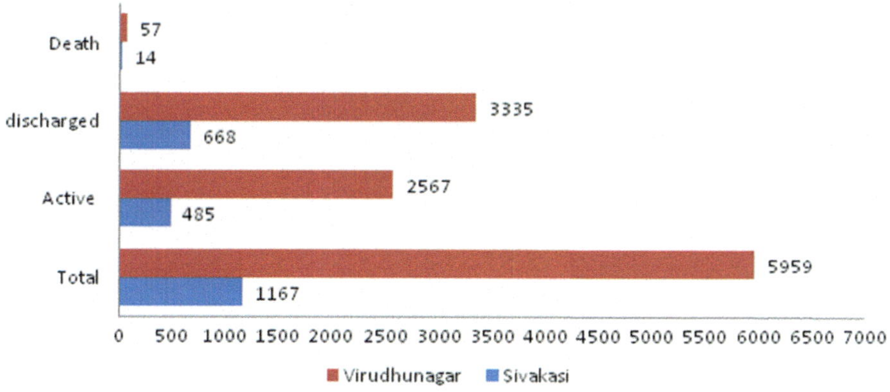

Fig. 10 Comparison of Covid- 19 cases of virudhunagar district and sivakasi as per 26 July 2020

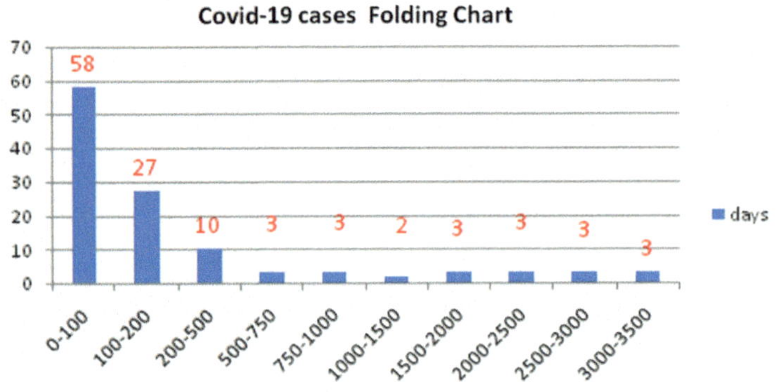

Fig. 11 Covid-19 infection rate folding chart between cases and days

After 500 cases the infection rate was very swift and growth phase was high. Every three days the infection rate was huge and reached to 500 cases (Fig. 11). At present the infection growth phase is peak in Sivakasi and Virudhunagar district.

4.3 Reasons and Outbreaks

People are not aware of social distancing, usage of mask and cleanliness. This could be the reason for swift of infection rate. Based on the geographical data the infection ratio of covid-19 in Virudhunagar was 0.01754074 (Table 4) and analyzed below,

Sivakasi area's outbreak

Based on the Sivakasi geographical data the infection ratio was 0.036643 as per 27 July 2020. When compared to the Virudhunagar district the aspect ratio was high in Sivakasi. In Sivakasi, Covid-19 spreading rate is fleet to 22.4725% and death rate 32.558% (Table 5).

Table 4 Covid-19 cases in Virudhunagar district as per 27 July 2020

Data	Virudhunagar
Population	2052365
Confirmed	2203
Recovered	2947
Deaths	43
Total	**5193**
Max	360
Density	450
Covid infection ratio (%)	**0.01754074**

Table 5 Covid-19 cases in Sivakasi up to 27 July 2020

Data	Sivakasi
Population	234700
Confirmed	668
Recovered	485
Deaths	14
Total	**1167**
Max	86
Density	458
Covid infection ratio (%)	**0.036643**

Comparison of Sivakasi and Virudhunagar

Figures 12 and 13 has been explained the Virudhunagar and Sivakasi during the period of 15 March 2020 and 27 July 2020. This has been furnished the overall data about confirmed corona cases, recovered cases and deaths of both areas.

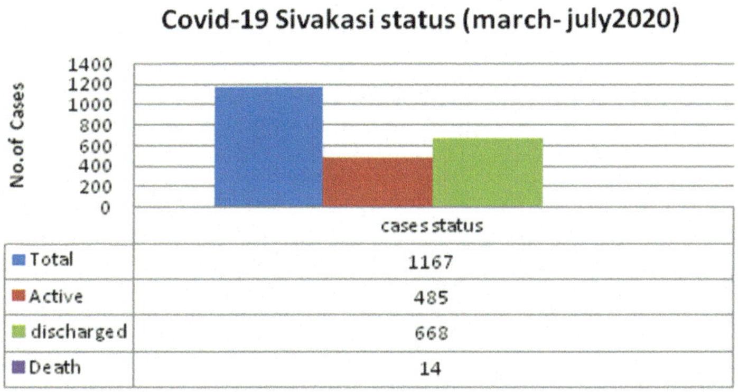

Fig. 12 Comparison of Virudhunagar and Sivakasi during 15 March 2020–27 July 2020

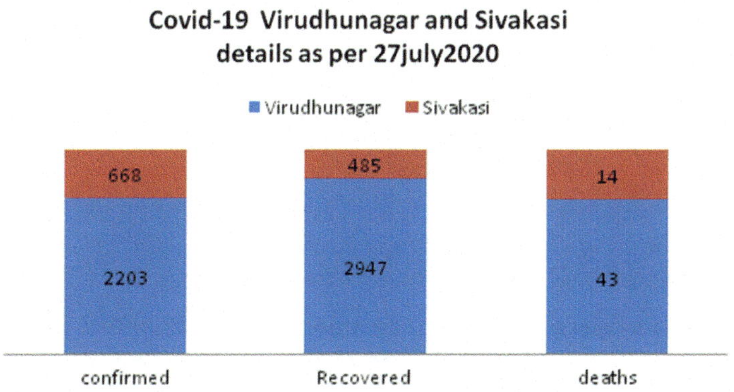

Fig. 13 Comparison of Virudhunagar and Sivakasi during proposed period

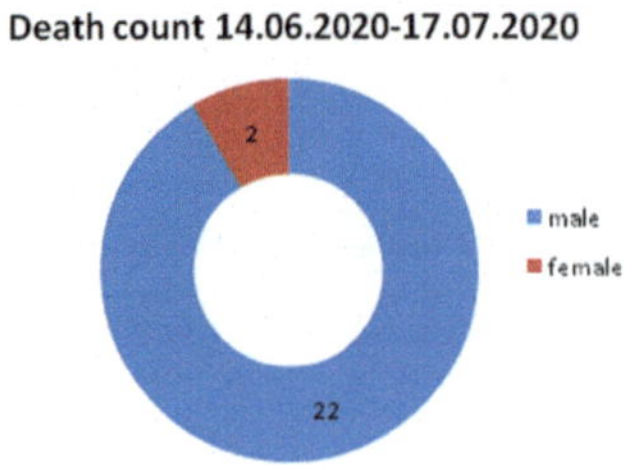

Fig. 14 Death Count in sivakasi on one month period of time

Gender wise analysis

For Gender wise data analysis, one month (14.06.2020–17.07.2020) data were taken and analyzed. These data were inferred the death rate of males higher than females (Fig. 14). The average age was **61.5**. Death happened due to respiratory, diabetics and weaker organs of the persons. Test was done in the late stage of covid-19 with and without symptoms. Few infected people died on the same day of the tested.

5 Conclusion

Covid-is flying in the count and augmenting every day. Researchers are exploring new and new sources every minute to support the public to get out from this pandemic situation. This prediction model depicted for remote place of Virudhunagar district and Sivakasi. These place are under notable condition due to amplification of an infections of covid-19. Finally, suggesting the model of oknn with the aminable result of predicting the infection rate of remote Sivakasi. The resultant outputs shown Sivakasi have more affected ratio than that of other taluks in Virudhunagar. This model can be implemented for all places to predict their panic situation.

This analysis gave warning message to Virudhunagar and Sivakasi peoples. As well as this could be one note to government officials to take defense on this issue. People have to concentrate on Safety measures.

Acknowledgements The first two authors would like to thank the organization of Kalasalingam Academy of Research and Education for offering fellowship to take out the research work.

References

1. Koff, W.C., Williams, M.A.: Covid-19 and immunity in aging populations—a new research agenda. New England Journal of Medicine 2020
2. Rafiq, D., Batool, A., Bazaz, M.A.: Three months of COVID-19: A systematic review and meta-analysis. Rev. Med. Virol., p.e2113 (2020)
3. WHO, Advice for Public, WHO Int.,2020. [Online]. Available: https://www.who.int/emergencies/diseases/novel-coronavirus-2019/advice-for-public. Accessed 27 Feb 2020

4. Corona virus latest: pandemic could have killed 40 million without any action. https://www.nature.com/articles/d41586-020-00154-w. Accessed 27 March 2020
5. Chang, S.C.: Raising clinical awareness for better dengue fever outbreak control. J. Formosan Medical Assoc. **114**(11), 1025–1026 (2015)
6. Indian government coronavirus upate.MHFW. www.mohfw.gov.in
7. Stage 3 begins, we are running out of time: Covid-19 task force. https://www.nationalheraldindia.com/flick-past/stage-3-begins-we-are-running-out-of- time-covid19-task-force. Accessed 1 April 2020
8. COVID19 Government Measures Datasetl ACAPS. https://www.acaps.org/covid19-governmentmeasures-dataset. Accessed 9 April 2020
9. Latest news on corona-19:www.health.gov.au
10. Coronavirus diseases 2019: Domestic travel during the covid-19 pandemic. https://www.cdc.gov/coronavirus/2019-ncov/travelers/travel-during-covid19.html
11. Prevention of coronavirus: https://www.who.int/health-topics/coronavirus#tab=tab_2. Accessed 9 April 2020
12. COVID-19 pandemic lockdwn in India: https://en.wikipedia.org/wiki/COVID-19_pandemic_lockdown_in_India
13. About Virdhunagar district. https://virudhunagar.nic.in/about-district/
14. Agrebi, S., Larbi, A.: Use of artificial intelligence in infectious diseases. In: Artificial Intelligence in Precision Health, pp. 415–438. Academic Press (2020)
15. Peiffer-Smadja, N., Rawson, T.M., Ahmad, R., Buchard, A., Pantelis, G., Lescure, F.X., Birgand, G., Holmes, A.H.: Machine learning for clinical decision support in infectious diseases: a narrative review of current applications. Clin. Microbiol. Infect. (2019)
16. Toğaçar, M., Ergen, B., Cömert, Z.: COVID-19 detection using deep learning models to exploit Social Mimic Optimization and structured chest X-ray images using fuzzy color and stacking approaches. Comput. Biol. Med., 103805 (2020)
17. Kathiresan, S., Sait, A.R.W., Gupta, D., Lakshmanaprabu, S.K., Khanna, A., Pandey, H.M.: Automated detection and classification of fundus diabetic retinopathy images using synergic deep learning model. Pattern Recognit. Lett. (2020)
18. Ogunleye, A.A., Qing-Guo, W.: XGBoost model for chronic kidney disease diagnosis. IEEE/ACM Trans. Comput. Biol. Bioinform. (2019)
19. Bishop, C.M.: A new framework for machine learning. In: IEEE World Congress on Computational Intelligence, pp. 1–24. Springer, Berlin, Heidelberg (2008)
20. Pham, Q.V., Nguyen, D.C., Hwang, W.J., Pathirana, P.N.: Artificial Intelligence (AI) and Big Data for Coronavirus (COVID-19) Pandemic: A Survey on the State-of-the-Arts (2020)
21. How to fight with COVID-19 with machine learning: https://www.datarevenue.com/en-blog/machine-learning-covid-19

Internet of Things and Covid-19 Safety Precautions: Roles of Information Communication Technology in Health Emergency Control for Global Development

Haruna Ishola Abdullahi, Adeola Latifat Odeniyi, and Sarafadeen Tunde Ganiyu

Abstract Internet of Things (IoT) as a modern tool which works as a global entity by interconnecting object especially in the health sector is also susceptible to various challenges. With the advent of IoTs, the safety precautions against COVID-19 could be enforced and monitored to minimize the global effects of the pandemic because health is wealth. Security and reliability are great issues during corona virus, COVID-19; there are established cases of poor compliance with the safety precautions which consequently increases the mortality rate of patients during emergency. Hence, this chapter addresses IoTs and COVID-19 safety precautions. This chapter adopts both quantitative and qualitative research methods, data were sourced secondarily through the content analysis of peered review journals, edited books and credible online resources. Findings showed that IoTs enhance safety precaution of COVID-19 pandemic. The study will be useful to individuals, organizations, non-governmental institutions, corporate bodies and scholars in the fields of computer sciences and criminology, security studies and health sciences.

Keywords IoTs · Security · Crimes · COVID-19 · Emergency · Safety · Precaution · ICT · Development

H. I. Abdullahi (✉) · S. T. Ganiyu
Department of Sociology, Federal University, Oye-Ekiti, Ekiti State, Nigeria
e-mail: harunism@gmail.com

S. T. Ganiyu
e-mail: tunde34@gmail.com

A. L. Odeniyi
Department of Computer Sciences, College of Natural and Applied Sciences, Chrisland University, Abeokuta, Ogun State, Nigeria
e-mail: odeniyilateefah95@gmail.com

D. Oliva et al. (eds.), *Artificial Intelligence for COVID-19*, Studies in Systems, Decision and Control 358, https://doi.org/10.1007/978-3-030-69744-0_19

1 Introduction

Internet of Things is the application of information communication technology to cover diverse areas of human activities. IoT was defined as the structure of interrelated devices and operations arranged with network elements such as; software, hardware, connectivity of the network, and any other required and related electronic and computer which ultimately makes them responsive by supporting in data exchange and compilation [12, 15, 20]. The term internet of Things (IoT) was first used in a presentation on Radio Frequency Identification (RFID) at Procter and Gamble (P&G) [4]. According to Haddad et al. [13], any object useful for monitoring of data after connection with the internet can work as Internet of things.

Conventional health care provider had since adopted the manual method of diagnosis and general treatment of patients especially during Covid 19 pandemic. The manual method may expose the health practitioners to risk and hazards due to direct exposure to infected patients. Internet of Medical Things (IoMT) as an organized and interconnection of robust and integrated principles and approach for medical and health domain overcomes human error as well as prevent exposure of health workers to hazards and diseases during diagnosis and treatment especially during Covid-19 pandemic.

The corona virus also known as COVID-19 is on-going pandemic that threatens global peace and security. According to Europeans Centre for Disease control, over eight million lives have been lost to COVID-19 pandemic in the world. The terrible aspect of the pandemic is that, it has no cure at the present. According to statistics from the World Health Organization over 800,000 thousand lives have been lost to the crisis. The COVID-19 confirmed cases are over 23,000,000 million globally. This outbreak of COVID-19 compelled governments all over the world to take drastic actions like lockdown of the economies and its concomitant insecurity crisis. The non- availability of clinically tested vaccines to combat the emergency, emphasized strict COVID-19 safety rules compliance. A number of safety precautions such as social distancing, wearing of face masks, imposition of curfew, washing of hands, avoiding crowds and others. In order to enforce the COVID-19 safety rules, some governments made and enforce laws. In African countries, the level of compliance is limited, therefore worsening the mobility and mortality of the crises. One modern method of ensuring compliance is the deployment of Internet of Things.

The application of internet of things could enhance flattening the COVID-19curves. One of the conventional measures put in place to combat COVID-19 is setting up of task force, mobilizing police at strategic checkpoints to arrest and prosecute COVID-19 safety precaution protocol defaulters. However, on the ground of massive corruption in the land. Most of the law enforcement agencies turned the opportunities to means of making money and extorting the masses. This worsens the insecurity created by COVID-19 and efforts put in place to reduce the crisis in Africa and other countries in the world. There are many studies on the Internet of Things(IoTs) and COVID-19, Sekehalti, Gotceli, Nilcolay, Zhmurou, GunesKarabuil, Kurt and Berma (2017) investigated IoT in Action: Design and

Implementation of a Building Evidence, in the work of Bia, Yang, Wang, Tong, Zhu, Bai (2019) investigated Chinese Experts Consensus on the Internet of Things-aided diagnosis and treatment of coronavirus disease. Singh et al. [19], examined internet of medical things for orthopedic in CIVID-19 pandemic; roles, challenges and applications. To the best of the ability of the authors, there is no study that have been conducted on IoT and COVID-19 safety precaution. Hence, this chapter address Iot and COVID-19 safety precaution. The specific objectives are; to examine the various IoTs tools used in COVID-19 safety precautions, to investigate the types of safety protocols and to assess the effects of COVID-19 pandemic.

2 Methodology

The chapter applied qualitative and quantitative research methods, data were sourced secondary through the content analysis of edited books, peer-reviewed journals and credible online sources. The systematic literature review was used to explore the meanings of IoTs, types of Iots, deployment and enforcement of COVID-19, types of COVID-19 safety protocols and how the IoTs assists in enforcing flattening the curves of COVID-19 protocols.

3 Review of Literature

Here is the work of other scholars, organizations on COVID-19.

4 History of IoT and IoMT

Internet of Things (IoT) was originated by Procter & Gamble in 1999. IoT was defined as the structure of interrelated devices and operations arranged with network elements such as; software, hardware, connectivity of the network, and any other required and related electronic and computer which ultimately makes them responsive by supporting in data exchange and compilation [12, 15, 20].

The major benefits of IoT and IoMT to health sector is mainly for technological control over patients treatment, monitoring of patient improvement and general oversee of patients recuperation or otherwise with little or no health professional intervention. Various technology have been applied in both IoT and IoMT which includes big data, cloud computing smart sensors, artificial intelligence, actuator, virtual reality and so on [11].

5 IoT and IoMT as a Technology-Based Tool for Treatment

Internet of Things (IoT) is a network of physical objects called "things" which are equipped with various software, sensors, computing elements and connectivity which allow the objects to work as a global entity for sending, receiving and processing of data. It is also an ecosystem of connected devices which communicate over distributed networks. Ravi et al. [21] defined Internet of Things as a well-defined scheme of interconnected computing tactics, digital and mechanical devices which have the capabilities of transmitting data over defined network without having any human involvement at any level. IoT is generally use and applied to every area of life especially health. IoT technology with the use of sensors can generate complete information of proper treatment of patients [3].

5.1 Internet of Medical Things (IoMT)

Internet of Medical Things (IoMT) is a well-organized and interconnected application of principles, elements, gadgets, tools and notion of integrated internet approach for medical and health sector. IoMT offers all possible treatments for patients generally in various parts of the body especially bones, tendons, ligaments, muscles etc. [21]. It is an advanced technology-based method of administering health care to patients in every aspect of health as well as continuous monitoring of patient through interconnected devices with less or no human intervention. It can as well accurately provide improvement in treatment, surgery, provide information and update about patient, educate patient about improvement on their status and also research and provide necessary solution where applicable to problems in health generally through IoMT. Figure 1 depicts the features of IoT in Covid-19.

6 Usefulness of IoT

Internet of Things (IoT) is of great importance to health domain especially during Covid-19 when mortality rate increases daily. The general features of IoT include artificial intelligence, interconnectivity, sensors application, active engagement tools and small device use. Reviews of the features are discussed below:

AI—IoT and IoMT essentially makes virtually anything and everything "smart" and ready for use actively which means that it enhances every aspect of life with the power of data collection with artificial intelligence algorithms, and networks availability. Its use is as simple as enhancing your television and table to detect when food items run low and need replacement. Such application is being adopted in health domain for diagnosing patients with various diseases and ailment especially Covid-19.

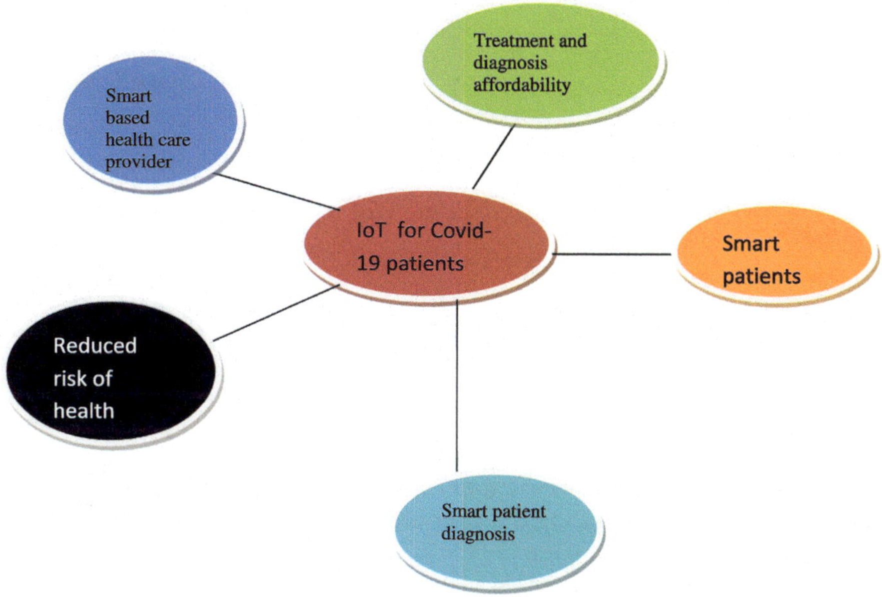

Fig. 1 Importance of IoT in treating Covid-19 patients usefulness of IOT

Connectivity—networking exists between the systems for easy integration. Networks can exist on a much smaller and cheaper scale while still being practical and useful. IoT and IoMT create small networks between its system devices.

Sensors—sensors is an important and transformation tool for bringing any tool within the network into limelight of an active tool capable of real world functional integration especially in IoMT. IoT loses its distinction without sensors. They act as defining instruments value without an active sensor.

Active Engagement—Much of present interaction with connected technology do occur via inactive contribution and engagement. IoT introduces a new paradigm for active content, product or service engagement.

Small Devices—Generally, devices as predicted, have become smaller, cheaper, and more powerful over time. IoT exploits purpose-built small devices to deliver its precision, scalability, and versatility.

7 Problems Faced by IoMT

Though IoMT delivers a tremendous and an impressive set of benefits but also has various set of challenges among which are:

Table 1 Global cases of Corona Virus by continents

Global	Cumulative cases	Fresh cases in the 24-hour	Cumulative total fatalities	Mortalities in the last 24-hrs
	28,329, 049	287,968	911,877	5,783
Percentage of Base Case	–	1.02%	3.22	0.63

Source World Health Organization (2020), https://covid19.who.int/table, as at 12 September 2020, 03: 48 pm

Security—IoMT creates an interconnection of devices that communicate over networks. The system offers little control despite any security measures which exposes users to various kinds of attacks.

Privacy—The sophistication of IoMT provides substantial personal data in extreme detail without user's active participation.

Complexity—Some people see IoMT as a complex system in terms of design, deployment, and maintenance given their use of multiple technologies and a large set of new enabling technologies.

Flexibility—Many are concerned about the flexibility of an IoMT system for easy integration to avoid conflicting or locked system

Compliance—IoMT, like any other technology in the realm of business, must comply with regulations. Its complexity makes the issue of compliance seem incredibly challenging when many consider standard software compliance a battle.

8 Corona Virus or Covid-19

The corona virus is deadly disease originated from China in the late 2019, before spreading to other parts of the world. According to the World Health Organization WHO (2020) and supported by Bai, Yang, Wang, Tong. Zhu, Bai et al. (2019). The latest statistics showed that COVID-19 affected 28,329,049 people and 911,877 deaths recorded so far. The pandemic affects socio-economic conditions over the world.

From Table 1, 28,329,049 had so far been affected globally, 911,877 deaths recorded. This shows the need to deplore IoTs to mitigate the crisis. And the next twenty-hour, 1.02% of fresh cases, cumulative fatalities for over 24-h.

9 Effects of Corona Virus

The following are the are the socio-economic effects of corona virus.

Mortalities. The most challenging aspects of COVID-19 are deaths and its social economic consequences on the world. Since 2019, over 28, 329,049 cases have been recorded globally and over 8,000,000 million lives claimed by the emergency [22].

Lockdown. One of the undesirable effects of COVID-19 is lockdown. This could be partial or full lockdown of the economies, thereby preventing the uncontrolled gathering of people. Lockdown is one of the means of enforcing stay home policy. In this policy; down to dusk curfews are imposed on particular places. However, the COVID-19 lockdown is unique in the sense that it cuts across a whole state or two or more in some circumstances [17].

Increased in Poverty Level. One of the side effects of emergency is the closed down of the productive sectors of an economies. Businesses were shut down and other critical sectors of economy were deactivated. This resulted in the crises of employment, most private institutions embarked on staff restructuring, reshuffling and re-alignment. Mass sack, reduction in salary, delayed salary are parts of the global challenges created by COVID-19 [26].

Increased in Crimes. Unemployment result in increase in crimes like burglary, theft, armed robbery, arson and other heinous crimes, domestic violence, online fraud, banditry and other anti-social behavior. Lack of robust national social safety net worsening these social problems imposed by COVID-19 pandemic [10].

Corruption. Aside mass unemployment, COVID-19 pandemic resulted in massive collection and disbursement of the palliatives. In the words of Transparency International (2020), the systemic corruption in most Third Word countries worsened the fatalities of COVID-19 pandemic. This creates serious crises in most African countries, there are allegations and counter allegations over misapplication of donations made towards COVID-19 relief materials [8].

Highhandedness. Corruption also produces highhandedness on the part security personal, taskforce and other agencies. COVID—19 emergency led to strict restriction of movement and enforcement of movement restriction laws. There are incidents of infringement on fundamental human right rights of citizens especially where the provision for well-being's of the citizens are poor. In most African countries, arrangement for welfare of the masses are poor to the extent that famine and other undesirable social variables worsen people conditions and forced them to struggle for their well-beings [23].

From Table 2, America took the first position among continents with confirmed COVID-19 pandemic with the 51.42% of total global confirmed cases. The second continent is South-East Asia recorded 18.63% of the cumulative confirmed cases. The Western Pacific is the least with 1.91% and Africa Continent has 3.93% of the global confirmed cases.

10 Safety Precautions During Covid-19

As opined by Elehattin, Nikolay, Gunes, and Berna (2017) the following are the safety precautions against COVID-19 pandemic.

Table 2 COVID-19 Cases by the Continents in the World

S/N	Continent	Total number of cases	Percentage of global cases
1	Americas	14,566,710	51.42
2	South-East Asia	5,275,943	18.63
3	Europe	4,747,273	16.76
4	Eastern Mediterranean	2,086,849	7.37
5	Africa	1,111,680	3.92
6	Western Pacific	540,594	1.91
	Total	28, 329,049	100

Wearing of Face Masks. The essence of wearing face masks is to prevent COVID-19 droplets from an infected person for uninfected ones. The pandemic has high morbidity and mortality rates. As part of efforts to enforce use of face mask; COVID-19 laws were made and enforced following the easing out of COVID-19 lockdown. However, the level of compliance varies from one area to another. In some African countries, the where there is weak respect for rule of law coupled with unimpressive law enforcement processes [27].

Physical Distancing. This is also known as social distancing; it is about two feet away from the next person or two arm's length. The safety precaution complements wearing of face masks.

Because wearing of face masks prevents droplets from COVID-19 infected persons to healthy persons. This is also challenging in terms of social and economic pressure. In the transport sector, vehicles owners were mandated to carry passengers up to 50 percent of their normal passenger capacity [17]. Therefore, for vehicle operators to maximize profits and remain in business, they were left with the option of hike in fare. In the banking halls, customers have to spend a whole day to complete banking transactions that could not take them more than two or three hours due to restriction on the number of customers over a period of time [19].

Avoidance of Gatherings. As opined by WHO (2020), corona virus gather strength in large human gatherings. This prompted government to impose restriction on social activities that attract large crowd. In most territories with high cases of COVID-19, schools, religious centers, viewing centers, sport activities, club houses and other crowd- attraction centers were shut. This action was greeted with public outcry. There are instances of violation of these rules by desperate citizens.

Washing of Hands under Alcoholic Sanitizer. Hand washing is another recommended way of checkmating corona virus infection. There are sanitizers that are recommended for the hand washing. During lockdown, everybody was admonished to embrace the principle of regular handwashing with recommended sanitizers. After the lockdown, in the words of WHO (2020), in the process of easing out of the lockdown, all social institutions were mandated to make adequate provision for handwashing in line with COVID-19 safety protocols [14].

Table 3 COVID-19 Cases in Five Affected Countries in Africa

S/N	Country	Global confirmed cases	Percentage of confirmed case	Mortality	Percentage of global mortality
1	South Africa	646,398	2.28	15,378	1.69
2	Ethiopia	63,367	0.22	986	0.11
3.	Nigeria	56,367	0.20	1,076	0.12
4	Algeria	47,752	0.102	1,599	0.18
5	Ghana	45,388	0.16	285	0.03 s

Source World Health Organization (2020) https://covid19.who.int/

Environmental and Personal Hygiene. Hygiene of any angle is needed as a prevention against any disease. Corona virus. Environmental cleanliness like cleaning of drainages, adequate disposal of waste, getting water source from approved places. Personal hygiene like washing of cutting of fingernails, washing mouth at appropriate time and other personal cleanliness [18].

From Table 3, across Africa, South Africa has the highest number of deaths, followed by Ethiopia and Nigeria.

Considering the high mortality rate, the enhanced method of application of IoT to the general safety precaution could give an improvement over the pandemic control.

Related Literatures on Measures to prevent Covid-19.

Enhanced smart glasses for preventing Covid-19: Enhanced IoT smart glasses is an optical and thermal based application which is useful in monitoring congested areas [2]. It has capability for detecting body temperature, capturing face identity for easy tracking of people with the help of google location history (Fig. 2).

Smart thermometer: Smart thermometer is highly important in prevention of COVID-19. It helps to constantly record body temperature for possible detection of coronavirus. The wearable thermometer was design with high technology application to report result of recorded body temperature to smart phone for easy record of tracking if necessary (Fig. 3).

IoT smart helmet: IoT smart helmet is a robust application with features such as thermal camera, high temperature detector, location detector through google location

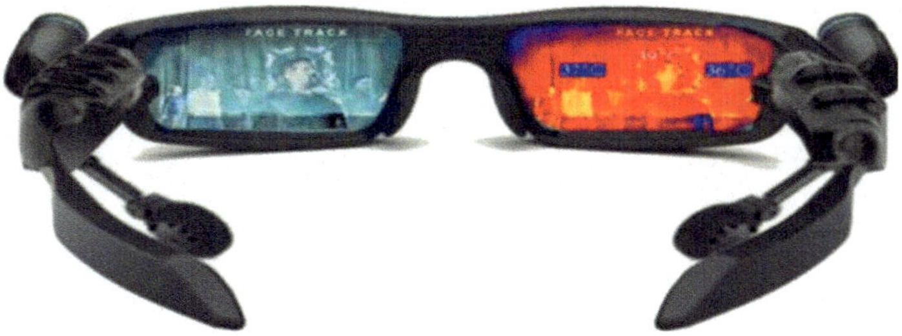

Fig. 2 shows image of Enhanced smart glasses (*Source* Abdulrasaq et al. [2])

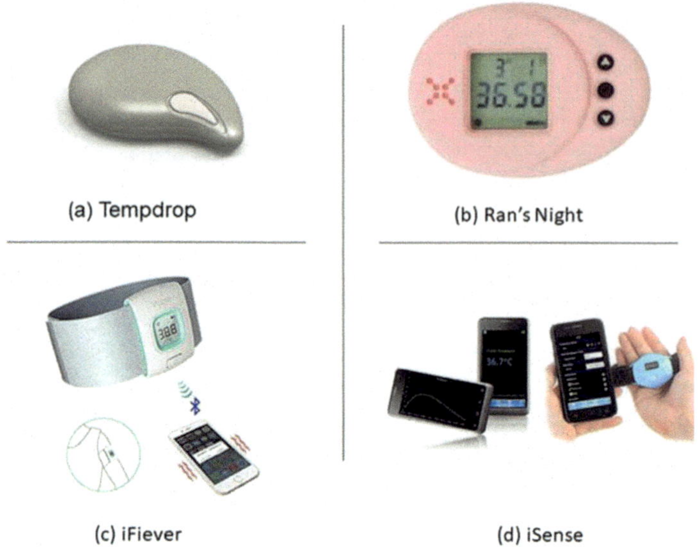

Fig. 3 Wearable thermometer (*Source* Tamura et al. 2018)

history, image capturing, facial recognition, people's personal information record detector and so on. Smart helmet is capable of detecting anybody with high temperature within crowd and will send alarming signal of the detectors image, temperature as well as location to the connected smartphone for immediate action (Fig. 4).

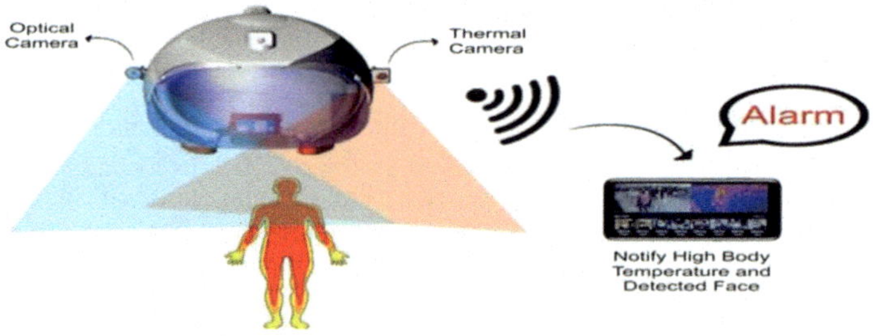

Fig. 4 IoT smart helmet (*Source* Abdulrasaq et al. [2])

Table 4 Literatures on application of IoT devices for preventing/reducing risk of coronavirus

Authors	Year	Technology used	Description of the technology	Preventive measure on Covid-19
AbdulRasaz et al.	2020	Enhance smart glasses	Its capable of image capturing as well as measuring wearers temperature	It enforces social distancing as well as detecting high temperature
Chamberlain **et al.** Tamura T., Huang, M., and Togawa T	2020 2018	Smart thermometer	For measuring temperature for possibility of Covid-119 infection	Everybody should put it on at all times to easily detect possibility of coronavirus
Abdulrasaq et al.	2020	IoT enhanced helmet	Capturing of face and location as well as capability of measuring temperature	Maintain social distancing and detection of body temperature
Tripathy et al.	2020	Smart and enhance wristband	Closeness detection through LED	Maintain social distancing

Source https://covid19.who.int/table, WHO(2020), 12 September 2020

11 IoT and COVID19 Safety Precautions and Global Development

Every nation has national development plans, the commitment to fulfillment of those plans enhances the space on growth and development. One aspect of COVID-19 emergency is disruption in global development plans. The role of economy in National development could not be underestimated. Outbreak of COVID-19 production local and international production to standstill. The operations of commerce and industry are partially of totally grounded. The impacts on informal sector in most economies are disgusting. It widens the gap between the rich and poor. The adoption of safety precautions will promote sustainable growth and development. Transportation as a veritable means of moving from one place to another has been disrupted and a result of COVID-19 pandemic. However, when IoTs are duly adopted in COVID-19 safety precaution the more economy recovery is attained for speedy global development (Table 4).

12 How IoT Influences COVID-19

The Internet of things influences the roles and commitments of various stakeholders in the health sector. The installed sensors will give signals if an infected person enters public domains. For instance, if COVID-19 patient boards public transport, the installed sensors will notify the authorities for an appropriate action. In the areas of compliance as precautions to curb the spread of COVID-19 pandemic. The Internet of Things, will definitely give signs if there is any breach of safety precautions. For instance, failure to wear face masks, inability to maintain physical distance, failure to wash hands under running water with soap will be captured and culprits be brought to book. The IOT will facilitate testing and treatment of COVID-19 patients [2].

13 Theoretical Framework

To shed more light on IoTs and COVID-19 safety precautions the following theories will be adopted. The first theory in the routine activity theory by Felson Marcus, as noted by the Marcus deviance behavior is a function of opportunity place. The scholar explain deviance based on three factors that must be available. The first one is a motivated offender, deviance or any act that contradict societal rules and regulation does not exist in a vacuum. So, someone who is ready to commit criminal activity must be present. The second factor according to Felson Marcus is a target. In this regard, a motivated offender aimed to take aware a particular property without the consent of owner. The third factor is the availability of reliable guardian, this prevents perpetration of deviant act. As per application of this theory to IoTs and COVID-19 safety precautions is that, every individual is liable to disregard COVID-19 safety precautions because of the harshness of some of the rules and strangeness. For instance, complete lockdown or imposition of curfew is strange to some majority of people, using of personal protective devices; like face masks, hand glove, regular handing washing, social distancing and not shaking of hands. The safety precautions in some regions caused serious clashes between people and the law enforcement agencies. The third factor is IoTs, COVID-19 emergency resulted strained demand on the physical security agents like police, armed forces, private security and paramilitary agencies, couple with inadequate personal to meet the demand of the emergency. Electronic security, like IoT, is necessary to address the issues of shortage of personal. The adoption of electronic security will ensure real-life and closed monitoring of various places and bring culprit to book. This promotes synergy between physical and electronic guardianship in enforcement of COVID-19 protocols. When people are aware that they their behaviour is under monitoring, they act as expected of them.

14 Findings and Discussions

From findings, IoT resources are very useful in monitoring compliance with COVID-19 safety protocols. The smart thermometer is one of the IoT devices that could be applied in monitoring people body temperature to further spread of the pandemic. The deployment of smart thermometer in various social gatherings will give people confidence as per their safety from corona virus pandemic. It also minimizes the community transmission of the disease. Smart helmet is another IoT technology that could be used to detect those people with COVID-19 crisis and isolate them for possible treatment. Aside mobility of these devices, smart thermometer and smart helmet are economical in view of high cost of administering COVID-19 tests. Another tool is enhanced eye-glasses, this type of device has inbuilt technology for real-life location monitoring of events. Thus, COVID-19 safety defaulters could be tracked and brought to book. This will reduce morbidity and mortality of the disease. The various safety precautions like social distancing, could be monitored with IoT eye glasses. The embedded technology like google location has capability of capture people from far distances. The physical control has limitation and that limitation could be addressed by applying smart security devices to monitor places that attract social gathering like churches, mosques, sport facilities, motor parks and other places. The activities in the various COVID-19 tests and care centers could also be monitored to ensure standardization of processes and protocols. Another aspect of COVID-19 is the area of national development, with effective application of IoTs to ensure compliance, stability will be restored to economy to facilitate speedy growth and development.

15 Conclusion

Internet of things has tremendous contribution in the areas of detection, prevention and treatment of COVID-19. The application of IoTs will go along way to reduce increased number of COVID-19 cases and subsequent mortalities. This will among other things restore global economic order. And make the life more meaningful to all. All hands must be on deck to extirpate the COVID-19 by taking responsibilities that is more expected. This study will be useful to individuals, government at various level, National Centre for Disease Control, European Centre for Disease Control, World Health Organization

16 Recommendations

The study recommends thorough public enlightenment on the usage of IoT technologies in every stage of COVID-19 administration. The prices of IoT devices should be subsidized to enhance their affordability and accessibility to all. One motivational factor to ensure people cooperation and compliance to provision reliable and effective social security systems for the people, as palliatives for harsh consequences of lockdown and other drastic measures for prevention of COVID-19 pandemic.

References

1. Abdulrazaq, N.M., Hazairin, N.A., Zuhriyah, H., Al-Zubaidi, S.S., Abdul Karim, S., Mustapha, S., Yusuf, E.: 2019 novel coronavirus disease (covid-19): Detection and diagnosis system using iot based smart glasses. Int. J. Adv. Sci. Technol. **29**(7), 954–960 (2020)
2. Abdulrazaq, N.M., Zuhriyah, H., Al-Zubaidi, S.S., Abdul Karim, S., Ramli, R., Yusuf, E.: Novel covid-19 detection and diagnosis system using iot based smart helmet. Int. J. Psychosoc. Rehab. **24**(4), 2296–2303 (2020)
3. Abid, H., Ibrahim, H.K., Mohd, J.: Internet of Things (IoT) Applications in orthopaedics. J. Clin. Orthopaed. Trauma. https://doi.org/10.1016/j.jcot.2019.07.003 (2019)
4. Ashton, K., et al.: That internet of things thing. RFID J. **22**(7), 97–114 (2009)
5. Bai, D., Yang, X., Wang, L., Tong, X., Zhu, C., Bai, et al.: Chinese experts' consensus on the Internet of Things-aided diagnosis and treatment of corona-virus disease (2019)
6. Chamberlain, S.D., Singh, I., Ariza, C.A., Daitch, A.L., Philips, P.B., Dalziel, B.D.: Real-time detection of covid-19 epicenters within the united states using a network of smart thermometers. med Rxiv (2020)
7. Christaki, E.: New technologies in predicting, preventing and controlling emerging infectious diseases. Virulence **6**(6), 558–565 (2015)
8. Davies, Sara E., Kamradt-Scott, Adam, Rushton, Simon: Disease Diplomacy: International Norms and Global Health Security. Johns Hopkins University Press, New York City (2015)
9. Elehattin, G., Nikolay, Z., Gunes, K.K., Berna, O.: IoT Action: design and implementation of building evaluation service. J. Comput. Netw. Commun. **13** (2017)
10. Fisk, D.: Cyber security, building automation, and the intelligent building. Intell. Build. Int. **4**(3), 169–181 (2012)
11. Haleem, A., Vaishya, R., Javaid, M., Khan, M.I.: Artificial Intelligence (AI) applications in Orthopaedics: an innovative technology to embrace. J. Clin. Orthopaed. Trauma. (2019). https://doi.org/10.1016/j.jcot.2019.06.012
12. Haoyu, L., Jianxing, L., Arunkumar, N., Hussein, A.F., Jaber, M.M.: An IoMT cloud-based real time sleep apnea detection scheme by using the SpO2 estimation supported by heart rate variability. Fut. Generat. Comput. Syst. **1**(98), 69e77 (2019)
13. Haddad Pajouh, H., Dehghantanha, A., Parizi, R.M., Aledhari, M., Karimipour, H.: A survey on internet of things security: requirements, challenges, and solutions. Internet of Things, p. 100129 (2019)
14. International Monetary Fund: Corona Virus more from over, https://www.vanguardngr.com/2020/09/coronavirus-crisis-far-from-over-more-support- needed -imf/ retrieved 08/09/2020 @ 2:30 pm (2020)
15. Luz, E., Silva, P.L., Silva, R., Moreira, G.: Towards an efficient deep learning model for COVID-19 patterns detection in X-Ray images. Apr 12. arXiv preprint arXiv: 2004.05717
16. Metcalf, D., Milliard, S.T., Gomez, M., Schwartz, M.: Wearables and the internet of things for health: Wearable, interconnected devices 'promise more efficient and comprehensive health care. IEEE Pulse **7**(5), 35–39 (2016)
17. Noweiri, M.: Novel Covid-19 detection and diagnosis system using iot based smart helmet. Int. J. Psychosoc. Rehab. **24**(7), 2296–2303 (2020)
18. Pillinger, M.: WHO Declare a Public Health Emergency about Zika's Effects Here are to Free takeaways. Washington Post (2016)
19. Pratap Singh, R., Javaid, M., Haleem, A., Vaishya, R., A.lS: Internet of medical things (IoMT) for orthopedic in COVID-19 pandemic: roles, challenges, and applications. J. Clin. Orthop. Trauma. The Use of IoT Technologies to Identity and Control the COVID-19 Pandemic in Urban Areas s (2020)
20. Rani, S., Ahmed, S.H., Talwar, R., Malhotra, J., IoMT Song, H.: A reliable cross layer protocol for internet of multimedia things. IEEE Internet Things J. **204**(3), 832e839 (2017)
21. Singh, R.P., Javaid, M., Haleem, A., Vaishya, R., Al, S.: Internet of Medical Things (IoMT) for orthopaedic in COVID-19 pandemic: Roles, challenges, and applications. J. Clin. Orthopaed. Trauma (2020). https://doi.org/10.1016/j.jcot.2020.05.011

22. Roy, D., Tripathy, S., Kar, S.K., Sharma, N., Verma, S.K., Kaushal, V.: Study of knowledge, attitude, anxiety & perceived mental healthcare need in Indian population during COVID-19 pandemic. Asian J. Psychiatry. **51** (2020)
23. Sood, S.K., Mahajan, I.: Wearable IoT sensor-based healthcare system for identifying and controlling chikungunya virus. Computer Ind. **91**, 33–44 (2017)
24. Tamura, T., Huang, M., Togawa, T.: Current developments in wearable thermometers. Adv. Biomed. Eng. **7**, 88–99 (2018)
25. Tripathy, A.K., Mohapatra, A.G., Mohanty, S.P. Kougianos, E. Joshi, A.M., Das, G.: Easyband: a wearable for safety-aware mobility during pandemic outbreak. IEEE Consumer Electron. Mag., 1–1 (2020)
26. Vaishya, R., Javaid, M., Khan, I.H., Haleem, A.: Artificial Intelligence (AI) applications for COVID-19 pandemic. Diabetes MetabSyndr. **14**(4), 337–339 (2020)
27. Yai, L., Yang, D., Wang, X., Tong, L.: Chinese experts' consensus on the Internet of Things-aided diagnosis and treatment of coronavirus disease 2019 (COVID-19) Clinical eHealth **3**(1), 7–11 (2020)

Big Data in COVID-19 Assistance—Concepts, Motivations, Advances and Applications in Real-World

Sukriti Tiwari and Ashwani Kumar

Abstract The first diseased coronavirus event (COVID-19) has been reported in the Hubei, China, December 2019. The COVID-19 epidemic has affected around 214 countries all over the world, that has severely impacted each and every piece of our day-to-day lives. While writing this chapter, the number of diseased cases reported and expiries still rise, and there is no hint of a controlled situation; e.g. worldwide, 4 September 2020, about 26,171,112 confirmed instances of COVID-19, plus 865,154 deaths, testified to WHO. Inspired by current advances and applications of big data in many research fields, this article focuses on accenting the data significance in retorting the COVID-19 outburst, also, averting the harmful consequences of the present situation. Besides, the application of big data is highlighted while comprehending this virus, along with real-world case studies. First of all, an outline of big data is presented, followed by applications intended for combating COVID-19 are recognized, succeeding challenges and problems related to the existing solutions are discussed. Lastly, recommendations are provided to stop the COVID-19 outburst effectually. It has been anticipated that this article offers researchers and groups with a compilation of accessible open resource of datasets in context to the COVID-19, new visions into all of the ways by which big-data revamp the COVID-19 scenario, and promotes additional research studies for ending this COVID-19 epidemic.

Keywords Big data · Datasets · Data framework · COVID-19

1 Introduction

COVID-19, a resultant of a novel coronavirus, has significantly reformed our world, in the health/medical care area, and various other facets of human life activities viz transportation, education, supply chain, politics etc. Disease-ridden COVID-19

S. Tiwari (✉) · A. Kumar
Department of Electrical Engineering, NIT Hamirpur, Hamirpur, Himachal Pradesh, India
e-mail: sukritiee0053@gmail.com

A. Kumar
e-mail: ashchandelin@nith.ac.in

D. Oliva et al. (eds.), *Artificial Intelligence for COVID-19*, Studies in Systems, Decision and Control 358, https://doi.org/10.1007/978-3-030-69744-0_20

persons generally report respiratory ailment that can improve with suitable treatment procedures. COVID-19 is fatal and can easily blowout compared to the other members of Coronavirus families, and also it has turn out to be very competent in person-to-person transmissions. While preparing this chapter, COVID-19 epidemic has already affected over 214 countries in the world. The USA presently accounts for the maximum COVID-19 instances. Other countries like India, Brazil, Spain and, Russia are extremely influenced too. Though, no medical vaccines are there to stop this COVID-19 virus, including explicit therapeutic procedures to battle this contagious viral disease.

The leaders in this fight with the new coronavirus viz the Centers of Disease Control and Prevention (CDC) and World Health Organization (WHO), provided a series of public instructions with technical procedures [1, 2]. The cooperation amongst and actions taken by central governments and big corporate houses are anticipated to condense risks imposed from the binge of COVID-19 epidemic competently. Google released a COVID-19 portal publicly, to get useful information, like latest statistics, coronavirus map, and most asked queries on the COVID-19. Amazon, IBM, Microsoft, and Google, with the involvement of White House, established a fast computing structure for research related to the new corona virus [3]. The data and statistics that are available now a days through various publications, websites etc. [4] have immensely led to the big data utility in several fields, like., computer science, agriculture, banking, and healthcare. For illustration, the medical statistics continues to expand quickly, medical information has grown up rapidly, and massive counts of medical gadgets have formed an unbelievable peril on existing hospital information servers and systems [5]. The arena of healthcare produces a wide variety of data on patient records, medical diagnosis, medication, treatment, etc. The actual fear is due to the inadequate data processing; the correctness of available information has an influence on the society of health care [6]. From that matter, the data is of no use without an exact result which should be derived from the efficient processing of these huge data [7, 8]. Big data visualization is not only important in the administration of the hospitals but then also aids in the reduction of medical wastes [9]. All these technologies can be expected to play imperative parts in the global fight counter to the COVID-19 epidemic.

In order to realize and lighten the COVID-19 rampant in a better way, numerous articles are published in the past few months. The foremost aim is to demonstrate the use of the big-data to contest with the COVID- 19 epidemic and analyze existing results by means of this technology. Moreover, some representative examples of big data-driven solutions are also elucidated for a good understanding. Main Challenges and issues related to prevailing big-data involved methods are studied, which inspired us to pen down some recommendations to the researchers and academicians, societies, and governments. The highlights of the contribution made by this article are as follows:

- Various applications for fighting a novel coronavirus by utilizing big data concepts are collected and described.

- This article offers researchers and groups with a compilation of accessible open-source of datasets.
- Real-world case studies that have been discussed enhance the understanding of the big data applications in COVID-19 aid.
- Set of recommendations have been provided at the end that can assist the researchers in battle against COVID-19 virus strongly.

This chapter is prepared as follows. In Sect. 2 essential understanding of COVID-19, big data is offered, and also prime impetuses behind the utilization of big data are elaborated. Subsequent, big data applications in combating the COVID- 19 epidemic, are studied and briefed in Sect. 3. Section 4 provides some examples of big data-driven agendas for battling the COVID-19 outbreak. Section 5 presents recommendations for research communities based on this study and also debates the challenges that should be unraveled in the upcoming times. Lastly, Sect. 6 concludes the work.

2 Fundamentals and Motivations

This segment provides the basics for COVID-19 and, the big-data. Here, also impetuses for the usage of big data in retort to COVID-19 epidemic are discussed.

2.1 COVID-19

The worldwide COVID-19 trend is shown in Fig. 1. Based on the seriousness of the situation caused by COVID-19 pandemic, WHO already amplified COVID-19 menace calculation to its peak level and has approved it as a global epidemic. For the best realization of structure of virus, pathogenesis, characteristics, along with current treatment advancement, the concerned readers can refer to the article [10]. Due to the

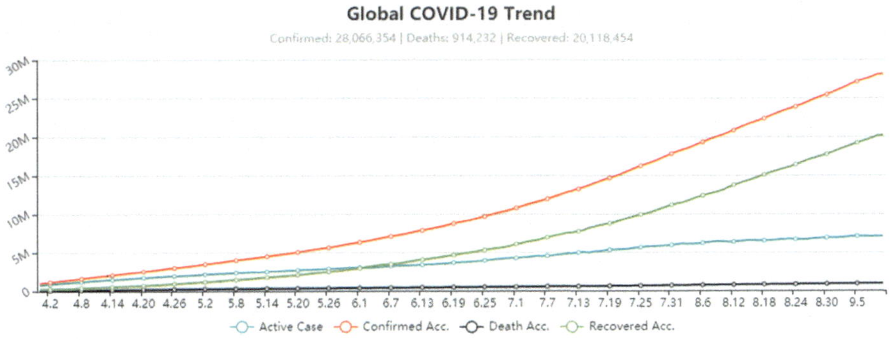

Fig. 1 Global COVID-19 trend [*Source* corona board]

serious impacts of COVID-19 in the world, efforts have been made to get solutions for continuing the battle with the COVID-19 outburst. Government's policies are mostly accountable to halt this pandemic, viz, locking down of the zone to hold the blowout of the infection, confirmation with the health care system has enabled them to handle the outbreak and offer crisis packages to improve virus impacts on the nationwide economic condition and approve adaptive plans rendering to COVID- 19 condition.

Meanwhile, inhabitants are stimulated to be healthy and watch others too by applying certain guidelines like wearing of the masks when in public places, washing of the hands recurrently, maintaining proper social distance, and inform the symptoms to the local health care centers. Besides, research regarding development applicable to the COVID-19 are on priority nowadays, and also have grabbed special consideration from numerous stakeholders, e.g., industries, governments, and academicians [11, 12]. In response to the world-wide challenge to find and produce an effective vaccine in COVID-19 treatment, computer-science scholars made early efforts to combat the COVID-19. Driven by this fabulous triumph of the big-data in many research fields, trending solutions using approaches built on the big-data for dealing with this COVID-19 virus, is presented.

2.2 Big Data

Definitions and Features:

The speedy growth of concept of Internet of Things (IoTs) led to the immense burst of the data produced by universal wearable equipment and the sensors [13]. The unparalleled growth of the data capacities allied with developments of the analytic practices vested by AI has caused the upsurge in a big data era [13]. These data have been used in a varied array of business application spheres, which also includes health sector where the electronic health records (EHRs) are scrutinized by means of smart analytics to enable medical services. Health data possibly assist patient's health scrutiny, diagnosis support, and the drug engineering [14]. Big-data may get produced from varied resources that constitute online societal graphs, mobile phones, IoT devices, and big public data [15] in several forms as video or text. Inside the framework of COVID-19 epidemic, big-data points of the patient-related information like X-Rays, medical history, a record of doctors plus nurses, and data from outbreak zones. Overall, big-data is the data asset categorized by quiet high capacity, and diversity to gain explicit technology, expertise and the analytical means for its conversion into the valuable information in order to assist the users, viz, digital twin technologies [16–18].

Big Data Role in COVID-19 Battle:

Big data have shown its competence to sustain the fight with transmittable viruses like COVID-19 [19, 20]. Big data has actually made available a good number of potential answers to help in combating COVID-19 over the globe. Its combination with AI analytics supports us to better comprehend the COVID-19 in regard to outbreak tracking facility, virus visualization, disease treatment, and also the vaccine manufacturing [21]. For instance, big-data linked with smart AI tools can produce intricate simulation models by making use of coronavirus data collection for epidemic estimation. This can help health care agencies in watching the corona virus spread and then preparing for improved precautionary measurements [22]. Models which are obtained from the big-data also assist in future prediction facility for COVID-19 pandemic by using its data collection capability to leverage the huge volume of data for initial detection. Likewise, big data analytics from various worldly resources together with infected patient's data can help apply largescale COVID-19 inquiries to finally develop inclusive medication solutions of high dependability [23]. This would also aid health providers to realize the new development of virus to improve response to the several processes for treatment and diagnoses.

On the basis of the above learnings, big data analytics is well-defined as a method of collection and investigation of the large size of data sets to determine hidden forms and further information, for instance., COVID-19 data realization. The potential applications and utility of this technology in battling COVID-19 pandemic is discussed in the subsequent sections with some practical scenarios as well.

2.3 Datasets

COVID-19 pandemic has jabbed eagerness for the large collection of data so as to track the spreading of the transmitting pathogen and to plan ailment prediction endeavours. Governments and Organizations overall are piling up the area info of a huge number of cell phone customers and web for the intimations on how the contamination blowouts and if the social eradicating measures are applicable. These actions break down vast information collections to disclose designs for individuals' development and their behavior over the extent of the outbreak. Researchers are now utilizing big data-based investigations to possibly grasp corona virus from many edges [24]. Recently, arrangements to gather large information are made available to help track the virus spread. For instance, the makers in [25] have used both huge data from spatial examination approaches and Geographic Information Systems (GIS) that could encourage linking of heterogeneous data from varied medical information resources, viz, patients, governments, labs and general population. Huge data plausibly gives several promising results and solutions for serving the fight against COVID-19 epidemic. Table 1 displays some of the accessible datasets associated to their references relating to other viruses.

Table 1 Some open access datasets and websites

S. No.	Dataset	Size	Data type	Link to access
1	COVID-19	–	Text values (Prevalence)	https://github.com/CSSEGISandData/COVID-19
2	COVID-19 image data collection	345	chest X-ray or CT images	https://github.com/ieee8023/covid-chestxray-dataset
3	COVID-CT-Dataset: A CT	398	CT images	https://github.com/UCSD-AI4H/COVID-CT
4	COVID-19-CT-Seg-Benchmark	525	CT images of Lungs	https://gitee.com/junma11/COVID-19-CT-Seg-Benchmark
5	COVID-19 CT	100	CT images	http://medicalsegmentation.com/covid19/ segmentation dataset
6	Segmentation dataset nr. 2	829	CT images	http://medicalsegmentation.com/covid19/
7	Apple Mobility Trends Report	–	Values (Mobility data)	https://www.apple.com/covid19/mobility
8	Google COVID-19	–	Community Values (Mobility data)	https://www.google.com/covid19/mobility
9	Our World in Data	–	Values (COVID-19 testing data)	https://www.acaps.org/covid19-government-measures-dataset
10	ACAPS	–	Text and Values (Management measures)	https://www.acaps.org/covid19-government-measures-dataset
11	COVID-19-TweetIDs	100 million	Text (Social media)	https://github.com/echen102/COVID-19-TweetIDs
12	CORONA VIRUS	30 million	Text (Social media)	https://doi.org/10.21227/781w-ef42

3 Applications: Big Data for COVID-19 Aid

Data analytics in COVID-19; mostly characterized by means of significant methods from concepts of big-data, like multi-domain data analysis (collective COVID-19 image-time sequences information), deep analysis (by Boltzmann machine, Markov model, hidden neural networks), high-dimension analysis (that is, 3- D COVID-19 pictures), and parallel computation. Here, we summarize about crucial big-data applications aided by this technique, with outburst prediction, coronavirus spread and tracking, virus diagnosis or treatment, also drug/vaccine discovery as given in Fig. 2.

3.1 Prediction of Outbreak

Big-data have an imperative part to play in battling COVID- 19 using its ability of forecasting the epidemic from comprehensive data analytics. The addressed work in [27] leveraged empirical world data obtained from the COVID-19 epidemic information in Italy to evaluate the likelihood of virus outbreak that has significance in planning efficient control strategies. Other than using a deterministic prototype built on human transmission [28], the researchers have come up with more intricate prototypes that can correctly frame the dynamics of the epidemic from the data of Italian Civil Protection resources. Alternative dataset resource for outburst forecast is community data that could be utilized in order to visualize the topographical regions with probable outbreak [29]. An initial trial in a study in Wuhan, targeting to check on the individual migrations to and from Wuhan city for the agencies based on health care can envisage the population sick with COVID-19 and their isolation.

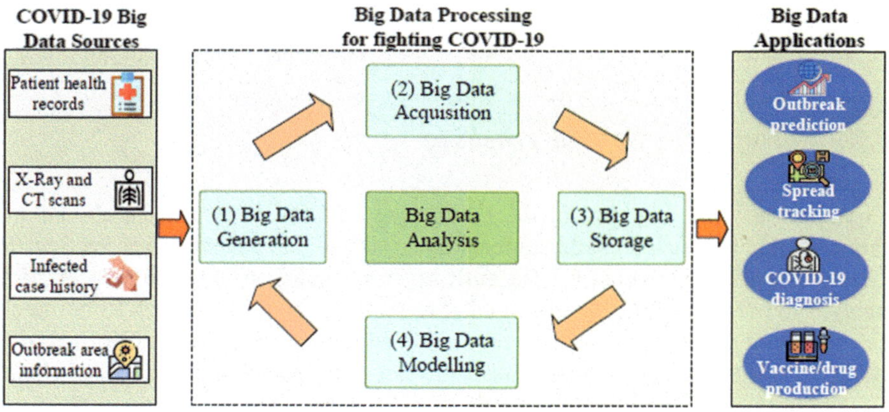

Fig. 2 Big data utilization flow for different applications [26]

In the meantime, the work presented in [30] utilized the COVID-19 data from authentic sources like the National, provincial and Health Commissions of China. These big data sources may support implementation of pandemic model to infer the growing numbers of diseased individuals, recovery cases in the different regions. More notably, it facilitates us to complete proper simulations to conjecture the blowout of the COVID-19 epidemic. Big data permits prediction of an outbreak at the global level. From the big-data science study point, the spread is projected exploiting existing data locations that can put to the accurateness of the fitting curve for dependable estimate under suspicion because of incomplete investigations. Accuracy of estimates may be subject to the various aspects, extending from the infected population, environments, living environments, etc. Motivated by the idea, researchers in [31] utilized large datasets from countries as China, Korea, to evaluate the disease on logistic modelling that can assert the consistency of the forecasts. On a similar line, other tests in [32] utilized Google Trends like a data-driven engineering tool for gathering of corona virus information in South Korea, China, Iran, and Italy. The reports by government obtained from the virus spread in South Korea, China, Iran, and Italy are analyzed in [33] with a new data optimization prototype, to generate the precise calculation of the sick cases on a daily basis, this has potentially long-lasting hold on the impending outburst.

Furthermore, the effort in [34] used datasets taken from John Hopkins University source, that contain statistics of the confirmed cases, recovered cases and death cases of from all the other countries, with the intension to develop the prediction models through data learning tools. The trials are executed for India, signifying that the given data should estimate the occurrence in the short intervals, like. two-week, possibly expanded to visualize bigger models for long duration forecasts. In the interim, alternative data process in [35] which is conducted in the USA using large datasets obtained from cities in America. The important persistence of this study is knowledge from the recently generated statistics to gauge prediction blunders so as to optimize and improve the big-data models for enhancing the reliability of future estimate, likely for pandemics like coronavirus.

3.2 Coronavirus Spread Tracking

The application of big data in the monitoring of COVID-19 is of a chief reputation for health-related establishments and also the governments in directing the virus pandemic effectively [36]. Recently emergent solutions by exploiting big-data analytics have been anticipated to facilitate the following of COVID-19 outbreak. For illustration, the work in [37] recommended a data-driven method for tracking of the COVID-19 binge. A huge dataset has obtained from Chinese National Health Commission stating 854,424 air travellers left 55 Wuhan Airports to go to 49 Chinese cities between Dec. 2019-Jan. 2020. The data analytic outcomes show a very high correlation among the positive contamination instances plus size of population. The researchers of [38] have done leveraging together big data for the spatial analysis approaches and the Geographic Information Systems (GIS) that would facilitate data procurement and the incorporation of varied data from health-related data sources.

The data knowledge and modelling formed the basis of a macroscopic growth law that assists in estimating the peak number of diseased patients inside a particular zone. Different to [39], the authors in [40] presented temperature-based modelling that assesses the connection among the total count of infected cases and the individual's body temperature in diverse countries which is essential for tracking of coronavirus.

The work in [41] recommended an unsupervised prototype for COVID-19 outbreak where tracking is done on the basis of online data. They chose a varied range of connected symptoms which has been identified and recorded by an inspection from the National Health Service (NHS) of the United Kingdom by integrating a basic mass media coverage metric related with those of the confirmed COVID-19 instances. Then, a transference learning method is presented for mapping of the supervised COVID-19 model from one to another country wherever the COVID-19 virus probably spreads.

3.3 *COVID-19 Virus Treatment*

The spread and tracking related applications of big data have the ability to assist COVID-19 analysis and treatment progressions. In fact, the existing potential of big data in diagnosing infectious viruses like COVID-19 is verified via recent achievements, from the very early diagnosis in [42], forecast of treatment consequences, and preparation of supportive tools for surgical treatment. In regard to COVID-19 diagnosis and proper treatment, big data in most of the cases has provided affirmative solutions as testified in the existing literature [43, 44].

Simultaneously, the authors of [45] employed the proteomics cells which gets infected by COVID-19 virus, for analysis. More precisely, data comprises of 6381 proteins inside human cells with COVID-19 contagion. Based on this reasoning, a supportive analysis of an influence pathway analysis along with network analysis is done to scrutinize the information collected from Kyoto Genes storage. The result in [46] leveraged existing mouse and nonhuman primate to derive the nonneural expression for SARS-CoV-2 entrance genes. Due to inadequate dataset, while performing COVID-19 analysis and treatment, extra information has been produced from experiments, in [47] in which all the six antigenic determinants (A, B, C, E, F/G and H) may encourage the body to make agreeing antibodies and produce explicit humoral immunity. Interestingly, the new work done in [48] offered a comprehensive guideline in addition to suitable tools to aid the analysis and treatment in case of COVID-19. The guideline entails the new guideline method, epidemiological features, population deterrence, diagnosis, treatment of COVID-19 virus.

3.4 Drug/Vaccine Discovery

New vaccine development is very vital for stopping the limitless global problem due to the COVID-19 epidemic. Big data give visions on vaccine encounter to deal with COVID-19 epidemic. Some efforts have been already made to test, develop and provide an appropriate drug for COVID-19 by means of big data within a short time span [49–51]. A vast dataset which has been obtained from the National Center of Biotechnology helped in enabling vaccine production [52]. Big data is capable of supporting policies for drug engineering to battle with COVID-19. For instance, a solution built on molecular docking has been proposed in [53] for drug research. More than 2500 molecules permitted the drug database that is firstly screened and then authenticated through a molecular dockage program called Glide. A big data supported drug transposition scheme did introduce by [54]. The main purpose of this project constituted the application of Machine Learning to combine the knowledge of graph and existing literature for development of COVID-19 drug.

4 Real-World Data Frameworks for Combating COVID-19

This segment gives some illustrations of data frameworks describing how big-data are at present assisting the fight with COVID-19 epidemic.

Mobile-based Solution for Contact Tracing and Surveillance

The new sign of progress in hardware skills, development of non-wired mobile infrastructures, and advent of edge computing have strengthened countless opportunities offered by mobile phones, throughout the outbreak, for e.g., outburst detection, diagnosis, good treatment, and disease eradication. Adopted from [55], we suggest a mobile-assisted basis for COVID- 19 surveillance. Wireless connectivity, like., WiFi, 3G, 4G, and 5G, have been expansively positioned in nearly all the major countries, such that each individual with a cell phones can link to Internet and can pursue various online activities. Data learning model can get trained within the cloud, as well as in server lumped at the edge of network, which is pushed to mobile phones after that for further purposes. By utilizing the photographic camera and sensors, a cell phone can gather individual's information, like, X-rays, CTs, cough sounds, and the heart rate, that might be protected with encryption and is trampled prior to sending it to the cloud for learning and training purposes [56, 57].

Conferring to the state-of-the-art yearly Internet reports by Cisco [58], by 2023 about 29.3 billion devices shall be introduced to Internet, where the mobiles and the tablets accounts around 23% and 3% correspondingly, and around 70% of the people in world would have the mobile connectivity. In spite of several possibilities, some challenges should be taken care for the triumph of AI and dataset-related mHealth [59]. The very initial limitation is imposed by the ability and reliability of software and hardware, which are utilized in mobiles for the medical research purpose. This limitation may get overcome by emerging standard mobiles with explicit computing or sensing mechanisms and chips. Another limitation ascends from the decorum to store or collect the diagnosis outcomes, and the means to enhance patients' belief, specially when, in reality, they usually choose a face-to-face conversation with the doctors. Lastly, the challenge in the commissioning of the mobiles for proper tracking and surveillance is just how to estimate clinical cost and its usefulness. This is realistic then the outcomes utilizing mobile frameworks are generally uncertain and not similar with those of direct trials.

China's Infrastructure for Surveillance to Track Exposed Individuals

China's surveillance arrangements have turn out to be very useful in the nation's response to COVID-19 situation. Thermal scanners are installed in railway stations to spot the increase in body temperatures—a possible indicator of infection. If temperature rise is sensed, then the person is held by the health officials to undertake corona virus testing. Next, if the corona virus test turns out to be positive, authorities would immediately warn every passenger who might have made an encounter with the virus so that they can quarantine themselves. The warning system has been enabled because of the nation's transportation rules which require every traveller who takes public transportation to reveal their real identities and travel with government-issued ID cards. The Chinese government too released a "Close Contact Detector" app that notified users if they are/were in interaction with somebody who has/had the virus. By assimilating the data obtained by China's surveillance system, the nation is capable of finding ways out to fight against the spread of this novel COVID-19 virus.

Risk Handling by Google

Big data can show an important role in investigating screening information of patients and connecting it with unspecified health issues of the hospitalized patients. The results of the analysis will support in determining the main risk factors. So, as data fed into huge data tools and programs is more and more, the accuracy of risk calculations will increase. Google's DeepMind artificial intelligence system utilizes big data to understand the virus by scrutinizing its corresponding characteristics. This can help doctors in developing drugs and treatment strategies.

5 Challenges, Solutions and Recommendations

From the previous sections, it can be observed that big-data have got excessive potentials around the globe to combat with COVID-19 epidemic. Besides the noticeable advantages, there are some challenges that should be essentially conferred and addressed in the coming future.

5.1 Challenges/Solutions

Absence of Standard and Reliable Datasets

To rely on big-data dashboards/collection platform for its applications and trustworthy solutions to contest the prevailing COVID-19 pandemic, a serious limitation ascends from the deficiency of typical and reliable datasets. Likewise, mostly datasets given in the existing works have been created due to separate efforts, for e.g., the concerned authors have merely collected some datasets accessible from the Internet, and then again modified them to make their particular datasets for validation of their algorithms. In order to avoid this task, giant firms, government, and health organizations like WHO, played a vital role as they are now working in unison for collection and quality maintenance of datasets (Table 2).

Security and Privacy Challenges

In the state of epidemic, the establishments may appeal to the people for sharing of their individual info, for instance, GPS location, scans, travel trajectory, reports, and routines, that is desirable to monitor the situation, to form up to- date strategies, and to approve straight actions. Data is central to establish that AI will be an effective tool in fighting against future epidemics. The fear is that the public health fears would trump data privacy apprehensions. Governments might want to continue the surveillance of the citizens even after the pandemic is ended. Consider some possible solutions [60–62], which can act as research directions in the near future.

5.2 Recommendations

Some commendations might be considered to endorse the coronavirus combat. First of all, big data employed procedures must be efficiently optimized so as to boost the accurateness and consistency of the big data and analytics for the improved COVID-19 diagnosis, treatment and handling. Secondly, data can be merged with innovative skills to bid new and effectual solutions in battling COVID-19. For instance, data analysis tools of the Oracle cloud computing are leveraged in designing and development of vaccine, an innovative vaccine applicant counter to the COVID-19 [63]. More stimulatingly, current studies displayed that 5G wireless types of machinery like drones, IoT, localization, can be employed to fight the COVID-19 epidemic [64] with applications, like distribution of test samples, goods transportation, social distancing, plus monitoring of movement of people for spread tracking. Finally, non-technology-based procedures viz social distancing restrictions also play an imperative role in retarding the virus blowout and therefore they are required to be executed efficiently under the supervision of government firms [65], directing to check and control the spread of COVID-19 epidemic in the coming future.

Table 2 Summary of some big data applications in COVID-19

Category	Reference	Contributions
Prediction of outbreak	[28] [32] [34] [35]	The complex models are developed that can accurately visualize the dynamics of the epidemic based on vast data sets from the Italian Civil Protection sources Google Trends as a data engineering tool is used to collect coronavirus-based information of China, Iran, South Korea, and Italy The datasets of John Hopkins University repository that are obtained from the confirmed cases, death and recovered cases of every country is used to build prediction models using machine learning This study has been done by learning from the recent data for computation and prediction of errors so as to facilitate efficient optimization of the data model for refining the value of future estimations, mainly for coronavirus-type situations
Coronavirus spread tracking	[38] [40]	Here, the leverage of big data for spatial investigation approaches and Geographic Information Systems (GIS) are considered, which might probably facilitate the acquisition of data and the incorporation of heterogeneous data sets from various health care database A novel temperature-based model is given that assesses the relationship amongst the infected cases and the body temperature in various countries essential for virus tracking
Covid-19 diagnosis and treatment	[44] [46] [48]	This research applied an atomic diagnostic technique for genomic analyses of SARSCoV-2 stresses, with an emphasis on reviewing Australia returned travellers having COVID-19 illness by means of genome information available at https://www.gisaid.org/. This solution leveraged the publicly accessible mouse and non-human primate for deriving the nonneural expression for SARS-CoV-2 genes The work presented a proper recommendation with convenient tools for diagnosis aiding and handling of COVID-19. Set of recommendation involves guideline scheme, epidemiological features, population diagnosis, and treatment for the fatal COVID-19 disease

(continued)

Table 2 (continued)

Category	Reference	Contributions
Drug and vaccine discovery	[51] [52]	The methods of reversing the vaccinology and immunity information science may be valuable to develop drugs for COVID-19. Big-data facilitated drug transposition structure is presented. Here, the main persistence of project included application of machine learning to put together the knowledge of graph and existing works for COVID-19 drug development

6 Conclusions

In this chapter, a study on the recent technologies and their results in the fighting of the COVID-19 epidemic are thoroughly presented. Firstly, a brief outline of the COVID-19 virus is provided, the required basics and impetuses of big-data for unravelling the effective and fast procedures that can effectually fight the COVID-19 virus is elaborated. The prevailing applications and approaches of big data for COVID-19 are reviewed, together with prediction of an outbreak, tracking of virus spread, diagnosis/treatment, and drug/vaccine discovery. Besides, a separate section presenting some real-world applications is given. Moreover, the challenges imposed by big-data in the times of COVID-19 like situation, are also discussed. Finally, a highlight of imperative recommendations for the research groups and authorities have been provided. More surveys and experiments are to be conducted on the basis of the big data congregated from the patients, and utilization of this data can decrease the spread/outbreak or if it is of worth saying, can aid in discovering an effective solution to this COVID-19 pandemic.

References

1. Coronavirus disease (COVID-19) pandemic, 2020. [Online]. Available: https://www.who.int/emergencies/diseases/novel-coronavirus-2019
2. Coronavirus (COVID-19), 2020. [Online]. https://www.cdc.gov/coronavirus/2019-nCoV/index.html
3. White House announces new partnership to unleash U.S. supercomputing resources to fight COVID-19, 2020, accessed date: March 23, 2020. [Online]. https://www.whitehouse.gov/briefings-statements/white-house-announces-new-partnership-unleashusupercomputing-resources-fight-covid-19/
4. arXiv announces new COVID-19 quick search, 2020. [Online]. https://blogs.cornell.edu/arxiv/2020/03/30/newcovid-19-quick-search/
5. Latif, J., Xiao, C., Imran, A., Tu, S.: Medical Imaging using machine learning and deep learning algorithms: a review. In: 2nd International Conference on Computing, Mathematics and Engineering Technologies (iCoMET), Sukkur, Pakistan, pp. 1–5 (2019)

6. Yang, Y., Chen, T.: Analysis and visualization implementation of medical big data resource sharing mechanism based on deep learning. IEEE Access. **7**, 156077–156088 (2019)
7. Zhao, H., Li, G., Feng, W.: Research on application of artificial intelligence in medical education. In: 2018 International Conference on Engineering Simulation and Intelligent Control (ESAIC). 340–342 (2018)
8. Al-Turjman, F., Nawaz, M.H., Ulusar, U.D.: Intelligence in the Internet of Medical Things era: a systematic review of current and future trends, Comput. Commun. doi:https://doi.org/10.1016/j.comcom.2019.12.030 (2019)
9. Chan, Y.-K., Chen, Y.F., Pham, T., Chang, W., Hsieh, M.Y.: Artificial intelligence in medical applications. J. Healthc. Eng.. https://doi.org/10.1155/2018/4827875 (2018)
10. Li, H., Liu, S.-M., Yu, X.-H., Tang, S.-L., Tang, C.-K.: Coronavirus disease 2019 (COVID-19): current status and future perspectives. Int. J. Antimicrob. Agents. **55**(5) (2020)
11. Ivanov, D., Dolgui, A.: Viability of intertwined supply networks: extending the supply chain resilience angles towards survivability: A position paper motivated by COVID-19 outbreak. Int. J. Prod. Res. **58**(10), 2904–2915 (2020)
12. Ivanov, D.: Predicting the impacts of epidemic outbreaks on global supply chains: A simulation-based analysis on the coronavirus outbreak (COVID-19/SARS-CoV-2) case. Transp. Res. Part E: Logist. Transp. Rev. **136** (2020)
13. V.R., Alazab, M., Srinivasan, S., Pham, Q.-V., Kotti Padannayil, S., Simran, K.: A visualized botnet detection system based deep learning for the internet of things networks of smart cities. IEEE Trans. Ind. Appl. (2020) in press
14. Priyanka, K., Kulennavar, N.: A survey on big data analytics in health care. Int. J. Comput. Sci. Inf. Technol. **5**(4), 5865–5868 (2014)
15. Cottle, M., Hoover, W., Kanwal, S., Kohn, M., Strome, T., Treister,N.: Transforming health care through big data strategies for leveraging big data in the health care industry. Institute for Health Technology Transformation. http://ihealthtran.com/big-data-in-healthcare (2013)
16. Barricelli, B.R., Casiraghi, E., Gliozzo, J., Petrini, A., Valtolina, S.: Human digital twin for fitness management. IEEE Access. **8**(26), 637–664 (2020)
17. Barricelli, B.R., Casiraghi, E., Fogli, D.: A survey on digital twin: definitions, characteristics, applications, and design implications. IEEE Access **7**, 167 653–671 (2019)
18. Rasheed, A., San, O., Kvamsdal, T.: Digital twin: Values, challenges and enablers from a modeling perspective. IEEE Access. **8**(21), 980–1012 (2020)
19. Chae, S., Kwon, S., Lee, D.: Predicting infectious disease using deep learning and big data. Int. J. Environ. Res. Public Health **15**(8) (2018)
20. Bansal, S., Chowell, G., Simonsen, L., Vespignani, A., Viboud, C.: Big data for infectious disease surveillance and modeling. J. Infect. Dis. **214**(4), S375–S379 (2016)
21. Eisenstein, M.: Infection forecasts powered by big data. Nature **555**(7695) (2018)
22. Buckee, C.: Improving epidemic surveillance and response: big data is dead, long live big data. The Lancet Digit. Health. **2**(5), e218–e220 (2020)
23. Chen, C.-M., Jyan, H.-W., Chien, S.-C., Jen, H.-H., Hsu, C.-Y., Lee, P.-C., Lee, C.-F., Yang, Y.-T., Chen, M.-Y., Chen, L.-S. et al.: Containing COVID-19 among 627,386 persons in contact with the diamond princess cruise ship passengers who disembarked in Taiwan: big data analytics. J. Med. Internet Res. **22**(5) (2020)
24. Xu, X., Jiang, X., Ma, C.: Deep Learning System to Screen Coronavirus Disease 2019. Pneumonia, arXiv:2002.09334 (2020)
25. Zhou, C., Su, F., Pei, T., Zhang, A., Du, Y., Luo, B., Cao, Z., Wang, J., Yuan, W., Zhu, Y.: COVID-19: Challenges to GIS with big data. Geogr. Sustain. (2020)
26. Pham, Q.V., Nguyen, D.C., Huynh-the, T., Hwang, W.J., Pathirana, P.N.: Artificial Intelligence (AI) and Big Data for Coronavirus (COVID-19) pandemic: a survey on the State-of-the-Arts. IEEE Access. **4** (2020)
27. Giordano, G., Blanchini, F., Bruno, R., Colaneri, P., Di Filippo, A., Di Matteo, A., Colaneri, M.: Modelling the COVID-19 epidemic and implementation of population-wide interventions in Italy. Nat. Med., 1–6 (2020)

28. Brauer, F., Castillo-Chavez, C., Castillo-Chavez, C.: Mathematical models in population biology and epidemiology. **2** (2012)
29. Chen, B., Shi, M., Ni, X., Ruan, L., Jiang, H., Yao, H., Wang, M., Song, Z., Zhou, Q., Ge, T.: Visual data analysis and simulation prediction for COVID-19. arXiv preprint arXiv:2002.07096 (2020)
30. Peng, L., Yang, W., Zhang, D., Zhuge, C., Hong, L.: Epidemic analysis of COVID-19 in China by dynamical modeling. arXiv preprint arXiv:2002.06563 (2020)
31. Tátrai, D., Várallyay, Z.: COVID-19 epidemic outcome predictions based on logistic fitting and estimation of its reliability. arXiv preprint arXiv:2003.14160 (2020)
32. Strzelecki, A.: The second worldwide wave of interest in coronavirus since the COVID-19 outbreaks in South Korea, Italy and Iran: A Google trends study. Brain, Behavior, and Immunity. (2020)
33. Long, Y.-S., Zhai, Z.-M., Han, L.-L., Kang, J., Li, Y.-L., Lin, Z.-H., Zeng, L., Wu, D.-Y., Hao, C.-Q., Tang, M., et al.: Quantitative assessment of the role of undocumented infection in the 2019 novel coronavirus (COVID-19) pandemic. arXiv preprint arXiv:2003.12028 (2020)
34. Gupta, R., Pandey, G., Chaudhary, P., Pal, S.K.: SEIR and regression model based COVID-19 outbreak predictions in India. medRxiv (2020)
35. Heroy, S.: Metropolitan-scale COVID-19 outbreaks: how similar are they? arXiv preprint arXiv:2004.01248 (2020)
36. Ienca, Vayena, E.: On the responsible use of digital data to tackle the covid-19 pandemic. Nature medicine. **26**(4), 463–464 (2020)
37. Zhao, X., Liu, X., Li, X.: Tracking the spread of novel coronavirus (2019-ncov) based on big data. medRxiv (2020)
38. Zhou, C., Su, F., Pei, T., Zhang, A., Du, Y., Luo, B., Cao, Z., Wang, J., Yuan, W., Zhu, Y., Song, C., Chen, J., Xu, J., Li, F., Ma, T., Jiang, L., Yan, F., Yi, J., Hu, Y., Liao, Y., Xiao, H.: COVID-19: challenges to GIS with Big Data. Geogr. Sustain. **1**(1), 77–87 (2020)
39. Castorina, P., Iorio, A., Lanteri, D.: Data analysis on coronavirus spreading by macroscopic growth laws. arXiv preprint arXiv:2003.00507 (2020)
40. Notari, A.: Temperature dependence of COVID-19 transmission. arXiv preprint arXiv:2003.12417 (2020)
41. Lampos, V., Moura, S., Yom-Tov, E., Cox, I.J., McKendry, R., Edelstein, M.: Tracking COVID-19 using online search. arXiv preprint arXiv:2003.08086 (2020)
42. Garattini, C., Raffle, J., Aisyah, D.N., Sartain, F., Kozlakidis, Z.: Big data analytics, infectious diseases and associated ethical impacts. Philos. Technol. **32**(1), 69–85 (2019)
43. Li, C., Debruyne, D.N., Spencer, J., Kapoor, V., Liu, L.Y., Zhou, B., Lee, L., Feigelman, R., Burdon, G., Liu, J., et al.: High sensitivity detection of coronavirus SARS-CoV-2 using multiplex PCR and a multiplex-PCR based metagenomic method. bioRxiv (2020)
44. Eden, J.S., Rockett, R., Carter, I., Rahman, H., De Ligt, J., Hadfield, J., Storey, M., Ren, X., Tulloch, R., Basile, K., Wells, R., Byun, J., Gilroy, N., O'Sullivan, M.V., Sintchenko, V., Chen, S.C., Maddocks, S., Sorrell, T.C., Holmes, E.C., Dwyer, D.E., Kok, J.: An emergent clade of SARSCoV- 2 linked to returned travellers from Iran. Virus Evol. **6**(1) (2020)
45. Ortea, I., Bock, J.-O.: Re-analysis of SARS-CoV-2 infected host cell proteomics time-course data by impact pathway analysis and network analysis. a potential link with inflammatory response. BioRxiv (2020)
46. Brann, D., Tsukahara, T., Weinreb, C., Logan, D.W., Datta, S.R.: Nonneural expression of SARS-CoV-2 entry genes in the olfactory epithelium suggests mechanisms underlying anosmia in COVID-19 patients. bioRxiv (2020)
47. Lon, J.R., Bai, Y., Zhong, B., Cai, F., Du, H.: Prediction and evolution of B cell epitopes of surface protein in SARS-CoV-2. bioRxiv (2020)
48. Jin, Y.-H., Cai, L., Cheng, Z.-S., Cheng, H., Deng, T., Fan, Y.-P., Fang, C., Huang, D., Huang, L.-Q., Huang, Q., et al.: A rapid advice guideline for the diagnosis and treatment of 2019 novel coronavirus (2019-ncov) infected pneumonia (standard version). Military Med. Res. **7**(1) (2020)

49. Ahmed, S.F., Quadeer, A.A., McKay, M.R.: Preliminary identification of potential vaccine targets for the COVID-19 coronavirus (SARSCoV-2) based on SARS-CoV immunological studies. Viruses **12**(3), 254 (2020)
50. Banerjee, A., Santra, D., Maiti, S.: Energetics based epitope screening in SARS CoV-2 (COVID 19) spike glycoprotein by immuno-informatic analysis aiming to a suitable vaccine development. bioRxiv, (2020)
51. Sarkar, M.A., Ullah, F.T., Johora, M.A., Taniya, Y.A.: The essential facts of wuhan novel coronavirus outbreak in China and Epitope-based vaccine designing against 2019-nCoV. BioRxiv (2020)
52. Abdelmageed, I., Abdelmoneim, A.H., Mustafa, M.I., Elfadol, N.M., Murshed, N.S., Shantier, S.W., Makhawi, A.M.: Design of a multiepitope-based peptide vaccine against the E protein of human COVID-19: an immunoinformatics approach. BioMed Res. Int. (2020)
53. Li, Z., Li, X., Huang, Y.-Y., Wu, Y., Zhou, L., Liu, R., Wu, D., Zhang, L., Liu, H., Xu, X., et al.: FEP-based screening prompts drug repositioning against COVID-19. bioRxiv (2020)
54. Ge, Y., Tian, T., Huang, S., Wan, F., Li, J., Li, S., Yang, H., Hong, L., Wu, N., Yuan, E., et al.: data-driven drug repositioning framework discovered a potential therapeutic agent targeting COVID-19. bioRxiv (2020)
55. Udugama, B., Kadhiresan, P., Kozlowski, H.N., Malekjahani, A., Osborne, M., Li, V.Y., Chen, H., Mubareka, S., Gubbay, J., Chan, W.C.: Diagnosing COVID-19: The disease and tools for detection. ACS Nano (2020)
56. Rao, A.S.S., Vazquez, J.A.: Identification of COVID-19 can be quicker through artificial intelligence framework using a mobile phone-based survey in the populations when cities/towns are under quarantine. Infect. Control Hosp. Epidemiol., 1–18 (2020)
57. Imran, A., Posokhova, I., Qureshi, H.N., Masood, U., Riaz, S., Ali, K., John, C.N., Nabeel, M.: AI4COVID-19: AI enabled preliminary diagnosis for COVID-19 from cough samples via an app. Inform. Med. Unlocked., 100378 (2020)
58. Cisco annual internet report (2018–2023). (2020) [Online]. Available: https://www.cisco.com/c/en/us/solutions/executive-perspectives/annual-internet-report/index.html
59. Wood, C.S., Thomas, M.R., Budd, J., Mashamba-Thompson, T.P., Herbst, K., Pillay, D., Peeling, R.W., Johnson, A.M., McKendry, R.A., Stevens, M.M.: Taking connected mobile-health diagnostics of infectious diseases to the field. Nature **566**(7745), 467–474 (2019)
60. Nguyen, D.C., Pathirana, P.N., Ding, M., Seneviratne, A.: Blockchain for 5G and beyond networks: A state of the art survey. J. Netw. Comput. Appl. **166**, (2020)
61. Kuo, T.-T., Kim, H.-E., Ohno-Machado, L.: Blockchain distributed ledger technologies for biomedical and health care applications. J. Am. Med. Inform. Assoc. **24**(6), 1211–1220 (2017)
62. Gao, H., Liu, C.H., Wang, W., Zhao, J., Song, Z., Su, X., Crowcroft, J., Leung, K.K.: A survey of incentive mechanisms for participator sensing. IEEE Commun. Surv. Tutor. **17**(2), 918–943 (2015)
63. Rees, V.: AI and cloud computing used to develop COVID-19 vaccine. (2020) [Online]. https://www.drugtargetreview.com/news/59650/ai-and-cloud-computing-used-to-develop-covid-19-vaccine/
64. Chamola, V., Hassija, V., Gupta, V., Guizani, M.: A comprehensive review of the COVID-19 pandemic and the role of IoT, drones, AI, Blockchain, and 5G in managing its impact. IEEE Access. **8**(90), 225–265 (2020)
65. Lewnard, J.A., Lo, N.C.: Scientific and ethical basis for social distancing interventions against COVID-19. The Lancet Infect. Dis. **20**(6), 631 (2020)

Two Layer Hybrid Scheme of IMO and PSO for Optimization of Local Aligner: COVID-19 as a Case Study

Mohamed Issa and Ahmed Helmi

Abstract Nowadays, meta-heuristic algorithm (MA) succeeded in optimizing many engineering problems. Ions motion optimization (IMO) algorithm is a MA that inspired its search strategy from ions attraction based on force law. IMO has good exploration capability but poor exploitation of the search space. The performance of IMO was tested for implementing fragmented local aligner technique (FLAT) which is a local aligner method for finding the longest common consecutive subsequence (LCCS) between pair of biological sequences. Due to the huge length of sequences FLAT based on IMO produce poor results due to the poor exploitation which need to be enhanced by adding particle swarm optimization (PSO) algorithm which has efficient exploitation capability. The enhanced version of IMO (IMO-PSO)was merged as two layer (bottom layer for exploration using IMO and the upper layer exploit the best solution founded from the bottom layer). This hybrid scheme increase the diversity of solutions which increase the quality of solutions. FLAT based on IMO-PSO was tested on real biological sequences gathered from NCBI versus IMO and the standard local alignment algorithm. Besides, COVID-19 was analyzed against other viruses to detect the LCCS between it. FLAT based on IMO-PSO produced an enhancement of the performance of IMO for finding LCCS between biological sequences.

Keywords Bioinformatics · Local sequence alignment · Meta-heuristics · Ions motion optimization (IMO) and particle swarm optimization (PSO)

1 Introduction

Meta-heuristic algorithms (MA) are stochastic search algorithms that finds the near optimal solution of an optimization problems [1]. It mimics the search methodology from physics, nature or human. Differential Evolution [2] and Genetic Algorithms [3] an example of MA that mimic its updating strategy from theory evolutionary.

M. Issa (✉) · A. Helmi
Computer and Systems Engineering Department, Faculty of Engineering, Zagazig University, Zazig, Egypt
e-mail: mohmed.issa@gmail.com

D. Oliva et al. (eds.), *Artificial Intelligence for COVID-19*, Studies in Systems, Decision and Control 358, https://doi.org/10.1007/978-3-030-69744-0_21

From physics, such as Sine-Cosine Algorithm (SCA) [4] which based on sine and cosine mathematical operators for updating the movement of the search agent toward the best solution founded through the search space.

Besides, Ions Motion Optimization (IMO) algorithm [5] which mimics the repulsion and attraction law of ions and there are other physical inspired meta-heuristic algorithms such as thermal exchange optimization algorithm [6], Electromagnetic Field Optimization [7], Lightning Attachment Procedure Optimization [8],Gravitational Search Algorithm (GSA) [9], Electron radar search algorithm [10], The Whirlpool Algorithm [11] and Squirrel Search Algorithm for optimization [12].

In addition, there are MA that mimics their updating strategy from animals and insects such as Moth-Flame Optimization (MFO) [13], Artificial Bee Colony (ABC) [14], Particle Swarm Optimization (PSO) [15], Lion optimization algorithm (LOA) [16], Artificial Feeding Birds (AFB) [17], Ant Lion Optimizer [18]. There are hundreds of MA since no one MA can solve all optimization problems with the same efficiency according to No-Free-Lunch (NFL) theorem [19].

IMO is a physics based MA that updates its solutions based on the concepts of attraction and repulsion of ions in the law of force [5]. It divides the solutions into two groups (anions and cations) where each search agent attracted to the best solutions with opposite signs. For example, an anion attracted to the best cation and the reverses.

IMO has been succeed in for optimizing many engineering applications such as load economic dispatch [20], short-term hydrothermal scheduling [21], breast cancer prediction [22], AGC investigation in [23], protein folding prediction [24], robotics [25] and cloud job scheduling [26].

The choice of using IMO due to its powerful exploration capabilities where it is based on two best solutions (best anion and best cation) which increase the exploration of the search space. Since, the huge length of sequences (search space) IMO explores the regions of it efficiently. However, it has poor exploitation (focus searching for optimal solution in very narrow region of the search space).

Hence, the performance of IMO is enhanced by hybrid another algorithm has efficient exploitation such as PSO in a two layer hybridization scheme [27] where bottom layer responsible for exploration the search space while the top layer intensify the best results found by the bottom layer.

Particle Swarm Optimization (PSO) algorithm [15] is a meta-heuristic algorithm its methodology inspired from the flying of particles to reach a specific destination. PSO has an efficient exploitation of the search space and there is motivation to use it due to its success to optimize the exploitation phase in a lot of meta-heuristics such as SCA [27], Grey Wolf Optimization (GWO) [28], Differential Evolution [29], Tabu Search [30], Gravitational Search Algorithm (GSA) [31], Swallow Optimization Algorithm (SOA) [32], Bacterial Foraging Algorithm (BFA) [33], Ant Colony Algorithm [34], [35], Genetic algorithms [36] and there are other trials of optimization other algorithms. It has efficient exploitation due to it move the solutions toward not only the best achieved solution but also toward the best positions founded by each solution.

The performance of IMO and the enhanced version (IMO-PSO) were tested for finding the longest common consecutive subsequences (LCCS) between two biological sequence that was determined by Fragmented Local Aligner Technique (FLAT) [27]. This problem was chosen to test the performance of enhanced version of IMO (IMO-PSO) due to it measure the exploitation performance of MA and its search space (length of sequences) is huge.

The performance of FLAT was tested using IMO, PSO, SCA and the enhanced the version (IMO-PSO). A set of biological protein data gathered from National Center for Biotechnology Information (NCBI) (https://www.ncbi.nlm.nih.gov/) the sequences to be aligned have a product of its lengths ranges from 250,000 to 9,000,000. Besides, COVID-19 protein was used as a case study to measure the LCCS between it and other viruses using various MA techniques of FLAT and the results are evaluated versus the accurate LCCS measured by SW algorithm [37].

The rest of chapter is organized as follows:

Section 2 describes FLAT procedure based on MA for finding LCCS between pair of sequences. In Sect. 3, the procedure of PSO and IMO is described. Section 4 presents the enhanced hybrid technique of IMO and PSO.

2 Fragmented Local Aligner Technique

Sequence Alignment is a basic operation in bioinformatics for aligning DNA, Protein and RNA sequences to measure its evolutionary relationships [38], protein secondary structure prediction [39], construction of phylogenetic trees [40] and DNA fragment assembly [41]. Two kinds of sequence alignments are pairwise sequence alignment which aligns pair of sequences and multiple sequence alignment which aligns more than two sequences.

This chapter focus on pairwise sequence alignment which categorize as global alignment and local alignment [38]. Global alignment aims to align the entire of sequences over the length of sequence [42]. Local sequence alignment aims to align portion of the sequences to find the longest common subsequence between two subsequences [37]. Figure 1 shows the comparison between global alignment and local alignment.

Smith-Waterman (SW) alignment algorithm [37] produces the accurate alignment between two sequences (finding the longest common consecutive subsequences).

It Based on dividing the alignment into sub-problems and solve it on accumulative manner using dynamic programming (DP). However, it consumes huge execution time due to the long of biological sequences. The main important usage of local sequence alignment operation are binding sites in the protein sequences for molecular docking process of drug design and finding the common features between biological sequences which aims to construct the phylogenetic tree of sequences.

Fragmented Local Aligner Technique (FLAT) [27] is an enhanced version of local sequence alignment based on using meta-heuristic algorithms. FLAT divides the long

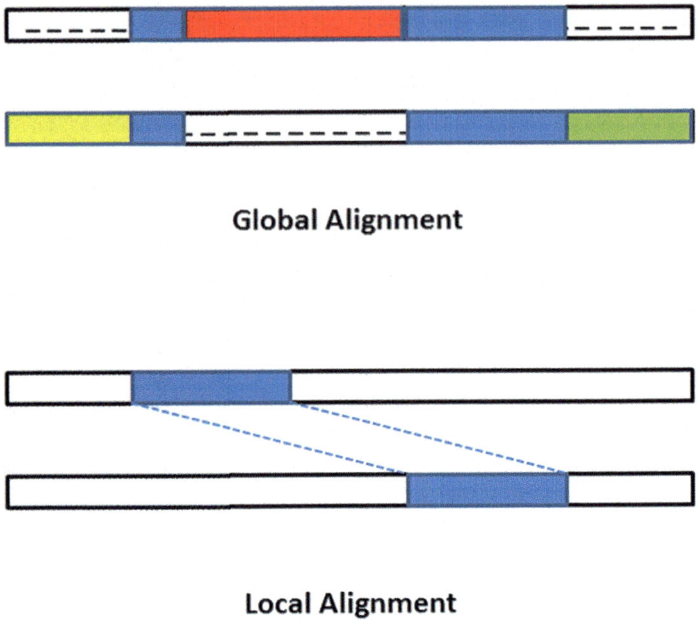

Fig. 1 Global alignment versus Local alignment

sequences into fragments with small lengths and these fragments are aligned using Smith-Waterman algorithm.

Hence, the execution time is reduced due to small length of fragments instead of the overall length of sequences. The rule of using meta-heuristic algorithm is determining the positions of cutting fragments to be aligned. Therefore, the solution is the position at which two fragments to be cut and aligns using SW algorithm and these solutions are updated to move toward the positions that have fragments produced the longest common subsequences.

SW alignment algorithm works as following to find LCCS between pair of sequences. First, a matrix with size (n + 1) X (m + 1) is constructedwhere the two sequences have lengths of m and n.

The cells of matrix are filled by the various alignment scores that are computed using Eq. 1.

$$\mathrm{Score}(\mathrm{i},\mathrm{j}) = \max\left\{\begin{array}{c} Score(\mathrm{i}-1,\mathrm{j}-1) + Similarity\left(\mathrm{Seq}_1(\mathrm{i}),\mathrm{Seq}_2(\mathrm{j})\right) \\ \max_{\mathrm{k}=1:\mathrm{i}-1}\left(\mathrm{Score}(\mathrm{i},\mathrm{k}) + \mathrm{g}_0 + \mathrm{k}\ \mathrm{g}_\mathrm{e}\right) \\ \max_{\mathrm{k}=1:\mathrm{i}-1}\left(\mathrm{Score}(\mathrm{k},\mathrm{j}) + \mathrm{g}_0 + \mathrm{k}\ \mathrm{g}_\mathrm{e}\right) \\ 0 \end{array}\right\} \quad (1)$$

where Seq $_1$ and Seq_2 are the sequences to be aligned and have lengths m and n in order. i and j represents the indices of row and column in order and i lies in the range from 1 to m and j lies in the range from 1 to n.

Similarity () is a function that score the similar and un-similar residues of protein. In some cases of partial alignment, it may be need to shifted until matching occur. For shifting a gap '---' can be inserted which is evaluated as a g_0 score for first gap and g_e for other k inserted consecutive gaps. Note that g_0 and g_e has a negative scores that reduce the alignment score. $(g_0 + k\ g_e)$ is a linear gap function is used for maximizing the alignment score instead of using individual scoring scheme due to g_0 has negative score lower than that of g_e [43].

The second step for computing the alignment is trace back stage which is started to construct the alignment of the two sequences after computing the scoring matrix. During the computation of the scoring matrix, another matrix is constructed to determine the trace back to construct the alignment between the sequences. Considering local pairwise alignment, for each cell in the scoring matrix if a maximum value is obtained from left or top cells then the corresponding cell in the trace back saves the symbol "L" or "T" respectively. While if the maximum value comes from the diagonal cell then the symbol "D" is kept.

To construct the local alignment (finding longest common substrings) we can trace back over the trace back matrix starting from the maximum alignment score in the scoring matrix until reaching score zero as following:

While the cell in the trace matrix contain a 'D' then align the two residues from the two sequences.

- While the cell contain a 'L' then align a residue from Seq_2 with a gap.
- While the cell contain a 'T' then align a residue from Seq_1 with a gap.

However, these method provide the accurate local alignment between two sequences but it consumes huge time since the computational complexity of this algorithm is $O(n^3)$ and the space complexity is $O(n^2)$, where n is the length of the two sequences to be aligned. This alignment method was optimized to speed up the execution time of alignment process especially for sequences for very long lengths [27].

The acceleration of SW algorithm based on fragment the longer sequences into short fragments that can be aligned in small time due to the short length. The question is where the fragment is cut and the is the rule of using MA to determine the position at which the fragments are cut. The LCCS are computed of all fragments and the positions are updated toward the position that produces the maximum LCCS founded.

As shown in Fig. 2, three positions are determined in each sequences and the LCCS between each pair of sequences are computed. All other positions updates their locations toward the (P_{A1} in Seq $_1$ and P_{B1} in Seq $_2$) since they produce the maximum LCCS.

To increase the diversity three ways to cut a fragment as shown in Fig. 3:

i. A Fragments with length LF are cut from (P_i) to $(P_i + L_F)$.
ii. A Fragments with length LF are cut from $(P_i - (L_F/2))$ to $(P_i + (L_F/2))$
iii. A Fragments with length LF are cut from $(P_i - L_F)$ to (P_i).

For the optimization of finding the location of fragments an objective function is used that evaluates the corresponding residues in the best two fragments found.

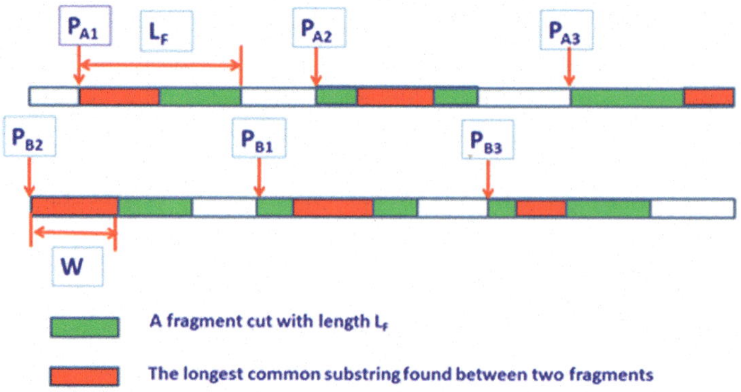

Fig. 2 Updating the positions of fragments of FLAT

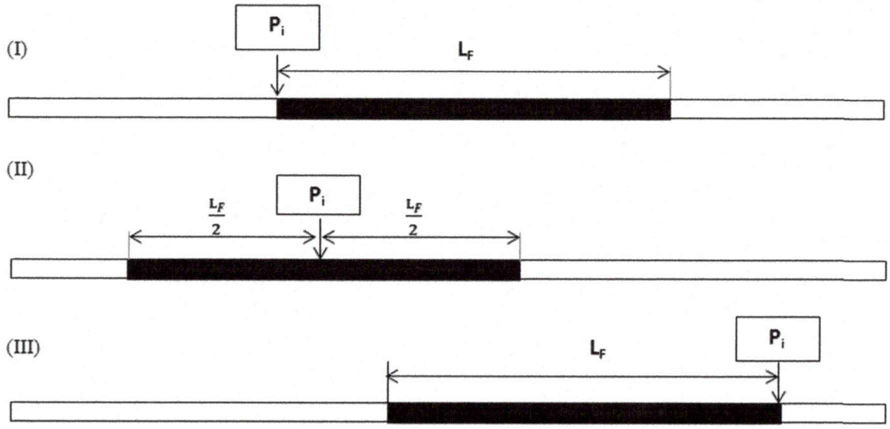

Fig. 3 Different ways to cut a fragment with length L_F

Equation 10 is used as an objective function that is used to control the movement of search agents and evaluate the finding alignments.

$$\text{Alignment}_{\text{Score}} = \sum_{i=1}^{L} \left\{ \begin{matrix} if\, A_i == B_i \; penalize(+1)score \\ otherwise penalize zero \end{matrix} \right\} \quad (2)$$

where A and B are the aligned sequences. The optimized fragmented pairwise local sequence alignment algorithm is presented in Algorithm (1).

Algorithm (1) FLAT Procedure

1. A K agents (P_i, i in the range (1, K)) are initialized randomly with a one position in each sequencesand is chosen in the range (1, length ((Seq_1 or Seq_1) − L_F)) where $L_F$represents the length of fragment.

2. A fragment has a length L_F is cut according to the three cutting method of Figure 3 and is chosen randomly to increase the diversity.

3. Each two fragments that are cut by each search agent are aligned using SW alignment aligns and Eq. 2 is used to estimate the alignment score as anfitness function.
4. The positions of solutions are updated according to the update mechanism of the MA used toward the position that have maximum LCCS founded.
5. Repeat the steps (from 2 to 5) for a number of iterations.

FLAT has a time of complexity $\left(T\ K\ L_F^2 C\right)$, where T, K and L_F are the number of iteration, number of search agents, the length of fragments and C is the cost time of updating equation of the MA in order.

2.1 Preliminaries

In the following subsections, the procedure of IMO and PSO and their searching mechanism are described in Sects. 3.1 and 3.2 in order.

3 Ions Motion Optimization (IMO) Algorithm

The IMO algorithm [5] is an algorithm that inspired from the properties of attracting of ions in physics. The candidate solutions of IMO algorithm are separated into two groups of cations (represents the ions with negative signs) and anions (represents the ions with positive signs). The basic idea of updating the solutions is attracting the anions to the best cation and cations to the best anion founded.

The algorithm execution is divided into two phases: the liquid phase and the solid phase. In liquid phase, the ions are updated to move free more than in the solid phase that give for high probability of exploration the search space more than exploitation. In the solid phase, the ions becomes in stable form where attraction forces between ions prevent it to be moved for big step.

The liquid and solid phases are described as follows:

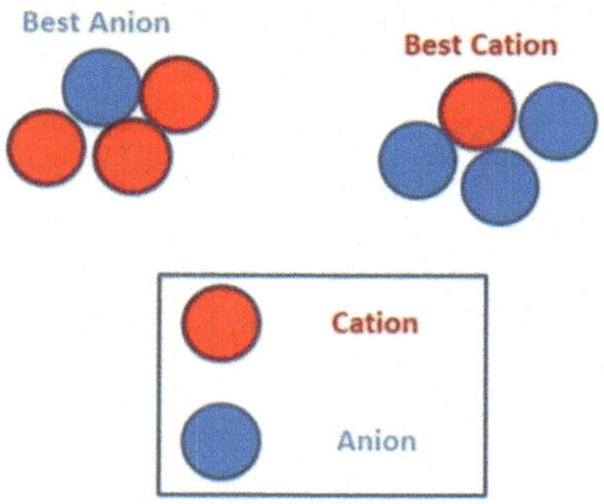

Fig. 4 Ions motion around an optimum in the solid phase

Liquid phase:

In the liquid phase each population of anions and captions updates its movement such that each anion move toward the best cation and each cation move toward the best anion as in Fig. 4. Equations 3 and 4 are used for updating theanions and the cation.

$$A_{i,j} = A_{i,j} + AF_{i,j} * \left(C_{bestj} - A_{i,j}\right) \quad (3)$$

$$C_{i,j} = C_{i,j} + CF_{i,j} * \left(A_{bestj} - C_{i,j}\right) \quad (4)$$

where j is the dimension, i is the index of ions,$C_{i,j}$ is the cation candidate solulution, $A_{i,j}$ is anion candidate solution. C_{bestj} is the best cation solution found, A_{bestj} is the best anion solution. $AF_{i,j}$ and $CF_{i,j}$ is the mathematical modeling that represents the distance between ions and cations as in Eqs. 5 and 6.

$$AF_{i,j} = \frac{1}{1 + e^{-\frac{0.1}{AD_{i,j}}}} \quad (5)$$

$$CF_{i,j} = \frac{1}{1 + e^{-\frac{0.1}{CD_{i,j}}}} \quad (6)$$

where $AD_{i,j}$ is $\left|A_{i,j} - C_{bestj}\right|$ and $CD_{i,j}$ is $\left|C_{i,j} - A_{bestj}\right|$.

Exploration can be guaranteed due to ions are attracted to the opposite charges ions. With increasing the iterations, more ions interact and converge toward the best ions with opposite charges and the exploration are gradually decreased. After iteration of execution, the ions enter the solid state phase where the ions becomes approximately fixed due to stability of attraction forces as in Fig. 5.

Solid Phase

In solid phase, ions have difficult move become in stable phase so an external force to be applied to the ions to give it energy to break the stable form and avoids local minima. Equations 7 and 8 are used for this purpose and to increase the diversity

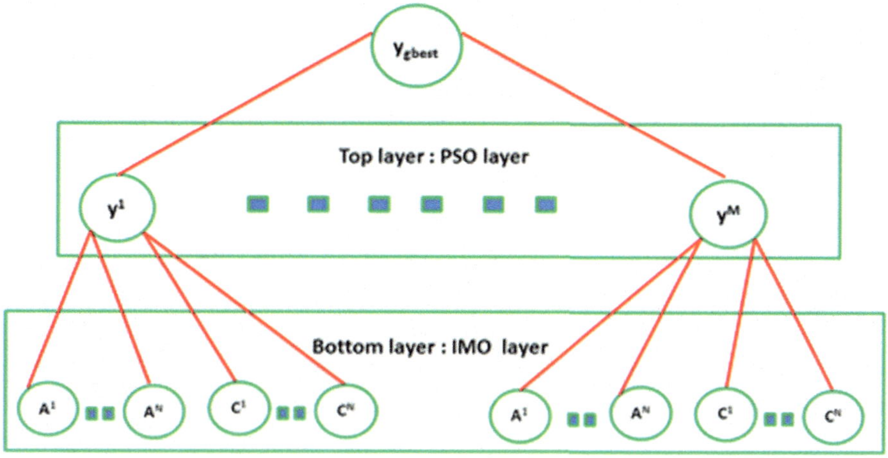

Fig. 5 The proposedhybrid scheme between PSO and IMO

of ions around search space there is a random initialization of some ions around search space. Hence, apply external force there is an important condition that must be satisfied first is the value of fitness of best ion of cations (and anions) is more than or equal the half of the worst value of cations (and anions) which means the ions are in stable case.

$$A_i = A_i + \alpha_1 * (C_{best}) \tag{7}$$

$$C_i = C_i + \alpha_2 * (A_{best}) \tag{8}$$

The Procedure of IMO algorithm arepresentedin Algorithm (2).

Algorithm (1) : IMO Procedure
1: Initialize K ions solutions ($A_{i,j}$, j=1,2,3…K/2) and ($C_{i,j}$, j=1,2,3…K/2), IMO parameters (α1 and α2)
2: Evaluate the fitness function based on anion and cationions.
3: Update ($A_i^{best}$and C_i^{best})
4: Repeat
5: for j=1 : K/2
6: Update ($A_{i,j}$ and $C_{i,j}$) according to Eq.3 and Eq.4for liquid phase and Eq.7 and Eq.8for solid phase.
7: Update (A_i^{best}, C_i^{best})
8: end for i
9: Until (T < maximum number of iterations)
10: Return the A_{best} if Fitness (A_{best}) is the better else return C_{best} as global best solution

IMO has a complexity of time is $O(R^{*}K^{*}(c_{Liquis} + c_{Solid}))$ where R is the number of iterations, K is the number of search agents and C_{Liquid} and C_{Solid} are the cost time of updating equations of one search agents in the liquid and solid phase in order.

IMO has advantages such as low computational complexity few number of parameters that to be tuned, and fast convergence. But the main limitation poor exploitation capabilities and trapping in local minima.

4 Particle Swarm Optimization (PSO)

PSO is a population based randomsearch method where its search strategy is based mainly on global communications between the candidates solutions. All the search agents update their movetoward the best global solution. The main advantage of PSO is it depends on the history which enhance its exploitation capabilities.

The updating movement equations of PSO are Eqs. 9 and 10 where (P^{gbest}) has the global best position between all candidates and the best personal position ($P^{i}best$) that each candidate found through the previous iterations.

$$v_i(t+1) = w^{*}\, v_i(t) + c_1 rand\left(P_i^{best} - P_i(t)\right) + c_2 rand\left(P^{gbest} - P_i(t)\right) \quad (9)$$

$$P_i(t+1) = P_i(t) + v_i(t+1) \quad (10)$$

where c_1 and c_2 are the local the global best position weight coefficient in order, v_i represents the velocity of the *i*th particle,. *w* is the coefficient of inertia that evaluates the control of the previous velocity on the new evaluated velocity. rand () is a random function generate values in the range (0–1). The steps of PSO are summarized in Algorithm (3).

Algorithm (3) : PSO algorithm
1: Initialize a set of population solutions (P_i), initial velocity (v_i) and algorithm's parameters (c_1, c_2 and w)
2: **Repeat**
3: Evaluate the objective function based on population solutions
4: Update the best local solution for each particle (P^{i}_{best})
5: Update the best global solution over all particles (P^{gbest})
6: Update the next position of population solutions using Eq. 10 and Eq. 11
7: **Until (T < maximum number of iterations)**
8: Return the best solution (P^{gbest}) obtained as the global optimum

PSO has a complexity of time is $O(T^{*}n^{*}c_{pso})$ where T is the number of iterations, n is the number of search agents and c_{pso} is the cost time of modifying position of one search agents.

PSO has many advantages information communication between search agents which give it more reliability to achieve near optimal solution with reasonable convergence speed besides robustness. PSO succeeded in solving many optimization problems such as solar cell design [44–46], electrical motor design [47] and surgical robot applications [48].

4.1 The Proposed Hybrid Scheme of PSO and IMO (PSO-IMO)

IMO has many advantages such as efficient exploration capabilities of the search space in addition to few number of parameter to be adjusted. However it has poor exploitation capabilities hence it suffers from trapping in local minima. Two main reasons which make IMO has good exploration but not the best efficient, the first is dividing the ions into two groups hence there are two global best solutions found during the search process which make there is a big chance for more exploration of the search space.

The second reason is the attraction law between ions make there are more diversification of the search space. Hence, the aim of this paper to enhance the exploitation process of IMO and benefiting from the good exploration capabilities of IMO. The improvement of IMO based on trying two approaches, merging IMO with PSO where PSO has good exploitation capabilities and the second one is adding a random variable and control its variable using chaotic maps where this approach gives more diversifications.

PSO is a meta- heuristic algorithm that has good exploitation process of the search space more than exploration capabilities which make it superior for enhancing the exploitation process of many meta-heuristic s such as Differential Evolution [29], SCA [27], Grey Wolf Optimization (GWO) [28], Tabu Search [30], Gravitational Search Algorithm (GSA) [31],, Bacterial Foraging Algorithm (BFA) [33], Ant Colony Algorithm [34, 35], Swallow Optimization Algorithm (SOA) [32], Genetic algorithms [36] and there are other trials of optimization other algorithms (Fig. 6).

An enhancement of IMO processed by merging PSO by let IMO perform the search operation for many iterations and then the last solutions of IMO will be the initialization of PSO to be start with and resume the search operation for another number of iterations. The idea here is to perform exploration first and the PSO exploit the solutions founded by IMO.

This hybrid scheme belongs to the class High (due to each algorithm is self contained), Relay (due to the two algorithms are executed in serial manner). Figure 7 explain the hybrid scheme between PSO and IMO as a two layer. In this hybridization, the solution found by IMO will become an initialization solutions for.

PSO. PSO need three solutions, the global best one which is determined from the best fitness of best anion and best cations. The personal best solution for each

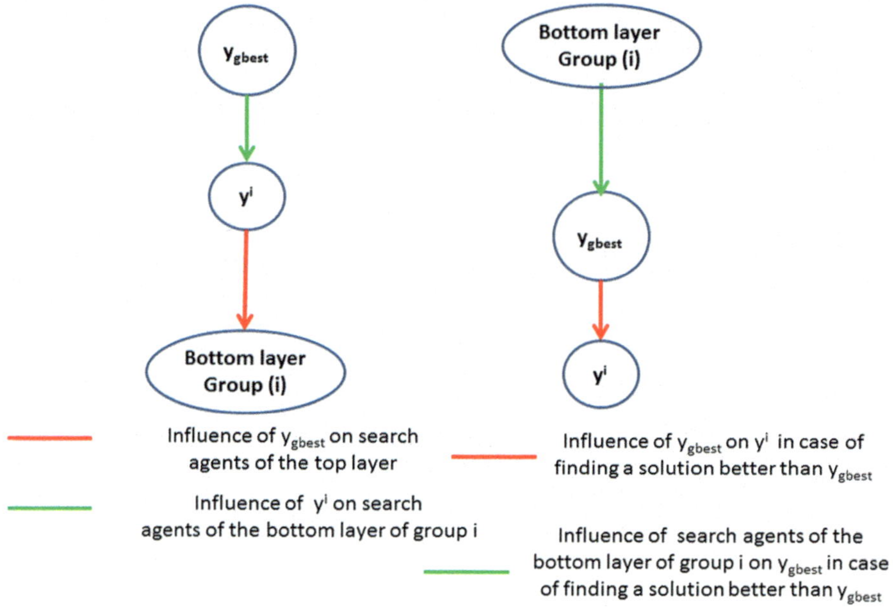

Fig. 6 The influence of search agents of bottom layer on that of upper layer and global best solution

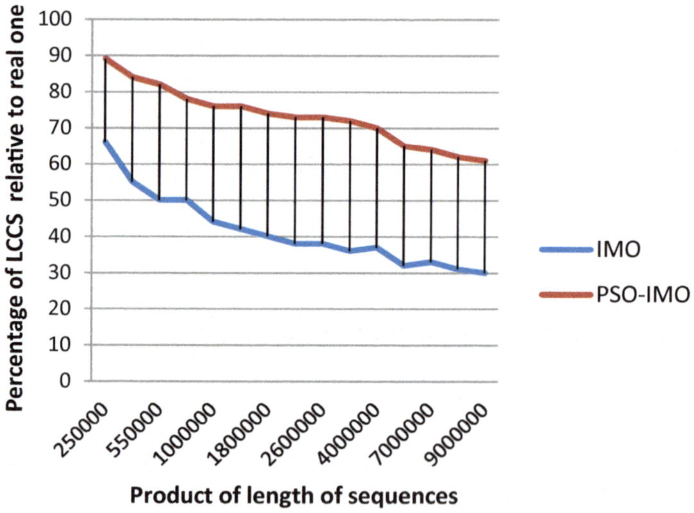

Fig. 7 The percentage of LCCS founded by FLAT relative to that of SW algorithm

solution is determined according to the best fit of each according ions of anion and cation and the other solution will become the solution of the search agents of PSO.

The movement of the search agents of bottom layer are controlled using the updating equations of IMO Eqs. 14–17. While the updating equation of the top layer is as Eqs. 12–13.

$$v^{t+1} = w * v^t + c_1 rand\left((y_i^{best})^t - (y_i)^t\right) + c_2 rand\left((y^{gbest})^t - (y_i)^t\right) \quad (11)$$

$$(y_i)^{t+1} = v^{t+1} + (y_i)^t) \quad (12)$$

$$A_{i,j} = A_{i,j} + AF_{i,j} * \left(C_{besti} or y_i - A_{i,j}\right) \quad (13)$$

$$C_{i,j} = C_{i,j} + CF_{i,j} * \left(A_{besti} or y_i - C_{i,j}\right) \quad (14)$$

$$A_{i,j} = A_{i,j} + \alpha_1 * \left(C_i^{best} or y^i\right) \quad (15)$$

$$C_{i,j} = C_{i,j} + \alpha_2 * (A_i^{best} or y^i) \quad (16)$$

While i denotes to the group number and j represent the index of search agent in the group i. In Eqs. 14 and 15 (for liquid states) and Eqs. 16 and 17 (for solid states) updates the anion and cation search agent toward the best cation or anion respectively or toward y_i based on the better fitness. The details of hybridization is described in Algorithm (4). Figure 6 shows the influence of bottom and upper search agents on each other.

Algorithm (4) : IMO-PSO algorithm

Initialize $M \times N$ ions solutions $(A_{i,j}, j=1,2,3...N/2)$ and $(C_{i,j}, j=1,2,3...N/2)$, IMO parameters (α_1 and α_2), PSO parameters (w, $c1$, $c2$).
Evaluate the objective function based on ions (A and C).
Update (A_i^{best} and C_i^{best})
Update y^i from (A_i^{best} and C_i^{best})
Find y_{gbest} as the solution produce best fit from the swarms (y^1 to y^M)
Repeat
for $i = 1 : M$
  for $j = 1 : N/2$
    Update ($A_{i,j}$ and $C_{i,j}$) according to Eq.14 and Eq.15 (Liquid state) and Eq.16 and Eq.17 (Solid state)
    Update (A_i^{best}, C_i^{best}, y^i and y_{gbest})
  end for j
  Update (y^i) according to Eq. 12 and Eq. 13
  Update (y_{gbest})
end for i
Until (T< maximum number of iterations)
Return the best solution (y_{gbest}) obtained as the global minimum solution

5 Experimental Results and Discussion

In this section the experimental results of testing the IMO and its developed versions for optimizing FLAT are presented. The objective function is to find the LCCS between pair of biological sequences. The test was performed on real biological protein sequences gathered from the National Center for Biotechnology Information (NCBI) where the product of length of sequences pair in the range from 250,000 to 9,000,000.

The experimental results were performed on a computer machine has a processor Core I3 (each processor was 2 GHz) and a RAM memory was 4GByte. The setting of parameters that was used for IMO, IMO-PSO and SW algorithms as shown in Table 1.

Table 2 shows the execution time of the IMO and enhanced version (IMO-PSO) versus that of SW alignment algorithm [37]. As shown in the table IMO and its enhanced version have very small execution time relative to that of SW algorithm over various length of sequences.

The performance of FLAT based on IMO and its enhanced version to find the LCCS with a percent related to that founded by SW algorithm was evaluated on a set of pair of sequences ranges from 250,000 to 9,000,000. Figure 7 shows the improvement of percentage of LCCS founded by the enhanced version of IMO over various lengths of sequences.

Table 1 The setting values for the parameters of MA used to implement FLAT

Algorithm	Parameter	Value
SW alignment	Match	+1.0
	g_e	−0.5
	g_o	−1.0
IMO–PSO	Inertia Coefficient	0.2
	Local coefficient (C1)	0.5
	Global coefficient (C2)	0.5

Table 2 Execution time comparison of FLAT based on IMO, IMO-PSO versus SW global alignment algorithm

m X n	SW	IMO	IMO-PSO
250000	11	4.7	6.04
350000	18	4.7	6.04
550000	37	12	12.7
750000	57	14.3	14.9
1000000	138	18.8	18.9
1400000	208	21.7	21.7
1800000	288	25	26
2200000	310	29	30.2
2600000	354	49.2	51.2
3000000	428	49.2	51.2
4000000	680	53.9	55.9
5000000	922	53.9	55.9
6000000	1275	53.9	55.9
7000000	1670	67	69.8
8000000	2134	78.9	83.7
9000000	2750	78.9	83.7

The virsues that were used for testing against COVID-19 virus are: Alveolar Proteinosis, Human Immunodeficiency, Hepatitis C, Influenza A, Influenza B and Trachea Infections. All the protein data of viruses were gathered from GenBank of NCBI (https://www.ncbi.nlm.nih.gov/).

As shown in Table 3, FLAT based on IMO-PSO beat the standard IMO to find the LCCS between COVID-19 and other viruses. SW alignment algorithm was used as a reference to find the exact LCCS. As shown in the table that IMO fail to find percent of exact LCCS while IMO-PSO can achieve despite low percent that is due to the huge length of COVID-19. Therefore, the enhanced version of IMO (IMO-PSO) succeded to enhance the performance of FLAT over than IMO where the PSO enhance the exploitation of IMO in addition the two layer execution (the bottom for exploration and the upper for exploitation) that increase the diversity of solution and enhance the qualtiy.

Table 3 Testing FLAT IMO and its enhanced version for finding LCCS of COVID-19 protein against other diseases

Virus protein	Method	Score	LCCS obtained
Alveolar Proteinases	SW algorithm	22	IDAMMFTSDLATNNLVVMAYIT
	IMO	4	GAVC
	IMO-PSO	4	AYIT
Human Immunodeficiency	SW algorithm	24	TYPSLETIQITSSFKWDLTAFGLV
	IMO	3	GAC
	IMO-PSO	5	TYPSL
Hepatitis C	SW algorithm	10	TSSGDATTAY
	IMO	3	SLL
	IMO-PSO	4	TTAY
Influenza A	SW algorithm	16	TGSSKCVCSVIDLLLD
	IMO	4	SLVP
	IMO-PSO	5	TGSSK
Influenza B	SW algorithm	24	FSTVFPPTSFGPLVRKIFVDGVPF
	IMO	4	KGRL
	IMO-PSO	5	FSTVF
Trachea Infections	SW algorithm	19	QQLRVESSSKLWAQCVQLH
	IMO	3	VPG
	IMO-PSO	4	VQLH

6 Conclusions and Future Work

This chapter presented an enhancement of IMO by adding PSO algorithm to enhance the exploitation of IMO. Besides, the two algorihms are executed in two layer hybrid scheme where the bottom layer was responsible for exploring the search space while the upper layer exploit the best solutions founded in the bottom layer. This hybrid mechansism increase the diversity of the solution which will produce a better quality of solutions.

The enhanced version (IMO-PSO) have small execution time such as IMO but very small than that of SW algorithm over various lengths of sequences (pair of sequences have a producr of its length ranges from 250,000 to 9,000,000). Besides, the percent of LCCS that founded by FLAT (using IMO and IMO-PSO) relative to the exact one founded by SW algorithm were measured where IMO-PSO presented an enahncement over than the performance of IMO.

In addition, COVID-19 was analyzed by FLAT based on IMO and IMO-PSO to measure the LCCS between it and other six viruses. The test verfied the enhancement of FLAT based on IMO-PSO where it finds LCCS have low percent of the exact one founded by SW algorithm while IMO finds other LCCS not relate to the exact one.

However, IMO-PSO presented an enhancement of performance of IMO for FLAT but it still need more enhancement in the future work to enahnce the percent of LCCS founded. An suggestion for more enhancement, a graphical processing unit (GPU) is used to increase the number of search agents of IMO-PSO ot be able to cover the huge length of biological sequences.

References

1. Talbi, E.-G.: Metaheuristics: from Design to Implementation, vol. 74. John Wiley (2009)
2. Storn, R., Price, K.: Differential evolution–a simple and efficient heuristic for global optimization over continuous spaces. J. Global Optim. **11**(4), 341–359 (1997)
3. Holland, J.H.: genetic algorithms. Sci. Am. **267**(1), 66–73 (1992)
4. Mirjalili, S.: SCA: a sine cosine algorithm for solving optimization problems. Knowl.-Based Syst. **96**, 120–133 (2016)
5. Javidy, B., Hatamlou, A., Mirjalili, S.: Ions motion algorithm for solving optimization problems. Appl. Soft Comput. **32**, 72–79 (2015)
6. Kaveh, A., Dadras, A.: A novel meta-heuristic optimization algorithm: thermal exchange optimization. Adv. Eng. Softw. **110**, 69–84 (2017)
7. Abedinpourshotorban, H., et al.: Electromagnetic field optimization: a physics-inspired metaheuristic optimization algorithm. Swarm Evol. Comput. **26**, 8–22 (2016)
8. Nematollahi, A.F., Rahiminejad, A., Vahidi, B.: A novel physical based meta-heuristic optimization method known as lightning attachment procedure optimization. Appl. Soft Comput. **59**, 596–621 (2017)
9. Rashedi, E., Nezamabadi-Pour, H., Saryazdi, S.: GSA: a gravitational search algorithm. Inf. Sci. **179**(13), 2232–2248 (2009)
10. Rahmanzadeh, S., Pishvaee, M.S.: Electron radar search algorithm: a novel developed metaheuristic algorithm. Soft Comput., 1–23 (2019)
11. Zou, Y.: The whirlpool algorithm based on physical phenomenon for solving optimization problems. Eng. Comput. (2019)
12. Jain, M., Singh, V., Rani, A.: A novel nature-inspired algorithm for optimization: Squirrel search algorithm. Swarm Evol. Comput. **44**, 148–175 (2019)
13. Mirjalili, S.: Moth-flame optimization algorithm: A novel nature-inspired heuristic paradigm. Knowl.-Based Syst. **89**, 228–249 (2015)
14. Karaboga, D., Basturk, B.: Artificial bee colony (ABC) optimization algorithm for solving constrained optimization problems. Found. Fuzzy Logic Soft Comput., 789–798 (2007)
15. Kennedy: Particle swarm optimization. Neural Netw. (1995)
16. Yazdani, M., Jolai, F.: Lion optimization algorithm (LOA): a nature-inspired metaheuristic algorithm. J. Comput. Des. Eng. **3**(1), 24–36 (2016)
17. Lamy, J.-B.: Artificial Feeding Birds (AFB): a new metaheuristic inspired by the behavior of pigeons. Advances in Nature-Inspired Computing and Applications, pp. 43–60. Springer, New York (2019)
18. Mirjalili, S.: The ant lion optimizer. Adv. Eng. Softw. **83**, 80–98 (2015)
19. Wolpert, D.H., Macready, W.G.: No free lunch theorems for optimization. IEEE Trans. Evol. Comput. **1**(1), 67–82 (1997)
20. Wang, M.-J., et al.: A load economic dispatch based on ion motion optimization algorithm. Advances in Intelligent Information Hiding and Multimedia Signal Processing, pp. 115–125. Springer, New York (2020)
21. Das, S., Bhattacharya, A., Chakraborty, A.K.: Quasi-reflected ions motion optimization algorithm for short-term hydrothermal scheduling. Neural Comput. Appl. **29**(6), 123–149 (2018)

22. Yang, C.-H., Wu, K.-C., Chuang, L.-Y.: Breast cancer risk prediction using ions motion optimization algorithm. J. Life Sci. Technol. **4**(2), 49–55 (2016)
23. Mohapatra, G., Debnath, M.K., Mohapatra, K.K.: IMO based novel adaptive dual-mode controller design for AGC investigation in different types of systems. Cogent Eng. (just-accepted), 1711675 (2020)
24. Yang, C.-H., et al.: Protein folding prediction in the HP model using ions motion optimization with a greedy algorithm. BioData mining **11**(1), 17 (2018)
25. Fong, S., Deb, S., Chaudhary, A.: A review of metaheuristics in robotics. Comput. Electr. Eng. **43**, 278–291 (2015)
26. Hassan, M., Yousif, A.: Cloud job scheduling with ions motion optimization algorithm. Eng. Technol. Appl. Sci. Res. **10**(2), 5459–5465 (2020)
27. Issa, M., et al.: ASCA-PSO: adaptive sine cosine optimization algorithm integrated with particle swarm for pairwise local sequence alignment. Expert Syst. Appl. **99**, 56–70 (2018)
28. Kamboj, V.K.: A novel hybrid PSO–GWO approach for unit commitment problem. Neural Comput. Appl. **27**(6), 1643–1655 (2016)
29. Zhang, W.-J., Xie, X.-F.: DEPSO: hybrid particle swarm with differential evolution operator. In: SMC'03 Conference Proceedings. 2003 IEEE International Conference on Systems, Man and Cybernetics. Conference Theme-System Security and Assurance (Cat. No. 03CH37483), 2003. IEEE
30. Shen, Q., Shi, W.-M., Kong, W.: Hybrid particle swarm optimization and tabu search approach for selecting genes for tumor classification using gene expression data. Comput. Biol. Chem. **32**(1), 53–60 (2008)
31. Jiang, S., Ji, Z., Shen, Y.: A novel hybrid particle swarm optimization and gravitational search algorithm for solving economic emission load dispatch problems with various practical constraints. Int. J. Electr. Power Energy Syst. **55**, 628–644 (2014)
32. Kaveh, A., Bakhshpoori, T., Afshari, E.: An efficient hybrid particle swarm and swallow swarm optimization algorithm. Comput. Struct. **143**, 40–59 (2014)
33. Abd-Elazim, S., Ali, E.: A hybrid particle swarm optimization and bacterial foraging for optimal power system stabilizers design. Int. J. Electr. Power Energy Syst. **46**, 334–341 (2013)
34. Holden, N., Freitas, A.A.: A hybrid particle swarm/ant colony algorithm for the classification of hierarchical biological data. In: Proceedings 2005 IEEE Swarm Intelligence Symposium, 2005. SIS 2005, 2005. IEEE
35. Pan, T.-S., Dao, T.-K., Chu, S.-C.: Hybrid particle swarm optimization with bat algorithm. Genetic and Evolutionary Computing, pp. 37–47. Springer, New York (2015)
36. Garg, H.: A hybrid PSO-GA algorithm for constrained optimization problems. Appl. Math. Comput. **274**, 292–305 (2016)
37. Smith, T.F., Waterman, M.S.: Identification of common molecular subsequences. J. Mol. Biol. **147**(1), 195–197 (1981)
38. Xiong, J.: Essential Bioinformatics. Cambridge University Press (2006)
39. Di Francesco, V., Garnier, J., Munson, P.: Improving protein secondary structure prediction with aligned homologous sequences. Protein Sci. **5**(1), 106–113 (1996)
40. Feng, D.-F., Doolittle, R.F.: Progressive alignment and phylogenetic tree construction of protein sequences. Methods Enzymol. **183**, 375–387 (1990)
41. Li, L., Khuri, S.: A Comparison of DNA Fragment Assembly Algorithms. in METMBS (2004)
42. Needleman, S.B., Wunsch, C.D.: A general method applicable to the search for similarities in the amino acid sequence of two proteins. J. Mol. Biol. **48**(3), 443–453 (1970)
43. Gotoh, O.: An improved algorithm for matching biological sequences. J. Mol. Biol. **162**(3), 705–708 (1982)
44. Khanna, V., et al.: Estimation of photovoltaic cells model parameters using particle swarm optimization. Physics of Semiconductor Devices, pp. 391–394. Springer, New York (2014)
45. Harrag, A., Daili, Y.: Three-diodes PV model parameters extraction using PSO algorithm. Revue des Energies Renouvelables **22**(1), 85–91 (2019)
46. Ishaque, K., et al.: An improved particle swarm optimization (PSO)–based MPPT for PV with reduced steady-state oscillation. IEEE Trans. Power Electron. **27**(8), 3627–3638 (2012)

47. Hannan, M., et al.: Optimization techniques to enhance the performance of induction motor drives: a review. Renew. Sustain. Energy Rev. (2017)
48. Wang, W., et al.: A universal index and an improved PSO algorithm for optimal pose selection in kinematic calibration of a novel surgical robot. Robot. Comput.-Integr. Manuf. **50**, 90–101 (2018)

Intelligent Monitoring System to Aid in the Proactive and Early Detection of People Infected by COVID-19

Saad Chakkor, Mostafa Baghouri, Ahmed El Oualkadi, Jalil Abdelkader El Hangouche, Jawhar Laamech, and Rachid Belfkih

Abstract In this research work, automated detection and a remote monitoring system for COVID-19 are suggested for use. This later is made up of a centralized network of intelligent communicating portable electronic devices based on biomedical sensors operating in IoT context in synergy with the wireless sensor network, telemedicine, and artificial intelligence technologies. The purpose of this system is the monitoring, detection, and early diagnosis of the COVID-19 disease in a population settling in a target area (city, region, country, etc.). This is done using an electronic device worn by each person (such as a bracelet or a chest strap). In fact, the designed device collects, in real-time, all the necessary biomedical measurements of a person, including their location, freeing them from any hospitalization or use of complex and expensive equipment. These informations are then transmitted, via a wireless connection, to the supervision center which takes care of its storage in a specialized database. This center processes the collected data for each person by

---

S. Chakkor (✉) · A. El Oualkadi
LabTIC, ENSA of Tangier, University of Abdelmalek Essaâdi, Route de Ziaten Km 10, Tanger Principale, Tangier B.P: 1818, Morocco
e-mail: s.chakkor@uae.ac.ma

A. El Oualkadi
e-mail: aeloualkadi@uae.ac.ma

M. Baghouri
Modeling and Control of Industrial Systems Team, Structural Engineering, Intelligent Systems and Electrical Energy Laboratory, ENSAM of Casablanca, University of Hassan II, Hassan, Morocco
e-mail: baghouri.mostafa@gmail.com

J. A. El Hangouche · J. Laamech
Faculty of Medecine and Pharmacy of Tangier, Laboratory of Physiology, B.P: 81, Route de Rabat, Km 15, Gzenaya, Tangier, Morocco
e-mail: elhangouche.jalil@gmail.com

J. Laamech
e-mail: j.laamech@uae.ac.ma

R. Belfkih
Department of Neurology, University Hospital Center of Tangier, Faculty of Medicine and Pharmacy of Tangier, Tetouan, Al Hoceima, Morocco
e-mail: belfkih.chutanger@gmail.com

D. Oliva et al. (eds.), *Artificial Intelligence for COVID-19*, Studies in Systems, Decision and Control 358, https://doi.org/10.1007/978-3-030-69744-0_22

running a decision-making algorithm using artificial intelligence and a fuzzy inference engine to detect accurately each possible abnormal change in the supervised quantities reflecting risk factors or indicating the appearance of symptoms characterizing COVID-19 disease. In this case, the control system triggers a warning alarm concerning this infected person and requests the intervention of the competent authorities to take the necessary measures and actions. Computer simulations with Matlab software and experimental test prove the satisfactory performance of the proposed system. Study findings show that the designed device is suitable for application in COVID-19 patient monitoring.

Keywords COVID-19 disease · Monitoring · E-health · Artificial intelligence · Embedded system · IoT · E-diagnosis · Decision algorithm · Fuzzy logic · Arduino · Wireless network · Cloud database

1 Introduction

This subject is in keeping with the critical and unparalleled circumstances facing the whole world and our country caused by the remarkable and rapid proliferation of COVID-19 declared as a pandemic of the global scope by the World Organization for Health (WHO). The latter urged government authorities to take preventive directives, measures, and recommendations aimed at fighting this pandemic. However, these procedures remain limited to fight effectively against this fatal disease especially given the long time taken for radiological and biological analyzes to confirm a suspected case. In this regard, some researchers have proposed techniques for monitoring infected people based on their geolocation maps extracted from the mobile networks to which their smartphones are connected. This is done in order not to share with these patients any locations they have visited, the objects they have touched and the paths they have taken. Other researchers have proposed applications on smartphones using Bluetooth wireless technology to ensure social separation between infected and uninfected people [1]. Indeed, the Moroccan authorities have developed a free application « Wiqaytna » [2], to be downloaded from Google Play or Apple store, which makes possible to follow contacts of people positive for the coronavirus in order to fight effectively against the spread of the virus. In fact, the notifications sent by « Wiqaytna » will allow rapid treatment of the infected person. This will help avoid complications and thus relieve the health system, but also limit contamination and therefore, reduce the circulation of the virus. It saves lives. Moreover, some researchers have leaned towards the development of an Artificial Intelligence audio smartphone application to aid in the early detection of COVID-19 from accurate discrimination between coughs of a potentially infected patient, and a normal cough [3–6]. This allows reducing the time required for the diagnosis of COVID-19. Furthermore, other researchers have used Deep Learning techniques to classify suspected cases based on COVID-19 X-Ray and CT Chest Images Dataset [7].

However, the first drawback of these techniques is that they assume that the person being monitored has a smartphone terminal connected to the internet and activating the GPS service. In addition, the second disadvantage is that the technique will only focus on the location of this person when it will be declared by the health authorities as being infected by the virus, and during this period the contamination risks increase greatly because this person remains out of control in front of an epidemic which spreads at a faster speed which follows an exponential law. Thirdly, note that infection with this disease is not always accompanied by dry cough because clinical medical studies have shown that there is a group of infected people who do not show symptoms of the disease. Figure 1 shows an estimation of coronavirus COVID-19 epidemic evaluation in Africa using the SIR model.

We observe that the trajectory of the COVID-19 pandemic begins with a phase of regular growth passing through a peak then ends with a final phase of gradual disappearance. Whereas, Fig. 2 illustrates the evolution statistics of the COVID-19 pandemic in Morocco.

Hence, there is an urgent need for a match between precautionary measures, examination, follow-up, and the search for other techniques to allow the flattening of the COVID-19 infection curve as shown in Fig. 3.

All in the absence of a medication or a vaccine that will permanently eliminate the virus which does not give us enough time to react when it contaminates our bodies. Certainly, this contribution is a challenge that responds to calls launched by governments, scientific organizations in order to propose and to develop solutions, tools, and methods based on research work allowing not only to minimize any danger

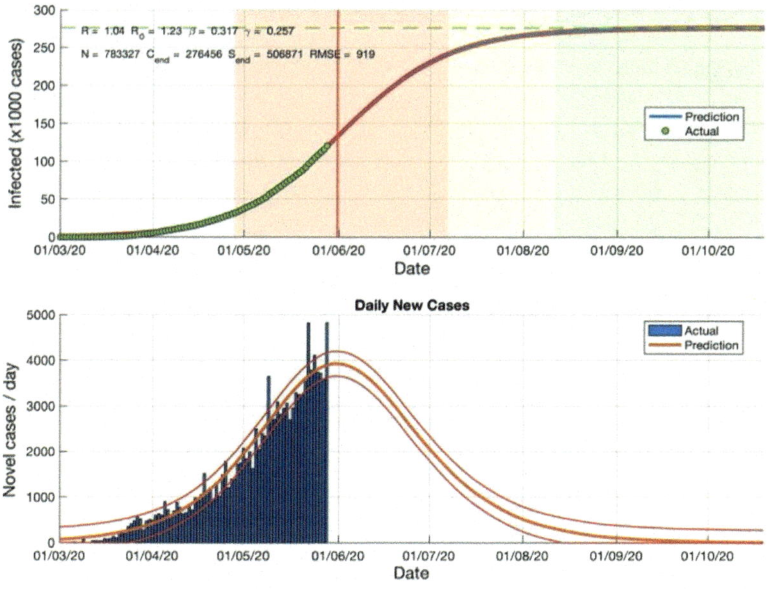

Fig. 1 Predicted and actual cases of COVID-19 (SIR model as of 28 May 2020 in Africa)

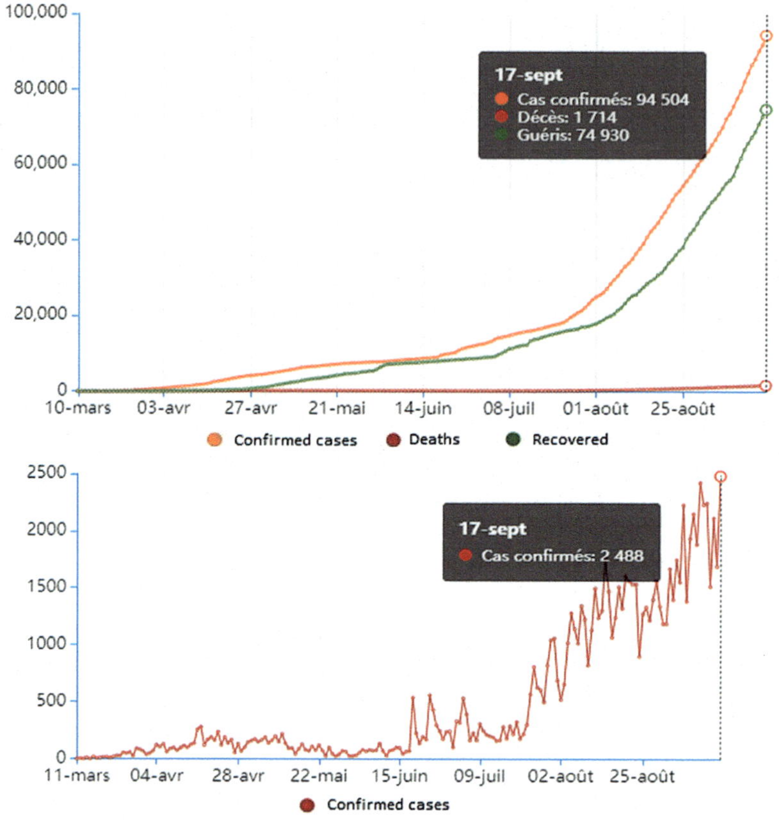

Fig. 2 Contamination curve of coronavirus COVID-19 epidemic in Morocco

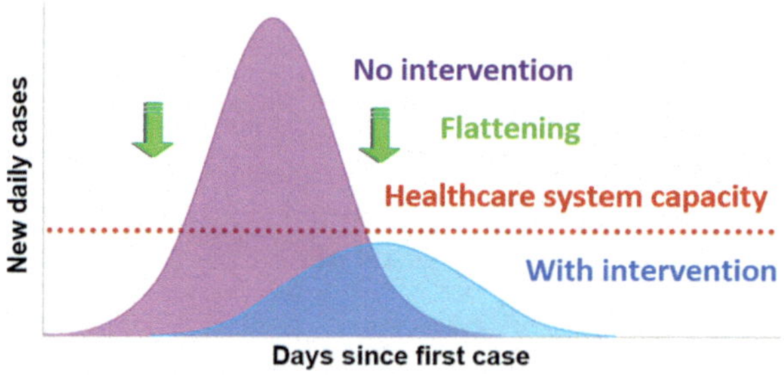

Fig. 3 Theoretical evolutions of an epidemic depending on the implementation, or not, of preventive measures

associated with this virus spread but also stop its span. The contribution of this proposal concerns the procedural side and not the therapeutic one, because it makes it possible to surround and reduce the rate of the virus spread.

2 Proposed Monitoring System and Network

The contribution of this proposal concerns the procedural side and not the therapeutic one, because it makes it possible to surround and reduce the rate of the virus spread. The suggested supervision system is a remote-control system made up of a centralized network of communicating and portable electronic devices based on smart sensors operating in the IoT context in synergy with wireless sensor network technologies, telemedicine (E-health), data mining, and artificial intelligence. Figure 4 illustrates the monitoring and control system architecture.

This system consists mainly of the following parts:

(1) Sensors for collecting the necessary biomedical measurements;
(2) Processing unit board which is an Arduino board;
(3) Wireless communication module;
(4) Remote monitoring center containing a server that manages a database (Big Data) and an intelligent decision-making algorithm;
(5) Power source: battery;

This network will be deployed to monitor a population settling in a target area (cities, regions, countries, etc.). The objective of this system lies in the detection and early diagnosis of the disease in people infected with the COVID-19 virus using a

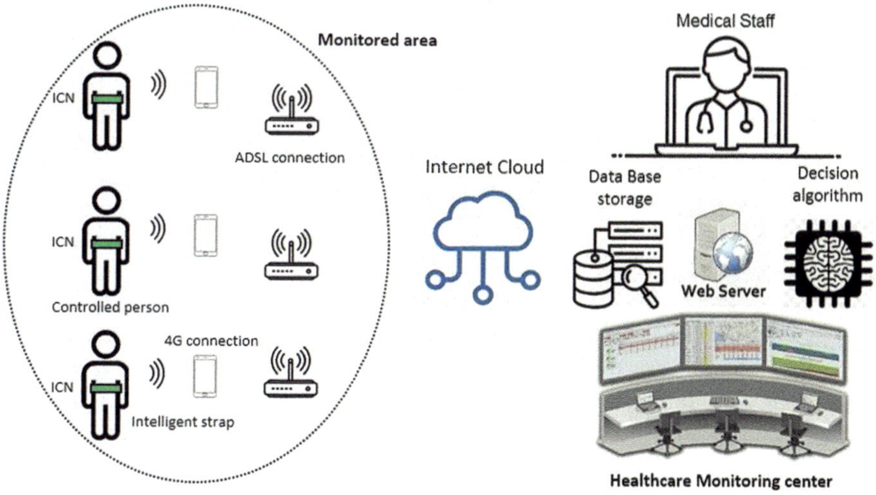

Fig. 4 Block diagram of the proposed monitoring system

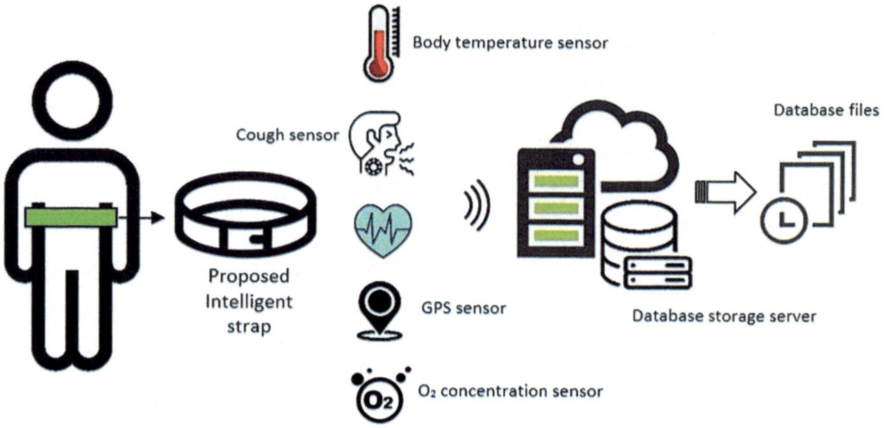

Fig. 5 Proposed healthcare control system architecture

device presented (in the form of a bracelet or strap) which will be distributed by local authorities and which will imperatively be worn by every citizen over the age of 14 years old (by law such as the protective mask) throughout the period of health emergencies. Figure 5 describes the components of the system.

The position of the electronic strap on the human chest is chosen carefully because this location offers a sampling of biomedical measurements with more precision compared to the other positions especially the sound acquisition by the mini microphone implemented on the Arduino Nano 33 BLE Sense board (which will be closer to the mouth which is the source of the cough) and the measurement of body temperature [8–11]. This healthcare application needs to acquire different types of sensor data [12]. This sensitive and valuable data must be collected in a precise and timely manner to avoid any possible loss in their transmission to the cloud database. Besides, the proposed system has other advantages. It is also used to remotely monitor the health state of the heart system of COVID-19 patients who follow the therapeutic protocol (Chloroquine, Azithromycin) knowing that these drugs cause sometimes undesirable side effects. This allows, on the one hand, minimizing the infection risk for the medical staff who will be in direct contact with these patients. On the other hand, this system offers the possibility of following these patients to their homes if their condition is not serious or critical and does not require resuscitation or artificial respiration. This frees up their hospital spaces for others with higher priority. Faced with the situation of total saturation of hospitals, the use of this system constitutes a good alternative. In addition, this system remains an effective and usable telemedicine tool even after the period of COVID-19, because it facilitates (by adding a few features) the follow-up and medical control of patients (who are in far and difficult rural areas.) with chronic diseases such as diabetes, cardiovascular diseases, diseases of high blood pressure. This intelligent device collects in real-time all necessary biomedical measurements of a person, including their location, freeing them from hospitalization and the use of complex and expensive equipment.

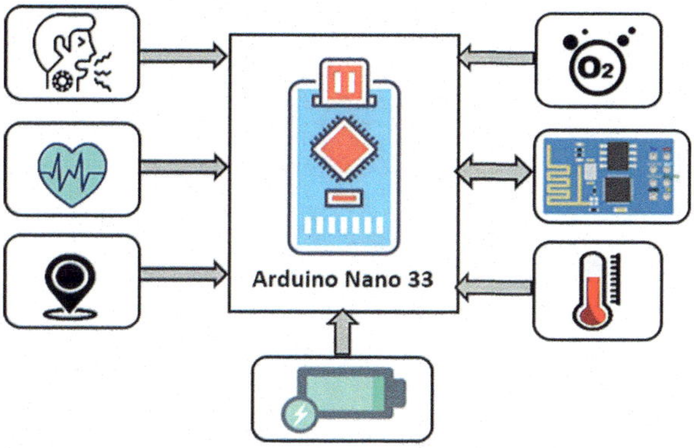

Fig. 6 Functional diagram of proposed strap

Each person will be recognized by the device and surveillance system through their national identity card number (ICN). The device transmits these informations via a wireless connection (using a gateway or an access point: Wi-Fi router or smart terminal offering a 4G internet connection) to the regional or national control center. This latter takes care, via a server (local, Big DATA or Cloud) using a Wi-Fi module connected to the internet, of the reception of all these data, their management, and their display (periodic storage of these data in a specialized database as the form of a daily files). The data were sent to a PHP script with GET method which were then translated onto the Web Page as values, graphs, and status conditions. The design diagram of this device is given in the following Fig. 6. In fact, the sensors are interconnected with an Arduino Nano 33 BLE Sense board combined to ESP8266 Wi-Fi module forming a miniature electronic circuit that facilitates wearing and portability of the suggested strap.

Furthermore, collected data is accessed either through the internet using a Web browser or either mobile application. Indeed, this device offers the possibility of connecting a smartphone to display, in real-time, collected data on its screen as shown in Fig. 7.

In addition, the supervision center displays the collected and saved measurements for each person on an interface as evolution curves form. It also processes them by running a decision-making algorithm using artificial intelligence (artificial neural networks, machine learning algorithms for real-time classification, and fuzzy inference engine for decision-making) to detect and recognizes in a precise manner each possible abnormal change in the supervised quantities reflecting risk factors or indicating the appearance of symptoms characterizing the COVID-19 disease. In this case, the control system triggers a warning alarm concerning this person and requests the intervention of the competent authorities to take the necessary measures and intervention actions (examination of the patient at home using the SpO_2 sensor for confirmation of his state of illness at the basis of which he will be hospitalized). The sensors used by the proposed device comply with the medical diagnosis

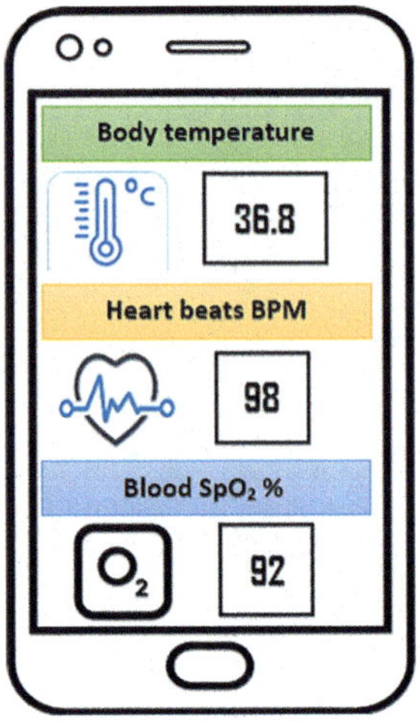

Fig. 7 Screen of mobile application

of COVID-19 disease symptoms which were determined by WHO [14–19]. The electronic device to be designed consists of the following units.

2.1 Arduino Nano 33 BLE Sense

The motherboard of the proposed strap is Arduino Nano 33 BLE Sense [9] shown in Fig. 8. It is a new board integrating a series of embedded sensors like a microphone: to capture and analyses sound in real-time, etc., and featuring a lot more powerful processor which includes other features like ultra-low power consumption modes.

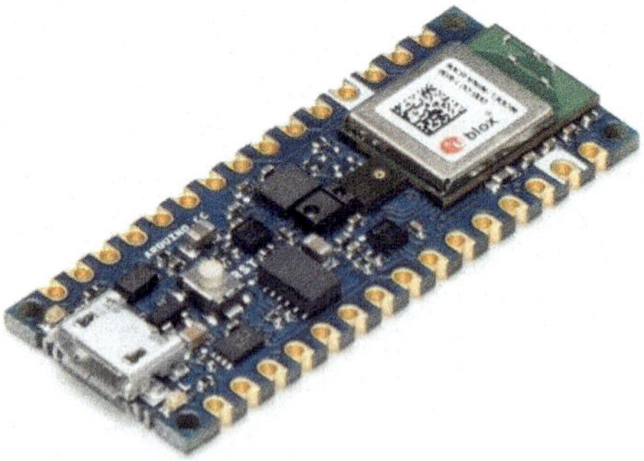

Fig. 8 Arduino Nano 33 BLE Sense board

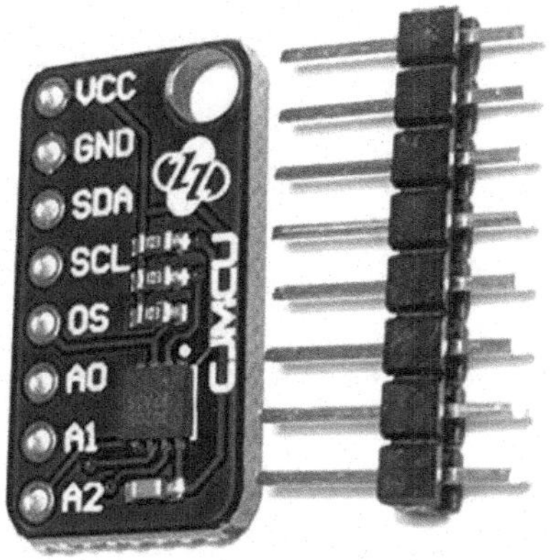

Fig. 9 MAX30205MTA body temperature sensor

The main feature of this board is the possibility of running Edge Computing applications (AI) on it using TinyML [10]. It allows create machine learning models using TensorFlow™ Lite and upload them to this board using the Arduino IDE.

2.2 *Body Temperature Sensor*

The body temperature information is collected using a specific sensor: Taidacent MAX30205MTA [11], shown in Fig. 9, which is a wearable human body temperature sensor that accurately measures temperature and provides an overtemperature alarm/interrupt/shutdown output. This sensor reads with an accuracy of "± 0.1 °C". It allows low-voltage operation which aids designers in meeting error and power budgets ("2.7 V" to "3.3 V" supply voltage range, low "600μA" supply current). This device converts the temperature measurements to digital form using a high resolution, sigma-delta, analog-to-digital converter (ADC). This sensor is available in an 8-pin TDFN package and operates over the "0°C" to "+50°C" temperature range.

2.3 *Cough Sensor*

The cough sensor is made by a cough detection system on Arduino Nano BLE Sense using TinyML and Edge Impulse [12]. Its objective is to sense the presence of coughing in real-time audio captured by a small built-in microphone on the Arduino Nano 33 board. To build accurately a cough training model, we must verify the following steps detailed in Fig. 10. The training phase is based on several datasets characterizing the cough related to COVID-19 [3–5].

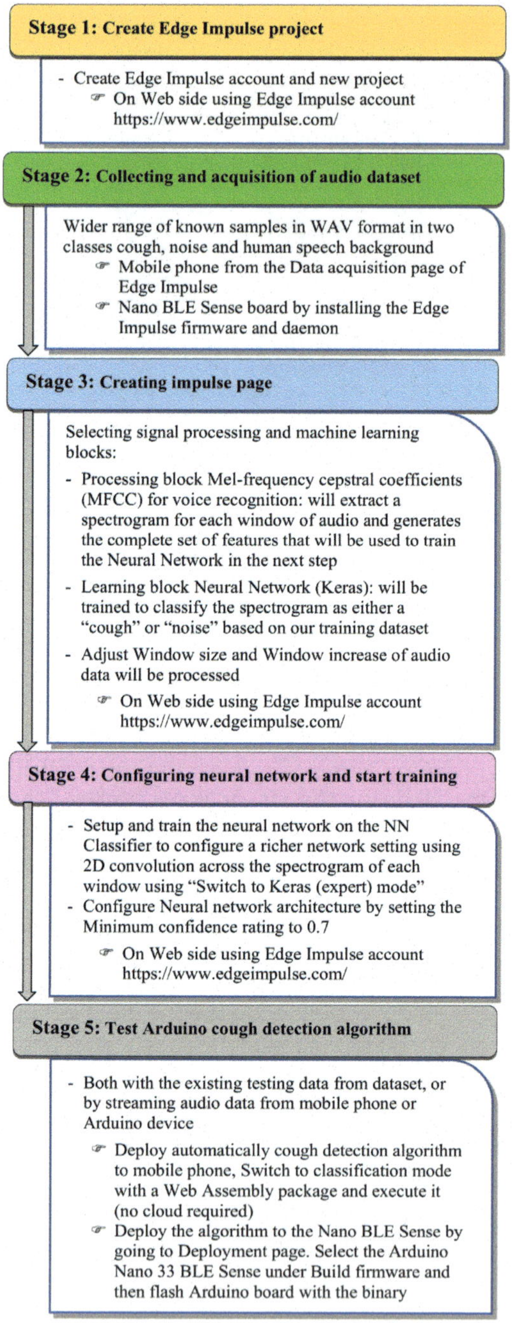

Fig. 10 Different stages for cough sensor training and testing

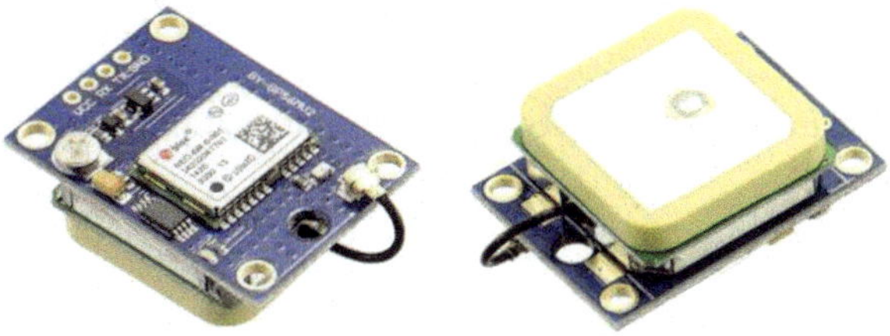

Fig. 11 GPS Neo-6 M module

2.4 GPS Location Sensor

The positioning device used in this medical strap is GPS Neo-6 M as illustrated in Fig. 11. It has a power supply range from "3.3 V" to "5 V". It collects all GPS data by satellites (longitude, latitude, date and time, speed of movement). The position of the antenna mounting is very crucial for the optimal performance of the GPS receiver. When using the patch antenna, it should be oriented parallel to the geographic horizon. The antenna must have a full view of the sky, ensuring a direct line of sight with as many visible satellites as possible.

For start using this module with Arduino Nano 33 BLE Sense, it is needed to download and install the "TinyGPS ++" library.

2.5 Heart Rate Variability Sensor

To collect live heart-rate data into our project with high sensitivity, we have using the MAX30102 pulse oximeter and a heart-rate sensor for wearable health appearing in Fig. 12. It is integrated pulse oximetry and heart-rate monitor module [20]. It is capable of recording heart rate and heart rate variability (HRV), and it can be plugged directly into the Arduino board. It has contact with your skin. This sensor uses PPG

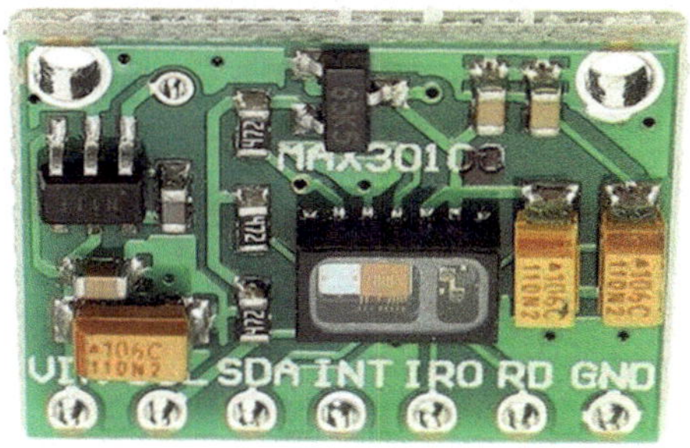

Fig. 12 MAX30102 heart rate pulse and oxygen saturation breakout sensor

(Photo Plethysmo Graphy) techniques [21]. This is a simple and low-cost optical technique that can be used to detect blood volume changes in the microvascular bed of tissues. It is relatively easy to detect the pulsatile component of the cardiac cycle according to this theory.

2.6 Arterial Oxygen Saturation Sensor

To measure arterial oxygen saturation (SpO_2), the above MAX30102 sensor module is used. The signal obtained from the pulse oximeter is known as the (PPG) waveform which shows the blood flow at the extremities [20, 21]. It should be noted that these pulse oximeters should be resistant to motion.

2.7 Radio Frequency Communication Module

We have chosen the Wi-Fi module ESP8266-ESP-01, illustrated in Fig. 13, as a circuit for a radio frequency communication circuit because it allows connecingt of any microcontroller (as long as it has a UART Rx/Tx) to a Wi-Fi network for a very low cost. It is a smaller module with fewer pins 8. It is supplied with 3.3 V and not 5 V. It offers low consumption of electrical energy.

3 Fuzzy Decision Algorithm for Covid-19 Diagnosis

In healthcare monitoring, we must consider the relationship between its input signals and its status indications. In most diseases, which have predictable symptoms or specific signs during their development, detection, and interpretation, only simple

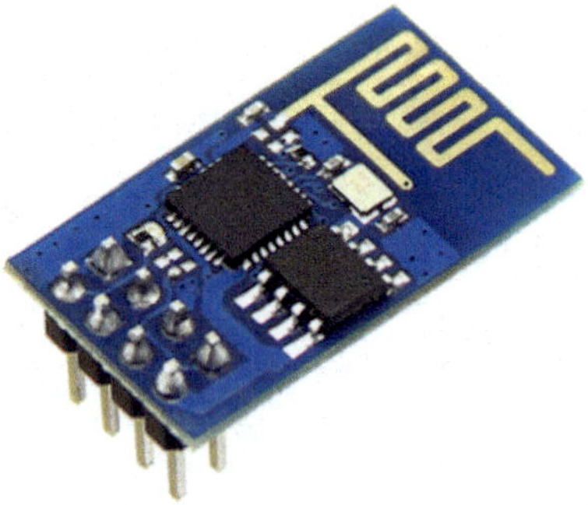

Fig. 13 ESP8266-ESP-01 Wi-Fi module

sensors are required. Contrariwise, the classification and diagnosis of the state of such illness and the determination of the severity evolution of its possible symptoms from its input signals are not an easy task, because they are affected by many factors. In front of this situation, the recourse to the computerized systems using artificial intelligence that mimicking human intelligence is necessary. In fact, fuzzy logic comes to formalize empirical methods, to generalize natural reasoning modes, to automate decision-making in their field, and to build artificial systems capable of performing the tasks usually taken care of by humans. The fuzzy approach allows meeting the requirements of a certain number of biomedical systems which are strongly nonlinear, complex, and difficult to monitor and diagnose automatically. This difficulty arises from:

- their non-linearity,
- the variation of their parameters,
- the quality of the measurable variables.

These difficulties have led to the advent and development of new fuzzy control and diagnostic techniques as long as there is no precise mathematical model of the process to be monitored which presents strong non-linearities or inaccuracies. In particular, the fuzzy control methodology appears useful when the processes are very complex to analyze by conventional techniques.

Fuzzy algorithms can indicate the precise health state of the patient by putting different probabilities of radical causes resulting in observed symptoms. They allow also making diagnoses and taking swift and consistent decisions. However, this requires a certain amount of knowledge and expertise on the relationship between the patient's health condition and its illness symptoms. The application of fuzzy logic offers very significant flexibility in making decisions compared to other methods. This logic allows reasoning from inaccurate input data to generate output results approximately or gradually uncertain [22, 23]. The use of this technique in our proposed diagnosis approach decision-making of COVID-19 detection is justified by the difficulty to make an explicit mathematical model or an analytical formulation of the decision especially when many inputs are used. So, it is possible to use an empirical model based on rules derived from human expertise in telemedicine and cardiology which can be incorporated. Determinant information can be exploited using fuzzy inference systems FIS to increase confidence and accuracy of diagnosis results.

3.1 Fuzzy Diagnosis Steps

The surveillance suggested to be applied in this work, based on fuzzy logic, proves to be more effective than traditional methods for several reasons: traditional medical diagnosis systems are not automated and having numerous continuous or discontinuous Inputs/Outputs and nonlinear responses which makes their modeling difficult or even impossible. Furthermore, for such systems, there are classes with poorly

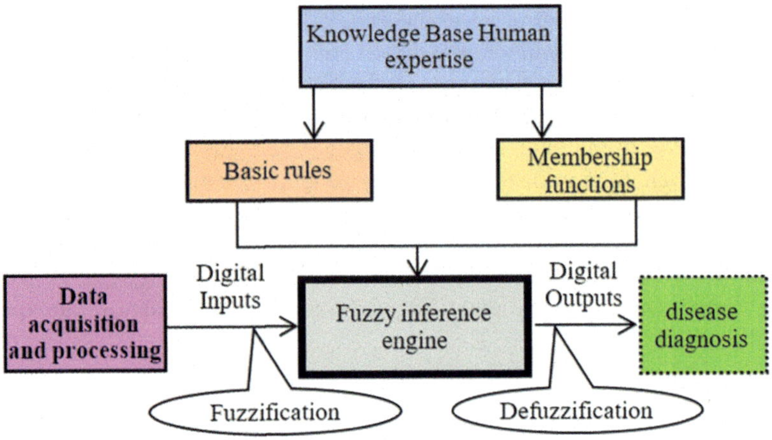

Fig. 14 Fuzzy classification block diagram

defined boundaries, whose confines cannot be specified precisely, or poorly separated categories that partially overlap. It is therefore possible to use fuzzy logic for classification, regression, and even extrapolation. The fuzzy rules and the functional steps of the proposed approach are applied under the following assumptions:

- The physical process is controllable;
- The existence of human expertise, qualitative and gradual;
- The inputs and outputs are measurable or observable quantities;

Figure 14 summarizes the fuzzy rules used in our approach. The fuzzification operation associates to each scalar value of real domain, one or more linguistic variables of the fuzzy area. This step involves evaluating the membership functions used in predicate rules. Whereas, the defuzzification combines the conclusion results of aggregation rules to infer the actual output value.

3.2 Proposed Approach

In our approach, the system contains various sensors, which measure some physical properties of a human body. Diagnosis is performed by studying several parameters of a human body known as symptoms and several symptoms are verified one after another before obtaining a deduction about a specific disease. In the diagnosis mode, the input signal, which is the sensor's signal in our case, is analyzed against any suspected signature or change. This later is previously obtained in the learning mode. The proposed algorithm generates decisions about disease diagnosis and patient health conditions by considering various fuzzy criteria and assumptions. We have suggested improving the diagnosis system by integration of a FIS because it seems necessary to make a decision without excessive loss of accuracy. This is justified by

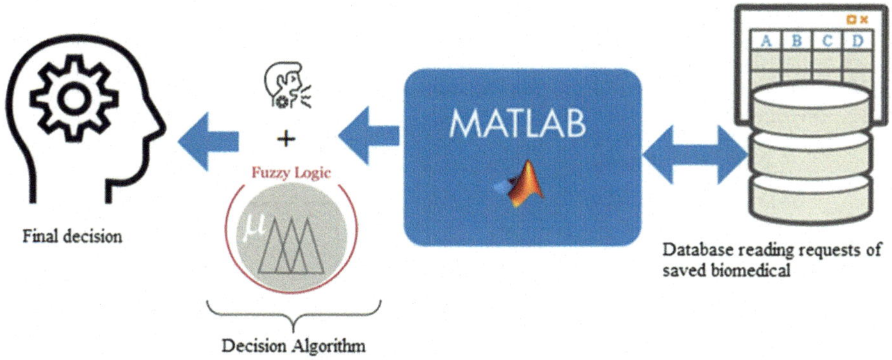

Fig. 15 Steps of final diagnosis decision

the benefits and capabilities that provide a FIS. The proposed diagnosis approach combines two techniques: intelligent cough detection and fuzzy classification of biomedical measurements. It contains multiple steps that must be executed to reach the final decision of diagnosis as shown in Fig. 15.

Initially, collecting, acquisition, and storage of the different sensor signals are carried out. Afterward, intelligent cough detection is applied to recognize the percentage of cough quantification. From the stored patient data in the cloud database and connecting MySQL database to Matlab using Database toolbox, knowledge is retrieved by matching the symptoms and their severity against the antecedent part of fuzzy rules. In the knowledge base, to make the decision as a disease name or a risk of the disease. The fuzzy decision value is defuzzified by the defuzzification component of the designed system to finally arrive at an accurate decision for the disease diagnosis.

4 Fuzzy Inference System

To evaluate the performance satisfaction of our proposed medical diagnosis system, an intelligent decision algorithm has been simulated with Matlab Fuzzy Logic toolbox. The employed FIS uses four inputs and generates a single output each having three different membership levels. The input variables considered are cough percentage, blood oxygen (SpO_2), body temperature, heart rate. Membership values are assigned to linguistic variables such as symptoms. Whereas, the output variable Risk-alarm shows the percentage of risk for the COVID-19 disease detection following the measured values of input parameters reflecting COVID-19 symptoms quantification. In Fig. 16, a detailed architecture description of this system is presented with Matlab software.

Moreover, in Table 1, the parameters and the methods used in this fuzzy inference system are illustrated. The selection of the trapezoidal membership functions for the

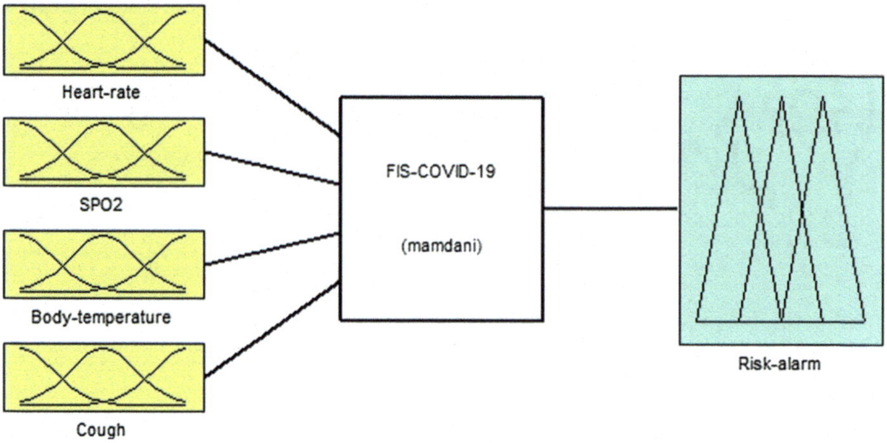

Fig. 16 Fuzzy inference system architecture

Table 1 FIS parameters

Parameter	Value
Fuzzy rules type	Mamdani
Input number	4
Output number	1
Rules number	63
AND Method	Min
OR Method	Max
Implication Method	Min
Aggregation Method	Max
Defuzzification Method	Centroid

fuzzy input variables is made by respecting the medicine expert doctors' instructions based on their statistical studies realized practically. This choice is also justified by the adaptation of these functions to the real numerical values needed in the diagnosis, in addition to their simplicity and their calculation rapidity of the membership value.

The selection of the following membership functions positions and theirs overlaps must respect certain rules to avoid indeterminate or dead zones and to avert problems of the controller instability or the flattening of the decision surface.

Figure 17, illustrates one input membership functions of the health parameters: Heart rate.

Bradycardia is a slower than normal heart rate. The hearts of adults at rest usually beat between 60 and 100 times a minute. In the bradycardia case, the heart beats fewer than 60 times a minute. Bradycardia can be a serious problem if the heart does not pump enough oxygen-rich blood to the body. Tachycardia is the medical term for

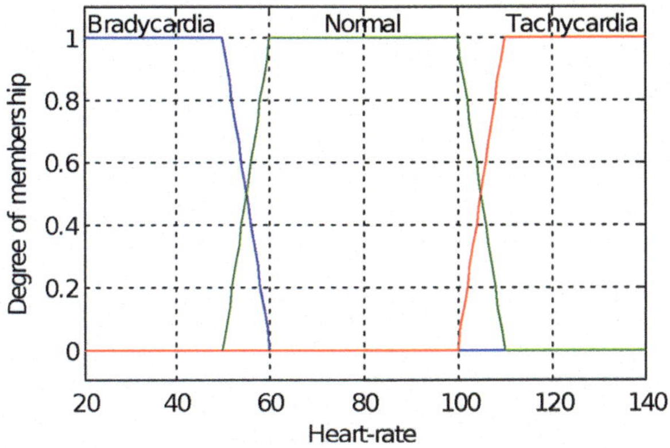

Fig. 17 Membership functions of the input1 fuzzy set

a heart rate of over 100 beats per minute. In tachycardia, the heart beats faster than normal due to conditions unrelated to normal physiological stress. Figure 18, shows the input membership functions of the oxygen percentage in the blood (SpO_2).

Hypoxemia can present due to impaired respiratory functions caused by COVID-19 viral load. Some patients do not necessarily have impaired oxygenation functions at the onset of infection but may manifest rapid deterioration in oxygenation over time. Therefore, continual monitoring of oxygen saturation is recommended. Oxygen therapy is not necessary for patients with oxygen saturation (SpO_2) of more than 93% or patients without obvious symptoms of respiratory distress. However, when oxygen saturation (SpO_2) drops below 88%, this indicates pulmonary respiratory failure [20, 21]. The membership functions for body temperature are shown in Fig. 19.

The initial presentation of the fever in COVID-19 in the first week, during the viral phase of this illness, is likely a manifestation of the body's immune response to

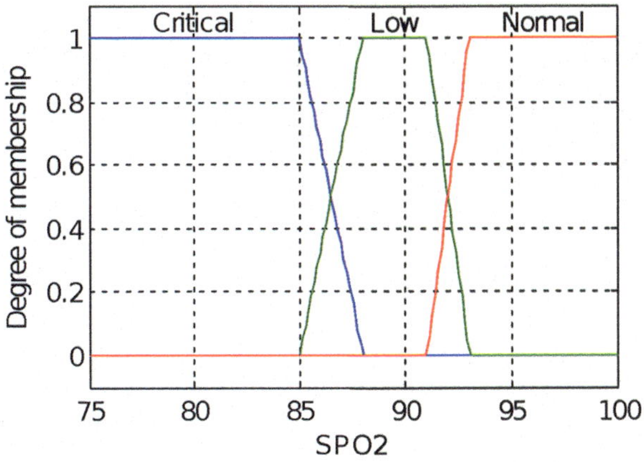

Fig. 18 Membership functions of the input2 fuzzy set

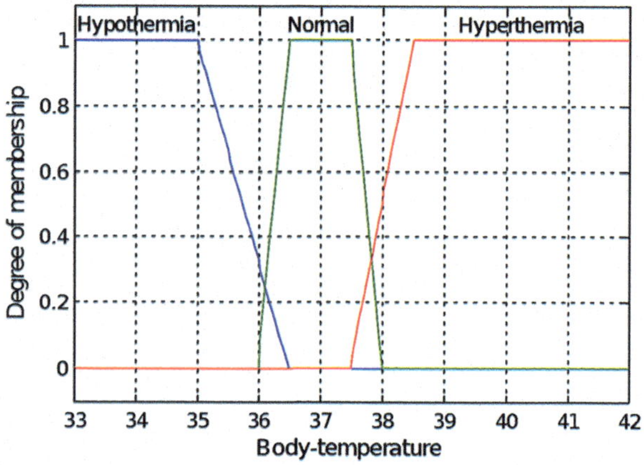

Fig. 19 Membership functions of the input3 fuzzy set

the viral replication to augment immunity. However, if the viral infection does not resolve in due course, the disease process is complicated by the viral triggered state of dysregulated inflammation described as cytokine storm heralded by unremitting fever. Body temperature remains a relevant indicator of changes in COVID-19 viral load in a patient's body. Normal body temperature is 37 °C but it may vary during the daytime, so a range between 36.5 and 37.5 °C is considered as normal body temperature. Figure 20 presents the membership functions of a patient's cough.

Coughing is a defining symptom of COVID-19. It is also a factor that determines transmission risk because the patient can spread infectious droplets to people around him, usually 5–10 days after being infected.

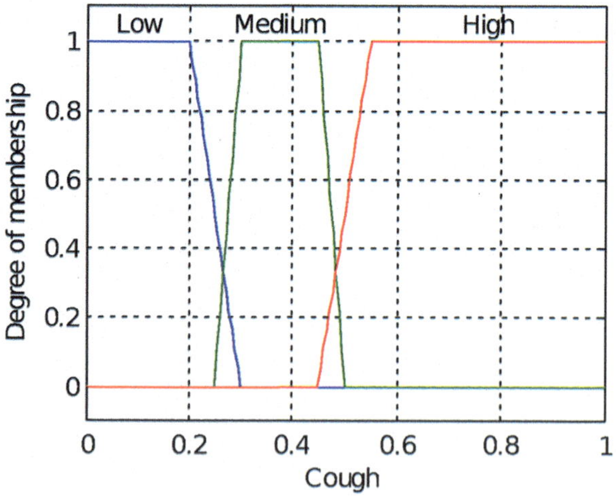

Fig. 20 Membership functions of the input4 fuzzy set

5 Fuzzy Rules and System Output

In this smart system, more than sixty fuzzy rules IF-THEN relating to symptoms of COVID-19 disease are formed. The rules are formulated using Matlab Fuzzy Toolbox editor. Effectively, the output from the FIS is used to detect if the risk detection of COVID-19 is Low, Medium, or High with, a well-quantified percentage, based on the submitted input parameters values. Depending on this fuzzy output, the actions and alerts are generated to alert the competent authorities and medical specialists by the obligation to intervene to examine each suspected case. The fuzzy expert system computes the probabilities and determines the output value in terms of the percentage of the risk alarm. Decisions are described through the output membership functions that are illustrated in Fig. 21. These functions determine whether the alert will be engendered or normal monitoring is sufficient.

The used IF-THEN rules are presented in Fig. 22. They can analyze all possible situations and generate accordingly the accurate output. In addition, to explain how these rules have been constituted and how does a rule work and execute, a set of sample rules is presented in Fig. 23. Rule 51 is described below. When the temperature sensor reads a Hyperthermia body temperature, and the MAX30102 sensor reads both Tachycardia and Low SPO_2 and the cough sensor detects a High cough level, it is indicated that the patient is contaminated by COVID-19 with a High level of Risk alarm equal to 79%.

To produce the Risk alarm, the FIS system passes through the defuzzification phase using the fuzzy centroid or gravity center technique and the Mamdani method. Indeed, the final decision, which is the FIS output, is equal to the gravity center abscissa of the resulting membership function surface. This later characterizes the fuzzy set formed after the aggregation of all conclusions. Therefore, the resulting membership function of the output variable is converted into digital quantity.

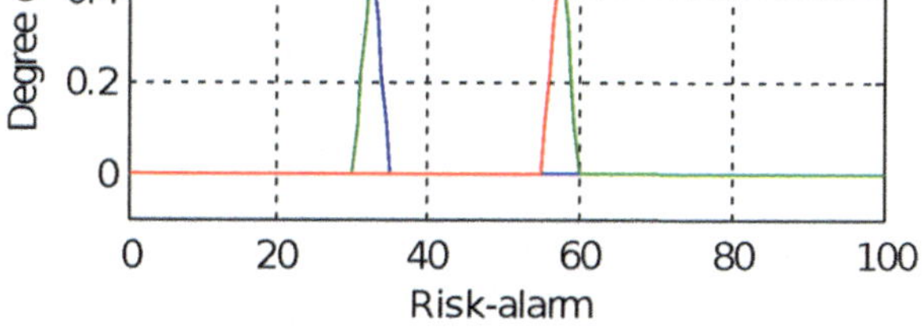

Fig. 21 Membership functions of the output fuzzy set

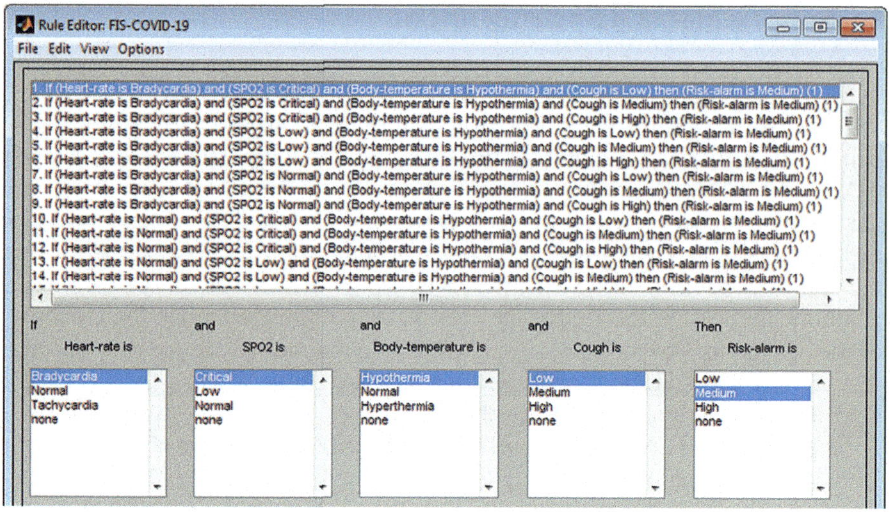

Fig. 22 COVID-19 FIS IF-THEN rules

In Figs. 24 and 25, the surface decisions are illustrated. It depends on each variable used in the employed FIS. It is observed that these decisions are in discontinuities, non-linear, flexible, and reflect human expertise in medical diagnosis.

In the event that the system generates a high-level alarm concerning a person infected with COVID-19, this system will search and identify, according to the GPS location coordinates saved in the cloud database, all the contact persons or all the people who are located close (within a radius of 5 m) of this infected and detected person. The system sends then alerts to the medical staff of the obligation to submit these people to a clinical examination and analysis. The algorithm of this search is illustrated in Fig. 26.

The proposed device makes it possible to maintain the social distancing of 1.5 m between people because it uses the Bluetooth technology with which the Arduino nano 33 BLE sense board is fitted to detect people in this neighborhood radius and trigger a beep sound alarm warning its wearer to not approach another person wearing a similar device as shown in Fig. 27.

Table 2 summarizes the meaning of each Risk-alarm level, the operating mode of the monitoring staff, and the procedure that has been associated facing the generation of each alarm level.

This intelligent supervision system offers another functionality using Big Data and Data mining techniques. In truth, it allows drawing automatically an accurate epidemiological map, following the statistics directly by regions, cities, and streets and classifying them into three groups: A high-risk geographical group that is likely to know a large increase in infected cases, which will require the authorities to take strict measures. A geographical group that exists in an unstable epidemiological situation with a fluctuating trend in daily-infected cases, which requires the authorities to maintain partial containment measures. A geographical group that is in a stable

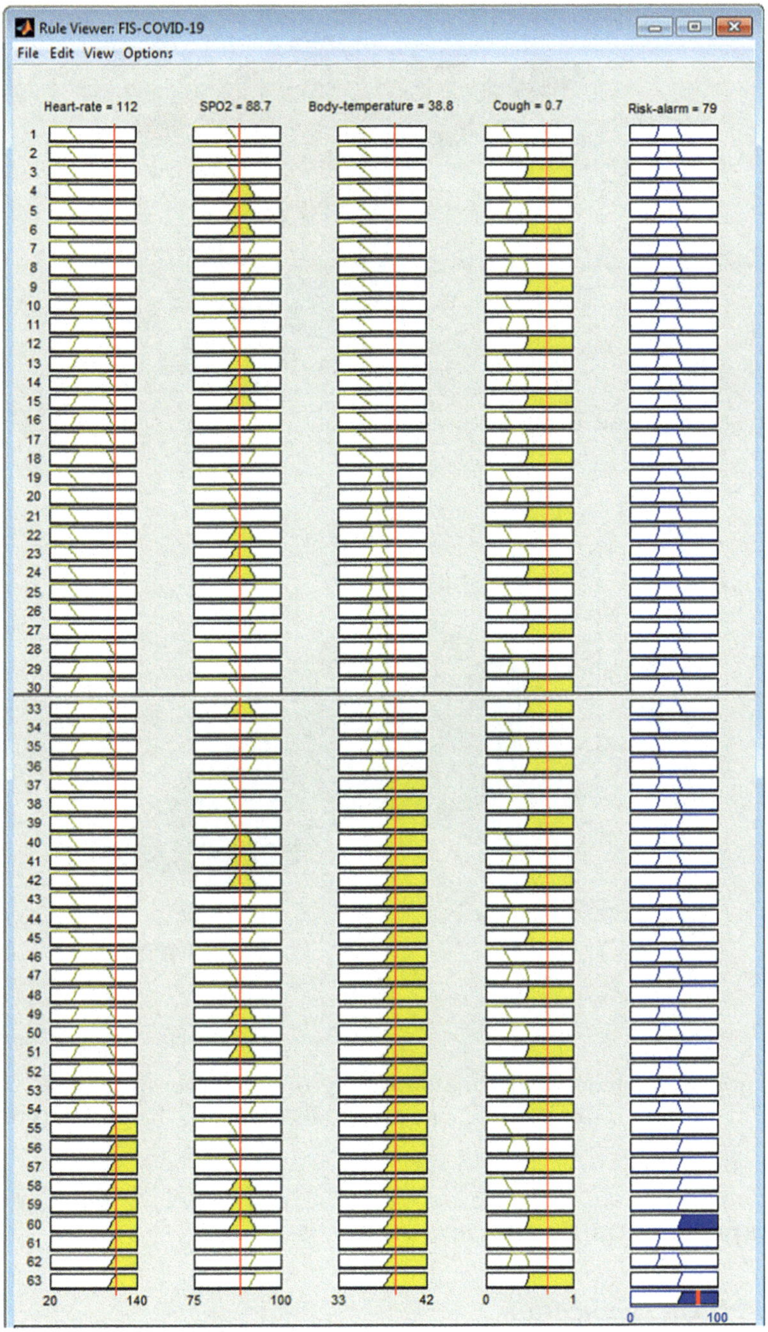

Fig. 23 Risk-alarm output determination

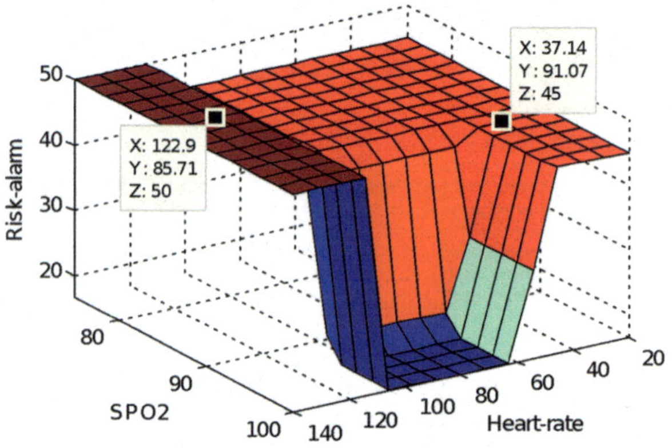

Fig. 24 SPO_2 and Heart rate versus Risk-alarm output

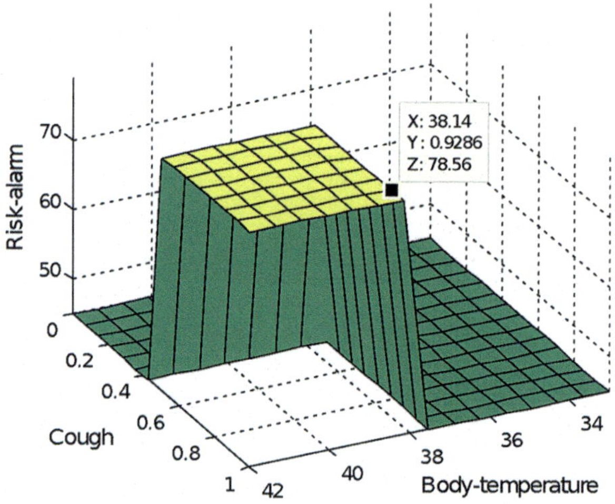

Fig. 25 Cough and Body temperature versus Risk-alarm output

epidemiological situation with the possibility of comprehensive control over the spread of the virus if self-protection measures, distancing and barriers are preserved.

6 Experimental Results and Analysis

6.1 System Application

All the communications between devices and the monitoring server are implemented through the application interface. A special application was designed and

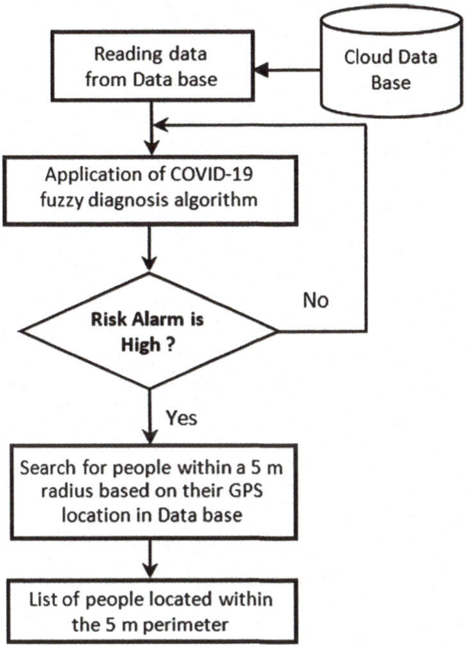

Fig. 26 Searching nearby people algorithm

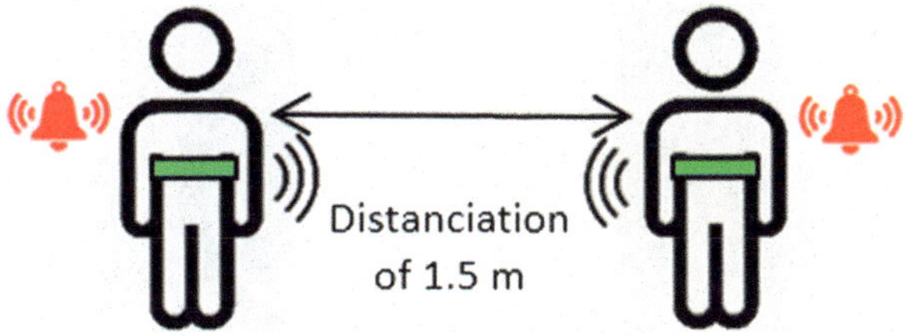

Fig. 27 Social distancing by Bluetooth technology

successfully ran for this particular purpose. This system's interface is the front-end control and monitoring platform used by system operators. It includes many different displays that allow system administrators to add, edit, and view patient information in the system. Figure 28 is displayed the Home page of the application. It is important to store some basic patients' personal information, which will be further used in the data processing part. Once the administrator enters his/her username and password, it directly goes to the Home Screen and he/she can add, delete or modify monitored areas, doctors, and People.

In the people section, each patient will be assigned a device ID number which is his ICN. So, each patient will have his/her own and unique identity in the system. Figure 29 shows the patient/doctor registration screen.

Table 2 Actions and procedures according to the risk level

Risk alarm level	Range	Associated Action
Low (Yellow)	[0, 35[%	• The operational is normal • No dangerous case detected and no alarm is activated
Medium (Orange)	[30, 60[%	• Notification that patient disease symptoms exceed the tolerance limits • Monitor closely this suspicious case • Triggering a warning alarm related to this case • Requirement of medical consultation
High (Red)	[55, 100[%	• Patient's symptoms develop into worrisome symptoms • System predicts an emergency condition and alerts doctors for an immediate intervention • Suspicious must be exanimated and should be confined and follow the associated treatment protocol

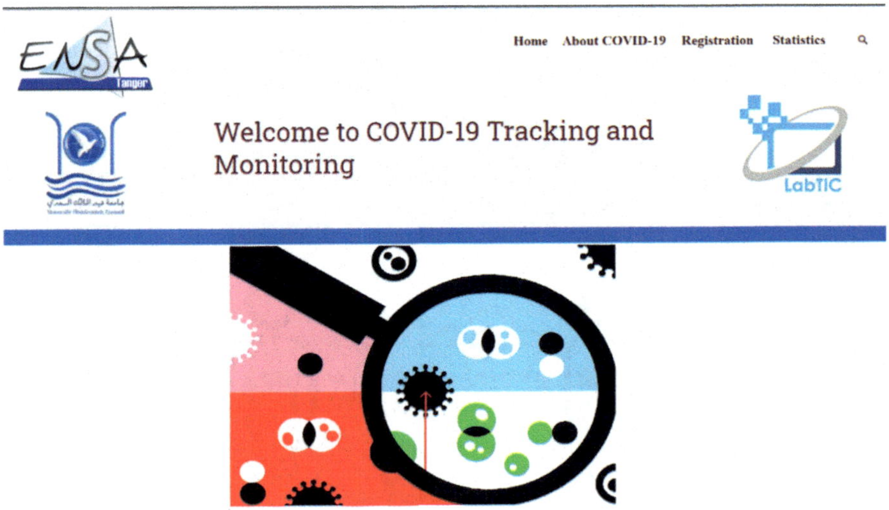

Fig. 28 Home page of the developed monitoring system platform

In the mobile patient monitoring system, we designed a web application that allows doctors and administrators to view real-time vital signs of patients. Using SQL/PHP Web/Cloud Database server based on APIs interfacing. Through this application, real-time data of patients can only be viewed; hence, data cannot be added, deleted, or modified. Figure 30 show also tracking and localization of monitored patients.

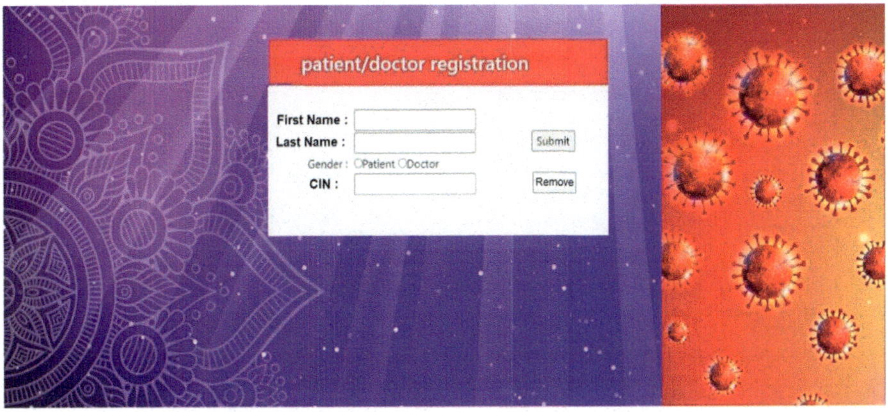

Fig. 29 Patient/Doctor Registering screen

6.2 Performance Parameters of Fuzzy Expert System

The main evaluation for this fuzzy model is to check whether the developed model can classify all the inputs given to the system. The model, which classifies the given inputs in correct and accurate classes, is said to be the best one. The error or accuracy can be calculated by comparing the observed output from the system with the target output, which is given by the professional of medicine.

Seventy tests were carried out to examine COVID-19 using the developed fuzzy expert system closely. The team of doctors also diagnosed each patient and gave a result for the same. After that, the results given by experts are compared with obtained results from the fuzzy expert system. By correlating the two results, 64 out of 70 tests were correctly classified, and hence the system showed 6 errors. A sample of tests is shown in Table 3.

By contrasting these tests, it is noticed that:

$$confidenceindicator = \left(\frac{Successnumber}{Totalnumberoftests} \times 100 \right) \quad (1)$$

where the number of successes = 64 and the total number of tests = 70. Using the above formula, it was examined that 91.42% of the results given by the fuzzy expert system are classified correctly by calculating the confidence indicator. Therefore, the developed fuzzy expert system can be used as an efficient tool for doctors in the diagnosis of COVID-19. The confusion matrix of the proposed FIS is shown in Table 4.

By calculating various parameters like accuracy, precision, specificity, and sensitivity, the performance of the developed medical expert system is evaluated as follow:

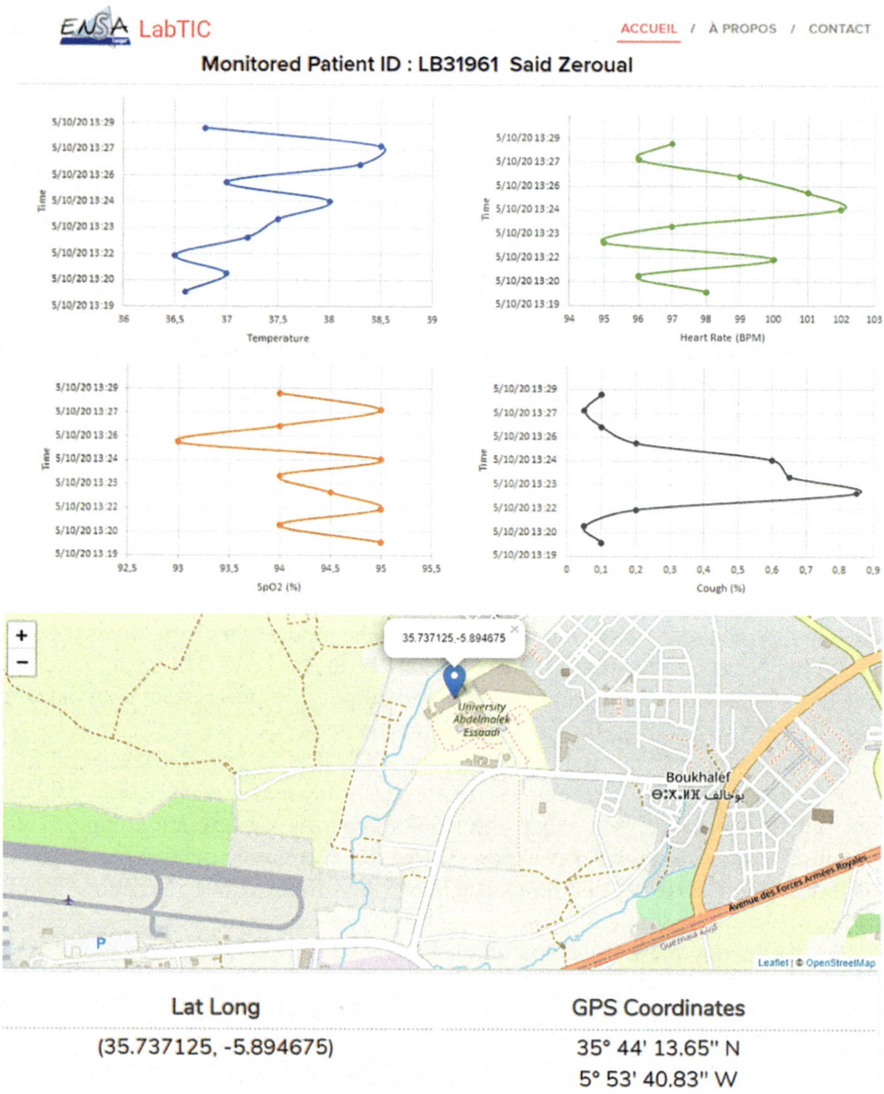

Fig. 30 Patient health status monitoring and tracking screen

- TP: true positive is 33
- FN: false negative is 04
- FP: false positive is 02
- TN: true negative is 31

$$Sensitivity = \frac{TP}{TP + FN} = \frac{33}{33 + 04} = 89.19\%$$

Table 3 A sample of tests performed with developed FIS

Test	Temperature	Heart rate	SpO_2	Cough	Doctors' team	FIS	Success
1	35.5	57	85	0.1	High	Medium	No
2	36	76	93	0.2	High	Medium	No
3	37.1	94	91	0.4	Medium	Medium	Yes
4	37.7	102	89.3	0.65	High	Medium	No
5	37.7	113	88	0.7	High	High	Yes
6	38.3	105	90.5	0.8	High	High	Yes
7	39	114	94	0.5	High	High	Yes
8	39	114	93.2	0.46	High	Medium	No
9	37.7	109	92	0.7	High	High	Yes
10	38.1	101	94	0.46	Medium	Medium	Yes

Table 4 Confusion matrix for COVID-19 FIS

Low	Medium	High	Class names
21	02	00	**Low**
00	20	00	**Medium**
00	04	23	**High**

$$Specificity = \frac{TN}{TN + FP} = \frac{31}{31 + 02} = 93.93\%$$

$$Precision = \frac{TP}{TP + FP} = \frac{33}{33 + 02} = 94.28\%$$

$$Classificationaccruracy = \frac{TP + TN}{TP + FP + TN + FN} = 91.42\%$$

These calculated parameters are shown in the form of a comparison histogram in Fig. 31.

7 Conclusion

This research deals with the problem of COVID-19 disease detection and monitoring. An intelligent algorithm for its accurate diagnosis has been studied to avoid this issue. The proposed solution approach is based on different technologies. Effectively, the suggested diagnosis approach correctly treats the problem with satisfactory performance. In addition, the proposed system constitutes an effort toward the design of an

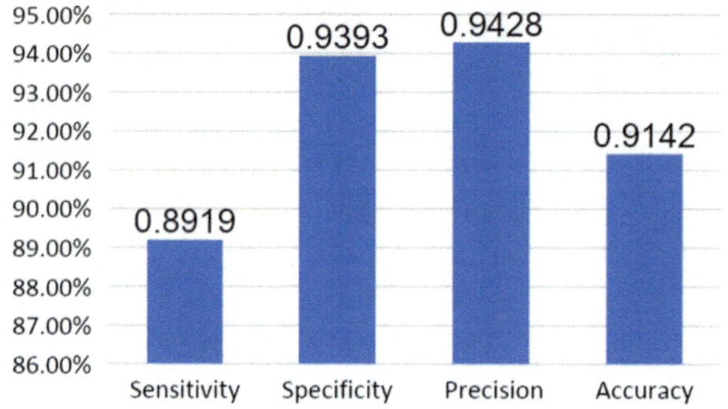

Fig. 31 Performance of the proposed system

intelligent, flexible, and integrated fuzzy logic-based home healthcare system. Simulation results prove the COVID-19 detection accuracy and the knowledge extraction feasibility. The exploitation of accurate medical knowledge or expertise can lead to enhance the performance of the whole system. Furthermore, it is concluded from the obtained outcomes that the proposed remote diagnosis task has been accomplished successfully in real-time. This promotes the experimental validation and evaluation of the system of the performance in a university hospital center with COVID-19 patients. As perspectives, we proposed to extend this work to establish a comparative study towards other types of fuzzy inference engine: Tsukamoto, Takagi-Sugeno, and ANFIS for an accurate diagnosis of COVID-19.

Acknowledgements The authors would like to express their gratitude to the University of Abdelmalek Essaâdi, Tetouan, Morocco for the financial support of this work.

References

1. Contact tracing and social distancing ecosystem, [Online]. https://create.arduino.cc/projecthub/mithun-das/tracex-contact-tracing-social-distancing-ecosystem-d46b62?fbclid=IwAR3IZa5RAYuO22-bsxmFONdhnhLsZtYMht_1WpQKMAfqpwkVyZZaDoRhG4Q
2. wiqaytna Application. [Online]. https://coronavirus.cgem.ma/wiqaytna-fr/https://www.wiqaytna.ma/Default_Fr.aspx
3. Gunvant Chaudhari et al, Virufy: Global Applicability of Crowdsourced and Clinical Datasets for AI Detection of COVID-19 from Cough Audio Samples, [Online]. https://arxiv.org/abs/2011.13320
4. COVID-19 cough dataset. [Online]. https://github.com/virufy/covid
5. Ali, I., et al.: AI4COVID-19: AI Enabled Preliminary Diagnosis for COVID-19 from Cough Samples via an App, arXiv:2004.01275v6 [eess.AS], 27 Sep 2020 [Online]. https://doi.org/10.1016/j.imu.2020.100378
6. The Institute's Editorial Staff, Doctors Can Track Patients' COVID-19 Symptoms with This App E-CoVig uses a cloud-based eHealth platform, https://spectrum.ieee.org, 10 Sep 2020 at 18:00 GMT

7. El-Shafai, W., Abd El-Samie, F.: Extensive and augmented COVID-19 X-Ray and CT chest images dataset, [Online]. https://data.mendeley.com/datasets/8h65ywd2jr/2
8. Heart rate monitoring using IoT, [Online]. https://create.arduino.cc/projecthub/technopaths/heart-rate-monitor-using-iot-ddafca?ref=similar&ref_id=343891&offset=3
9. Arduino Nano 33 BLE Sense. [Online]. https://store.arduino.cc/arduino-nano-33-ble-sense
10. Warden, P., Situnayake, D., Tiny, M.L.: Machine Learning with TensorFlow Lite on Arduino and Ultra-Low-Power Microcontrollers, O'Reilly books, 1st edn. (2019)
11. MAX30205 Human Body Temperature Sensor Datasheet, 2016 Maxim Integrated Products, Inc., 19–8505; Rev 0; 3/1, http://www.maximintegrated.com/
12. Cough detection. [Online]. https://create.arduino.cc/projecthub/edge-impulse/cough-detection-with-tinyml-on-arduino-417f37?f=1
13. Majumder, Sumit., et al.: Wearable sensors for remote health monitoring, review, Sensors. MDPI **17**, 1–45 (2017). https://doi.org/10.3390/s17010130
14. Liang, T., et al.: Handbook of COVID-19 Prevention and Treatment, The First Aliated Hospital, Zhejiang University School of Medicine Compiled According to Clinical Experience (2020)
15. Tobin, M.J., et al.: Why COVID-19 silent hypoxemia is baffling to physicians. Am. J. Respir. Crit. Care Med. **202**(3), 356–360 (2020). Published online 2020 Aug 1. https://doi.org/10.1164/rccm.202006-2157cp, PMCID: PMC7397783, PMID: 32539537
16. Dondorp, A.M., et al., Respiratory Support in COVID-19 patients, with a focus on resource-limited settings. Am. J. Trop. Med. Hyg. **102**(6), 1191–1197 (2020). Published online 2020 Apr 21. https://doi.org/10.4269/ajtmh.20-0283, PMCID: PMC7253105, PMID: 32319424
17. Gul, M.H., Htun, Z.Mar, Inayat, A.: Role of fever and ambient temperature in COVID-19. Expert Rev. Respir. Med. (2020). https://doi.org/10.1080/17476348.2020.1816172
18. Scientific Brief, Criteria for releasing COVID-19 patients from isolation. [Online]. https://www.who.int/newsroom/commentaries/detail/criteria-for-releasing-covid-19-patients-from-isolation]
19. Cho, R.H.W., et al.: COVID -19 viral load in the severity of and recovery from olfactory and gustatory dysfunction, The Laryngoscope, September 2020, https://doi.org/10.1002/lary.29056, PMID: 32794209, PMCID: PMC7436903
20. Madhan, M., et al.: Measurement of arterial oxygen saturation (SpO2) using PPG optical sensor. In: 2016 International Conference on Communication and Signal Processing (ICCSP), https://doi.org/10.1109/iccsp.2016.7754330 (2020)
21. MAX30102 High-Sensitivity Pulse Oximeter and Heart-Rate Sensor for Wearable Health Datasheet, 2018 Maxim Integrated Products, Inc., 19-7740; Rev 1; 10/18, http://www.maximintegrated.com/
22. Didier, D., et al.: Fuzzy-set based logics—an history-oriented presentation of their main developments, Handbook of the History of Logic, vol. 8, pp. 325–449, https://doi.org/10.1016/s1874-5857(07)80009-4
23. Özger, M.: Comparison of fuzzy inference systems for streamflow prediction. Hydrol. Sci. J. Sci. Hydrolog., **54**(2), 261–273 (2009)

Online Learning in the Low Internet Area, Planning, Strategies and Problems Faced by Students During the Covid-19 Period

Fitria Sartika, Mahyudin Ritonga, Ahmad Lahmi, Aguswan Rasyid, and Suci Ramadhanti Febriani

Abstract • Reveal planning that done in low internet areas in following online learning. • Get information about strategy done by students and college student following the online learning. • Finding problems and offering possible solutions can be a reference for students, college students or teachers in experiencing learning in areas of the low internet. **Objectives:** Areas with low internet need special attention from various parties especially in the condition of covid-19 which require that activities be held online as well as education. Through this research is expected to inform about the planning, strategy as well as the problems faced and solutions offered for the continuity of education in low internet areas. **Method:** This research was conducted in two sub-districts in Solok Regency, West Sumatra, Indonesia, data collection techniques are surveys, and observations, data sources are students and college students and teachers who are at the research location. Data analysis this researcher performed qualitative data analysis procedures, namely reducing data, displaying data, clarifying, and drawing conclusions. **Findings:** the local government which has low internet area has not done enough planning to support the continuity of online learning for the community, the implementation of online learning activities in low internet areas requires different preparation, less maximum implementation, and various difficulties or obstacles that can not be avoided such as the cost of online learning a lot, WiFi signal is not strong, electricity is often extinguished. As a result of this condition, students and college students living in low-internet areas have to struggle to find specific locations that are reached by signal, affordable locations must be reached for 15 min by motorcycle.

Keywords Low internet · Learning problem · Planning · Covid-19

F. Sartika · M. Ritonga (✉) · A. Lahmi · A. Rasyid · S. R. Febriani
Muhammadiyah University of West Sumatera, Padang, Indonesia
e-mail: mahyudinritonga@gmail.com

F. Sartika · M. Ritonga · A. Lahmi · A. Rasyid
UIN Maulana Malik Ibrahim Malang, Malang, Indonesia

D. Oliva et al. (eds.), *Artificial Intelligence for COVID-19*, Studies in Systems, Decision and Control 358, https://doi.org/10.1007/978-3-030-69744-0_23

1 Introduction

The use of information technology media is increasingly in demand in various aspects of life today, especially in the field of education [9, 15]. The use of information technology media in the world of education has become important for humans in recent decades, due to the increasingly rapid and varied technological developments. To develop education in Indonesia, information technology is also increasingly being studied, this reality is evidenced by the high public interest in choosing information technology majors. [12, 17]. Because living in this digital era, all human beings are required to be able to adapt quickly and intelligently to existing technological developments, especially to carry out education.

The need for information technology in education was increasingly felt when it happened The Covid-19 pandemic, which requires education personnel to transition to a rapid learning implementation model with distance learning [2, 8], or carry out learning from home, so that the use of information technology has become a necessity for interaction for every teacher and learner in order to carry out the learning process every day [11]. During this learning, it is also called learning online or online, which allows learners to take lessons from anywhere as long as they have an internet connection. Where learners concentrate their learning activities outside the institution, and accept or submit assignments online through various applications and platforms available in technology media [18]. The learning model that was originally centered in the classroom and the addition of tasks carried out at home or homework, while currently being reversed, learning is centered at home, while in class it is only as an acceptance and collection of assignments and explanations related to assignments given by educators only, that class either online or online. This reverse learning model is now known as flipped classroom or flipping e-learning [3, 18, 19].

Currently, learning through online or online media has become a daily meal for Indonesian students and students, both those living in urban and rural areas, all of whom must enjoy [5], the implementation of online learning aims to cut the spread of the endemic virus [4, 10]. So that the same thing must also be followed and carried out by students who come from rural areas without cellular networks or are in low internet areas. Where the area has not been covered by the cellular network as a whole, in the sense that the network can only be obtained at certain points. So that to provide an internet network you have to go through paid wifi, where the quality of the internet network cannot be said to be good when used due to various obstacles. The limitations of this cellular network and internet network make students and students in these areas experience joys and sorrows that are different from those in urban areas or other areas with good network coverage.

Based on the results of the research that the researchers stated above as well as the reality of the struggles of students and students in searching for internet networks, this research will focus on three main aspects, namely, first, preparation that should be made for learning during areas with difficult internet networks, second, strategy. students and students in low internet areas in participating in during learning, and third, the limitations and difficulties faced by students and students in during learning.

2 Method

This research is in the form of field survey research using a qualitative approach, namely research conducted to find out and understand the realities that occur in society regarding learning during the during the Covid-19 pandemic. The technique of collecting this data is through observation and interviews with informants in the field, then the information obtained is temporarily recorded in the researchers' notes.

Sources of data were obtained from 10 students and students representing various levels of education, namely junior high school, senior high school, and public and private universities, where they are implementing online learning in one of the rural areas in Solok Regency, West Sumatra province, Indonesia. Where this area is an area that is far from cities or crowds, so that it only gets permanent electricity, and has not been reached by cellular networks let alone the internet. To analyze the research data, the researcher performed qualitative data analysis procedures, namely reducing data, displaying data, clarifying, and drawing conclusions. To test the validity of the research data, researchers verified and reconfirmed informants.

3 Research Results and Discussion

Preparation for low internet areas to support the implementation of online learning for students and students during the Covid-19 period

Learning in various forms requires careful preparation, without serious planning it is certain that the learning that will be carried out will not get maximum results, according to the results of research and expert opinion it can be seen that areas with weak internet networks can do several things to support smooth operation. during the learning process. The preparations intended can be seen in Table 1:

From the table above, it can be seen that there are at least four categories prepared by both the community and the parents of each student, namely first, providing wifi stalls. In accordance with the results of surveys and interviews conducted with students, it is known that to be able to take part in learning during the Covid-19 period they took a ride to a cafe that provided an internet network. The provision of internet networks for learning in various countries has become a habit, because for

Table 1 Preparation of low internet areas to support learning during the Covid-19 period

No.	Preparation form	Party providing
1	Provide Wifi stalls	Cafe owner
2	Wifi network configuration	Cooperation between shop owners and residents' houses
3	Additional voucher quota	Parents
4	Buy android	Parents

people who have a shop, when the internet network is available, it is also a means of promotion for shop customers [20].

The development of digital technology can be used professionally in the world of education as a means of interaction between students and their educators [13, 16]. The use of this technology in distance learning must involve the internet as a liaison or a means of interacting in learning.

The need for an internet network in several regions in Indonesia is not in line with the facilities available as a network connection device, so cellular or internet networks cannot yet be obtained. Cellular networks can be reached only from certain points, such as hills or houses at high altitudes. So to get an internet network it is necessary to connect a wifi from outside the area which is more than 30 km away.

From the results of the interview, it is known that this wifi is provided by the shop owner who collaborates with wifi users who are in a smooth network area, the wifi user pairs a network capture device at certain points before entering the area without the network. Then install a special tool to catch the wifi network in a place that will be used for wifi stalls. This wifi shop is used by students and university students to carry out daily learning activities during the Covid-19 pandemic.

Furthermore, secondly, from the results of the interview, it is known that there are efforts from the community to configure the internet network between wifi stalls and residents' homes, this effort is carried out because in one village only two wifi stalls are available, these two stalls work together to facilitate learning activities for students and students. configure a wifi network between the two stalls. So that students and students can buy vouchers at one of the existing wifi stalls, and can use them at another shop, or choose the nearest and convenient shop for them. This also helps, because the vouchers are available in selected packages, and the amount at each shop is not the same.

Apart from planning as above, thirdly, increasing the quantity of vouchers or internet quota. In accordance with the results of interviews with informants, it is known that in order to prepare for learning during the Covid-19 period in areas where the internet is weak, parents have to spend quite a lot of money, because in addition to having to prepare package fees, it is also transportation to places that sell internet packages.

The place that sells internet data packages is 30 km away from the residents' residence, and according to the results of observations of package sellers, it is known that internet packages were not sold well in the area at first, but since online learning was implemented, internet packages have been selling well. So that the quantity must be increased. The choice of packages on the voucher is also added, packages are available per week and hourly. 2 h package for Rp. 5000, -, 5 h package for Rp. 10,000, -, and packages a week at a price of Rp. 40,000, -.

In this aspect, the research findings show that learning carried out online requires quite expensive financing, parents of a number of students and students prior to Corona virus can be said to not need to purchase internet packages but with Covid-19 they have to add expenses that were previously considered secondary needs. be primary.

Another finding from the planning carried out by students and students in taking part in learning during the Covid-19 period is that their parents have to buy an android, even though their area is not covered by the internet network and even cellular networks, but the need for android is increasingly felt, this is because students and students every time Today you have to bring your android to a certain location that is accessible to the network in order to get learning material sent by teachers and lecturers to the WhatsApp group.

3.1 Implementation of Online Learning by Students and Students in Low Internet Areas

The implementation of online learning is basically a flipped classroom learning model, where the center of learning activities is in each house, while the class is an addition to learning activities in the form of acceptance and collection of learning assignments. However, this learning model cannot be carried out completely the same by students and students who are in areas without cellular networks and low internet areas.

The center of learning activities for them is not at home, but in a special place that has an internet connection as a means of online learning. This place is called a wifi shop. Of course, not all students and students can reach this wifi shop quickly, especially those who live in villages without the support of transportation. The only way for them to get to the wifi shop where to learn online is by walking, so it takes a relatively long time.

The distance is not close to making students and students have to prepare breakfast and lunch from home before going to study online, this is the same as going to school when they were at the Elementary School level several years ago. Apart from breakfast and lunch, they also prepare chargers and fees to buy internet vouchers as the main media for online learning.

The implementation of online learning is generally the same as that followed by other students, namely through applications and platforms available in information technology, such as WhatsApp Group (WAG), Google Classroom, Video Call, and Zoom. Only a few people have institutions where they learn to implement offline learning by submitting assignments directly to school once a week, and even then they have to understand the material using Google's help too, because there are so many teaching materials that they cannot understand themselves.

According to them, the learning outcomes that have been carried out cannot be said to be satisfactory, because their understanding of the material is very minimal due to the lack of smooth implementation of learning due to inadequate network quality, as well as difficulty understanding the material without direct teacher guidance. They also feel their eye health has decreased than usual, because they have to deal with an Android screen every day for quite a long time.

The findings above show that learning during the covid-19 period is not the same as the demands of the slogan against Covid, namely learning from home (LFH), [7, 14], because in areas with low internet and difficult cellular networks, learning during requires them to leave the house to find a location that is affordable to the internet network. Along with the drastic development of technology in this modern century, the world of education must be able to compete in its use in various aspects of learning [1]. Learning that is done with technology can be through the help of celluler or with the smart technology known as smartphones today. In this case, user environmental problems should also be a concern.

Problems and Solutions for Continuity of Learning During Low Internet Areas

Some areas that are still weak cellular and internet networks are faced with various problems related to learning during the Covid-19 period, according to the survey results it is known that the problems faced by students and students in participating in learning during the Covid-19 period in weak areas of the internet are cellular networks which difficult, expensive, frequent power cuts and poor network quality.

Cellular network is a means of connecting to communicate via mobile phones. Along with its development, cellular networks have been utilized for internet connections, so that this makes it easier for mobile phone users to access the internet smoothly, which is now known as smartphones or androids. Simply by activating the celluler data package, the internet network can be connected to the cellphone.

However, it is different for some residents of this country, where they have not been able to enjoy the main cellular network. Not only was the internet unconnected, they couldn't enjoy the network to make calls and text messages. In some areas, celluler networks can be found at certain points, for example on hills, in fields, or in people's homes at high altitudes. So that communication via electronic media is minimal in the area.

Since the pandemic hit, students and students who come from areas without this network have felt tremendous difficulties. Their communication with friends and teachers or lecturers is not smooth, because usually they communicate via WA or social media using the celluler network for internet packages on Android. In carrying out their learning, they cannot be as good as those on the network smoothly. For online learning that must be followed every day, they can only take advantage of internet vouchers sold at wifi stalls.

The existence of a wifi shop is quite helpful in the implementation of online learning for students and students, but the distance between their house and the wifi shop is also not close. There is also no means of public transportation in that area, and not all of these people have private vehicles. Private vehicles can only be owned by those whose economies have improved, so that many students have to walk to be able to get an internet network in a wifi shop. Everyday fatigue in studying online is inevitable.

Online learning to do from a wifi shop costs a lot of money. The wifi internet package voucher is only available in 3 choices. Students and students must pay Rp. 5,000 to enjoy the wifi network for 2 h, Rp. 10,000 for 5 h, and Rp. 40,000 for a week. This price is not a cheap price when compared to internet packages and vouchers in areas with good networks. If calculated the costs that must be spent per month, students and students have to pay a fee ranging from Rp. 160,000-200,000, per month for studying only, not including pocket money that must be prepared more every day, because the average duration of study time is 8 h, meaning for those who do not prepare food from home,

In the economic downturn caused by the pandemic, urban communities are experiencing difficulties in fulfilling their daily needs [6]. This is especially true for rural communities, which in fact are at an economic level which is still concerning, only a small proportion of them are in the middle-level economy. In general, the income of rural communities is from agricultural or plantation products. During the pandemic, the selling price of foodstuffs is getting cheaper, while the needs of the community continue to increase, because they have to equip and prepare various forms of medical equipment to prevent the spread of the plague. So, with the increase in the cost of education for their children, it will make the community's economy more difficult and this cannot be denied.

Based on the research of Holzweiss and his friends, the large cost of online learning in a crisis situation can make the economic decline of rural communities which will cause many children to drop out of school [5]. This is also a concern for students who are in areas that are still weak with internet networks.

Another problem faced by people in low internet areas in online learning is that electricity often goes out. Wifi that is connected to reach rural areas is wifi that depends on electric power. So that electricity is also the main source in carrying out online learning for students and students in low internet areas. If the electricity suddenly goes out, learning online can no longer be continued, so students and students have to wait for the electricity to return to be able to continue their studies. During this pandemic, the electricity in the area often goes out, so learning online that requires a full internet connection in learning makes learning disrupted and not optimal.

Another complaint from students and students who live in areas that are difficult to network is a weak internet network or poor network quality. The large number of students and students who use wifi networks to study online at the same time, makes the network run slow. So that they cannot smoothly participate in learning, even though they have tried their best. Sometimes even within a day or two the wifi network doesn't work, this makes them unable to learn at all as long as the wifi is completely dead. There is no other choice for them to carry out online learning other than in a wifi shop, making their learning not work as expected, and not being able to achieve its learning goals optimally.

4 Conclusion

From the presentation of the discussion above, it can be concluded that the implementation of online learning for students and students who come from low internet areas can not be said to be carried out smoothly and optimally. Preparations for learning that can be done have not been able to provide a comprehensive solution for learning activities, so the implementation of online learning is often constrained. The obstacles or difficulties faced are the absence of a celluler network, the existing wifi internet network is also not smooth, the quality of the wifi network is not good, the price of vouchers is expensive, the electricity often goes out, the wifi stalls are a bit far and must be reached without a vehicle, if a laptop or The smartphone used in online learning is damaged, so the place for electronic service is also far away. Other than that, students and university students also feel tired in studying online that must be done every day. As a result of interacting with electronics that are connected to the internet network every day making them feel tired and dizzy, their learning concentration is also felt to decrease than usual, many subject matter is poorly understood. This makes the struggles of students who come from low internet areas requiring greater sacrifice and the experience of online learning during the Covid-19 pandemic is different from those from cities or areas that are well networked. learning concentration is also felt to be lower than usual, many subject matter is poorly understood. This makes the struggles of students who come from low internet areas requiring greater sacrifice and the experience of online learning during the Covid-19 pandemic is different from those from cities or areas that are well networked. learning concentration is also felt to be lower than usual, many subject matter is poorly understood. This makes the struggles of students who come from low internet areas requiring greater sacrifice and the experience of online learning during the Covid-19 pandemic is different from those from cities or areas that are well networked.

References

1. Ahmadi, M.R.: The use of technology in english language learning: a literature review. Int. J. Res. English Educ. (IJREE) **3**(2), 115–125 (2018). www.ijreeonline.com
2. Ali, W.: Online and remote learning in higher education institutes: a necessity in light of COVID-19 pandemic. High. Educ. Stud. **10**(3), 16–25 (2020). https://doi.org/10.5539/hes.v10n3p16
3. Angelina, P.: The effects of flipped learning implementation on the students' achievements in language teaching media course. In: Companion Proceedings of the SEADRIC 2019 (2020). Yogyakarta: Sanata Dharma University, pp. 92–97. https://doi.org/10.24071/seadr.2019.13
4. Djalante, R., et al.: Review and analysis of current responses to COVID-19 in Indonesia: Period of January to March 2020. Progr. Disaster Sci. **6**, 1–9 (2020). https://doi.org/10.1016/j.pdisas.2020.100091
5. Holzweiss, P.C., et al.: Crisis planning for online students: lessons learned from a major disruption. Online Learn. **24**(2), 22–37 (2020). doi:https://doi.org/10.24059/olj.v24i2.2135
6. Honey-Rosés, J., et al.: The impact of COVID-19 on public space: a review of the emerging questions, 2020(April), pp. 1–20. https://doi.org/10.31219/osf.io/rf7xa
7. Huang, R., et al.: Guidance on Active Learning at Home During Educational Disruption: Promoting Student's Self-Regulation Skills in COVID-19 Outbreak. Smart Learning Institute of Beijing Normal University, Beijing (2020)
8. Johnson, N., Veletsianos, G., Seaman, J.: U.S. Faculty and Administrators' experiences and approaches in the early weeks of the COVID-19 pandemic. Online Learn. J. **24**(2), 6–21 (2020)
9. Martínez, S.J.R., et al.: Attitudes toward technology among distance education students: validation of an explanatory model. Online Learn. J. **24**(2), 59–75 (2020)

10. Meng, L., Hua, F., Bian, Z.: Coronavirus Disease 2019 (COVID-19): emerging and future challenges for dental and oral medicine. J. Dental Res **99**(5), 481–487 (2020). https://doi.org/10.1177/0022034520914246
11. Nieuwoudt, J.E.: Investigating synchronous and asynchronous class attendance as predictors of academic success in online education. Austr. J. Educ. Technol. **36**(3), 15–25 (2020)
12. Reynolds, G.W.: Ethics in Information Technology. Cengage Learning, Boston (2015)
13. Ritonga, A.W., et al.: E-learning process of Maharah Qira'ah in higher education during the Covid-19 pandemic. Int. J. High. Educ. **9**(6), 227–235 (2020). https://doi.org/10.5430/ijhe.v9n6p227
14. Ritonga, M.: Learning From Home (LFH) dan Kerinduan yang Mendalam. Inovasi Pembelajaran Era Covid-19 Pengalaman & Pengamatan Selama Pandemi Covid19, pp. 80–83. Yogyakarta, Cv Markumi (2020)
15. Ritonga, M., Nazir, A., Wahyuni, S.: Pembelajaran Bahasa Arab Berbasis Teknologi Informasi dan Komunikasi. Arabiyat: Jurnal Pendidikan Bahasa Arab dan Kebahasaaraban **3**(1), 1–12. doi:http://dx.doi.org/10.15408/a.v3i1.2879
16. Smith, E.E., Kahlke, R., Judd, T.: Not just digital natives: Integrating technologies in professional education contexts. Austr. J. Educ. Technol. **36**(3), 1–14 (2020)
17. Sutton, B.: The effects of technology in society and education. Education and Human Development Master's Theses., (192). http://digitalcommons.brockport.edu/ehd_theses/192
18. Tekin, P.Ş., et al.: Flipping e-learning for teaching medical terminology: a study of learners' online experiences and perceptions. Online Learn. **24**(2), 76–93 (2020). doi:https://doi.org/10.24059/olj.v24i2.2030
19. Tomas, L., et al.: 'Are first year students ready for a flipped classroom? A case for a flipped learning continuum. Int. J. Educ. Technol. High. Educ. **16**(5), 1–22 (2019)
20. Tosun, N.: Social networks as a learning and teaching environment and security in social networks. J. Educ. Train. Stud. **6**(11), 194–208 (2018). https://doi.org/10.11114/jets.v6i11a.3817

Internet of Things (IoT) Enable Designs for Identify and Control the COVID-19 Pandemic

H. M. K. K. M. B. Herath

Abstract Coronavirus disease 19 or also known as COVID-19 is a highly transmittable and pathogenic viral infection triggered by Severe Acute Respiratory Syndromes Coronavirus 2 (SARS-CoV-2), which originated across the world from Wuhan, China. The current global COVID-19 pandemic challenge has crossed the limits of national, progressive, philosophical, cultural, financial, and pedagogy. The healthcare system enabled by the Internet of Things (IoT) is useful for the proper monitoring of COVID-19 patients by using an interconnected system. Hospital admission rates are growing as a result of COVID-19, and patients interact with healthier people within hospitals causing immense problems. Once COVID-19 has been identified, there is a high need for health precautions to prevent spread within hospitals. This chapter topic aims to investigate, design an IoT-based system to detect and control the COVID-19 pandemic inside the hospital environment. The proposed design has composed of the detection of COVID-19 patients with thermal images, IoT solution for social distancing, and Chatbot for the COVID-19 consultant which is functions as a single IoT solution in the hospital environment. We were aimed to highlight the IoT enabled wearable technologies with promising outcomes and the potential to identify COVID-19 cases to eliminate the spread by alerting the government authority.

Keywords COVID-19 · Chatbot · Epidemics · Internet of things (IoT) · Network · Pandemic · SARS-CoV · Social distance · Thermal image

1 Introduction

Pandemics are identified as an outbreak of a disease that becomes widely spread as a result of the growth of human-to-human infection. The term "Pandemic" derived from the Greek, Pan meaning by "all" and demos meaning by "the people". This term is widely used as a response to a global infectious disease outbreak in a country

H. M. K. K. M. B. Herath (✉)
Faculty of Engineering Technology, The Open University of Sri Lanka, Colombo, Sri Lanka
e-mail: kasunherathlive@gmail.com

D. Oliva et al. (eds.), *Artificial Intelligence for COVID-19*, Studies in Systems, Decision and Control 358, https://doi.org/10.1007/978-3-030-69744-0_24

or one or more continents in the same period (Honigsbaum, 2009) [1]. Historically, several epidemic outbreaks and pandemics have existed including Spanish Flu, Hong Kong Flu, SARS, H7N9, Ebola, Zika (WHO, 2011b) (Rewar, Mirdha, & Rewar, 2015) (Maurice, 2016). Many medical texts have not described the word "pandemic", but there are some main features of a pandemic which helps to understand the concept. The main features include wide geographical extension, movement of diseases, novelty, severity, high attack rates and explosiveness, low population immunity, infectiousness, and contagion.

Coronaviruses belong to the Betacoronavirus family which contains crown-like spikes on the virus's outer surface. Coronaviruses are 65–125 nm in diameter in size and containing a single-stranded RNA as a nucleic filament [2]. According to the recent study led by Shi Zhengli at Wuhan Virology Institute (WIV), the novel coronavirus seems to have originated from horseshoe bats and the probability cannot be ruled out that it could have arrived from Southeast Asian countries outside of China. They also mentioned that, after analyzing all known bat CoVs in China, the novel coronavirus likely derived from a class of viruses originating in horseshoe bats. Coronaviruses are a wide family of viruses that can cause serious illness to humankind. The first documented major infection is Severe Acute Respiratory Syndrome (SARS) which emerged in 2003, while the second severe disease outbreak started with the Middle East Respiratory Syndrome (MERS) in Saudi Arabia in 2012 [3].

Yadav and his research team at the University of Calgary in Canada have indicated that the novel coronavirus (SARS-CoV-2) [4] had leaped into humans from animals [5]. A community of researchers at the University of Calgary state that after 2013 at least, the COVID-19 virus has been spread among the human population. COVID-19 has spread quickly across the world after discovering the patient zero, with nearly 31.3 million confirmed cases and more than 965,000 deaths that are recorded in 215 countries and regions as of September 2020 (Fig. 1) [6]. People can get the infection by close contact with an individual who has symptoms of the virus which includes cough and sneezing. Coronavirus was usually distributed through zoonotic droplets which were conveyed by the air. The virus replicated in the ciliated epithelium that caused cellular damages at the site of infection [7]. COVID-19 influences the different

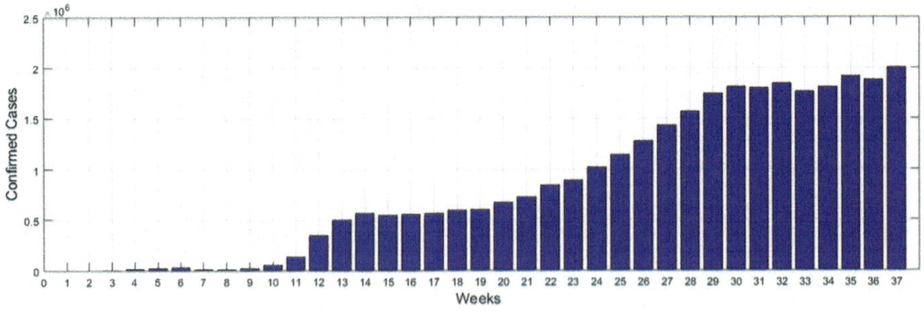

Fig. 1 COVID-19 confirmed cases as of September 2020

individuals in multiple respects. Most people who are infected will develop mild to moderate disease and recover without hospitalization.

The Internet revolution in recent decades has shown that all aspects of business can be affected by new technologies. Nowadays, ubiquitous communication is always possible with the aid of new technologies such as network connections, wireless communication, and sensors. IoT aims to empower the objects to connect anytime, anywhere, with anything and whoever gets the perfect use of any route, service, or network. The Internet of Things reflects a modern technological evolution in the world. IoT is a new technology that focuses on the effect on the environment and addresses a variety of wireless and wired connections that communicate with each other [8]. The objects surrounding our environments connect in one form or another with the Internet. It would integrate the physical and ICT worlds together, giving a vision beyond the realm of traditional networks [9].

Recently a growing interest in body wearable sensors has emerged as powerful tools for healthcare applications, and various devices are currently commercially available for various purposes including personal healthcare, activity awareness, and fitness. Researchers have also introduced new therapeutic uses of these technologies for remote health management systems that provide long-term status tracking functionalities, and diagnostic exposure to patient physiological knowledge [10–12]. IoT uses a large number of interconnected devices to build a connection to a smart health management system network. It warns about and tracks all kinds of illnesses to improve patient's safety. It captures the patient's data and information digitally without having any interaction between humans [13].

2 IoT and Its Background for COVID-19

IoT guarantees that health-care facilities are customized by creating a digital profile for each patient. Due to the lack of easy access to treatment services, numerous health conditions in traditional healthcare facilities have gone undetected [14]. Through IoT based healthcare, various distributed devices collect, process, and transfer medical information to the cloud through real-time, allowing vast data streams to be captured, processed, and analyzed in many new ways and context-dependent alarms to be enabled. This groundbreaking data collection approach allows continuous and invisible control to medical equipment through the internet from every connected device [15–17]. Mobile computing provides IoT services through the use of mobile phone devices, software, or m-health care [18]. The m-health contributes to the IoT by offering different services such as compactness, IP connectivity [19], low power consumption, and protection. After the research in the fields of gynaecology and pediatrics, smartphone applications allow patients to learn about their illnesses.

IoT is an advanced system that guarantees isolation for all contaminated individuals as a consequence of this infection. It is helpful for a proper monitoring system during the quarantine period. All patients at high risk are conveniently monitored using the Internet-based network. This technique is used for bio-metric measures such as blood pressure, heart rate and, glucose level [20]. Humans are generally interacting with others through voice, although it can also be used to illustrate different characteristics such as facial expression and gestures. Recognition [21] of hand movement in healthcare is generally agreed for IoT, particularly for deaf people [22].

Event recognition is recently accomplished through the introduction of machine learning algorithms to the data obtained by mobile sensors [23]. It senses such things as jumping, ascending, stepping, walking, driving, and cycling. The program is equipped with data patterns of using data that are collected by sensors while conducting certain tasks [24]. Many health and wellness apps are being developed to maintain a continuous track of a person's health using smartphones [25]. These keep track of the physical activity, diet, workouts, and lifestyle of the users to assess the level of fitness and send user feedback accordingly.

Wang and his research team described a smartphone-based mobile Application. They used it to assess a college student's overall mental health and performance. An activity detection (accelerometer) and GPS data were used to monitor the location and activities in which the student is involved. The accelerometer and light sensors were used to keep track of how long the student sleeps [26].

Mohammed and his team suggested a device design capable of automatically detecting the coronavirus from the thermal image using a smart helmet with a mounted thermal imaging system. The system is fitted with facial recognition technology; it can also view personal details of the pedestrian that can acquire temperatures from the pedestrians automatically [27].

Yang and others [28] have proposed some improvements to the Challenge-response based RFID authentication protocol for the development of an algorithm for a distributed database environment. They made it better suited for the IoT system control environment.

Souza, Srivatsava, Prithika and Sahana collaborated to build an inexpensive smart wheelchair by incorporating an IoT and microcontroller-based health monitoring device [29]. EEG based control systems for disabled people are widely accepted [30] in IoT. Remote control robots are suggested for the COVID-19 prevention due to the limited human involvement, especially in the laboratory environment. IoT has recently adapted efficiently and easily to the EEG and other biosignal based control systems for performing tasks.

According to a report by the Massachusetts Institute of Technology (MIT), it will help epidemiologists classify individuals who have met the infectious patients by superimposing geographic information systems (GIS) on IoT mobile data. The system will also better track high-risk conditions and to provide the healthcare staff with valuable data. Scientists at the IIT Istituto Italiano di Tecnologia have created sensorized suits that can track parameters of the human body and warn users when their body temperature has risen by more than 37.5 degrees. In China, bracelets and rings are used combined with AI platforms that have continuous tracking of vital signs, including temperature, pulse rate, and amounts of oxygen in the blood.

Majumder and his research team [31] have proposed a method to design and development of an advanced smart IoT device with a low-power communications module to capture heart rates and body temperatures discreetly utilizing a smartphone without impeding daily life. This work explores the usage of signal processing and machine learning methods for sensor data mining to extremely reliably recognize expected or unexpected cardiac arrests.

Table 1 depicts the different IoT applications and usage of each application during the COVID-19 pandemic.

From a systematic study, it has been found that several IoT solutions can be used to prevent COVID-19 in the hospital environment.

This study aims to investigate and design an IoT-based system to detect, monitor, and prevent the effect of COVID-19 disease on the hospital environment. The main objective is to alert the government authorities after the detection of COVID-19 patients in hospitals. The proposed system is composed of,

1. Identification of COVID-19 patients with thermal images
2. IoT approach for social distancing
3. Chatbot for the COVID-19 consultant

Table 1 Major applications of IoT for COVID-19 pandemic

IoT Application	Description
Internet connected hospitals	IoT deployment to help pandemics such as COVID-19 includes a robust integrated network inside hospital premises [12]
COVID-19 treatment	Patients should take advantage of the services provided without bias and favors. The collection of treatment approaches is efficient and helps to manage the cases properly
Automated laboratory process	During the COVID-19 diagnosis, IoT is linked via the internet with all medical instruments, devices that convey the details in real time during the procedure
Chatbots consultation	This allows the care accessible in distant areas to the vulnerable through the use of well-connected chatbots to consult patients
COVID-19 patient recognition and tracking	Different authentic software can be built on devices, and will render the identification process easier and more successful. The impactful monitoring of patients eventually strengthened the care agencies to manage the cases more intelligently
Forecasting of virus	The usage of any predictive approach will also help to forecast the condition in the coming years, depending on the data reports available. This would also help to plan for a healthier job environment for the community, physicians, educators, etc. [12]
Remote control wheelchair, beds etc.	Remote control wheelchair, chairs, trolley, and other equipment help keep COVID-19 disease from spreading throughout the pandemic

3 Proposed Design

The basic layered of IoT architecture that is a protocol depended may be either 3-Layer architecture or 5-Layer architecture. The 3-Layers architecture [32], which are the levels of Perception, Network, and Application describes the core concept behind the Internet of Things but does not have enough details for the IoT analysis. That is why more layers are added to provide the 5-layered architecture. Figure 2 illustrates the proposed IoT architecture of this study.

The perception layer consists of physical objects that are monitored, controlled by sensor and actuator devices. The main objective of the perception layer is collecting the sensor data and control actuation. The sensor data is then transmitted via the network layer to the data processing layer, which can be characterized by multiple network technologies. Information processing is performed in the processing layer where the received information can be stored and analyzed using advanced data analytics methodologies. Using with the application layer, the collected, analyzed knowledge will be addressed to an end-user, who may then use it to monitor the overall program. Finally, the business layer enables system administrators to authorities and control the overall functionality of the IoT platform strategically [33, 34].

The perception layer dedicated to this study are sensors for measuring blood pressure and heart rate, thermal camera for detection of COVID-19 patients using

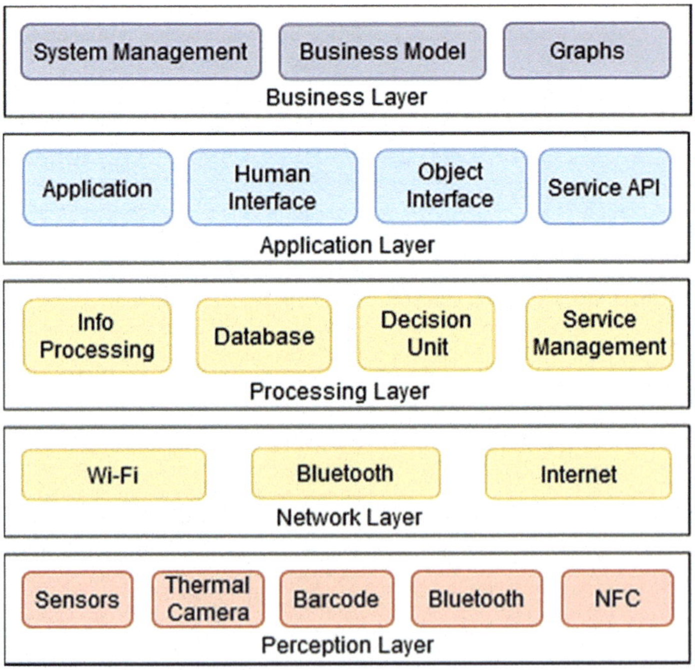

Fig. 2 Proposed IoT server architecture

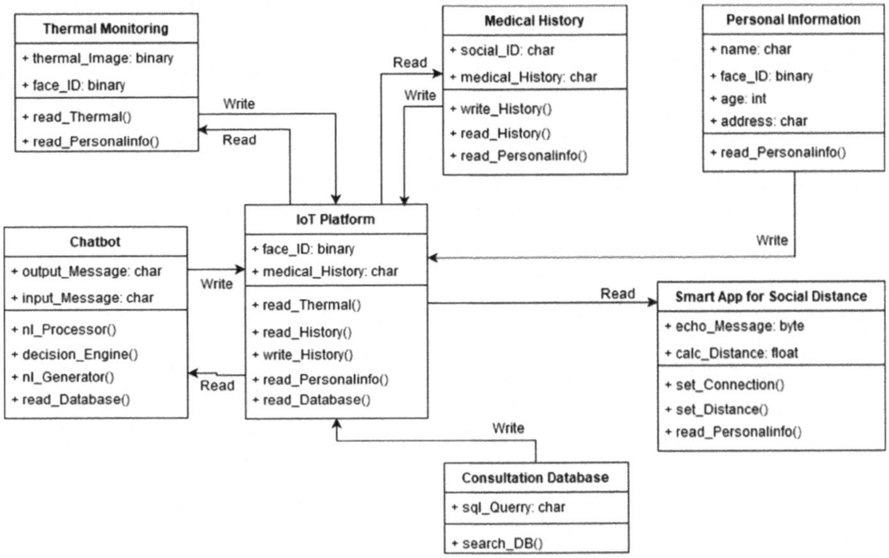

Fig. 3 Proposed IoT platform for the COVID-19 detection and monitoring

thermal images, Barcode reading for the medicine selection, Bluetooth for the social distancing measures and NFC (Near Field Communication) for the authentication requirements such as pass IDs. A layer associated with the functionalities of the data transfer was enabling the different networks participating in the IoT to be interconnected. In this case, we have introduced an appropriate architecture for a modern Internet infrastructure based on the Internet Protocol (IP), which can then be used between wired or wireless devices on the one side and software, services on the other.

The proposed IoT platform communicates with the personal information which registered with the service and medical history of the consumer. This interconnection helps to track patients and predict medical status based on the user's medical history. In Fig. 3 illustrates the proposed IoT platform that is a combination of a thermal monitoring system, smart app for social distancing, and chatbots for the consultation of COVID-19 patients.

3.1 *Identification of COVID-19 Patients with Thermal Images*

The most reliable instruments for measuring temperatures are those used to determining fever in medical patients, such as thermometers for the mouth, ear, and rectum. Such tools include an instruction to use correctly to put patients into close contact with a device that must then be washed before it can be used again. Thermal cameras are now being introduced as a way of tracking individuals with fever-like symptoms as they return to high-traffic locations such as hospital entrances, shopping malls, office complexes, and even mass attendance of activities. People that tend to have elevated temperatures can instead be led to further assessment and advise to separate themselves to help curb COVID-19 spread.

The proposed design of the thermal image detection system includes a thermal camera to determine body temperature. The thermal camera was used for hot body identification and recognition by following the high-temperature variations within the scanned region as opposed to other objects. If the thermal camera visualizes the high-temperature structure, it can then produce large rates of infrared spectra. Figure 4 reflects the layout of the algorithm for thermal control. According to the flowchart, if the spectra of the produced thermal images exceeded more than 37.5° of the device, the person is identified as a suspect. After producing the face ID, the thermal monitoring device is sending details to the IoT Platform (face ID and status of suspect). As a result, The IoT Platform gathers information from the databases and alerts the hospital (government) authority to take further action.

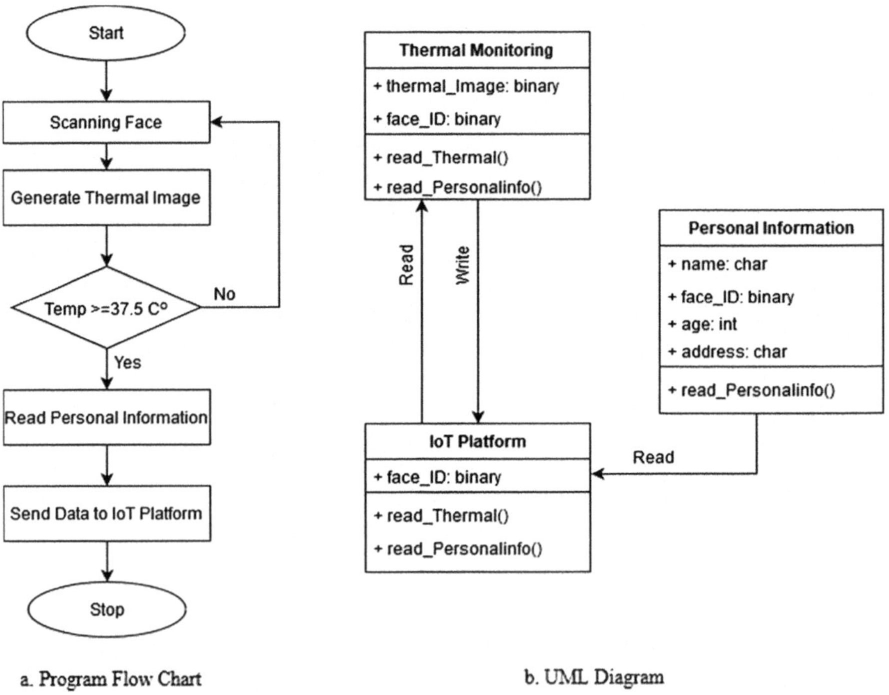

Fig. 4 Program structure of the thermal monitoring algorithm

3.2 IoT Based Smart App for Social Distancing

COVID-19 spreads over prolonged times mostly to peoples who are in near touch such as about 6 feet away. Spread develops as an infectious person coughs, sneezes, speaks, and droplets from their mouth or nose are released into the air, resulting in people's mouths or noses nearby [35]. They will even inhale droplets through the lungs. Since peoples are spread the infection before they know that they are sick, it is extremely important to stay at least 6 feet away from each other, even though there are no symptoms at all. Social distancing is especially necessary for people at increased risk for serious COVID-19 illness. In this section, we suggested a method for the development of an algorithm to preserve social distance focused on IoT approach and Bluetooth technologies.

Bluetooth is a wireless communication protocol used to transmit data between fixed and mobile devices over short distances utilizing short-wavelength UHF radio waves from 2,402 to 2,480 GHz in commercial, research, medical radio bands, and to help to create personal area networks (PANs). Class 3 radios typically have a range of up to 1 m (3 ft), Class 2, most usually used in mobile devices, 10 m (33 ft), and Class 1, mostly for commercial uses, 100 m (328 ft) [36]. We proposed class 2 radios for the contact between devices, due to the necessity of 6 feet measurement. Figure 5 illustrates the Bluetooth network developed within 10 m range using smart mobile phones or tablet computers. BB represents a mobile phone connected to the Bluetooth network.

Figure 6 demonstrates the program flow chart and UML diagram for the development of an algorithm for social distancing service. The software uses the IoT framework to set up the system. It would help to customize the software and collect user details from cloud repositories. When mounted, it will be attached to the whole system within a range of 10 m. Since smartphones are linked to Class 2 radio bands,

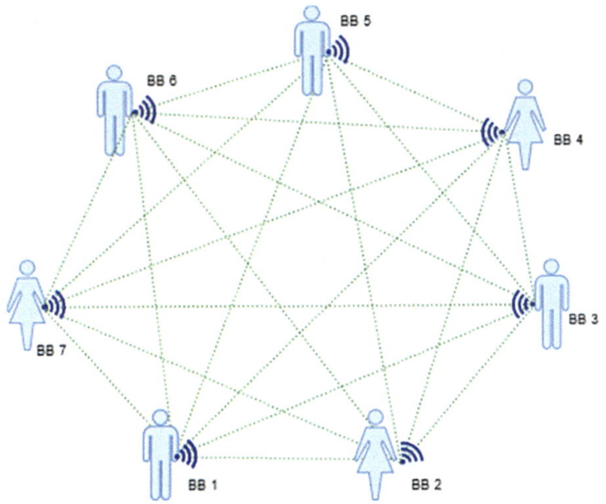

Fig. 5 IoT based social distancing system using bluetooth network

Bluetooth only detects a range of 10 m. The software transmits an echo signal to all users and, after the signal has been received, measures the gap between each device based on transmitting and receiving time. When the distance is less than 1.2 m, the mobile phone may continue to vibrate or sound the alarm.

3.3 Chatbot for the COVID-19 Consultant

With the pandemic, peoples and organizations are seeking to learn how and when the diseases propagate. Individuals want to avoid being sick and organizations such as clinics or local governments require information-based strategies to improve efficiency and prepare social programs. Chatbots may be best suitable for pandemic symptom monitoring, since individuals with anxiety frequently delay accessing health treatment and education [37]. Chatbots may be especially helpful in the case of a pandemic, but problems in information dissemination, symptom management, behavioral improvement, and mental wellbeing care are worthy of consideration.

Figure 7 illustrates the proposed architecture of the Chatbot consultant for the COVID-19. Once the consumer enters a query, it goes into the Natural Language Processing (NLP). Using Natural Language Processing, the machine translates the

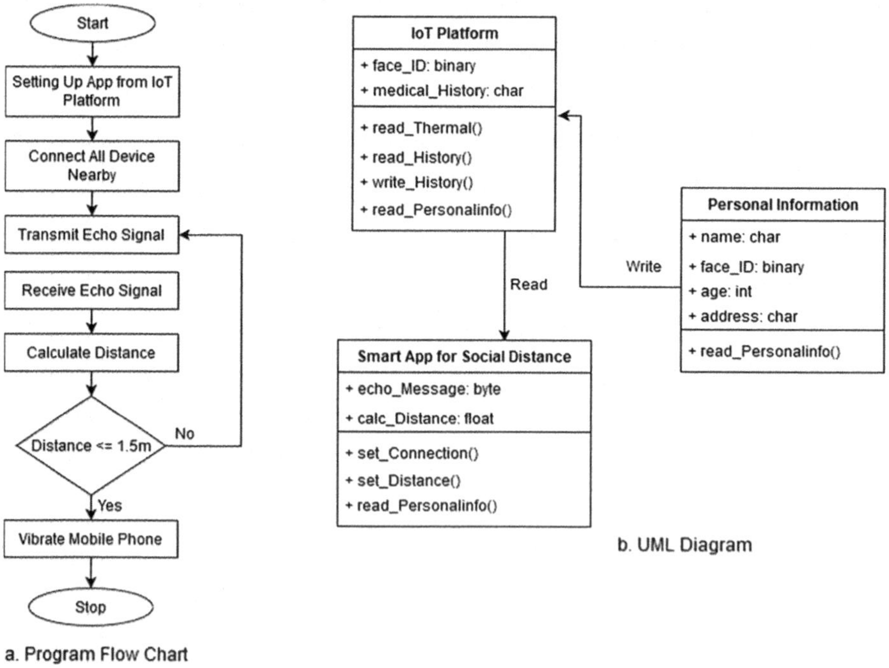

Fig. 6 Program structure of the social distance algorithm

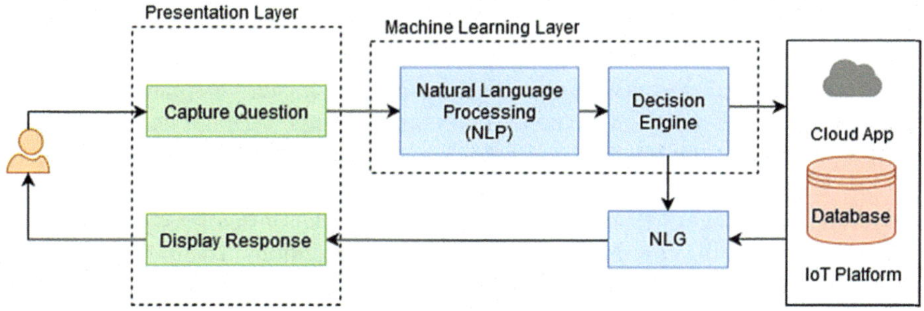

Fig. 7 The architecture of the proposed Chatbot consultant service

user's plain text message to interpreted commands on its own. The Chatbot transfers the data generated to the decision-making system. The decision-making process emerges from a rational judgment based on prior actions and tests.

Nowadays, several cloud platforms have bot infrastructure where we can build the bot and distribute it to each of the clouds. There are several cloud systems that provide various features apart from the bot software, such as built-in artificial intelligence, computational resources, etc. In this section, we proposed the Microsoft Azure cloud framework for the development of a Chatbot. The Microsoft Bot System consists of the Bot Creator, the Connector App, and the App Catalog. This even has a simulator where we can check the function of the bot. The Bot creator of the SDK is used with

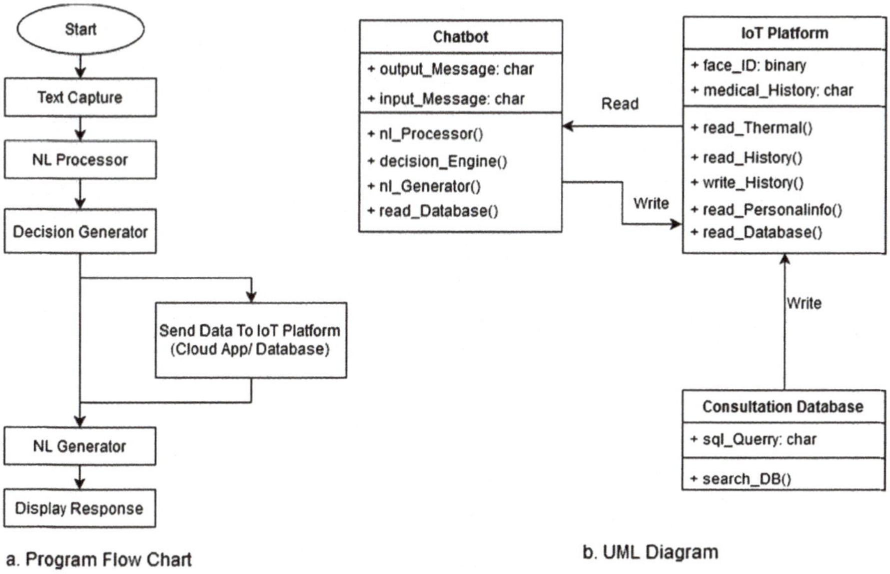

Fig. 8 Program structure of the Chatbot consultant algorithm

the Node. js to create the bot. Figure 8 illustrates the program flow chart and the UML diagram of the Chatbot algorithm.

These proposed designs are specifically intended for the hospital environment. The person who is enrolled in the system is taken to the hospital and tracked by a thermal camera at the hospital entrance. Once the body temperature of the person has hit more than 37.5 °C, the system will suggest that the person is suspected of developing COVID-19 infection. Once the COVID-19 has been identified, the system will notify the government authority for further actions. The IoT system would then be connected to the patient using the Chatbot service to instruct the patient to prevent interact with others. Chatbot also provides health facts, safety precautions, and health status, such as heart rate, blood pressure based on data received from wearable sensors. The IoT system also tracks the distances between patients within the hospital. Once the COVID-19 patient has been detected, the system will calculate the distances between the COVID-19 patient and the others. Distances are calculated with the use of Bluetooth technology. Once a person has breached distance controls, the system will alert the person using mobile phones.

4 Conclusion

IoT comes up with the facilities that required mitigating the effects of the novel COVID-19 virus. The goal of this chapter is to investigate and design of an IoT based system for detecting and controlling the COVID-19 inside the hospital environment. Proposed designs are highlighted to wearable sensors and mounted devices such as thermal cameras, sensors, mobile phones, and smart watches. Moreover, three major cases were identified and proposed a single solution for the detection and monitoring of COVID-19 patients. The proposed design is composed of identification of COVID-19 patients using thermal cameras, IoT solution for social distancing, and Chatbot consultation for the COVID-19 patients. This proposed design is suggested as a solid solution to prevent the spread of the novel COVID-19 virus.

References

1. Qiu, W., Rutherford, S., Mao, A., Chu, C.: The pandemic and its impacts. Health, Cult. Soc. **9**, 1–11 (2017)
2. Shereen, M., Khan, S., Kazmi, A., Bashir, N., Siddique, R.: COVID-19 infection: origin, transmission, and characteristics of human coronaviruses. J. Adv. Res. **24**, 91–98 (2020)
3. Punn, N., Sonbhadra, S. Agarwal, S.: COVID-19 epidemic analysis using machine learning and deep learning algorithms. MedRxiv, 1–10 (2020)
4. Brintnell, E., Gupta, M., Anderson, D.: Detailed phylogenetic analysis of SARS-CoV-2 reveals latent capacity to bind human ACE2 receptor. Biorxiv, 1–26 (2020)
5. Yadav, P., Katiyar, N.: A review Corona Virus (Covid-19): origin, history and transmission. Int. J. Pharmaceut. Sci. Health Care **5**(10), 1–7 (2020)

6. Who.int.: Coronavirus Disease (COVID-19) – World Health Organization. [online]. https://www.who.int. Accessed 20 July 2020
7. Kumar, D.: Corona Virus: a review of COVID-19. Eurasian J. Med. Oncol. **4**(1), 8–25 (2020)
8. Alansari, Z., Soomro, S., Belgaum, M., Shamshirband, S.: The Rise of Internet of Things (IoT) in Big healthcare data: review and open research issues. Adv. Intell. Syst. Comput., 675–685 (2017)
9. Abdul-Qawy, S., Pramod, J., Magesh, E., Srinivasulu, T.: The Internet of Things (IoT): an overview. Int. J. Eng. Res. Appl. **1**(5), 71–82 (2015)
10. Hassanalieragh, M., Page, A., Soyata, T., Sharma, G., Aktas, M., Mateos, G., Kantarci, B., Andreescu, S.: Health monitoring and management using Internet-of-Things (IoT) Sensing with Cloud-Based Processing: Opportunities and Challenges. 2015 IEEE International Conference on Services Computing, pp. 285–292 (2015)
11. Azzawi, M., Hassan, R., Bakar, K.: A review on Internet of Things (IoT) in healthcare. Int. J. Appl. Eng. Res. **11**(20), 10216–10221 (2020)
12. Singh, R., Javaid, M., Haleem, A., Suman, R.: Internet of Things (IoT) applications to fight against COVID-19 pandemic. Diabetes Metabol. Syndrome: Clin. Res. Rev. **14**(4), 521–524 (2020)
13. Farooq, M., Waseem, M., Mazhar, S., Khairi, A., Kamal, T.: A review on Internet of Things (IoT). Int. J. Comput. Appl. **113**(1), 1–7 (2015)
14. Kodali, R., Swamy, G. Lakshmi, B.: An implementation of IoT for healthcare. 2015 IEEE Recent Adv. Intell. Comput. Syst. (RAICS), **10**, 411–416 (2015)
15. Nazir, S., Ali, Y., Ullah, N., García-Magariño, I.: Internet of Things for healthcare using effects of mobile computing: a systematic literature review. Wirel. Commun. Mobile Comput. **2019**, 1–20 (2019)
16. Almotiri, S., Khan, M., Alghamdi, M.: Mobile Health (m-Health) system in the context of IoT. 2016 IEEE 4th International Conference on Future Internet of Things and Cloud Workshops (FiCloudW), pp. 39–42 (2016)
17. Karaca, Y., Moonis, M., Zhang, Y., Gezgez, C.: Mobile cloud computing based stroke healthcare system. Int. J. Inf. Manage. **45**, 250–261 (2019)
18. Nisha, N., Iqbal, M., Rifat, A., Idrish, S.: Mobile health services. Int. J. Asian Bus. Inf. Manage. **6**(1), 1–17 (2015)
19. Nandana, W., Mel, W., Priyankara, H.: Online remote laboratory for open distance learning. In: First International Conference on Open and Distance e-Learning. pp. 1–10 (2012)
20. Mohammed, M., Syamsudin, H., Al-Zubaidi, S., Sairah, A., Yusuf, E.: Novel COVID-19 detection and diagnosis system using IoT based smart helmet. Int. J. Psychosoc. Rehabil. **24**(7), 2296–2303 (2020)
21. Madhusanka, B., Sureswaran, R.: Implicit intention communication for activities of daily living of elder/disabled people to improve well-being. In: IoT in Healthcare and Ambient Assisted Living, pp. 1–20 (2020)
22. Madhusanka, B., Sureswaran, R.: Recognition of daily living activities using convolutional neural network based support vector machine. Int. J. Sci. Eng. Res. **11**(6), 526–528 (2020)
23. Ogbuabor, G., La, R.: Human activity recognition for healthcare using smartphones. In: Proceedings of the 2018 10th International Conference on Machine Learning and Computing - ICMLC 2018, pp. 1–6 (2018)
24. Lima, W., Souto, E., El-Khatib, K., Jalali, R., Gama, J.: Human activity recognition using inertial sensors in a smartphone: an overview. Sensors **19**(14), 3213 (2019)
25. Seifert, A., Schlomann, A., Rietz, C., Schelling, H.: The use of mobile devices for physical activity tracking in older adults' everyday life. Digit. Health **3**, 1–12 (2017)
26. Wang, R., Chen, F., Chen, Z., Li, T., Harari, G., Tignor, S., Zhou, X., Ben-Zeev, D., Campbell, A.: StudentLife: assessing mental health, academic performance and behavioral trends of college students using smartphones. In: Proceedings of the 2014 ACM International Joint Conference on Pervasive and Ubiquitous Computing, pp. 1–12 (2014)
27. Kurkute, S., Ahirao, N., Ankad, R., Khatal, V.: IoT Based smart system for the helmet detection. SSRN Electron. J., 1711–1716 (2019)

28. Yang, J., Pang, H., Zhang, X.: Enhanced mutual authentication Model of IoT. J. China Univ. Posts Telecommun. **20**, 69–74 (2013)
29. DSouza, D., Srivatsava, S., Sahana, R.: IoT based smart wheelchair for healthcare. Int. J. Recent Technol. Eng. **8**(2), 533–539 (2019)
30. Herath, K., Mel, W.: Electroencephalogram (EEG) controlled anatomical robot hand. In: The Open University of Sri Lanka, Proceedings of FET Student Academic Conference 2018. p. 73
31. Majumder, A., ElSaadany, Y., Young, R., Ucci, D.: An energy efficient wearable smart IoT system to predict cardiac arrest. Adv. Hum.-Comput. Interact. **2019**, 1–21 (2019)
32. Hinai, S., Singh, A.: Internet of Things: architecture, security challenges and solutions. In: 2017 International Conference on Infocom Technologies and Unmanned Systems (Trends and Future Directions) (ICTUS), pp. 1–4 (2017)
33. Antao, L., Pinto, R., Reis, J., Goncalves, G.: Requirements for testing and validating the Industrial Internet of Things. In: 2018 IEEE International Conference on Software Testing, Verification and Validation Workshops (ICSTW), pp. 110–115 (2018)
34. Zheng, X., Julien, C.: Verification and validation in cyber physical systems: research challenges and a way forward. In: 2015 IEEE/ACM 1st International Workshop on Software Engineering for Smart Cyber-Physical Systems, pp. 15–18 (2015)
35. Huremović, D.: Social distancing, quarantine, and isolation. Psychiatry Pandemics, 85–94 (2019)
36. Hernandez-Orallo, E., Manzoni, P., Calafate, C., Cano, J.: Evaluating how smartphone contact tracing technology can reduce the spread of infectious diseases: the case of COVID-19. IEEE Access **8**, 99083–99097 (2020)
37. Miner, A., Laranjo, L., Kocaballi, A.: Chatbots in the fight against the COVID-19 pandemic. NPJ Digit. Med. **3**(1), 1–4 (2020)

Modelling and Analysis the Population Density Effect on the Infectiousness Rate of COVID-19 Novel Virus and the Mortality Rate Percentage Regarding Oxford's Stringency Index Model of Governmental Response in MATLAB

Amira Mofreh Ibrahim, Nour El Hoda Mohamed Bishady, Samar Hassan Elghalban, Nagham Nessim Mostafa, Mohab Mohamed Eid, and Khaled Mohamed Abdelhamid

Abstract Numerical data on fifty pioneer adopting countries of Covid-19 novel pandemic has been put into study each on their first month of the virus's spread. Ten groups were created with each including the countries of around the same average population density. This was meant to study the difference between each group's growth of infected cases in addition to their mortality percentage rates (MPR). Modeling was done for each group with the use of MATLAB; for the growth rate, the exponential growth equation was considered, and for the mortality rate percentage, the equation was modeled over the span of the first chosen thirty days of the virus's spread. An analysis was done with the consideration of Oxford's Stringency Index Model (SIM) of government responses for each day in order to understand the effect of such taken regulations in the virus's spread and fatality for different groups of population densities. Eventually, it was found that population density is not a significant factor in the virus's infectiousness and mortality percentage rates; Instead, taking

A. M. Ibrahim · N. E. H. M. Bishady (✉) · S. H. Elghalban · N. N. Mostafa · M. M. Eid · K. M. Abdelhamid
School of Engineering and Applied Sciences, Nile University, Giza, Egypt
e-mail: no.saad@nu.edu.eg

A. M. Ibrahim
e-mail: amofreh@nu.edu.eg

S. H. Elghalban
e-mail: s.elghalban@nu.edu.eg

N. N. Mostafa
e-mail: n.nessim@nu.edu.eg

M. M. Eid
e-mail: moh.eid@nu.edu.eg

K. M. Abdelhamid
e-mail: k.abdelhamid@nu.edu.eg

D. Oliva et al. (eds.), *Artificial Intelligence for COVID-19*, Studies in Systems, Decision and Control 358, https://doi.org/10.1007/978-3-030-69744-0_25

governmental responses of appropriate stringencies is found to be the key solution for control and protection.

1 Introduction

This chapter aims to illustrate and diagnosis the growth of Covid-19 in sample of countries using numerical methods and Oxford's Stringency Index Model (SIM) which will make it easier for rest of the community to predict the behavior of viruses infection and help in decision making in such pandemic events.

Corona virus disease 2019 is one of Betacoronavirus species which is classified as one of the coronaviruses genres [1]. Coronavirus is a complex incased positive-strand RNA virus that affects the human respiratory system and has the ability of many hosts of species infection. COVID-19 can be transmitted from animals to human so, the regular interaction between huma jons and animals makes them a main zoonotic infection source. The first discovered COVID-19 patients were three adults Chinese bronchoalveolar-lavage cases from Wuhan [2]. Coronaviruses are large viruses' group that belongs to Nidovirales order that consists of Roniviridae, Arteriviridae, Coronaviridae, and Mesoniviridae families. The Coronaviridae family consists of two subfamilies, one of them is the Coronavirinae subfamily which includes beta, alpha, delta, and gamma genres. Betacoronavirus has 5 species MHV, BCoV, SARS-CoV, MERS-CoV [3]. So, to demonstrate, their structure will be illustrated more.

The six versions of the TGEV M^{pro} in the asymmetric unit of the crystal can be reformed into a well-defined electron density (Fig. 1), as it surrounds the 302 amino acid residues of each monomer. The difference between the five and six chains were the disappearance of the two C-terminals residues. There is also a leakage in electron density for residue 300 in monomers A, E and F [4].

The design contains 1798 amino acid residues and 1006 water molecules, as well as 27 sulfate ions, nine dioxane molecules and six 2-methyl-2, 4-pentanediol (MPD) molecules from the crystallization medium. The sophistication joined to a final R-factor of 0.210 and an R_{free} [5] of 0.256, with good stereochemistry. The most ideal areas of Ramachandran plot are where 88.4% of the amino acid residues, and 10.8% is in allowing regions. Residues Asn70, Asn71 and Ser279 were in regions only generously allowed, but had a clear electron density. After discussing the structure, which is interested in microscopic level of the virus, the symptoms of the virus will be posited.

It takes an average of 5.2 days of the appearance of COVID-19 symptoms which represents the incubation period of the virus [6]. The virus appears for 14 days on average with a range of 6 to 41 days, including the incubation period, the symptom appearance and the attacking of the immune system which leads to virus death [7]. This period varies according to patient age and his immune system status [7]. COVID-19 can be detected according to following symptoms are fever, cough, and fatigue, while other symptoms include sputum production, headache, haemoptysis, diarrhoea, dyspnoea, and lymphopenia [7–10]. The examination, which based on

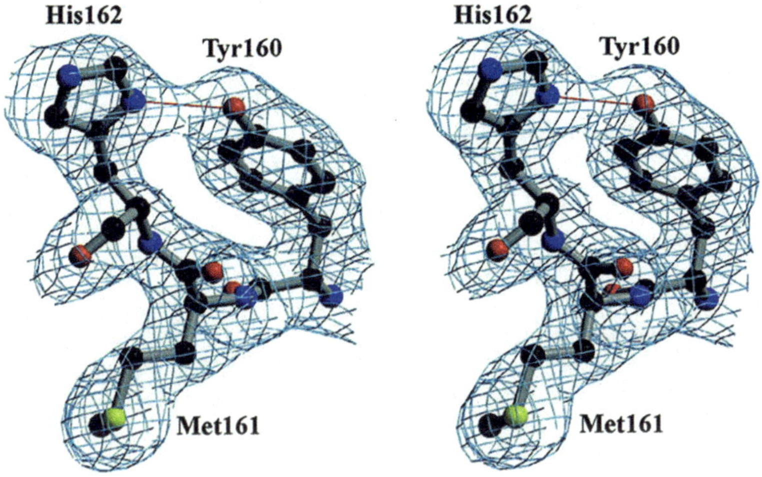

Fig. 1 Stereo view of a representative part of the electron density map. The $2|F_o| - |F_c|$ electron density map (1.96 Å resolution, contoured at 1σ above the mean) corresponds to M^{pro} residues 160–162 (Tyr–Met–His), a conserved motif in coronavirus main proteinases. The strong hydrogen bonding interaction between the Tyr160 hydroxyl group and His162 $N^{\delta 1}$ is indicated [4]

chest CT scan presents the virus as pneumonia, although it has abnormal characteristics such as RNAaemia, acute respiratory distress syndrome, acute cardiac injury, and incidence of ground-glass opacities that led to death [9]. For some patients, the multiple peripheral ground-glass opacities are appearing in subpleural regions of both lungs [11] which leads to both systemic and localized immune response that cause the increased inflammation. Unfortunately, there is no medical improvement of some causes using interferon inhalation, in the other side, the condition of the patient become worse by developing pulmonary opacities [11] (Fig. 2). Next, the history of these symptoms will be discussed to know the origins of coronavirus.

The first characteristic of coronavirus case was in the 1960 s, as in 1965 Tyrrell and Bynoe have discovered a virus called B814 in the embryonic tracheal organ of an adult respiratory tract. Hamre and Procknow have grown a virus named 229E that has infrequent properties in the tissue culture. Other viruses were discovered later on that had the same properties, so they were added to a new group of viruses called coronavirus. In 2002–2003, SARS virus has appeared in southern China affecting the human respiratory system. In 2004, another virus called NL63 was discovered in the Netherlands. HCoV-NH virus has appeared in Newhaven, 2005 [12]. In Saudi Arabia, a virus termed as MERS has appeared in the year 2012. Finally, a new outbreak of the respiratory system in Wuhan, 2019 that caused by COVID-19 coronavirus [13] (Fig. 3).

The chapter will discuss the previous work in this field and describe how scientific community deals with Covid-19 as a pandemic, then the methodology of growth prediction will be illustrated in 2 parts (SIM and growth prediction based on population density) which both depends on numerical methods. After that, the results and

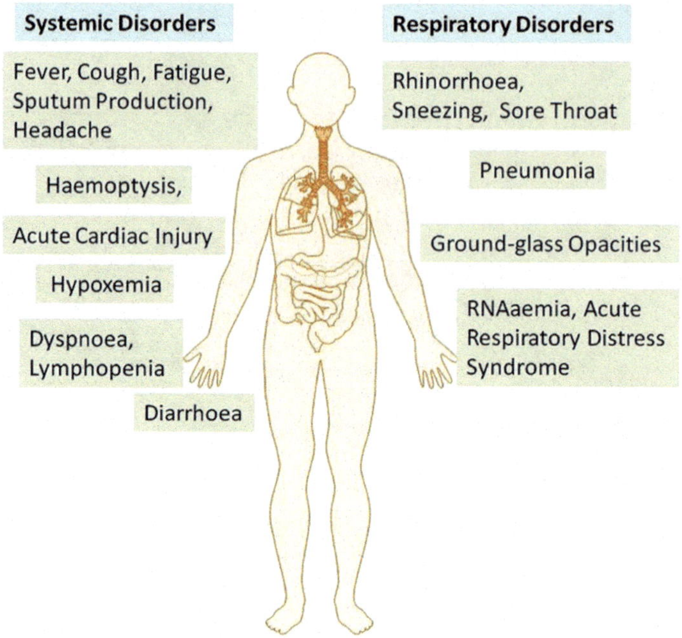

Fig. 2 The systemic and respiratory disorders caused by COVID-19 infection [11]

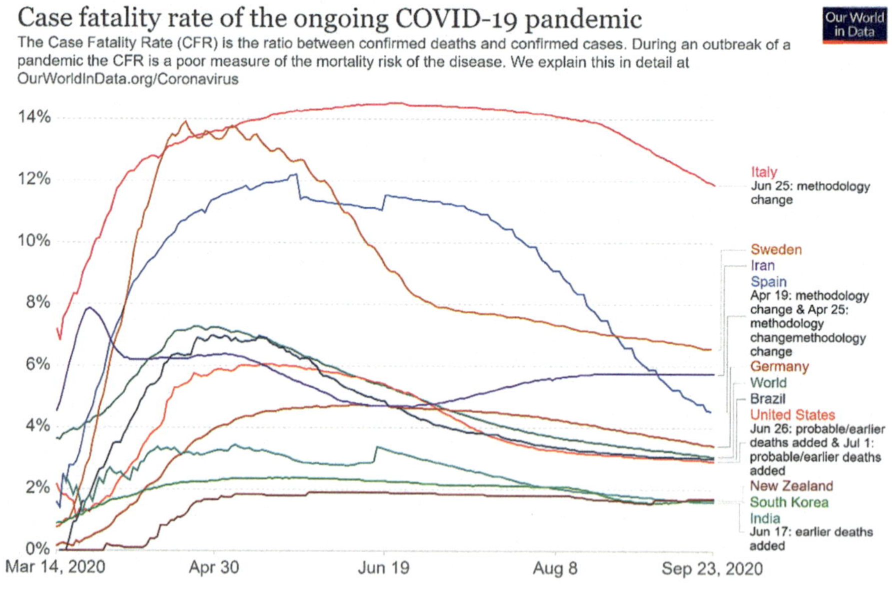

Fig. 3 Shows CFR of COVID-19

observation will be presented visually and by mathematical models for each country. Finally, the conclusion will summarize the results to be used in decision making if there is another such event occurs.

2 Literature Review

This chapter focuses on the argument that Covid-19 initial spread is significantly affected by the population densities of adopting countries. This Thesis has been proven for multiple diseases before, such as for a measles epidemic [14] and Diphtheria [15]. However, some recent papers have shown a relation between population density and Covid-19 such as the work of K. T. L. Sy, L. F. White, and B. E. Nichols in which an association between population density and the basic reproductive number of COVID-19 has been shown. After doing a cross-sectional analysis and with the usage of linear mixed models, fixed slopes and random interceptions, their paper concluded that when the population density is high, the interaction between infectious and susceptible individuals is potentially high and causationally the spread of the virus [16]. Dave Babbitt Patrick Garland and Oliver Johnson also investigated the relation using a new model of population density distribution which they called "the lived population density" [17] Their work was a continuity of the detailed distribution and organizational model adopted by Hasan Samdani and his team in 2014 which shows a slight effect of population density only for groups living in dynamic crowded areas in a country [18].

In contrary, some other papers found that higher population densities can aid in controlling covid-19 such as the work shown by Shang and Wahba [19]. However, their conclusion might not be generalized worldwide as it was noticed that their argument was based on a wealthy sample of dense-in-population countries which made them more privileged in providing enough sources to bear with the epidemic. By the same token, and as demonstrated by Desai [20], countries with high population densities are completely capable of controlling Covid-19 as shown with China, Singapore and South Korea.

Given the above findings and due to the contradictions featured when reviewing the literature of the population density factor, It became a motive for us to represent a recent study of the population density effect on the first month of Covid-19 spread with the usage of MATLAB curve fitting, exponential growth equation and for the first time, the stringency index model. The stringency index model is a systematic cross-national, cross-temporal measure [21] that evaluates the government responses taken each day since the emergence of the novel coronavirus and its data will be used in this chapter as an input for our analysis. In brief, this chapter tries to further investigate the hypothesis that the larger the population density of a country is, the more difficult it becomes to control the virus's initial spread and the stricter the government response should be.

Calculation of severity rate or mortality rate of COVID-19 has been difficult for the World Health Organization (WHO). Countries showed broad variations in estimations of their case fatality rate (CFR) which may be misleading. Fatality rate of the virus is important to be calculated since it helps identifying the at-risk populations, understand the severity, and reevaluate the healthcare system quality. Doing so, WHO used two measures, the infection fatality rate (IFR) and CFR [22].

On the timeline between January 22nd and September 23rd, more than 30 million cases were confirmed of having corona virus. On the other hand, there were around 1 million deaths. The sudden and fast break out of the virus began after March 3rd, when the exponential curve began to gain its shape. After this date, cases were confirmed to be thousands per day and in some countries, tens of thousands.

The first, IFR, estimates the proportion of total deaths of only the infected individuals. The other, CFR, estimates the proportion of deaths of only identified and confirmed cases; their equations can be found below [22]:

$$IFR(in\%) = \frac{Totaldeaths}{Totalinfected} \times 100 \quad (1)$$

$$CFR(in\%) = \frac{Totaldeaths}{Totalconfirmedcases} \times 100 \quad (2)$$

During the early outbreak, studies tend to concentrate of those symptomatic patients while asymptomatic cases are not that likely to be detected, thus it leads to an overestimation of the CFR which decreases as active case findings increase. On the other hand, during the ongoing epidemic itself, active cases may encounter deaths leading to underestimation of the CFR, so a modified equation is used to calculate the CFR during the ongoing epidemic, and it can be found below [22]:

$$CFR(in\%) = \frac{Totaldeaths}{Deathsfromdisease + Recoveredfromdisease} \times 100 \quad (3)$$

An updated CFR graph demonstrated by the European CDC could show the history of the virus and how it affects the populations, and it is shown below:

An often confusion is the difference between the CFR and the crude mortality rate. The crude mortality rate is sometimes called the crude death rate as it measures the probability of any individual in the population might die from the disease [2]. Its equation can be found below:

$$Crudemortalityrate = \frac{Totaldeaths}{Totalpopulation} \times 100 \quad (4)$$

To differentiate between the CFR of COVID-19 and other outbreaks, one should be aware of the measurements taken to interpret and estimates the CFR, so the below table is to compare COVID-19 CFR with other diseases like MERS-COV and seasonal flu [23] (Table 1).

Some studies used a different approach to estimate the mortality rate. One is called Patient Information Based Algorithm (PIBA). It will predict death rates in the near

Table 1 Shows a comparison between the CFR of different diseases

Disease	Estimated case fatality rate (CFR)
SARS-CoV	10% [24, 25]
MERS-CoV	34% [25]
Seasonal flu (US)	0.1 to 0.2% [26]
Ebola	50%, 40% in the 2013-16 outbreak [27, 28]

future based on real-time data, meaning that it uses patients' data in the early stages of the disease to count the average number of being hospitalized until death.

PIBA calculation uses a number of deaths per a given day and divide it by the number of possible patients on the same day the patients have just showed symptoms of the disease. It is considered one the most reliable way to calculate the mortality rate since it uses the actual number of deaths and patients on specific dates.

Steps to calculate the mortality rate using PIBA can be summarized as follows [29]:

First: patient's data from the initial admission to a hospital must be gathered.

Second: calculate the average number of days of hospitalization till death.

Third: calculate two standard deviation intervals.

Fourth: use the previous parameters to calculate the mortality rate per day.

Fifth: prediction of mortality of the disease in the near future, then these numbers is compared to real mortality for testing and collecting the correct model data.

Sixth: modification of data takes place.

3 Methodology

The methodology and process of the chapter aims to reach and model the relation between the growth of Covid-19 in the scale of the first thirty days of adopting the epidemic and the PD (population density) in a sample of countries. The data has been collected from the world bank website [30] and the United Nations population and Vital Statistics Report that has been accessed in mid-April 2020 [31] This chapter was developed using multiple stages which are as follows:

3.1 Choosing the Countries that Will Be Suitable as Dataset for the Research

The dataset filtration proceeded during April 2020, so the following method depends on the data provided during this period. The top 50 countries with high Covid-19 infection have been selected for this study, excluding Singapore only due to its high PD (8358/km^2) Which may lead to an outlet and affect the models negatively. The countries have been divided into 10 sectors, according to their intervals of PD (3 to 16, 17 to 26, 45 to 51, 57 to 72, 79 to 99, 102 to 111, 118 to 136, 144 to 223, 235 to 301, 320 to 512) p/km^2. Each sector contains 4-6 countries, according to the previous interval.

3.2 Recording the Growth of Covid-19 Cases in Each Country

The procedure was implemented to reduce error as much as possible. The data started to be recorded after the day that the country hit 20 Covid-19 cases or above; to avoid the ignorance of governments that may lead an error in data. To plot a graph for every sector, data gathered from day 1 to day 30 in each country in the dataset. And it has been plotted in the sectors with the countries in the same interval.

3.3 Curve Fitting for Each Country Plotted Points

A graph is created by MATLAB for each sector containing from 4 to 6 fitted curves as every country has a fitted curve. An excel file is created for each sector, in which the file includes the everyday growth of each country in the sector. In each graph an excel file is imported then the data of each country in the excel file imported independently, so that the growth and the days saved as column vectors in the MATLAB. After that a code is written to make a curve fitting to each country in the graph, then the fitted curves start to be plotted on the same graph. The curve fitting is done according to an exponential equation:

$$y = ae^{bx} \tag{5}$$

where 'a' is the graduation rate in growth and 'b' is the flattening rate of the curve. The exponential growth function is chosen to represent the growth of COVID-19. Exponential growth defined as increasing the quantity with a proportional rate to its current size grows exponentially, and that represents the way of COVID-19 growth as it spreads continuously as people meet each other's as the infected people will infect others, so that people are infected with proportional rate to the size of the infected people, which makes an exponential growth, and here's a link for the MATLAB codes.

3.4 The Classification of the Stringency Index Model Rates

According to work of Oxford Covid-19 Government response tracker team [21], The stringency index model is based on the eight containment and closure indicators (C1:C8) besides a sole Health index; The public health awareness campaigns (H1).

The stringency index model rating is system composes of 100 ranks, 100 being the strictest and 0 for no measurements taken at all. We take in our analysis is (100:90) for extremely strict measurements, (90:70) for stronger regulations, (70:50) as upper intermediate responses and (60:40) as moderate ones and anything beyond 40 is considered unrestrained.

3.5 Mortality Rate Calculation

The mortality rate calculation is very important as it is considered as an indicator for the disease if it is risky that could cause a pandemic and be a public concern [29]. In this chapter, the mortality rate is calculated according to the classical death rate calculation. The mortality rate was calculated for each country along the 30 days using the mortality equation:

$$mortalityrate = \frac{numberoftotaldeaths}{numberoftotalcases} \tag{6}$$

Then, the mortality percentage was calculated using the mortality percentage equation:

$$mortalityrate = \frac{numberoftotaldeaths}{numberoftotalcases} \times 100 \tag{7}$$

The two equations were added in new two columns in the 10 excel sheets that contains the countries groups data to calculate the mortality of each country along the specified 30 days, so that each excel sheet contains the total number of cases, population density, new deaths, population, total number of deaths, stringency index, days, mortality rate, and mortality percentage to facilitate the modeling, plotting, and analysis.

3.6 Plotting the Mortality Rate Per Day

Ten graphs were created using the MATLAB plotting tool, each graph contains from 4 to 6 curves as the countries are distributed according to their population densities. The number of deaths per day was collected from [32], then the data required, which is the deaths of the first 30 days of having 20 COVID-19 cases in the chosen 53 countries were added in 10 excel sheets in which every excel sheet contains from 4 to 6 countries according to the population density, then the mortality rate was calculated by Eq. (6) in the excel sheet. A MATLAB code was created to plot the mortality rate in each country per day, where the x-axis of the graphs represents the days and the y-axis represents the mortality rate. The mortality rate per day in each country were imported from the excel sheet to the MATLAB as a column vector, after every plotted curve the plotting is hanged on to add the data for plotting another curve in the same graph.

4 Results and Discussion

Proposed hypothesis

The larger the population density of a country is, the more difficult it becomes to control the virus's initial spread, the more fatal the first month's effect is and the stricter the government response should be.

4.1 Group One: Average Population Density of (4) PD/ km^2 (Canada, Australia, Saudi Arabia, Finland, Argentina, Russia)

As shown in Figs. 4 and 5, Australia follows our theory for being the country with the least population density and shows the most flattened curve; however, its mortality rate percentage is one of the highest in this group. We can also see that Saudi Arabia, Finland and Argentina have the same population density; however, Finland, shows the most flattened curve of them all and the rest to show the same graduation of growth though differ in MRP which Argentina soared the most in. Moreover, Russia

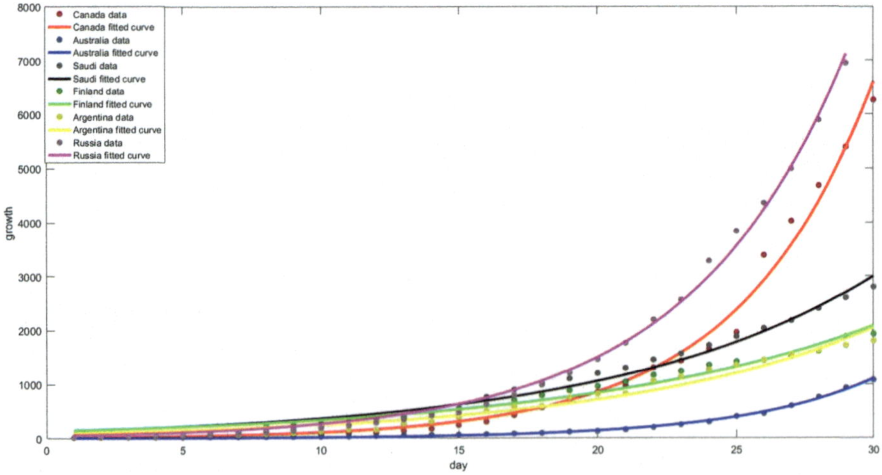

Fig. 4 Shows the daily growth of infected cases over the first month of spread for the first group

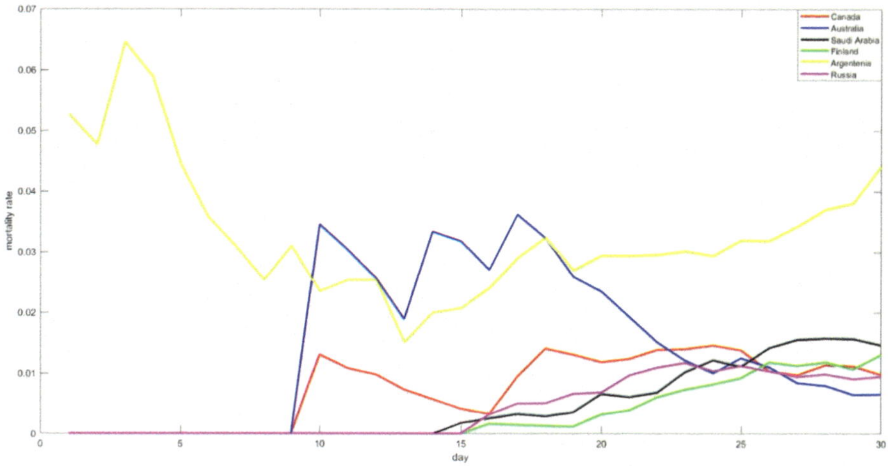

Fig. 5 Shows the mortality rate over the first month of spread for the first group

Table 2 Data of the first group

Country	Population density	Equation = $(A)e^{(B)x}$	Mortality rate percentage (MRP)	Stringency index
Canada	4	$(342)e^{(1.797)x}$	[0.3, 1.45]	[2.78, 72.69]
Australia	3	$(55.71)e^{(1.81)x}$	[0.64, 3.4]	[19.44, 44.44]
Saudi Arabia	16	$(662)e^{(0.9169)x}$	[0.18, 1.57]	[30.56, 91.67]
Finland	16	$(560.2)e^{(0.797)x}$	[0.11, 1.29]	[19.44, 60.19]
Argentina	16	$(448.9)e^{(0.9187)x}$	[1.5, 6.4]	[25, 100]
Russia	9	$(632.2)e^{(1.471)x}$	[0.3, 1.17]	[31.94, 85.19]

in this group is the most recorder of cases and shows a high mortality rate percentage, although not being the highest in population density. 80% C (Table 2).

4.2 *Group Two: Average Population Density of (4) PD/ km^2 (Brazil, Norway, Sweden, Peru, Chile)*

As shown in Figs. 6 and 7, Although Brazil and Chile have the same population density, Brazil shows a higher growth and mortality rate. In contrast to our theory, Peru; the densest country in population shows a controlled approach in handling the pandemic; however, its mortality rate reached the highest in this group which confidently can be put over its weak stringency index rate. Norway and Sweden on the other hand are showing a similar predicted peak point in Fig. 7, though Norway, the country with the least population density, shows a less flattening tendency. A very

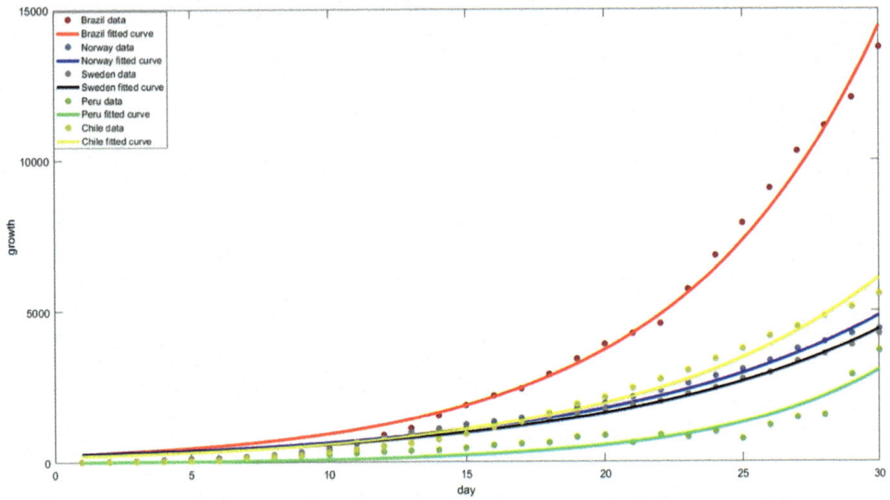

Fig. 6 Shows the daily growth of infected cases over the first month of spread for the second group

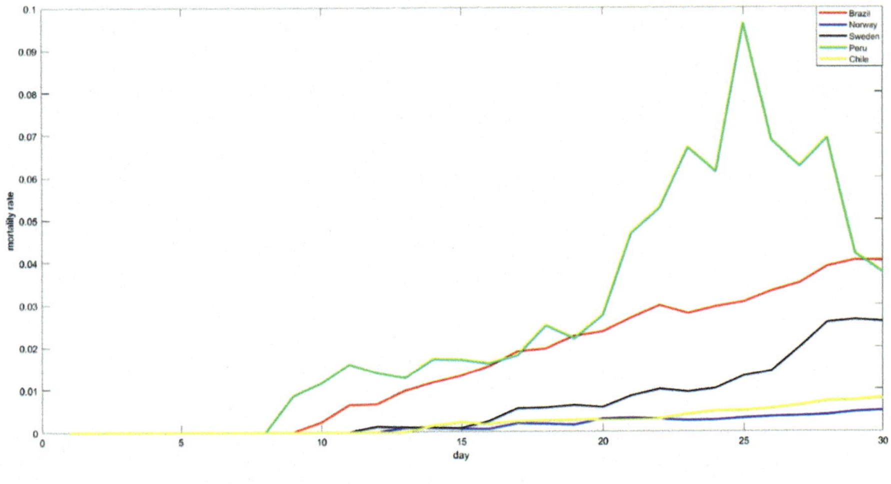

Fig. 7 Shows the mortality rate over the first month of spread for the second group

interesting tendency was found in this group which is Norway and Chile, countries with the least and largest population tendencies showed an almost identical mortality rate percentage and followed the same strong stringency index rates. 60% C (Table 3).

Table 3 Data of the second group

Country	Population density	Equation = $(A)e^{(B)x}$	Mortality rate percentage (MRP)	Stringency index
Brazil	25	$(2020)e^{(1.194)x}$	[0.2, 4.03]	[11.11, 74.54]
Norway	17	$(1147)e^{(0.8757)x}$	[0.1, 0.4]	[11.11, 79.63]
Sweden	22	$(1035)e^{(0.8777)x}$	[0.08, 2.63]	[11.11, 35.19]
Peru	26	$(264.4)e^{(1.486)x}$	[0.86, 9.86]	[44.44, 94,44]
Chile	25	$(1152)e^{(1.009)x}$	[0.13, 0.775]	[11.11, 73.15]

4.3 *Group Three: Average Population Density of (49) PD/km^2 (Iran, Belarus, Colombia, South Africa)*

As shown in Figs. 8 and 9, Iran fulfills our theory in being the country with the densest population, the highest spread rate and MRP. This might be the caused by the weak governmental response taken in this country, according to its stringency index model. Moreover, a very notable trend is found in Belarus, that though its stringency index rate is the weakest in the group, it has the most flattened growth curve and a very low mortality rate that started high but kept decreasing. On the other hand, Colombia being the least populated country in the group shows a very flattened growth curve and moderately low MRP although the country's stringency index rate is the strictest in the group. 80% C (Table 4).

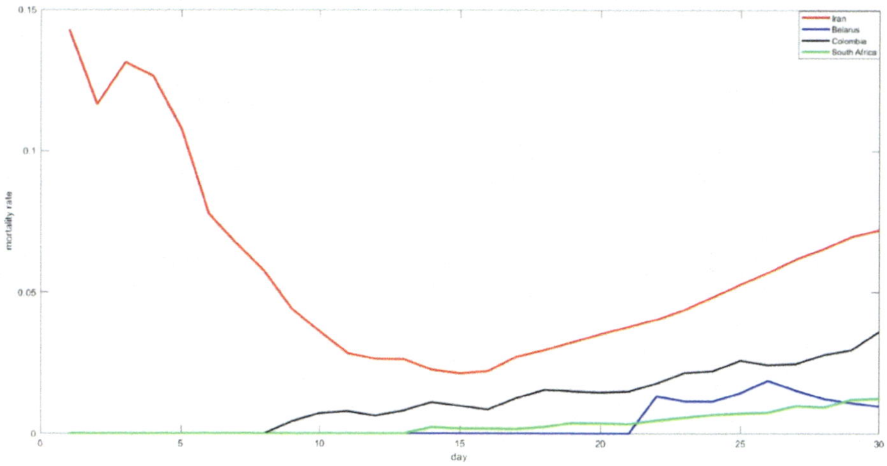

Fig. 8 Shows the daily growth of infected cases over the first month of spread for the third group

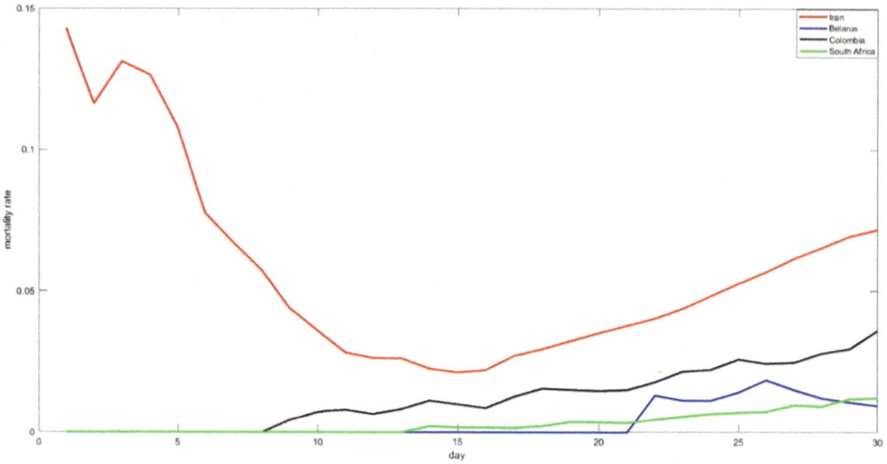

Fig. 9 Shows the mortality rate over the first month of spread for the third group

Table 4 Growth data and population of third group

Country	Population density	Equation $= (A)e^{(B)x}$	Mortality rate percentage (MRP)	Stringency index
Iran	51	$(5647)e^{(0.8894)x}$	[2.1, 14.285]	[11.11, 57.41]
Belarus	46	$(51.53)e^{(2.195)x}$	[0.95, 1.86]	[8.33, 19.44]
Colombia	45	$(654.6)e^{(0.9242)x}$	[0.43, 3.602]	[34.26, 87.96]
South Africa	49	$(792.9)e^{(0.6476)x}$	[0.15, 1.23]	[13.89, 87.96]

4.4 Group Four: Average Population Density of (66) PD/ km^2 (Mexico, Panama, Ukraine, Ireland, Ecuador)

As shown in Figs. 10 and 11, Contradicting our theory, Ecuador being the second least dense country in the group, it shows the most peaking curve in both the cases growth and the MRP graphs. What makes this case questionable is when looking to the country's stringency model, we see that it has been following a very good range of regulations. In the other hand, Panama is following our theory, as being the least dense country did it well in handling the pandemic that it showed the most flattened curve in growth and a very low range in MRP. Supportingly, the country adopted very strict regulations that its stringency index scored considerably high rates. Furthermore, Ukraine being the densest country of this group shows the hit the highest MRP and followed the strictest national regulations as our theory suggested. The country also scored the third in cases which also support the thesis prediction. 95% C (Table 5, Fig. 12).

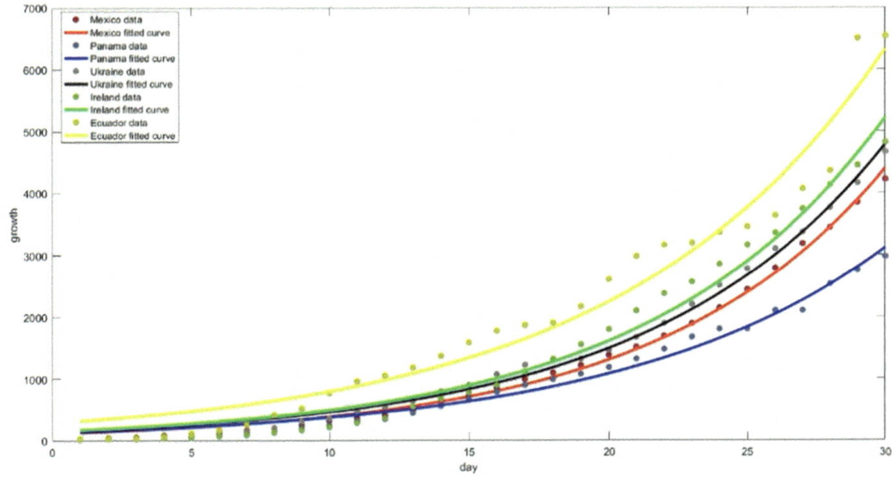

Fig. 10 Shows the daily growth of infected cases over the first month of spread for the fourth group

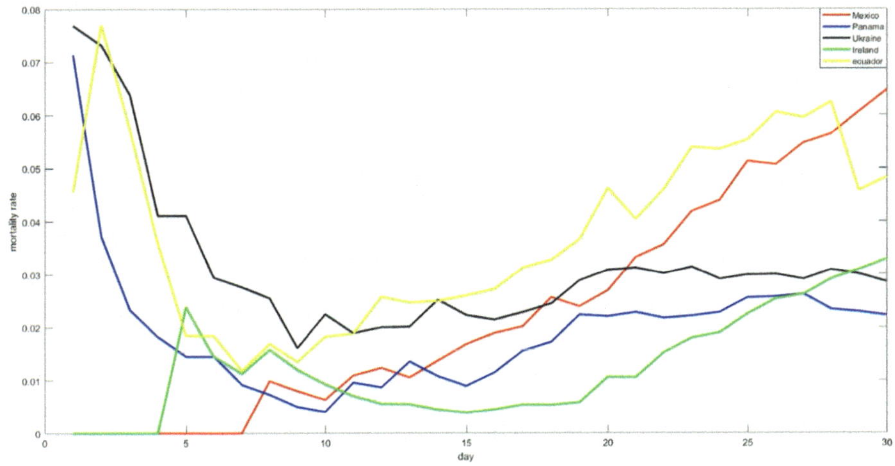

Fig. 11 Shows the mortality rate over the first month of spread for the fourth group

Table 5 Data of third group

Country	Population density	Equation = $(A)e^{(B)x}$	Mortality rate percentage (MRP)	Stringency index
Mexico	66	$(754.1)e^{(1.069)x}$	[2.78, 82.41]	[0.63, 6.5]
Panama	57	$(670.2)e^{(0.9323)x}$	[0.41, 2.57]	[19.44, 90.74]
Ukraine	72	$(885.3)e^{(1.024)x}$	[1.61, 7.69]	[88.89, 92.59]
Ireland	70	$(946.2)e^{(1.036)x}$	[0.38, 3.28]	[11.11, 90.74]
Ecuador	64	$(1403)e^{(0.9187)x}$	[1.17, 6.24]	[36.11, 93.52]

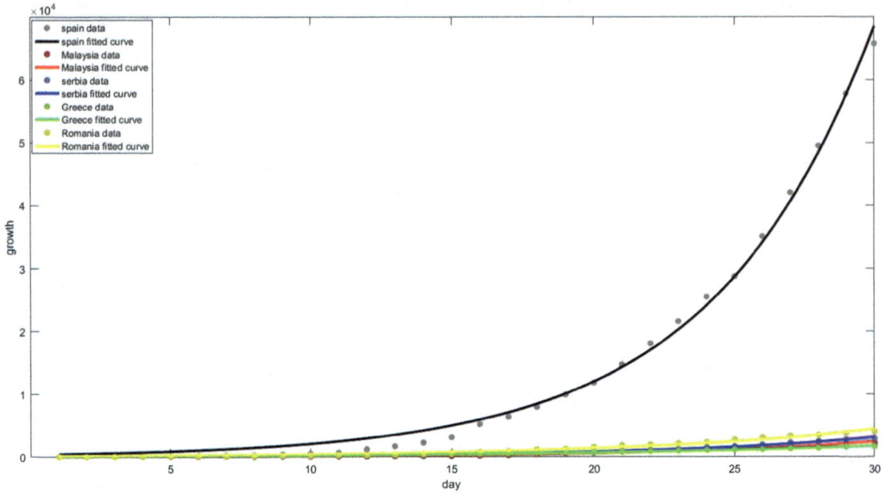

Fig. 12 Shows the daily growth of infected cases over the first month of spread for the fifth group

4.5 Group Five: Average Population Density of (81) PD/ km² *(Spain, Malaysia, Serbia, Greece, Romania)*

As shown in Fig. 13, In different with our theory, Although Spain is not the densest country in the group, that did not help in flattening its growth curve nor securing it a low MRP range. Spain's stringency index rate was quite moderate; thus its outbreak could not be justified due to weak regulations. Contradicting our thesis,

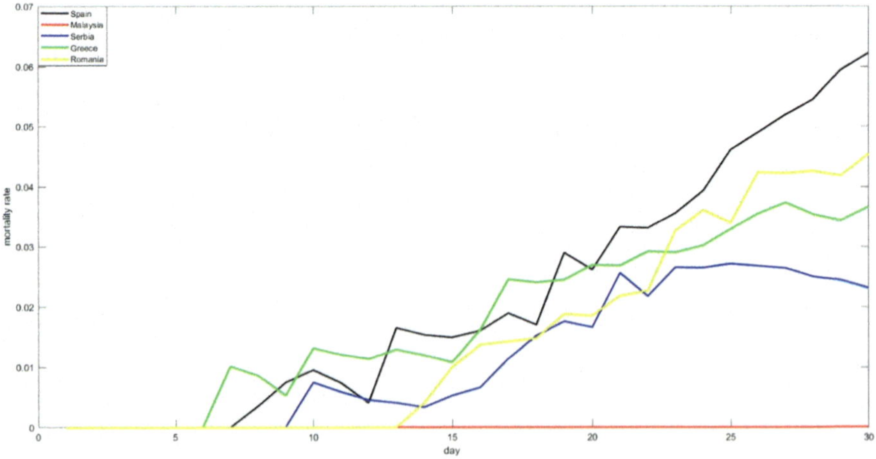

Fig. 13 Shows the mortality rate over the first month of spread for the fifth group

Table 6 Data of fifth group

Country	Population density	Equation = $(A)e^{(B)x}$	Mortality rate percentage (MRP)	Stringency index
Spain	92	$(5489)e^{(1.532)x}$	[0.35, 6.2]	[11.11, 71.76]
Malaysia	98	$(329.1)e^{(1.197)x}$	0	[19.44, 31.48]
Serbia	99	$(438.7)e^{(1.184)x}$	[0.33, 2.71]	[25, 100]
Greece	79	$(457.4)e^{(0.8079)x}$	[0.52, 3.729]	[28.7, 84.26]
Romania	81	$(829.1)e^{(1.018)x}$	[0.4, 4.53]	[36.11, 87.04]

Serbia showed the most flattened curve in growth and scored the lowest range in MRP despite being the densest country in the group and regardless of following a strong range of regulations as shown in its stringency index model rates. On the other hand, Greece being the least dense country here showed a quite controlled growth graph; however, a soaring MRP. A last interesting observation found here is that despite being one of the highest in PD in this group, Malaysia showed a zero-mortality rate along the month of our investigation 0% C (Table 6).

4.6 Group Six: Average Population Density of (107) PD/ km^2 (Turkey, Egypt, Portugal, Austria)

As shown in Figs. 14 and 15, Confirming our theory, Turkey being the most populated country showed a tremendous increase in its growth-rate curve; however, the country

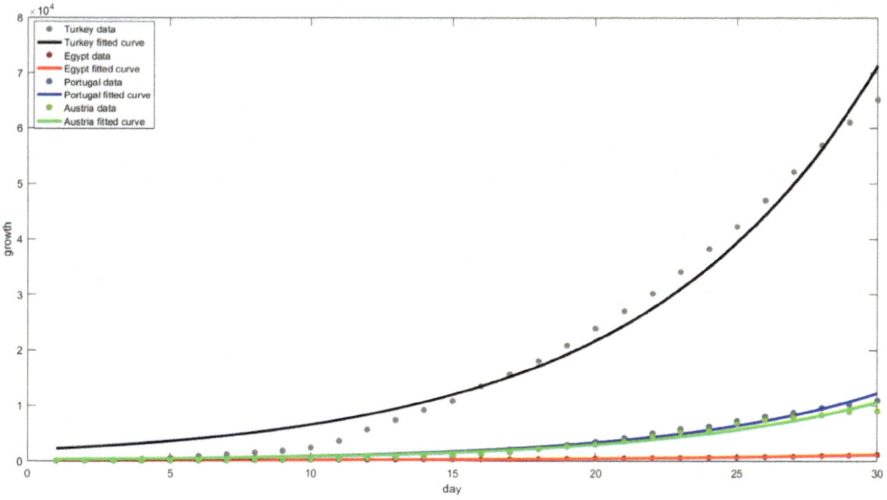

Fig. 14 Shows the daily growth of infected cases over the first month of spread for the sixth group

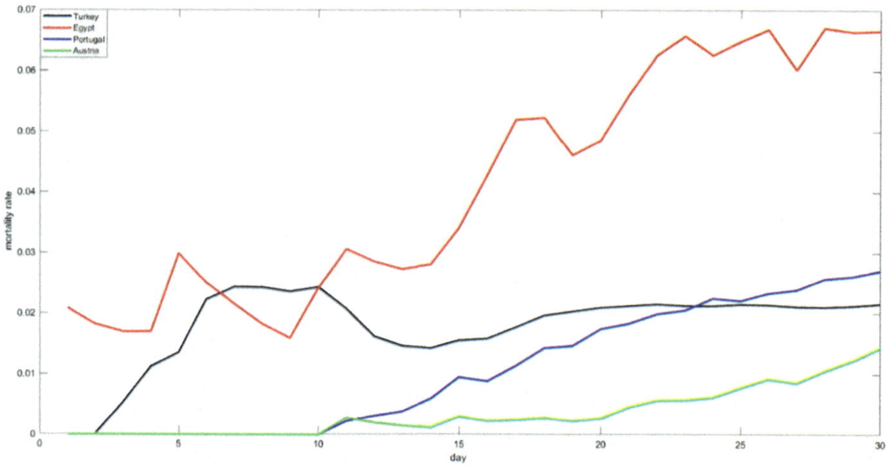

Fig. 15 Shows the mortality rate over the first month of spread for the sixth group

did not show the most severe MRP range and followed a considerably strict stringency index approach. In the other hand, Portugal being the country with the least populated cases showed a very moderate growth in confirmed cases, followed a very strict stringency index model and, in favor to our theory, scored the second least in MRP which Austria, one of the densest country of the group, scored the least in. A very interesting observation can be also seen in Egypt as being the least populated country didn't prevent it from contradicting our theory in reaching the highest MRP range despite showing a mild and obviously linear increase in growth rate. What is more interesting is that Egypt followed a very strict stringency index model which raises skepticism that the country only reported death cases of the virus. 80% C except for Egypt (Table 7).

Table 7 Data of group six

Country	Population density	Equation $= (\boldsymbol{A})\boldsymbol{e}^{(\boldsymbol{B})\boldsymbol{x}}$	Mortality rate percentage (MRP)	Stringency index
Turkey	108	$(1.273e+04)e^{(1.046)x}$	[0.5, 2.15]	[52.78, 75.93]
Egypt	102	$(297)e^{(0.8374)x}$	[1.69, 6.7]	[11.11, 84.26]
Portugal	111	$(1869)e^{(1.138)x}$	[0.22, 2.7]	[11.11, 82.41]
Austria	107	$(1688)e^{(1.112)x}$	[0.11, 1.42]	[11.11, 85.19]

4.7 Group Seven: Average Population Density of (127) PD/km² (Denmark, Czechia, Thailand, France, UAE, Poland)

As shown in Figs. 16 and 17, In extreme contrary to our theory, France is one of the two least in population density played the outlet of this group; it showed a soaring increase in cases and the highest range in MRP despite the fact of following very strict stringency index approach. On the contrary, although UAE and France possess the

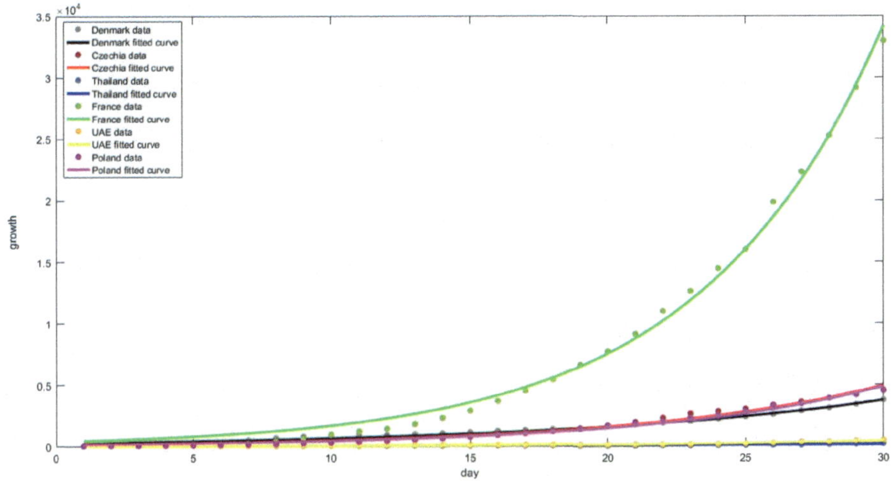

Fig. 16 Shows the daily growth of infected cases over the first month of spread for the seventh group

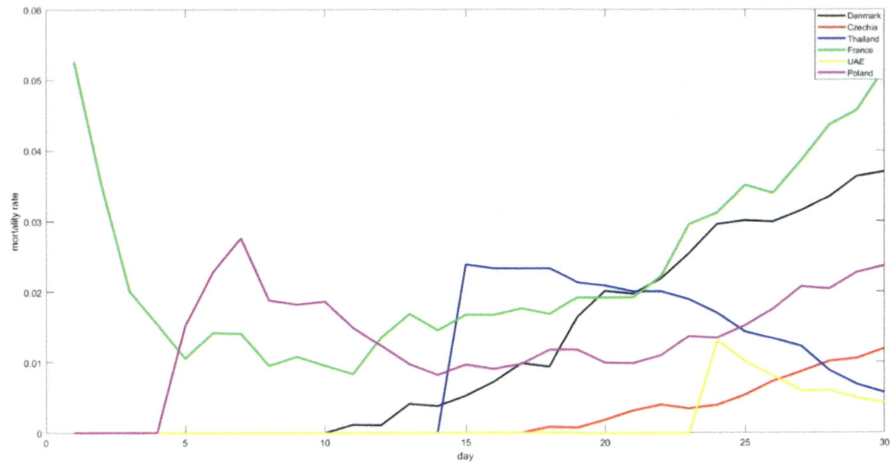

Fig. 17 Shows the mortality rate over the first month of spread for the seventh group

Table 8 Data of group seven

Country	Population density	Equation = $(A)e^{(B)x}$	Mortality rate percentage (MRP)	Stringency index
Denmark	134	$(1070)e^{(0.7589)x}$	[0.11, 3.69]	[25.93, 72.22]
Czech	136	$(941)e^{(1.003)x}$	[0.07, 1.185]	[19.44, 82.41]
Thailand	136	$(42.57)e^{(0.6729)x}$	[0.56, 2.38]	[16.67, 52.31]
France	118	$(3811)e^{(1.332)x}$	[0.83, 5.26]	[16.67, 90.74]
UAE	118	$(70.34)e^{(1.115)x}$	[0.42, 1.3]	[8.33, 84.26]
Poland	121	$(856.6)e^{(1.052)x}$	[0.81, 2.7]	[13.89, 81.48]

same PD, UAE perfectly followed our theory by showing the most flattened growth of cases, the least MRP range; however, followed a strong lockdown policy. On the other hand, Thailand, and Check, being the highest in PD, showed very controlled growth curves, considerably mild MRP ranges and followed moderate regulation in stringency. 40% C only UAE followed our theory (Table 8).

4.8 Group Eight: Average Population Density of (185) PD/km^2 (Italy, China, Switzerland, Indonesia, Dominican Republic)

As shown in Figs. 18 and 19, In contrary to our theory, Indonesia, the least populated country of the group, showed the most range of MRP in the group. And what is

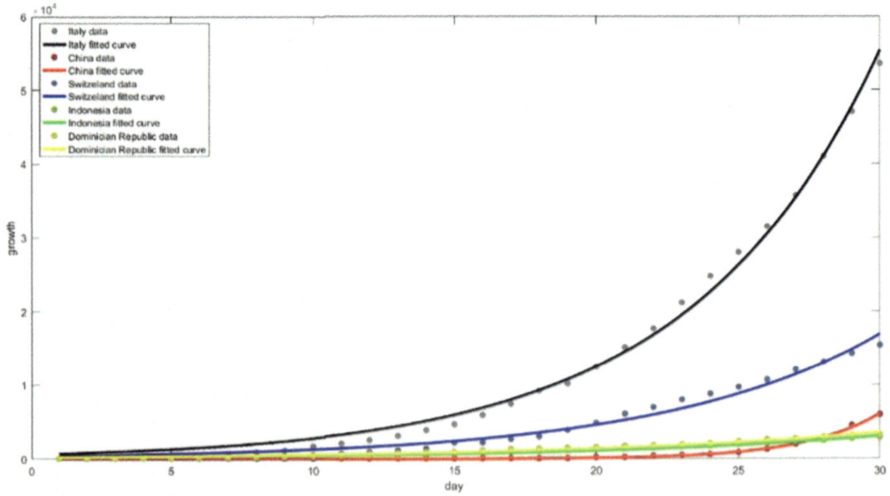

Fig. 18 Shows the daily growth of infected cases over the first month of spread for the eighth group

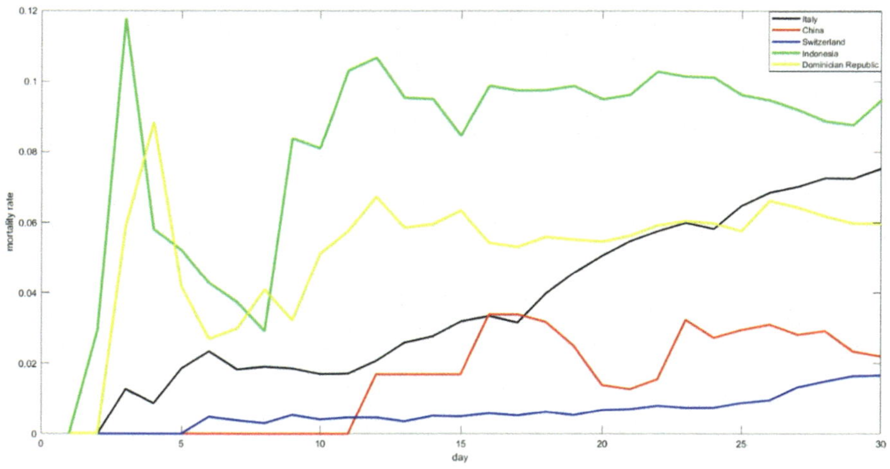

Fig. 19 Shows the mortality rate over the first month of spread for the eighth group

more interesting is that Indonesia replicated the same growth trend of the Dominican Republic even though the least is the densest country in group eight. However, when looking to both countries stringency index ranges, it is obvious that Indonesia's high mortality rate can be caused by the country's quite weak regulations being followed. Moreover, the Dominican Republic followed the strictest approach in SIM which can be the reason for its controlled spread and MRP. Italy on the other hand played the outlet of the group despite possessing a moderate PD. It also showed a high range in MRP and followed the strongest SIM in the group; However, that did not help in maintaining the country a controlled adoption of the virus in its first month of spread. 50% C, following the correct stringency model helps in controlling any spread (Table 9).

Table 9 Data of group eight

Country	Population density (PD)	Equation = $(\boldsymbol{A})e^{(\boldsymbol{B})x}$	Mortality rate percentage (MRP)	Stringency index model (SIM)
Italy	201	$(6360)e^{(1.314)x}$	[0.87, 7.52]	[27.78, 91.67]
China	148	$(28.5)e^{(3.259)x}$	[1.27, 3.23]	[2.78, 69.91]
Switzerland	210	$(2580)e^{(1.141)x}$	[0.3, 1.66]	[19.44, 73.15]
Indonesia	144	$(718.6)e^{(0.8916)x}$	[2.94, 11.76]	[37.04, 71.76]
Dominican Republic	223	$(923.8)e^{(0.8279)x}$	[2.67, 6.71]	[70.37, 89.81]

4.9 Group Nine: Average Population Density of (185) PD/km^2 (USA, UK, Qatar, Luxembourg, Germany, Pakistan)

As shown in Figs. 20 and 21, there is a rapid German and American growth in cases despite being the least and the most in PD respectively. In contrary to our theory, Germany showed the most growth in cases; however, the least range in MRP and followed the second strictest SIM regulations. USA on the other hand, showed the highest range in MRP and followed one of the lowest approaches in SIM. This

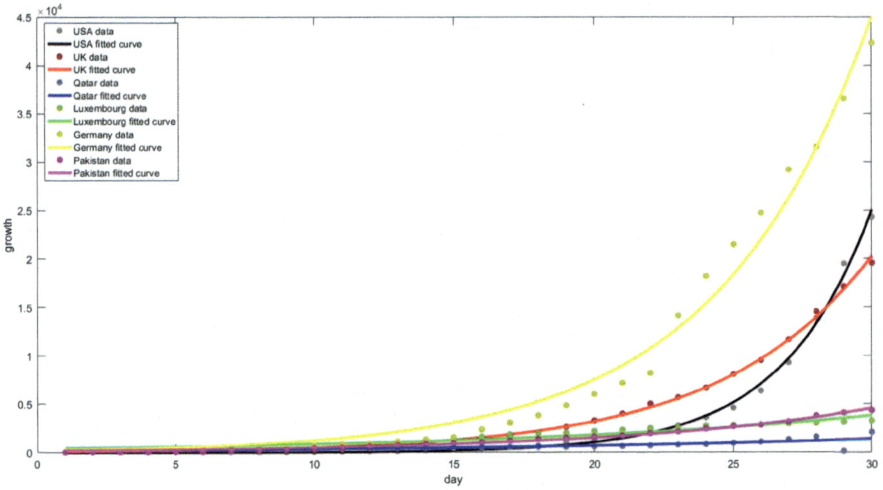

Fig. 20 Shows the daily growth of infected cases over the first month of spread for the ninth group

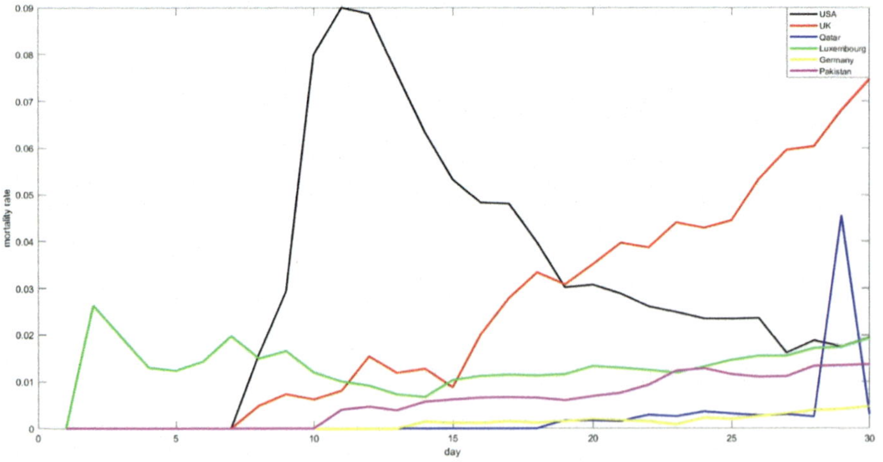

Fig. 21 Shows the mortality rate over the first month of spread for the ninth group

Table 10 Data of group nine

Country	Population density (PD)	Equation = $(A)e^{(B)x}$	Mortality rate percentage (MRP)	Stringency index (SIM)
USA	301	$(255.2)e^{(2.785)x}$	[1.58, 8.87]	[5.56, 72.69]
UK	279	$(1397)e^{(1.621)x}$	[0.48, 7.45]	[11.11, 75.93]
Qatar	249	$(513.5)e^{(0.5902)x}$	[0.15, 4.5]	[25, 86.11]
Luxembourg	242	$(1282)e^{(0.6571)x}$	[1, 2.63]	[42.59, 79.63]
Germany	235	$(3366)e^{(1.573)x}$	[0.09, 0.47]	[16.67, 73.15]
Pakistan	250	$(926.6)e^{(0.9577)x}$	[0.39, 1.36]	[28.7, 96.3]

observation can clearly show us the positive results of following the appropriate SIM regulations regardless of the PD numeric. 50%C, the stringency index model is the strongest factor affecting both MRP and growth in cases (Table 10).

4.10 *Group Ten: Average Population Density of (395) PD/km^2 (Belgium, Netherlands, Philippines, Israel, South Korea, Japan)*

As shown in Figs. 22 and 23, An unexpected growth curve is shown by the densest country in the group, Korea. Adding to our surprise, the country possessed the least MRP range and followed a very moderate and fast SIM regulations. This country's statistics can mean that they have been reporting all possible cases and following

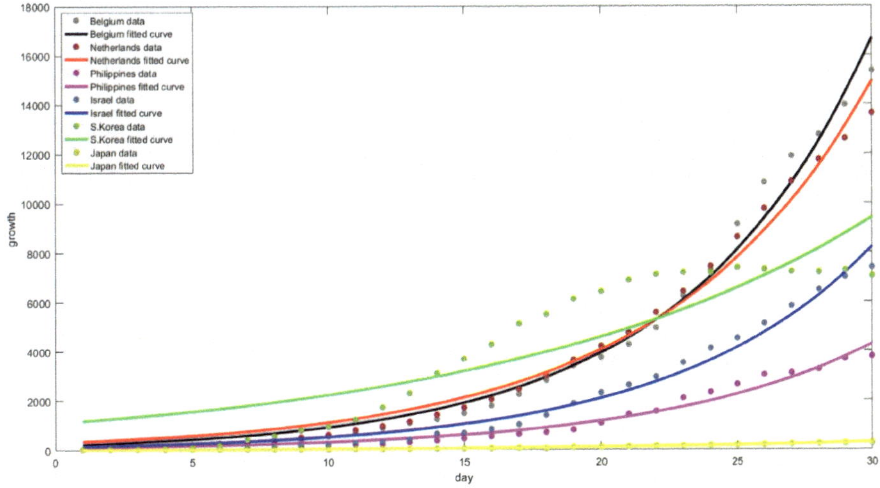

Fig. 22 Shows the daily growth of infected cases over the first month of spread for the tenth group

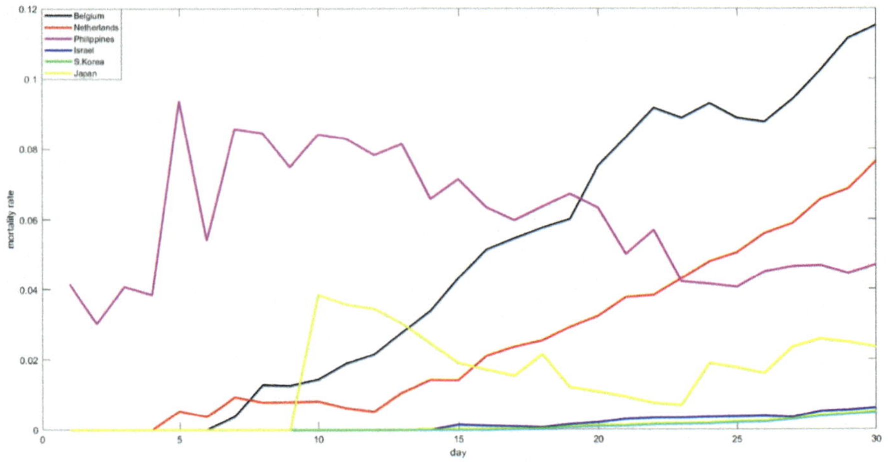

Fig. 23 Shows the mortality rate over the first month of spread for the tenth group

Table 11 Data of group ten

Country	Population density (PD)	Equation = $(A)e^{(B)x}$	Mortality rate percentage (MRP)	Stringency index (SIM)
Belgium	380	$(2060)e^{(1.27)x}$	[0.37, 11.5]	[13.89, 81.48]
Netherlands	409	$(2259)e^{(1.146)x}$	[0.377, 7.63]	[1.85, 79.63]
Philippines	320	$(655.3)e^{(1.139)x}$	[3.03, 8.57]	[34.26, 100]
Israel	417	$(1129)e^{(1.205)x}$	[0.07, 0.62]	[33.33, 87.96]
Korea	512	$(3311)e^{(0.6325)x}$	[0.02, 0.49]	[27.78, 55.56]
Japan	335	$(59.14)e^{(0.9419)x}$	[0.68, 3.84]	[19.44, 43.52]

dynamic and precise SIM regulations. In the other hand, we can see that although the Philippines is the least dense country in the group, it did not show the most flattened curve, its MRP scored the highest ranges ever although the country followed the highest SIM regulations. Instead, Japan took this honor showing the second most flattened curve after South Korea and its SIM regulations aligned with the timely raise in its MRP range. 50% Precise dynamic and timely mannered SIM regulations work the best for denser countries (Table 11).

5 Conclusion and Future Work

Reflecting on our hypothesis; the larger the population density of a country is, the more difficult it becomes to control the virus's initial spread, the more fatal the first month's effect is and the stricter the government response should be. Our results show that despite the vast infectiousness of the Covid-19 epidemic, controlling the novel virus within the first month does not significantly depend on the population density. In other words, and according to the stringency index model we used in our analysis, countries with larger population densities can handle the first cycle very well and even prevent a second cycle of spread only by taking appropriate and precise governmental responses early enough. Furthermore, it is noticed that as we study groups of larger population densities, severity of outbreaks raises and a dynamic and time-dependent approach in SIM is most effective. Since now a great relation could be found between the stringency index model, the growth of covid-19 cases, and the MPR range in a quite sufficient portion of countries, it is planned to study the effect of each SIM rank on the basic reproductive number of the disease while overcoming population density as a factor. Thus, hopefully there would be a chance to confidently tell which and when to take a measurement of a certain stringency and precisely determine the effect of each SIM rank on both the MRP and the growth reproductive number.

References

1. Chen, KH., Chan, W.H., Woo, P.C.K., Yuen, K.Y.: Genetic characterization of Betacoronavirus lineage C Viruses in bats reveals marked sequence divergence in the spike protein of Pipistrellus Bat Coronavirus HKU5 in Japanese Pipistrelle: implications for the origin of the Novel Middle East Respiratory Syndrome Coronavirus. J. Virol. **87**(15) (2013)
2. Phan, T.: Novel coronavirus: from discovery to clinical diagnostics. Infect. Genet. Evol. **79**, (2020)
3. Fehr, A.R., Perlman, S.: Coronaviruses: an overview of their replication and pathogenesis. Methods Mol. Biol. **1**, 1–23 (2015). https://doi.org/10.1007/978-1-4939-2438-7_1
4. Anand, K.: Structure of coronavirus main proteinase reveals combination of a chymotrypsin fold with an extra alpha-helical domain. EMBO J. **21**(13), 3213–3224 (2002)
5. Brünger, A.: Free R value: a novel statistical quantity for assessing the accuracy of crystal structures. Nature **355**(6359), 472–475 (1992)
6. Li, Q., Guan, X., Wu, P., Wang, X., Zhou, L., et al.: early transmission dynamics in Wuhan, China, of novel coronavirus-infected pneumonia. N. Engl. J. Med. **382**(13), 1199–1207 (2020)
7. Wang, W., Tang, J., Wei, F.: Updated understanding of the outbreak of 2019 novel coronavirus (2019-nCoV) in Wuhan, China. J. Med. Virol. **92**(4), 441–447 (2020)
8. Ren, L., Wang, Y., Wu, Z., Xiang, Z., et al.: Identification of a novel coronavirus causing severe pneumonia in human. Chin. Med. J., 1 (2020)
9. Huang, C., Wang, Y., Li, X., Ren, L., et al.: Clinical features of patients infected with 2019 novel coronavirus in Wuhan, China. The Lancet **395**(10223), 497–506 (2020)
10. Carlos, W., Dela Cruz, C., Cao, B., Pasnick, S., Jamil, S.: Novel Wuhan (2019-nCoV) Coronavirus. Am. J. Respir. Critical Care Med. **201**(4), 7–8 (2020)
11. Lei, J., Li, J., Li, X., Qi, X.: CT imaging of the 2019 Novel Coronavirus (2019-nCoV) pneumonia. Radiology **295**(1), 18–18 (2020)
12. Kahn, J.S., Mcintosh, K.: History and recent advances in coronavirus discovery. Pediatric Infect. Dis. J. **24** (2005)
13. Andersen, K.G., Rambaut, A., Lipkin, W.I., et al.: The proximal origin of SARS-CoV-2. Nat. Med. (2020). https://doi.org/10.1038/s41591-020-0820-9
14. Tarwater, P.M.C.: Effects of population density on the spread of disease. Complexity **6**(6), 29–36 (2001)
15. Li, R., Richmound, P.: Effect of population density on epidemics. Physica A: Stat. Mech. Appl. Elsevier **501**(c), 713–724 (2018)

16. Therese, K.L., White, L.F., Brooke, N.: Population density and basic reproductive number of COVID-19 across United, Medix. 12 June 2020. https://www.medrxiv.org/content/10.1101/2020.06.12.20130021v1.full.pdf. Accessed 15 June 2020
17. Babbit, D., Garland, P., Johnson, O.: Lived population density and the spread of COVID-19. arXiv, 3 May 2020. [Online]. https://arxiv.org/pdf/2005.01167v1.pdf. [Accessed 12 May 2020]
18. Tarwater, P.M., Martin, C.F.: Effects of population density on the spreadof disease. Complexity **6**(10), 29–36 (2000)
19. Wahba, S., Fang, W.: World Bank blogs. WorldBank, 20 April 2020. [Online]. https://blogs.worldbank.org/sustainablecities/urban-density-not-enemy-coronavirus-fight-evidence-china. Accessed 22 April 2020
20. Desai, D.: ORF Occasional paper: urban densities and the Covid-19 pandemic: upending the sustainability myth of global megacities, May 2020. [Online]. https://www.orfonline.org/wp-content/uploads/2020/05/ORF_OccasionalPaper_244_PandemicUrbanDensities.pdf. [Accessed 25 May 2020]
21. Hale, T.N.A.B.K.A.: Variation in Government Responses to Covid-19. Blavatnik School of Government Working Paper, vol. 6.0, May, 2020
22. Estimating mortality from COVID-19. [Online]. https://www.who.int/news-room/commentaries/detail/estimating-mortality-from-covid-19. Accessed 20 Sept 2020
23. Mortality Risk of COVID-19 - Our World in Data. [Online]. https://ourworldindata.org/mortality-risk-covid. Accessed 20 Sept 2020
24. Venkatesh, S., Memish, Z.A.: SARS: the new challenge to international health and travel medicine. East. Mediterranean Health J. **10** (2004)
25. Munster, V.J., Koopmans, M., van Doremalen, N., van Riel, D., de Wit, E.: A Novel Coronavirus Emerging in China — Key Questions for Impact Assessment. New England J. Med. **382**(8), 692–694 (2020)
26. Estimated Influenza Illnesses, Medical visits, Hospitalizations, and Deaths in the United States - 2018–2019 influenza season. Centers for Disease Control and Prevention, 08-Jan-2020. [Online]. Available: https://www.cdc.gov/flu/about/burden/2018-2019.html. [Accessed: 02-May-2021]
27. Ebola virus disease.: World Health Organization. [Online]. Available: https://www.who.int/en/news-room/fact-sheets/detail/ebola-virus-disease. [Accessed: 02-May-2021].
28. Shultz, J.M., Espinel, Z., Espinola, M., Rechkemmer, A.: (2016) Distinguishing epidemiological features of the 2013–2016 West Africa Ebola virus disease outbreak. Disaster Health **3**(3):78–88
29. Wang, L., Li, J., Guo, S., Xie, N., Yao, L., Cao, Y., Day, S.W., Howard, S.C., Graff, J.C., Gu, T., Ji, J., Gu, W., Sun, D.: Real-time estimation and prediction of mortality caused by COVID-19 with patient information based algorithm. Sci. Total Environ. 08-Apr-2020. [Online]. https://www.sciencedirect.com/science/article/pii/S0048969720319070?fbclid=IwAR0CN_EESCnz5In0PO3J-XZVYxXNeA85k7clsP2UyvItWBjWGcXSZMKZuF4. Accessed 23 Sept 2020
30. T. W. Bank. [Online]. https://data.worldbank.org/indicator/EN.POP.DNST. Accessed 15 April 2020
31. S. d. United Nations, Population and Vital Statistics Report, United Nations, April 2020. [Online]. https://unstats.un.org/unsd/demographic-social/products/vitstats/. Accessed 2020 April 2020
32. Ritchie, H., Roser, M., Giattino, C., Macdonald, B., Hasell, J., Mathieu, E., Beltekian, D., Ospina, E.O.: Coronavirus (COVID-19) Deaths - Statistics and Research," Our World in Data. [Online]. https://ourworldindata.org/covid-deaths. Accessed 17 Sept 2020

Forecasting of COVID-19 Using Modified SEIR, Logistic Growth and Holt's Models

Touka M. A. Mahmoud, Norhan Mohsen ElOcla, Mohamed S. A. Abu-Tafesh, and Ahmed S. A. Mohamed

Abstract Understanding the transmission dynamics of the novel coronavirus is the concern that attracted many researchers nowadays. In this chapter, three mathematical models, modified SEIR, logistic growth and double exponential smoothing, were implemented in Matlab to predict the transmission of COVID-19 in Egypt, Oman, Nigeria and South Africa. To estimate the models' parameters, the reported data were used to fit the models using Nelder-Mead, Levenberg-Marquardt, Trust-Region-Reflective, and MultiStart object with Interior-Point optimization algorithms. Then, a sensitivity analysis was made to understand the effect of different parameters on the models' prediction. The application of the three models on the reported data was compared despite their different nature. It was shown and verified that the three models are highly dependent on the parameters' values, referring to the importance of determining their estimates using an optimization algorithm. It was found out that the most dominant parameter is the one denoting the rate by which susceptible people are protected, which emphasizes the effect of social distancing and quarantine.

Keywords COVID-19 · Logistic growth model · Mathematical modeling · Optimization · SEIR model · Holt's model · Sensitivity analysis

T. M. A. Mahmoud · N. Mohsen ElOcla · M. S. A. Abu-Tafesh
Zewail City of Science and Technology, Giza 12578,, Egypt
e-mail: S-touka99-mohamed@zewailcity.edu.eg

N. Mohsen ElOcla
e-mail: S-norhanmohsen@zewailcity.edu.eg

M. S. A. Abu-Tafesh
e-mail: S-mohamedsaadahmed98@zewailcity.edu.eg

A. S. A. Mohamed (✉)
University of Science and Technology, Applied Math, Zewail City of Science and Technology, Faculty of Engineering, Cairo University, Giza 12613, Egypt
e-mail: aashiry@ieee.org

D. Oliva et al. (eds.), *Artificial Intelligence for COVID-19*, Studies in Systems, Decision and Control 358, https://doi.org/10.1007/978-3-030-69744-0_26

1 Introduction

Coronavirus disease (COVID-19) is an infectious disease caused by severe acute respiratory syndrome coronavirus 2 (SARS-CoV-2). The infection with the COVID-19 virus results in respiratory illness which is mild or moderate that most people can recover without special treatment. However, this infection can cause serious illness to people with medical conditions like diabetes, cardiovascular diseases, and chronic respiratory diseases [1, 2].

WHO (World Health Organization) received detailed information about its outbreak in Wuhan, China on 11 and 12 January 2020. After then, the number of cases has increased outside China in 114 countries as well as the number of people that have lost their lives. Therefore, this outbreak was characterized as a pandemic [3, 4].

The reason behind this outbreak is that the virus can spread easily and sustainably from one person to another. It is thought to be spread by respiratory droplets of a patient, or through contaminated surfaces. Therefore, maintaining social distance, washing hands, and disinfecting surfaces are very important to help reduce the spread of this virus [5].

In the face of COVID-19, mathematical infection models are used to faithfully describe the COVID-19 development and estimate its spread. Based on this estimation, the government health agencies and decision-makers act accordingly to this development. Mathematical modeling of an infectious disease aims to evaluate its transmission so that it can provide control measures and help to tailor intervention strategies.

For avoiding biased results of a single mathematical model, three different common models, which are the modified susceptible-exposed-infectious-removed (SEIR) model, the logistic growth model and the double exponential smoothing model (Holt's method), were employed so that the results could be compared to reach an objective estimation.

The SEIR model depends on a set of ordinary differential equations that describe the epidemic dynamics. However, adjustments were made to measure the effort of the government through the effect of precautionary measures, such as changes in the education system and lockdown policies. The SEIR model and its modified forms have been widely used to estimate the growth of the epidemic in many countries such as Indonesia, Italy, and India [6–8]. Moreover, improvements were done using a stochastic approach that increases the prediction reliability as it enhances the fitting of the model parameters [7].

The logistic function was first devised by the Belgian mathematician Verhulst in 1838 for population growth description. Then, it became an essential tool in the bioassay field [9]. Its importance lies in the description of the dynamic evolution of the infected people with the control of population capacity and growth rate. In addition, it was used to describe the COVID-19 proliferation in China and India [10, 11].

The Exponential smoothing model is considered to be one of the popular techniques to obtain a smoothed time series that was proposed and formulated in the late

1950s [12–14]. Its main idea is to give more importance to the recent observations by increasing the weights exponentially as the observations become more recent. There are three main forms for the exponential smoothing techniques which are single, double, and triple exponential smoothing [15].

Double exponential smoothing (Holt's method) was extended from simple exponential smoothing by Holt in 1957 [13]. It was chosen as it is exponential smoothing to time series characterized by showing local level and trend changes (as that shown in the time series of corona virus data) since it works to adjust them at each period end [15].

The three models are used to predict the spread of COVID-19 epidemic in Egypt, Oman, Nigeria and South Africa to compare their results and have a deeper understanding of the proposed models.

2 Data

To estimate the values of parameters in the equations describing the three models under study, the reported data of total, active and removed cases are used for fitting the models, and thus finding the optimum parameters' values. These data are taken from the Worldometer website until 20th of July [16], for Egypt, Oman, Nigeria and South Africa. The initial date was chosen for each country to be the day when the total cases exceeded 1000 cases, which is 4 April for Egypt, 16 April for Oman, 24 April for Nigeria and 27 March for South Africa. This choice proved to produce more realistic results, either in the model fitting or in the accuracy of the model prediction when it was compared with the actual data. This is because the data at the beginning of the virus spread are usually inaccurate due to the few number of performed tests and the less public awareness towards it, making it mislead the model as it was noticed.

More updated data sets were also entered into the models to better understand its dynamic behaviors. For the modified SEIR model, data were used until 5th of August for Egypt, and 10th of August for South Africa. For the logistic growth model, more data were entered until 18th of September for Egypt and 21st of August for Nigeria. Finally, four different data sets were used with Holt's model for each country that end at 10 July, 20 July, 31 July and 10 August, as will be discussed in the next sections.

3 Modified SEIR "SS_pEIR" Model

The basic $SEIR$ model is a compartmental model that divides the population into four groups. "S", "E", "I" and "R" represent the susceptible, exposed, infectious, and removed compartments respectively, where the removed group includes both recoveries and deaths by the infection. It does not consider new births or deaths, or any applied control measures. Therefore, different modifications were made by adding more compartments, resulting in more complex forms of the model. Even though these complex models that consider more biological factors are more realistic, they can be inaccurate due to the lack of enough data. In other words, they contain a larger number of unknown parameters that need to be estimated using the limited available data sets, leading to a greater uncertainty in the results [17].

Therefore, to get the most use of the available data and still have a more realistic model, we used a modified version of it, in which one more group for the protected population was added. This group was necessary after the decisions of schools and universities closure, and even a complete lock-down in some countries. Therefore, S_p represents the portion of S that is either confined or protected using face masks and other control measures. Equations 1–5 are the five nonlinear coupled ordinary differential equations that govern this model [7, 18].

$$\frac{dS(t)}{dt} = -\beta\frac{S(t)I(t)}{N} - pS(t) \tag{1}$$

$$\frac{dS_p(t)}{dt} = pS(t) \tag{2}$$

$$\frac{dE(t)}{dt} = \beta\frac{S(t)I(t)}{N} - \alpha E(t) \tag{3}$$

$$\frac{dI(t)}{dt} = \alpha E(t) - rI(t) \tag{4}$$

$$\frac{dR(t)}{dt} = rI(t) \tag{5}$$

where β is the infection rate by which a susceptible person becomes exposed, while p is the rate by which s/he is protected, and thus insusceptible. Then, the exposed person takes an incubation period to develop symptoms and move to the infectious group by an incubation rate α, which is the inverse of the incubation period in days. In other words, it is the inverse of the latency period, since the exposed group is assumed to be noninfectious unless they move to the infectious group. Finally, they either recover or die by the removal rate r. Here, N is the total population, that is the sum of all these compartments, i.e., $N = S(t) + S_p(t) + E(t) + I(t) + R(t)$.

3.1 Parameters Estimation

Nelder-Mead "simplex direct search", Levenberg-Marquardt, and Trust-Region-Reflective optimization algorithms were used to fit the proposed model to the given data by getting least square error between them, using Matlab functions "fminsearch" and "lsqnonlin" respectively. However, the formulated optimization problem needs

Table 1 Optimal parameters for SS_pEIR model

Country	p	β	α	r
Egypt	0.0204	0.5258	0.0714	0.0151
Oman	0.0138	0.3631	0.0714	0.0461
Nigeria	0.0107	0.2555	0.4677	0.0208
South Africa	0.0005	0.3758	0.0714	0.0514

an initial guess for each parameter that is going to be optimized, so an initial guess was made for each.

In the SS_pEIR Model, α is the reciprocal of the incubation period that is around 6 days [19], thus α is given an initial guess of $\frac{1}{6}$. For the removal rate r, it is estimated by getting the reciprocal of the average time that the infected person takes to recover or die. It is reported that the average time for recovery is either two weeks, or four and a half weeks, depending on the case [19]. Therefore, by taking the average of both numbers, r is given an initial value of $\frac{1}{22.75}$. On the other hand, different initial guesses were tried for p and β since they do not have fixed reported values, and can vary according to the country.

On using "fminsearch" function, it produced the same results on varying the initial guesses of p and β, unlike "lsqnonlin" function, with Levenberg-Marquardt algorithm, that was highly sensitive to the initial guesses. Therefore, the results of the first function were used to enter good initial values to the second one, and fortunately, it produced the same results, in addition to being much faster.

However, the problem needed some constraints to ensure that the values of the optimal parameters are in the acceptable range. Therefore, "lsqnonlin" function was finally used with the Trust-Region-Reflective algorithm, to give suitable upper and lower limits for the parameters. α was enclosed between $\frac{1}{14}$ and 1, while the other ones are ensured to be positive numbers. The values of the SS_pEIR parameters after the optimization are given in Table 1.

Furthermore, the system of differential equations of SEIR model is solved numerically using "ode45" Matlab function. Therefore, it is also crucial to put good initial conditions. The initial value of S is the total population minus the initial values of the other groups. For the protected compartment, we assumed that its initial value is the portion of the total population that is confined according to the decisions of each country. Therefore, the percentage of children, students, and elderly people is calculated. Then, $S_p(0)$ is the estimated percentage of confined people multiplied by the total population. Moreover, both $I(0)$ and $R(0)$ are taken as the reported data on the initial date. For $E(0)$, it is estimated by adding the new cases of the next 6 days, assuming that this is the incubation period as mentioned before. The initial conditions are given in Table 2.

Table 2 Initial conditions for SS_pEIR model

Country	$S(0)$	$S_p(0)$	$E(0)$	$I(0)$	$R(0)$
Egypt	42, 159, 980	60, 172, 629	724	758	312
Oman	3, 210, 451	1, 894, 557	595	839	180
Nigeria	67, 611, 853	138, 525, 802	837	855	240
South Africa	27, 280, 535	32, 026, 693	292	1, 137	33

3.2 Results

Results of applying the modified $SEIR$ model on Egypt, Oman, Nigeria and South Africa are shown in Figs. 1, 2, 3, 4, 5, 6, 7 and 8.

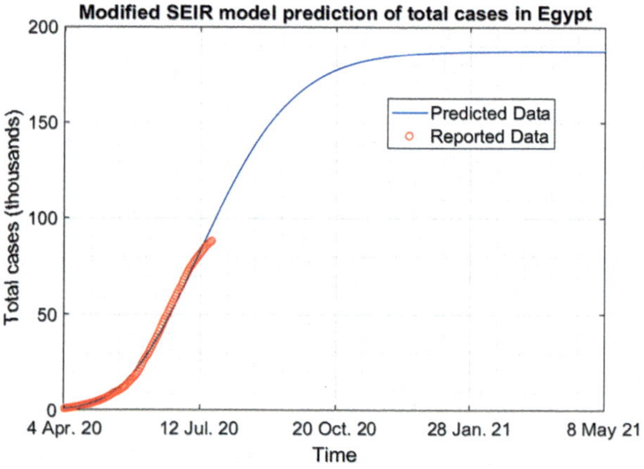

Fig. 1 SS_pEIR model prediction of total cases in Egypt

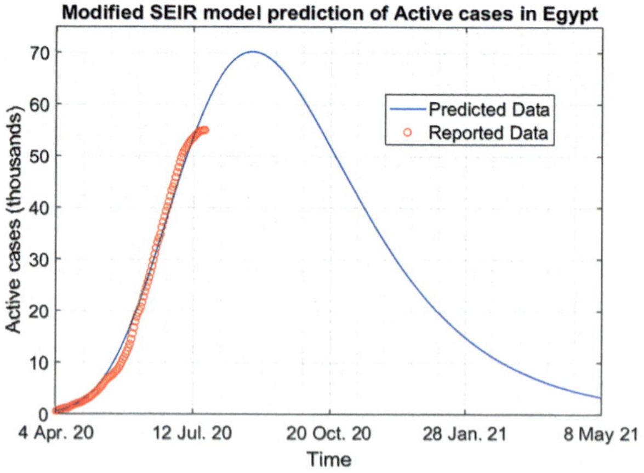

Fig. 2 SS_pEIR model prediction of active cases in Egypt

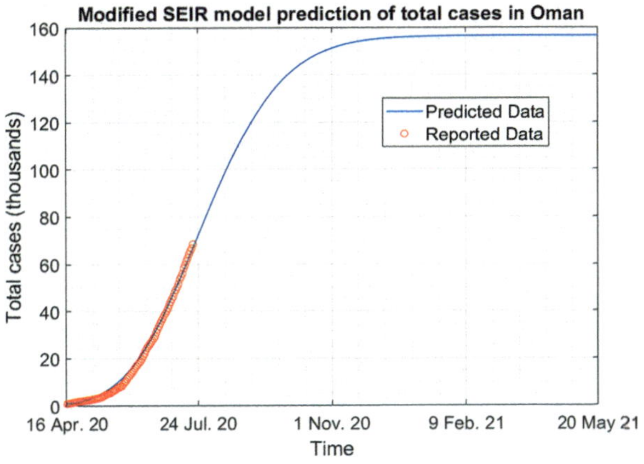

Fig. 3 SS_pEIR model prediction of total cases in Oman

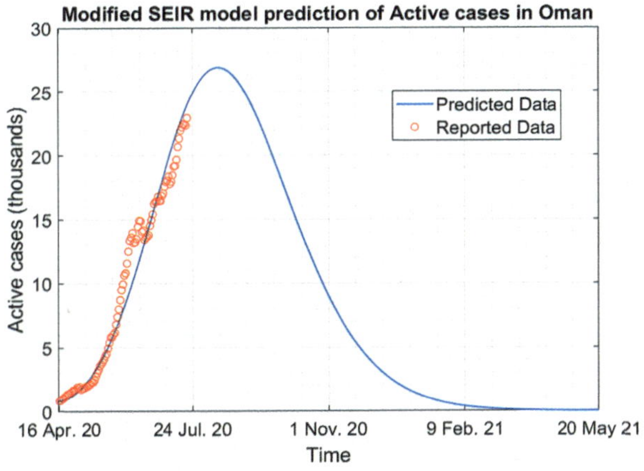

Fig. 4 SS_pEIR model prediction of active cases in Oman

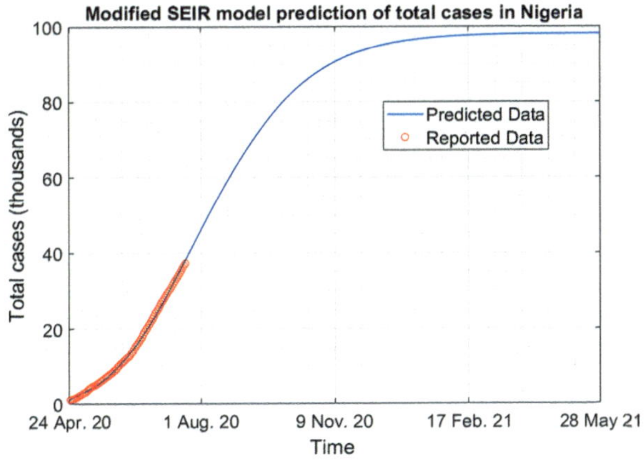

Fig. 5 SS_pEIR model prediction of total cases in Nigeria

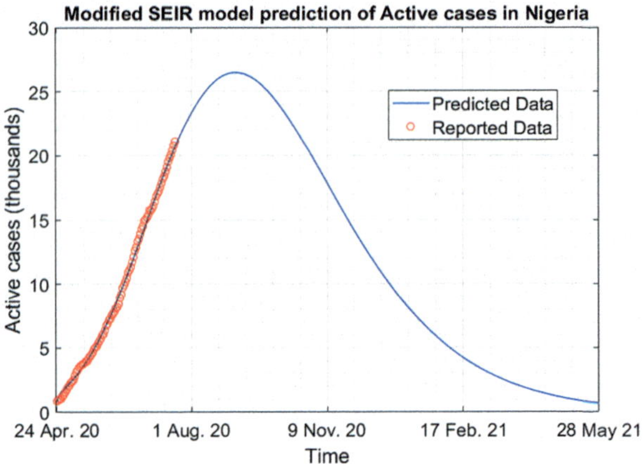

Fig. 6 SS_pEIR model prediction of active cases in Nigeria

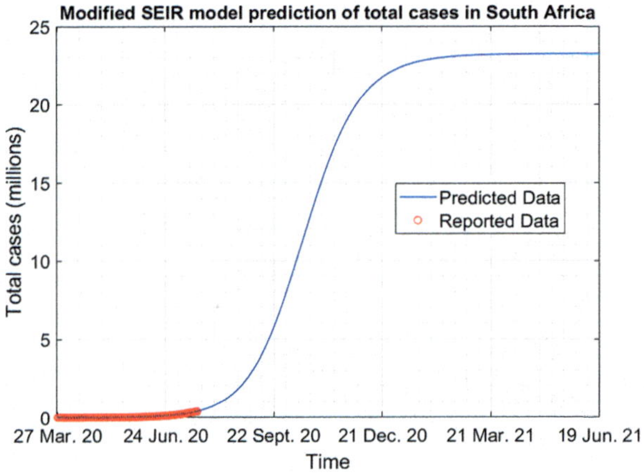

Fig. 7 SS_pEIR model prediction of total cases in South Africa

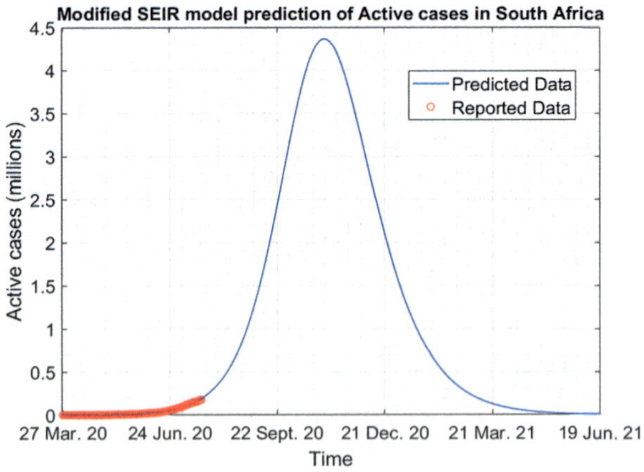

Fig. 8 SS_pEIR model prediction of active cases in South Africa

Table 3 Results of the SS_pEIR model

Country	Peak time	Active cases (peak)	End time	Total cases
Egypt	23 Aug. 20	70, 240	21 Mar. 21	187, 500
Oman	12 Aug. 20	26, 860	18 Mar. 21	156, 500
Nigeria	1 Sept. 20	26, 450	13 Apr. 21	98, 000
South Africa	31 Oct. 20	4, 359, 100	14 May 21	23, 220, 000

Table 4 Results of SS_pEIR model using different data sets

Country	Data set	Peak time	Active cases	End time	Total cases
Egypt	4 Apr. to 15 July	30 Aug. 20	78, 400	27 Apr. 21	219, 400
Egypt	4 Apr. to 25 July	18 Aug. 20	64, 560	23 Feb. 21	165, 900
Egypt	4 Apr. to 5 Aug.	6 Aug. 20	54, 940	18 Jan. 21	134, 800
South Africa	27 Mar. to 10 Aug.	11 Oct. 20	378, 400	28 May. 21	3, 355, 000

Table 3 summarizes the results of the modified $SEIR$ model, showing the predicted time and value for the peak and the end of SARS-COV-2 in the four countries, based on the reported data sets until 20th of July.

For a deep understanding of the modified $SEIR$ model, three additional data sets for Egypt were entered into the model to observe their effect on the results. They are of the same initial date as the first data set, but one of them ends on 15th of July, another one ends on 25th of July, and the third ends on 5th of August. Moreover, a more updated data set was used for South Africa that ends on 10th of August. Results are summarized in Table 4.

As it is shown in Figs. 1, 2, 3, 4, 5, 6, 7, 8 and Table 3, the model is applied on four countries with different conditions such as phase of virus spread and different population size, which implies the validity of modified $SEIR$ model. It predicts different results for the four countries, either in the maximum active or total cases, because it depends on the actual data that varies for each one. For Oman, the population is much smaller than the others, making the initial number of the susceptible group, which the infectious population comes from, much smaller. Moreover, it is noticed that the number of active cases in Oman was less than half the number of active cases in Egypt, and was much less than that of South Africa. Therefore, both the entered data and the initial conditions produced a relatively low infection rate, thus the peak and end of the virus dates for Oman are predicted to be earlier than Egypt and South Africa with smaller number of cases, using the SS_pEIR model.

On the other hand, Nigeria is predicted to have the smallest number of cases despite having the largest population. This is because the entered reported data has a very small number of cases relative to the susceptible people, causing the infection rate to be the least among the mentioned countries.

For South Africa, it has the largest number of total and active cases in Africa, making the rate by which people are protected very low, which justifies its results. However, these results can be less pessimistic on entering more data. We entered more of the actual data for which it predicted huge values, so that it is fitted again, producing smaller numbers, as shown in Table 4.

Table 4 indicates that the more updated data-sets are, the closer to reported cases the results are.

4 Logistic Growth Model

Conventionally, the number of confirmed cases can be estimated as a function of time. At the beginning of the epidemic, cases are increasing with a high infection rate due to the lack of personal protection measures which approaches an exponential rate. After a significant time, the rate of infection decreases continuously due to control measures imposed by governments until no new reported cases. In other words, the curve reaches a maximum number called the carrying capacity (N_{max}). This is called a logistic growth model (LGM) with a result of an "S" shape curve [10, 11, 20].

The logistic growth model (LGM) is commonly used in dynamic modeling in various fields, such as ecology, statistics, chemistry, and machine learning [21–23]. For an epidemic outbreak in a specified population, the change of confirmed cases ($\Delta \mathrm{N}_{Log}$) relative to the change in time (t) can be expressed in the form of a first-order differential equation, as shown in Eq. 6 [24].

$$\frac{dN_{Log}}{dt} = r_0 N_{Log}(1 - \frac{N_{Log}}{N_{max}}) \tag{6}$$

where r_0 is the growth rate, N_{max} is the carrying capacity or maximum number of infections, with $N_0 = N_{Log}(t_0)$, which is the initial number of infections.

Equation 6 is a separable DE that can be solved as in Eq. 7 [24].

$$N_{Log}(t) = \frac{N_{max}}{1 + (\frac{N_{max}}{N_0} - 1).e^{-r_0(t-t_0)}} \tag{7}$$

4.1 Parameters Estimation

For the logistic model, only two parameters need to be optimized, which are N_{max}, and r_0. To improve the results of this model, the last few data points were given a higher weight than the rest of the fitting points, as the cases on the following days are more influenced by the last few days, much more than the early data.

Table 5 Optimal parameters for the logistic growth model

Country	r_0	N_{max}
Egypt	0.061	101, 153
Oman	0.054	113, 166
Nigeria	0.055	51, 159
South Africa	0.054	1, 155, 365

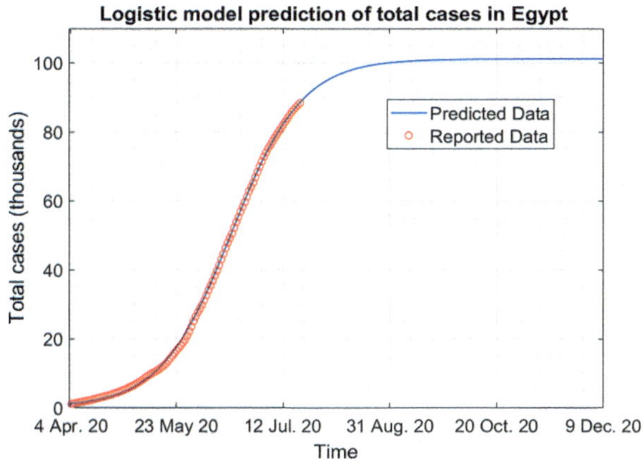

Fig. 9 Logistic growth model prediction of total cases in Egypt

Table 6 Results of the logistic growth model

Country	End time	Final total cases
Egypt	21 Oct. 20–11 Jan. 21	101, 101–101, 153
Oman	27 Nov. 20–23 Feb. 21	113, 100–113, 166
Nigeria	2 Nov. 20–27 Jan. 21	51, 101–51, 159
South Africa	31 Dec. 20–22 Apr. 21	1, 155, 002–1, 155, 365

On trying both optimization functions, they both produced the same results, that are shown in Table 5, even with the different initial guesses for both parameters. However, "lsqnonlin" took only 42 function evaluations, while "fminsearch" took 316 to reach the same tolerance, with Egypt data.

4.2 Results

Results of applying the logistic growth model on Egypt, Oman, Nigeria and South Africa are shown in Figs. 9, 10, 11 and 12.

Results of the logistic growth model using the data sets until 20th of July are summarized in Table 6.

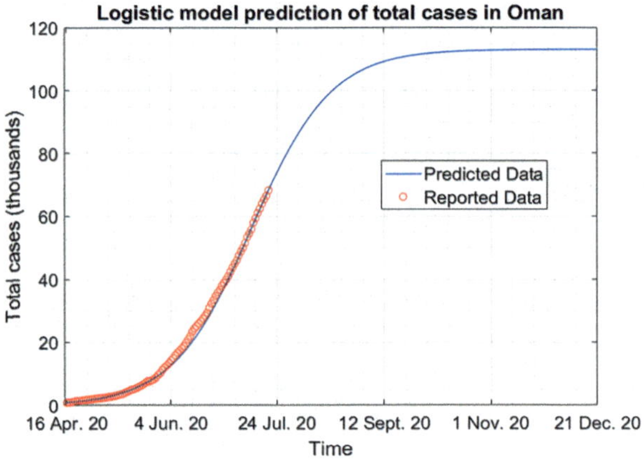

Fig. 10 Logistic growth model prediction of total cases in Oman

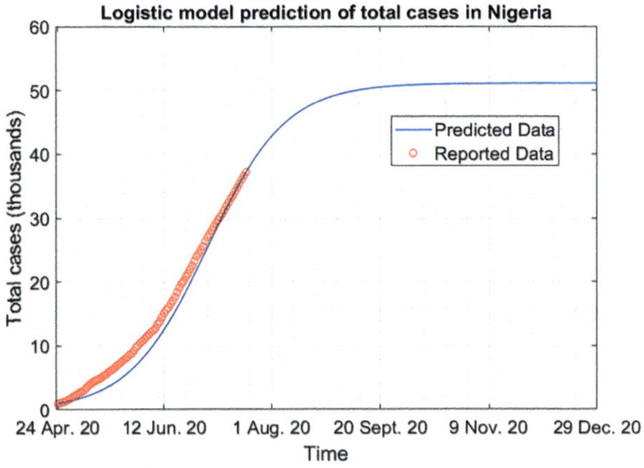

Fig. 11 Logistic growth model prediction of total cases in Nigeria

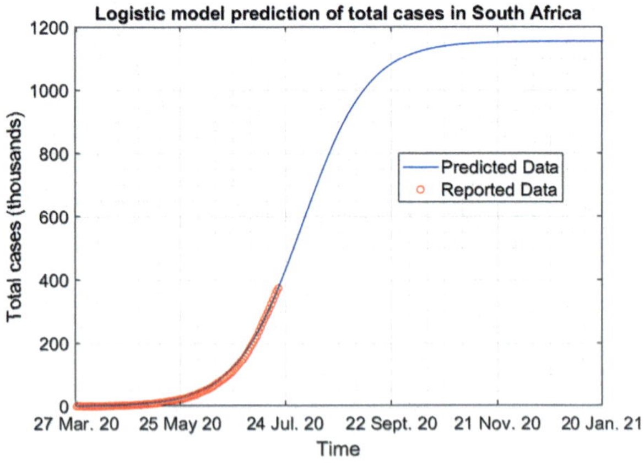

Fig. 12 Logistic growth model prediction of total cases in South Africa

Table 7 Results of the logistic growth model using updated data sets

Country	Data set	End time	Final total cases
Egypt	4 Apr. to 14 Sept.	8 Nov. 20–28 Jan. 21	101, 702–101, 747
Egypt	4 Apr. to 18 Sept.	2 Nov. 20–24 Jan. 21	102, 000–102, 058
Nigeria	24 Apr. to 21 Aug.	3 Dec. 20–9 Mar. 21	60, 700–60, 779

Results of the logistic growth model using more updated data sets are shown in Table 7.

On the contrary to the modified SEIR model, the logistic growth model produced larger numbers for Oman than Egypt, despite the mentioned differences between the countries. This is because the logistic model does not consider the total population number or even the active cases. It only takes the cumulative cases number, which was still rising in Oman. For South Africa, the entered total cases number was much larger than the other countries, so the model prediction was also much larger. On the other hand, its prediction for the cases in Nigeria was the smallest, due to its entered data that have relatively small number of cases, with respect to the other three countries.

However, it can be seen that the predicted final number of total cases in both Egypt and Nigeria has been reached earlier than expected and lager numbers of cases were reported. Therefore, an updated data set was employed for Egypt until 14th of September, which is the day it exceeded the model prediction, as shown in Table 7. Then, the new prediction was also exceeded on 18th of September, hence it was again updated. For Nigeria, the model prediction was exceeded on 21st of August, therefore, an updated data set until 21st of August was used to produce the new results in Table 7. It can be indicated that the entered data set should be updated frequently to have a better prediction on the long term.

Table 8 shows the prediction of the logistic model for the next 10 days as well as the reported numbers in Egypt using the data set until 20th of July, referring to its good accuracy on the short term too.

5 Double Exponential Smoothing "Holt's Model"

Equations 8–9 show adjusting level and trend of the data at the end of each period [15, 25].

$$L_t = \sigma X_t + (1 - \sigma)(L_{t-1} + T_{t-1}), \quad 0 \leq \sigma \leq 1 \tag{8}$$

$$T_t = \gamma(L_t - L_{t-1}) + (1 - \gamma)T_{t-1}, \quad 0 \leq \gamma \leq 1 \tag{9}$$

L_t and T_t are the level and trend, respectively, which are estimated at the end of each period by smoothing the values of data. σ and γ are the level and trend smoothing

Table 8 Logistic model prediction of total cases versus reported total cases in Egypt

Date	Reported cases	Predicted cases	Absolute Percent Error (APE)
21/7	89078	89187	0.1224
22/7	89745	89812	0.0746
23/7	90413	90408	0.0054
24/7	91072	90977	0.1048
25/7	91583	91518	0.0708
26/7	92062	92034	0.0307
27/7	92482	92524	0.0458
28/7	92947	92991	0.0473
29/7	93356	93434	0.0840
30/7	93757	93856	0.1052

parameters, respectively, and both of their values are between or equal to 0 and 1. Finally, this method is used in forecasting at time t through Eq. 10 [25].

$$F_{t+h} = L_t + hT_t, \quad h = 1, 2, 3, \ldots \tag{10}$$

where h is the forecast steps number.

5.1 Parameters Estimation

The two smoothing parameters of Holt's model are also optimized with considering the given constraints, where $0 \leq \sigma, \gamma \leq 1$. Both the Trust Region Reflective and the Interior Point optimization algorithms were tried, and they both showed that the optimal value of gamma is highly sensitive and dependent on the initial guesses. However, the interior-point algorithm produced close results for gamma in all trials. To reach the best value, the MultiStart solver was used with 1,000 custom starting points, using fmincon function and the interior-point algorithm.

Different data sets were entered to the model to check the effect of data on the forecasts, and each data set was used to forecast the total cases in the next 20 days. The estimated parameters for each data set are shown in Table 9, which demonstrates that the best value for σ is 1 in all cases, while γ optimal values are between 0.4 and 0.6. These values reflect that the most recent data should be considered for a good prediction.

Table 9 Optimal parameters for Holt's model using different data sets

Country	Data set	σ	γ
Egypt	4 Apr. to 10 Jul.	1	0.5351
	4 Apr. to 20 Jul.	1	0.5410
	4 Apr. to 31 Jul.	1	0.5429
	4 Apr. to 10 Aug.	1	0.5420
Oman	16 Apr. to 10 Jul.	1	0.5010
	16 Apr. to 20 Jul.	1	0.4774
	16 Apr. to 31 Jul.	1	0.4992
	16 Apr. to 10 Aug.	1	0.5029
Nigeria	24 Apr. to 10 Jul.	1	0.4611
	24 Apr. to 20 Jul.	1	0.4677
	24 Apr. to 31 Jul.	1	0.4763
	24 Apr. to 10 Aug.	1	0.4782
South Africa	27 Mar. to 10 Jul.	1	0.5290
	27 Mar. to 20 Jul.	1	0.5305
	27 Mar. to 31 Jul.	1	0.5847
	27 Mar. to 10 Aug.	1	0.4583

5.2 Results

Results of applying Holt's model on Egypt, Oman, Nigeria and South Africa are shown in Figs. 13, 14, 15 and 16.

As shown in figures, the model has very good accuracy on the short term prediction using specific data sets more than the others. In Egypt, using data set 2, that ends on 20th of July, to predict the next 5 days produced forecasts with MAPE of only 0.0635%, while a MAPE of 0.381% for 10 days prediction. This is because there was

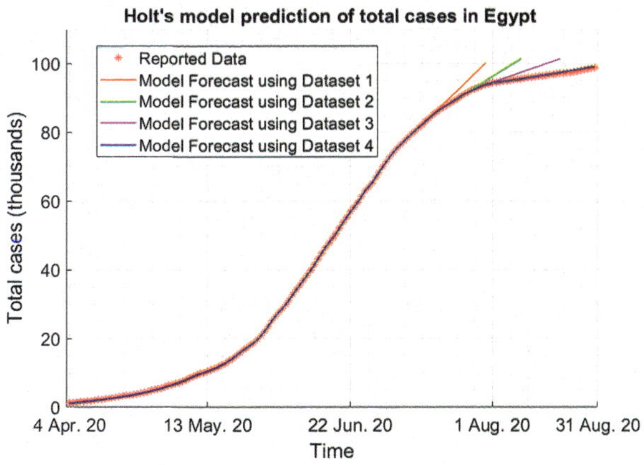

Fig. 13 Holt's model prediction of total cases in Egypt

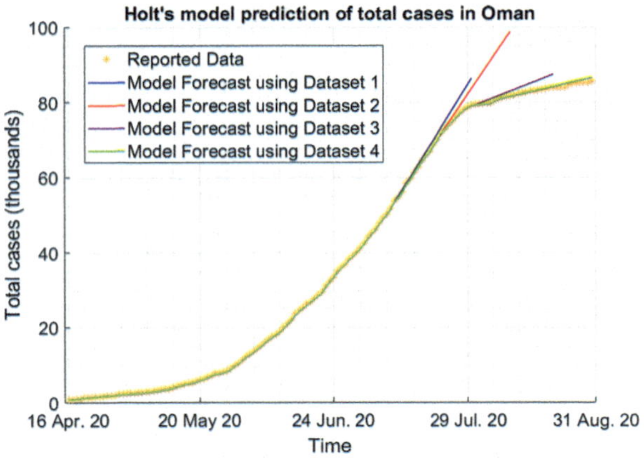

Fig. 14 Holt's model prediction of total cases in Oman

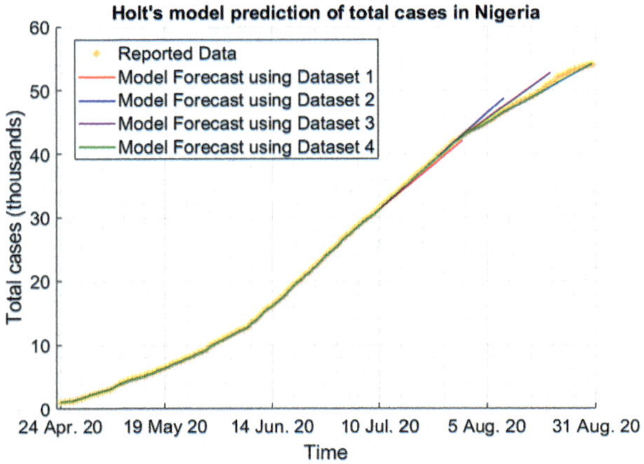

Fig. 15 Holt's model prediction of total cases in Nigeria

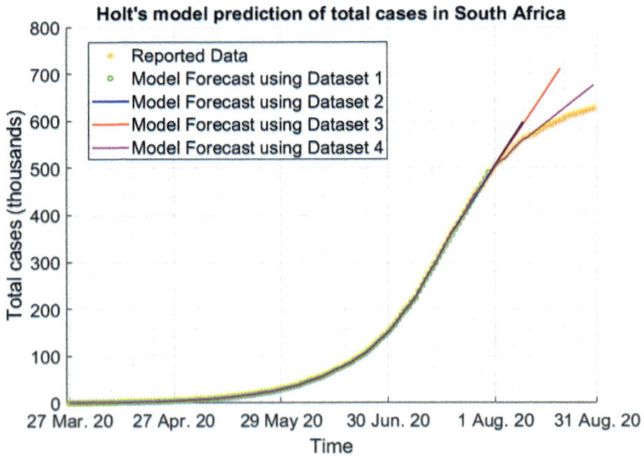

Fig. 16 Holt's model prediction of total cases in South Africa

a change in its trend as it started to diverge after 5 days, and the number of total cases became more stable in this time interval. On using the fourth data set, that ends on 10th of August, it shows a good accuracy with MAPEs of 0.0891% and 0.206% for the 5 and 10 days prediction, respectively. On the other hand, using the two remaining data sets is not recommended because the next interval was exhibiting a change in its trend, even though data set 3 is greater than data set 2. The same observation is for Oman, as it is obvious that the second data set did not produce good results for the next days because there was a transition in the trend of its total cases, unlike the fourth data set that produced the least MAPE reached for the two countries, that is 0.0366% and 0.1978% for the 5 and 10 days forecasts, respectively, because of the increased actual data used for the optimization as expected.

Moreover, for South Africa, there were many changes in its trend. Accordingly, despite the increased number of actual data used for optimization, it is found that the first data set was the most accurate one. Finally for Nigeria, the second data set is better than the first one as they have MAPEs of 0.0938 and 0.5612, respectively, for the predicted five days. Also, it shows that the change in the trend caused an increment in the error value as it increased for the third data set to become 0.9558, despite taking more actual data for the optimization.

In general, we concluded that Holt's method depends on two important factors which are the number of actual data used for the optimization of the different data sets and the most significant fact that it highly depends on the characteristics of the trend itself, which at the end it makes this method more suitable for the short term prediction.

Table 10 shows the model's prediction in Egypt for the next 10 days, using data set 2, which indicates how the APE for the first few days was very small, then increased by time.

Therefore, it is crucial to decide when and how to use Holt's model. It is best used in a time interval that exhibits the same trend, such as at the beginning or at the end of the virus spread.

6 Models Comparison

After presenting and discussing each model in the previous sections, here, the results of the three models are compared. Then, the parameters affecting the results of each model are further explored in the next section.

6.1 Logistic Growth Model Versus Modified SEIR Model

For Egypt, the logistic growth model produced more optimistic results. It predicts that around 21st of October, the total cases are almost stable with a value of 101, 101 cases. Then, very few cases are encountered along the next three months, reaching

Table 10 Holt's model prediction of total cases versus reported total cases in Egypt, using data set 2

Date	Reported cases	Predicted cases	Absolute Percent Error (APE)
21/7	89078	89048	0.0333
22/7	89745	89695	0.0561
23/7	90413	90341	0.0797
24/7	91072	90987	0.0930
25/7	91583	91634	0.0552
26/7	92062	92280	0.2367
27/7	92482	92926	0.4803
28/7	92947	93573	0.6730
29/7	93356	94219	0.9243
30/7	93757	94865	1.1820

a maximum of 101, 153 total cases on 11th of January 2021. On the other hand, the SS_pEIR model predicts that the active cases will still rise until reaching 70, 240 cases on 23rd of August. Then it begins to decrease until the total cases reach the maximum value of 187, 500 cases after 352 days from our chosen initial date. However, this result does not agree with the reported data, especially at the end of July, that shows that Egypt has already reached the peak with less value than what is expected by the SS_pEIR model. This is due to the nature of the model that depends on different factors deriving this result, other than the fitting data. In addition, by considering the population number, the model has more dynamics, as it moves the population between 5 compartments in a more realistic way. It can also be more flexible by adding other compartments and modifying the equations to better describe reality. Accordingly, its cross-correlations can even expect the unreported cases, which can explain the larger numbers it produces. On the other hand, the logistic growth model mainly depends on the total number of cases and the growth rate. They are entered into only one equation, which is assumed to describe the epidemic growth. Since it does not contain many parameters and dynamics such as the modified $SEIR$ model, it produces closer results to the reported data, especially on the short term, as shown in Table 8.

It is important to mention that all these results are predicted unless a second wave of the epidemic is encountered.

On trying to utilize Egypt data until 15th of July only into the SS_pEIR model, the predicted final total cases exceeded 200, 000 cases, which is almost double that of logistic model. However, on updating the data till 25th of July, it predicted 165, 900 cases, which is getting closer to logistic model prediction. Accordingly, it is noticed that the SS_pEIR model results approach that of the logistic model as we use more data. This is because the larger data set has more influence on the model. Although the three data sets are only 5 days apart, this small change has greatly affected the results and highlighted this relation. Therefore, on entering the data until 5th of August, the peak value and date became much closer to the peak of reported data, and the total cases are near to the logistic model prediction, as shown in Table 4.

6.2 Modified SEIR Model Versus Basic and Generalized SEIR Models

The modified $SEIR$ model has also solved the basic $SEIR$ model problem, which is being highly unrealistic in this situation, as it produced a peak value higher than 12 million active cases in Egypt, using the same data set and initial conditions. The reason is that the basic $SEIR$ model moves the population between only 4 compartments in one direction. It means that the population has no opportunity to survive from the epidemic because they must move from the susceptible to the exposed and then to the other groups, which is not the real case. Therefore, the advantage of our chosen model is that it adds another direction for susceptible people, in addition to the infection direction. Due to government decisions and control measures such as social distancing and wearing face masks, besides the increase of people awareness, the protected population increased by time, which is simulated in the S_p compartment. Moreover, this model is not as complicated as the generalized $SEIR$ model that contains more compartments, making it difficult to estimate all its parameters or find the needed fitting data [17]. Therefore, our chosen modified model has shown good results in simulating the situation, proving that it is a relatively simple and accurate model.

6.3 Logistic Growth Model Versus Holt's Model

As it is previously mentioned, both the logistic and Holt's models are good in the short term prediction. Therefore, different data sets were used for the four countries to predict the following days by the two models. It is shown in Tables 11 and 12 that both models have a small MAPE in most of the cases. However, when they were used to predict the next 5 days only, the MAPE for Holt's model prediction was less than that of the logistic model in 11 out of 16 cases. The MAPE values for Holt's model range from 0.0366 to 1.7484, while that of the logistic model range from 0.0409 to 3.0442. On the other hand, when the MAPE was calculated for the forecasts of the following 10 days instead of only 5 days in each of the cases, Holt's model was better in 8 out of 16 cases, as well as the logistic model. Moreover, the MAPEs of the forecasts of 20 days were also calculated, showing that Holt's model was better in only 7 out of 16 cases, while the logistic model was better in 9 cases.

Accordingly, a general observation can indicate that Holt's model is better in forecasting very short intervals, 5 days for example, unlike the logistic model that is

Table 11 Holt's model versus logistic growth model for short term prediction using Egypt data sets

Data Set	Predicted days	MAPE (Holt's)	MAPE (Logistic)
4 Apr. to 10 Jul.	5 days	0.2411	**0.1386**
	10 days	0.7077	**0.1157**
	20 days	2.4782	**0.1657**
4 Apr. to 20 Jul.	5 days	**0.0635**	0.0756
	10 days	0.3814	**0.0691**
	20 days	2.0910	**0.5273**
4 Apr. to 31 Jul.	5 days	**0.5901**	0.5962
	10 days	1.1710	**0.9563**
	20 days	2.3091	**1.7364**
4 Apr. to 10 Aug.	5 days	0.0891	**0.0592**
	10 days	0.2060	**0.1431**
	20 days	**0.3532**	0.5116

better on longer intervals up to 20 days. This is because Holt's model assumes that the data have a constant trend, which is usually not the case in the COVID-19 data on the long term. On the other hand, COVID-19 total cases data usually takes shape of the logistic growth model, which explains why it is better on a relatively longer term. Since the accuracy of these two models depend on the data, this observation is not always the case, as there might be some longer interval that has the same trend, thus following Holt's model more than the logistic curve. This is why each model fits in different applications either on the short or long term, depending on the time series data. For COVID-19 total cases, it is shown that using both models can lead to better forecasts, since the logistic model can produce good results on a longer term and can show the general trend of the data, from which we can predict the intervals on which it is better to apply Holt's model, and thus having good results also on the short term.

7 Sensitivity Analysis

Since the three models have different parameters that determine their outputs, it was important to show the effect of small changes in their values. Therefore, each parameter was given a set of values other than the optimum one, while keeping the other parameters constant, and the model output, using the data set that ends on the 20th of July for Egypt, was plotted in these cases, as shown in Figs. 17, 18, 19, 20, 21, 22 and 23.

For the modified SEIR model, Fig. 17 shows that increasing the parameter p by a very small value affects both peak time and value dramatically. This is because the

Table 12 Holt's model versus logistic growth model for short term prediction using different data sets

Country	Data set	Predicted days	MAPE (Holt's)	MAPE (Logistic)
Oman	16 Apr. to 10 Jul.	5 days	**1.0253**	1.4099
		10 days	**1.4709**	2.2752
		20 days	**3.2783**	3.4027
	16 Apr. to 20 Jul.	5 days	0.5897	**0.3515**
		10 days	2.0519	**1.2524**
		20 days	8.2155	**5.4882**
	16 Apr. to 31 Jul.	5 days	**1.0037**	3.0442
		10 days	**1.2533**	3.9095
		20 days	**2.1980**	5.3486
	16 Apr. to 10 Aug.	5 days	**0.0366**	0.0409
		10 days	0.1978	**0.0537**
		20 days	0.6596	**0.2664**
Nigeria	24 Apr. to 10 Jul.	5 days	**0.5612**	1.4999
		10 days	**0.9127**	2.7948
		20 days	**1.3073**	5.6773
	24 Apr. to 20 Jul.	5 days	**0.0938**	0.2515
		10 days	**0.2395**	0.6791
		20 days	1.6819	**1.0963**
	24 Apr. to 31 Jul.	5 days	0.9558	**0.8631**
		10 days	1.4378	**0.9178**
		20 days	2.3059	**0.7364**
	24 Apr. to 10 Aug.	5 days	**0.2351**	0.3895
		10 days	**0.3145**	0.8170
		20 days	**0.5153**	2.1008
South Africa	27 Mar. to 10 Jul.	5 days	**0.3617**	0.9061
		10 days	**0.6885**	2.5014
		20 days	**0.7522**	10.071
	27 Mar. to 20 Jul.	5 days	**0.6397**	2.4606
		10 days	**0.6473**	4.4332
		20 days	**2.1545**	9.7213
	27 Mar. to 31 Jul.	5 days	1.7484	**0.6782**
		10 days	3.3878	**0.9966**
		20 days	8.3126	**2.7319**
	27 Mar. to 10 Aug.	5 days	**1.0901**	1.5798
		10 days	**1.8377**	2.1486
		20 days	3.8257	**3.0291**

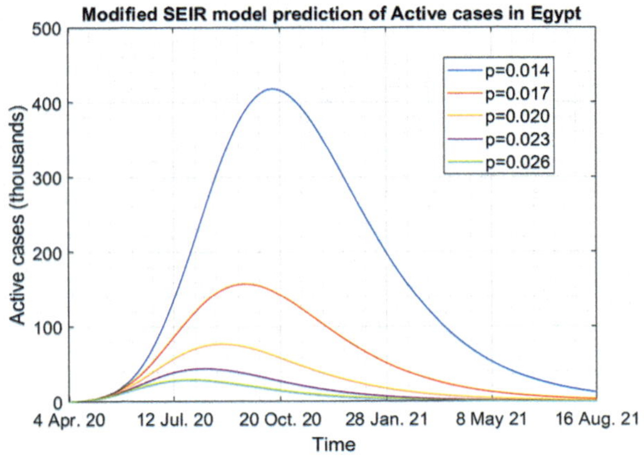

Fig. 17 Sensitivity analysis of p in the SS_pEIR model

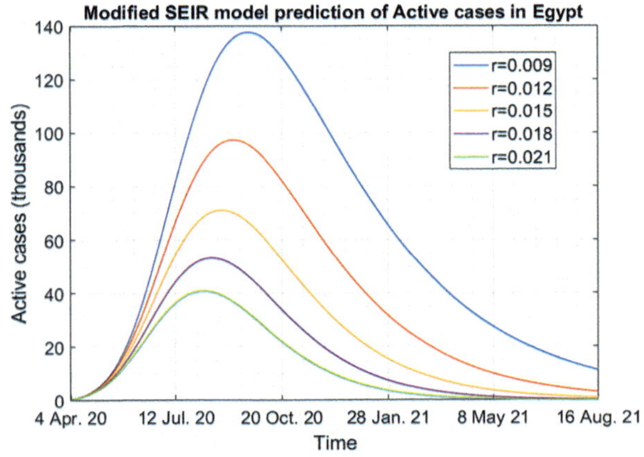

Fig. 18 Sensitivity analysis of r in the SS_pEIR model

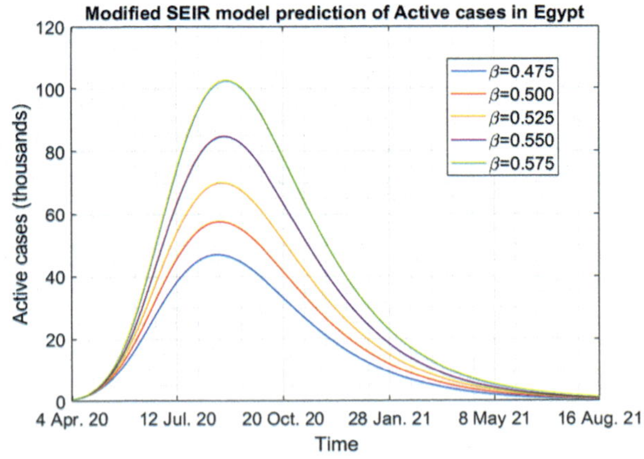

Fig. 19 Sensitivity analysis of β in the SS_pEIR model

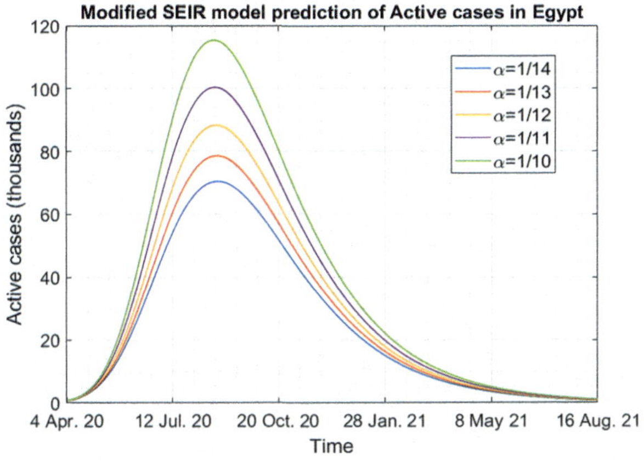

Fig. 20 Sensitivity analysis of α in the SS_pEIR model

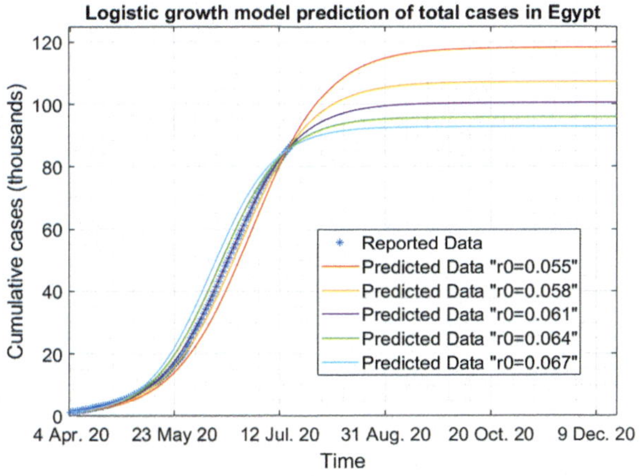

Fig. 21 Sensitivity analysis of the growth rate r_0 in the logistic model

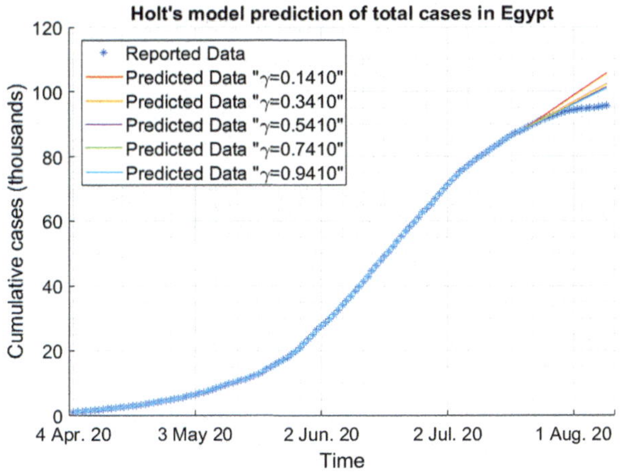

Fig. 22 Sensitivity analysis of the smoothing parameter γ in Holt's model

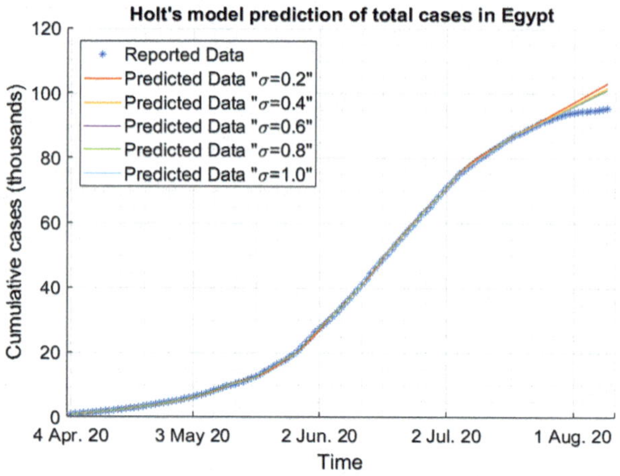

Fig. 23 Sensitivity analysis of the smoothing parameter σ in Holt's model

increase of awareness and thus the rate by which people go to the protected group decreases the infected population and ends the virus spread earlier. Similarly, as the removal rate r increases, the infected population decreases, as well as the peak time, as shown in Fig. 18. On the other hand, as the infection and incubation rates increase, the infected population increases, as in Figs. 19 and 20. Since the infection rate is the transmission probability multiplied by the number of close contacts, then it can be increased due to either of these two terms. Therefore, if the number of close contacts decreases, the infection rate and accordingly the peak value can be decreased, emphasizing the effect of social distancing on the spread of the virus.

For the logistic growth model, Fig. 21 shows how it is very dependent on the value of the growth rate r_0, as the number of cumulative cases greatly increased by decreasing r_0.

In case of the double exponential smoothing model (Holt's method), Figs. 22 and 23 show the effect of changing both trend and level smoothing parameters γ and σ. It indicates how much increased weight given to the latest data. While keeping the optimized value of σ constant, we changed the value of γ and vice versa as shown in figures. It was found that using small values of the parameters, the predicted data are more deviated from the actual data. This is justifiable because as we decrease the values of the parameters, the weight given to the latest data is decreased. Therefore, the higher deviation shows that the new data are more affected by the latest data points, due to the change in trend. However, larger values of the smoothing parameters lead to almost similar predicted values to that obtained from the optimized one, with a relatively good accuracy. This can be shown in the figures as the curves are almost coincident and closer to the reported data.

8 Conclusion

COVID-19 trends in Egypt, Oman, Nigeria and South Africa have been predicted based on the available data using three different models. On the long term, the logistic model results were closer to the reported data, while the modified SEIR model produced larger numbers due to its different nature. However, both models produce better results on entering more fitting data frequently. On the short term, both Holt's and the logistic models have a good accuracy. However, Holt's model is mostly better on the very short term, that exhibits constant trend, while the logistic model is usually better on a longer term.

Therefore, it is concluded that using the three models together can lead to a more accurate prediction and a deeper understanding of the virus spread. Where the logistic model can help know the intervals that have a constant trend so that we can use Holt's model, thus having an accurate short and long term prediction for the total cases, in addition to the active and removed cases by the modified SEIR model.

This study demonstrated how data fitting and optimization are crucial for giving good parameters' estimates and thus producing a more realistic prediction. It is also shown and verified that Levenberg–Marquardt algorithm is much faster than Nelder-Mead algorithm, which are both used for the logistic model, while the Trust-Region-Reflective algorithm is usually employed to produce optimal parameters between certain limits, thus using it for the SS_pEIR model. However, the MultiStart object with the Interior-Point algorithm could work better in case of Holt's model due to being very sensitive to the initial guesses.

Since using optimization algorithms is highly dependent on the initial guess, especially when dealing with a large number of parameters, it is recommended to have a parametric study in advance to pick a good initial point and also to employ a hybrid optimization algorithm to reach the optimal values of the model parameters with less computational effort. In this context, exploring metaheuristic, intelligent and nature-inspired optimization algorithms are worth to be investigated in future work.

Through the current study, parameters are tuned to investigate the effect of small changes in their values, and it can be indicated that the parameter p has the most dominant effect on the results of the modified SEIR model. Consequently, it highlights the great impact of the imposed quarantine and other social distancing measures. Stochastic algorithms will better analyze these variations and need further investigation in the future.

References

1. Naming the coronavirus disease (COVID-19) and the virus that causes it. https://www.who.int/emergencies/diseases/novel-coronavirus-2019/technical-guidance/naming-the-coronavirus-disease-(covid-2019)-and-the-virus-that-causes-it
2. Coronavirus. https://www.who.int/health-topics/coronavirus#tab=tab_1

3. Novel Coronavirus–China. https://www.who.int/csr/don/12-january-2020-novel-coronavirus-china/en/
4. WHO Director-General's opening remarks at the media briefing on COVID-19-11 March 2020. https://www.who.int/dg/speeches/detail/who-director-general-s-opening-remarks-at-the-media-briefing-on-covid-19. (11 Mar 2020)
5. How Coronavirus Spreads. https://www.cdc.gov/coronavirus/2019-ncov/prevent-getting-sick/how-covid-spreads.html
6. Rustan, R., Handayani, L.: The Outbreak'S modeling of coronavirus (Covid-19) using the modified seir model in Indonesia. Spektra: Jurnal Fisika dan Aplikasinya. **5**, 61–68 (2020)
7. Godio, A., Pace, F., Vergnano, A.: SEIR modeling of the Italian epidemic of SARS-CoV-2 using computational swarm intelligence. Int. J. Environ. Res. Public Health **17**, 3535 (2020)
8. Pai, C., Bhaskar, A., Rawoot, V.: Investigating the dynamics of COVID-19 pandemic in India under lockdown. Chaos Solitons Fractals **138**, 109988 (2020)
9. Cramer, J.S.: The early origins of the logit model. Stud. Hist. Philos. Sci. Part C Stud. Hist. Philos. Biolog. Biomed. Sci. **35**, 613–626
10. Shen, C.Y.: Logistic growth modelling of COVID-19 proliferation in China and its international implications. Int. J. Infect. Dis. **96**, 582–589 (2020)
11. Malavika, B., Marimuthu, S., Joy, M., Nadaraj, A., Asirvatham, E.S., Jeyaseelan, L.: Forecasting COVID-19 epidemic in India and high incidence states using SIR and logistic growth models. Clin. Epidemiol. Global Health (2020)
12. Brown, R.G.: Statistical Forecasting for Inventory Control. McGraw-Hill (1959)
13. Holt, C.C.: Authors retrospective on "Forecasting seasonals and trends by exponentially weighted moving averages." Int. J. Forecast. **20**, 11–13 (2004)
14. Winters, P.R.: Forecasting sales by exponentially weighted moving averages. Manag. Sci. **6**, 324–342 (1960)
15. Double Exponential Smoothing. https://www.itl.nist.gov/div898/handbook/pmc/section4/pmc433.htm
16. Coronavirus Cases. https://www.worldometers.info/coronavirus/coronavirus-cases/
17. Roda, W.C., Varughese, M.B., Han, D., Li, M.Y.: Why is it difficult to accurately predict the COVID-19 epidemic? Infect. Dis. Model. **5**, 271–281 (2020)
18. De-Camino-Beck, T.: A modified SEIR model with confinement and lockdown of COVID-19 for Costa Rica (2020)
19. Report of the WHO-China Joint Mission on Coronavirus …. https://www.who.int/docs/default-source/coronaviruse/who-china-joint-mission-on-covid-19-final-report.pdf
20. Pell, B., Kuang, Y., Viboud, C., Chowell, G.: Using phenomenological models for forecasting the 2015 Ebola challenge. Epidemics **22**, 62–70 (2018)
21. Mckendrick, A.G., Pai, M.K.: XLV.—the rate of multiplication of micro-organisms: a mathematical study. In: Proceedings of the Royal Society of Edinburgh. vol. 31, pp. 649–653 (1912)
22. Yin, X., Zelenay, P.: (Invited) Kinetic models for the degradation mechanisms of PGM-free ORR catalysts. ECS Trans. **85**, 1239–1250 (2018)
23. Gershenfeld, N.A.: The Nature of Mathematical Modeling. Cambridge University Press, New York (1999)
24. Liang, K.: Mathematical model of infection kinetics and its analysis for COVID-19, SARS and MERS. Infect. Genet. Evolut. **82**, 104306 (2020)
25. Marera, D.-H.S.-V.: An application of exponential smoothing methods to weather related data

An Hybrid Therapeutical Framework Based on Chatbots and Classic Psychotherapy for Mental Issues Raised from the Extended Pandemic Originated by COVID-19

Estefanía A. Hernández-Carvajal and Danny A. J. Gómez-Ramírez

Abstract We describe in a contextualized manner the indirect and evident correlation that the strong quarantine's conditions, originated by the global spread of COVID-19, possess with respect to mental health of people. In particular, we analyse this correlation with mental deceases like depression, stress, anxiety and bipolar and mood disorders. Specifically, we focus on the relation between the former phenomena and the modified workflow and structure of verbal communication among the quarantine. Moreover, we describe the most fundamental features and abilities that chatbots can simulate and stimulate in communication with people. Based on the former results we proposed hybrid therapeutic directions combining chatbots and human therapists for improving the mental health of people cognitively affected by the pandemic and with pronounced shy behaviour.

1 General Introduction

Although there are news of the COVID-19 virus since the first reported case in December 2019 in Asia, it was in February 2020 that the need to implement health measures in countries like Colombia began to be considered. Even more, such a measures were explicitly applied concretely since March where a national quarantine began to be carried out in order to control the outbreak of the pandemic, while the country's medical service was strengthened. Preventive isolation in Colombia were initially shown to be a temporary situation, something that would only last 14 days, with a maximum of two months of duration. However, the months passed and the pandemic began to be noticed as an unprecedented event, which is not known when or how it is going to finish. Preventive isolation measures forced the country's population

E. A. Hernández-Carvajal
Institución Universidad Pascual Bravo, Medellìn, Colombia
e-mail: estefania.hernandez183@pascualbravo.edu.co

D. A. J. Gómez-Ramírez (✉)
Parque Tech at the Institución Universitaria Pascual Bravo (Medellìn, Colombia) Visión Real Cognitiva S. A. S. (Itagüí, Antioquia, Colombia) and Instituto Tecnológico Metropolitano (ITM), Medellín, Colombia

D. Oliva et al. (eds.), *Artificial Intelligence for COVID-19*, Studies in Systems, Decision and Control 358, https://doi.org/10.1007/978-3-030-69744-0_27

to spend five months mainly in their homes, which has turned common work and study days into remote work and virtuality. Furthermore, there was a phenomena of closure of companies that cannot support payroll or pay the rents of their premises. The cause was that the COVID-19 crisis was not in the strategic plans of any brand for 2020, or for the informal vendors, that are about half of the working-age population in Colombia, and who have had difficulties to be at home during the pandemic. All of the above was evidenced in July when it was confirmed that the unemployment figure in the country was already 20.2% [8].

Mandatory preventive isolation has changed the routine of the vast majority of Colombians, who in addition to having to move away from their social and family circle (in some cases), lost their jobs, lost their financial security, got infected with the virus, saw how the COVID-19 takes their family, friends or colleagues. Moreover, the people dealt with an avalanche of information and misinformation that increases fear among the population, generating little energy, sleeping problems, lack of motivation to do the same routine activities, and physical and mental impairments [7]. It is not surprising that the chances of suffering from mental disorders associated with social, economic, family and personal factors may increase during the pandemic and the transition to the "new normal" way of living [20].

In this paper, we will propose to study the trends in mental health during mandatory quarantine around the globe, with a particular focus in Colombia. We will evaluate the technological applications related with human-machine interfaces that have been developed before and during the pandemic in order to support the population from a psychological point of view. After this, we will present effective blended preventive and (potentially) therapeutic guidelines for dealing with cognitive issues originated by prolonged quarantines, which could originate permanent isolation and overuse of virtual communication. Such a guidelines are based on a suitable combination of chatbots based technologies and classic psycho-therapeutic support.

2 Mental Health

Mental health is a psycho-emotional stability that demands a continuous effort to maintain balance in the face of new circumstances. Mental health is an optimistic concept in which it is sought to promote and generate well-being for all in social, labor, educational, cultural and religious aspects. Some of the causes of mental illnesses are generated by dramatic, social circumstances, disappointments, abandonment and even failures in the adaptation mechanisms. Some mental illnesses can also be caused by brain injury or poor brain function. It is necessary to perform a physical examination for the correct diagnosis of mental illness, since it can be confused with an infectious process or a change in some organic function, hormonal, adrenal and thyroid problems that can trigger similar symptoms. Special attention is required when evaluating abnormal movements, looks, language or understanding problems, deviant or antisocial behaviors, addictions, suicidal ideation, eating disorders, among others. Absolute silence, incoherent language, insomnia, drowsiness, lack of motivation, apathy, are warning signs for possible disorders of a mental illness.

It is common to find acquaintances, relatives or people around us who suffer from some type of mental disorder, that is, we are surrounded by a population that constantly faces a crisis of depression, anxiety or personality disorders. The most common of the above is to see how the importance of mental health monitoring is ignored and the need to find help to deal with them is underestimated. Depression, anxiety, post-traumatic stress disorder, bipolar disorder, and schizophrenia are known to be mental illnesses that affect more than one in five people globally. Since 2001, it has been established that some of the most common mental disorders in the world are unipolar depression, bipolar depression, post-traumatic stress disorder, panic disorder and primary loss of consciousness. It is necessary to clarify that mental health in our society is handled as a taboo, since the importance of it has always been underestimated, discriminating against the people who suffer from them and their closest social and family circle.

In Colombia the situation is not indifferent, an important part of medical attention is dedicated to treating mental disorders. Some studies have shown that the prevalence of any of these disorders sometime in life is 10.1%, 10.1%, [12]. Mental disorders can be produced by inheritance, also from our individual development and behavior and other factors such as nutritional, social, cultural, economic, political and environmental.

2.1 Mental Health in Colombia

According to the National Study of Mental Health carried out in 2014, it is determined that two out of every five Colombians present some time in their life some mental disorder and of these the most frequently identified were anxiety disorders in 19.3%, followed by 15% of mood disorders and psychoactive substance use disorders by 10.6% [9].

- Depression: Depression is a mental disorder characterized by the fact that the person suffering from it presents sadness, loss of interest, feelings of guilt or low self-esteem, among others. Emotions presented during depression can transform into physical patterns with no apparent cause. This disorder can be suffered by children, young people or adults and is one of the main causes of disability worldwide, affecting more than 264 million people around the world, with a higher prevalence in women than in men [26].
- Bipolar affective disorder: this disorder is characterized by alternating between manic and depressive episodes, also presenting a decrease in the need for sleep, this disorder affects around 45 million people around the world [26].
- Anxiety: It is a mental disorder that appears persistently to the stimuli that apparently trigger it and is characterized by feelings of fear, fear, and restlessness that may worsen over time [13].

2.2 *COVID-19 and Its Relationship with Mental Health in the World*

Mental illnesses or disorders are conditions that impact people's thinking, feeling, mood, and behavior. At the moment it has not been possible to associate the alteration of mental health as one of the sequel of COVID-19, however various studies have been carried out in which the emotional and mental state of not only people who have been infected with the virus, but also from the general population that has kept the mandatory isolation required in different countries. In this section of the document, some studies that were carried out from specialized surveys to determine stress, anxiety, depression, among others, will be reviewed and the correlation between quarantines and mental disorders such as depression, anxiety and personality disorders.

Public	Study method	Results
898 American young adults	Survey	18.3% of the surveyed population who stated that they had not been previously diagnosed with a mental illness show depression, 20.4% symptoms of anxiety and 13.8% post-traumatic disorder [19]
44,447 Chinese students	Survey	Prevalence of anxiety symptoms in 7.7% and depression in 12.2%. 42% of the people surveyed sought psychological care [32]
2,237 people in Shenzhen, China	Survey	6.21% of the undiagnosed COVID-19 population that was quarantined in Shenzhen, China demonstrated prevalence of depression symptoms [23]
435 US adults	Survey	An increase in depression was observed in 118 people during compulsory isolation [21]
3,676 participants from Wuhan City, China	Survey	19.2% showed moderate—severe symptoms of depression, while 20.3% showed moderate - severe symptoms of secondary trauma [33]
1,036 participants (ages 6–15) from Guiyang City, China	Survey	11.78% showed depression, 18.92% anxiety and 6.56% of respondents showed depression and anxiety [11]
290 citizens over 60 years of age in the north of Spain	Survey	8.2% of those over 60 show signs of moderate depression, 17.3% of anxiety and 14% of stress [28]
976 people from the Basque Autonomous Community (from 18 to 61 years of age)	Survey	48% of people between 18 and 25 years old showed moderate depression, 61% of them showed moderate anxiety and 45% of the same moderate stress [27]
4,459 Australians of which 1,292 respondents with personality disorders 3,167 respondents without any report of mental disorder	Survey	Psychological distress increased in the group with mood disorder compared to the group without mental disorder, and stress and depression were further elevated in respondents with bipolar disorder compared to those with depressive disorder [31]

The table above allows us to see that regardless of the location where the surveys were conducted and the age of their participants, it was not uncommon for them to show some affectations, and it also shows that one of the most common mental disorders that has been associated with the pandemic is depression [23]. This leads us to think that in addition to strengthening health systems in the face of COVID-19, it is important to keep cognitive health in mind because, although no alteration of emotions or cognitive functions has been determined as a direct effect of the virus on the brain [29], COVID-19 could lead to an epidemic of clinical depression that must be addressed by phone, email or video-conference.

2.3 COVID-19 and Its Relationship with Mental Health in Colombia

A report presented in May by Profamilia (a Colombian non-profit organization) shows the study of a sample of the Colombian population and the way in which their mental health has been affected while going through the consequences of the pandemic.

Public	Study method	Results
3,549 people over 18 years of age	Survey	More than 70% of the population surveyed shows nervousness, restlessness and fatigue for no reason. 56% are concerned about falling into anxiety and depression during isolation. 18% of the respondents (or one of their relatives) has presented mental health problems in the last six months [7]

Many of the factors that affect the mental health of Colombians are associated with economic insecurity, since 58% of the people surveyed do not have savings in money at the present time and 32% do not receive any type of income from work [7]. In countries like Colombia, more important than social distancing or the needs to improve the health system is the economy, since the economic effects of the pandemic are stronger than those of the 2008 crisis [30]. While in countries like the Netherlands, its inhabitants did not have strong emotional changes given that the government has a good health system and unemployment benefits, among others, which made it easy for people to stay in their homes during the mandatory quarantine. In addition to this, the inhabitants migrated the physical distancing and changed it for the contact by internet, which guaranteed that they did not have this type of mental problems [30].

2.4 Chatbot and Mental Health Support

Chatbots have been developed since the 60s that allow simulating a psychological accompaniment for users, such as the one developed in 1966 by Joseph Weizenbaum. Its name was 'Eliza', a program that allowed simulating in some aspects a conversation with a psychologist. Some of chatbots under these lines are:

- ELIZA (The First Chatbot): developed by MIT in 1966. It was designed to mimic a humanistic psychologist, one of the best-known therapies in psychology.
- KARIM: designed by X2AI mainly to help Syrian refugees with the emotional problems that may arise from their situation. It is also often used to accompany problems such as childhood diabetes.

- THERACHAT: developed as a tool used by psychologists whose users can interact from home, allowing a complete record of the conversations done.
- ELLIE: designed to detect psychological problems according to the text entered, the tone of voice and body expressions, detected by video-conference.

During the COVID-19 pandemic, there has been an increase in the download of different applications that provide psychological support, because in addition to not being subject to the scope of the health service, it has also been noted that when users are aware that they are interacting with a bot, they express their emotions more easily and do better in the process.

For example, in South Korea a study was carried out in which 41 patients were chosen from a psychiatric clinic and 21 patients were randomly assigned to talk to a chatbot and 20 patients to be in a control group. During this four-week exercise, it could be seen that panic disorder decreased significantly in the chatbot group, but not in the control group. The social phobia score decreased significantly, although the control impotence score increased significantly in the chatbot group compared to the control group [17].

One of the most popular bots used during the time of compulsory isolation was the one developed by Alison Darcy, a clinical psychologist at Stanford University called Woebot, this bot proposes conversations to users by constantly asking their mood, the user can also resort to him when he needs help and, at the same time, the app follows him up [5].

The chatbot Yana was developed in Mexico and was designed by Andrea Campos. It is based on cognitive behavioral therapy (it works to modify the perception of our emotions) and has reached more than 7,100 users in Mexico. The chatbot uses tools of Natural Language Processing and machine learning (ML) to respond correctly to the user [22].

It is important to be certain that at no time is a chatbot going to replace professional support, since it is possible that the users are not completely honest with their emotions or thoughts during their interaction. Thus, they make the application believe that they are well, while professionals are trained to understand the incongruities between people's non-verbal and verbal language [15].

3 Chatbots and Their Daily Cognitive Effect on Humans from a Linguistic Perspective

Since the 60's, work has been done on developing software programs that interact with users using natural language, better known as chatbots [6]. Chatbots are virtual machines with artificial intelligence capable of imitating human intelligence at a certain level and although the advances have been representative, it is still possible to detect that you are interacting with a machine. The foregoing is not an impediment to the fact that thousands of platforms are currently migrating the first customer service filter to bots, which allow to attend to defined basic needs, reducing costs in customer service areas and reducing waiting times for specialized care.

The interaction between chatbots and humans is the object of constant evaluation based on the Computers Are Social Actors (CASA) [2]. This paradigm, that is, people show social tendencies with machines similar to how they interact with another human Some studies show, among others , the following advantages:

- Bots, being machines, cannot make value judgments according to the information given to them, that is why there are people who prefer to hold conversations with bots than with humans [16]
- Chatabots are available 24 h a day, seven days a week, this provides peace of mind in the face of immediate response when seeking the attention of the bot, they also create the feeling of understanding and patience when interacting [10]
- Interactions with bots can be done in different modalities such as text, visual and speech [14]
- Chatbot users are eager to have frequent interactions with these machines in the future [6]

The previous affirmations on the advantages of the interaction bots-humans have opened the doors to support the mental health of the patients with chatbots and therefore the demand in this aspect has increased. In addition, people are increasingly seeking support for their mental health in bots while fighting the stigmas associated with the population with mental problems [18]. Chatbots have been used for various mental disorders and purposes. Healthcare providers should compare chatbots found in this review to help guide potential users to the most appropriate chatbot to support their mental health needs [1].

In Abd-alrazaq's studio et al. [1], analyzed 17 chatbots used to support mental health needs, showing that the most used are the chatbots used for therapy, training and detection, the most popular being the one used for cognitive-behavioral therapy, followed by depression and anxiety, training focused on people with autism and improvement of social skills for job interviews. While chatbots used as detection tools were also analyzed, which mainly focused on depression, dementia and post-traumatic stress disorder.

As an example of the benefits of this interaction, you can consider:

- The chatbot "Wysa" that uses several evidence-based therapies (e.g. cognitive behavioral therapy, behavioral reinforcement, and mindfulness) to target symptoms of depression for users [1].
- LISSA is another chatbot that provides training for people with autism in order to develop their social skills [1].
- Replika is used by orientation for general conversation and enables us to study social support from artificial agents in everyday contexts rather than only as a response to very stressful and health-related events [3].
- Woebot was designed to help combat depression [25].
- Vincent is based on the usage of limited pre-set responses was to continue its' narrative whilst allowing participants a choice between relevant responses (Woe-

bot also interacted with its users in a similar fashion). This allowed for greater comparability between participants in each condition [25].

Chatbots have also been implemented to accompany adolescents with special health needs to make their transition to adults, creating awareness of their medical problems and required medical treatments. In this case, the analysis of the pre- and post-project surveys revealed an increased patient participation in many important activities needed for successful health care transitions, like managing medications, ordering prescription refills, and proactively contacting providers about health-related concerns [4].

In the pandemic generated by COVID-19, the use of chatbots to support mental health's needs derived from social isolation has become common popular among the population. The main reason is that it has been noted that this interaction can mitigate psychological damage, although it is clear that not interacting with humans, disclosing concerns and receiving emotional support responses can reduce the damage from isolation, trauma and depression related to the pandemic [24].

4 Hybrid Therapeutic Directions for the Mental Effect of the Extreme Quarantine Conditions Originated by COVID-19 Based on a Blending Between Chatbots and Human Therapists and General Conclusions

In the current conditions of selective or mandatory isolation, it is possible to provide bots supported by health specialists through mobile applications. In this section, we will provide a global schematic description of hybrid (preventive) therapeutic directions for mental health involving a suitable combination of chatbots and human therapists. This is based and inspired by the former analysis of several study cases varying over a wide methodological spectrum of possibilities and evidencing different weakness and strengths.

These (chatbot) applications, after requesting authorization for the handling of personal data and the collection of information, analyzes the user's tastes and initiates conversations. Subsequently, the bot will obtain information from the user in order to characterize their personality according to surveys developed by psychologists that will provide basic information for the treatment that the bot must handle with the user and an initial rating of the risk level of the state of their mental health.

The chatbot is designed to initiate conversations with the user, proposing conversation topics related to the user's tastes and posing the options to keep social life active from virtuality. The development of the conversations generated between bots and humans will be supervised anonymously by psychologists or psychiatrists, who will provide therapies to users that will create conditions to make future interaction with other humans enjoyable.

During the first three months of using this application, only one interaction between bots and the users will be handled. From around the third-fourth month of use of the application (depending on the patient) and based on the information collected by the bot through interactions and analysis of user tastes, feedback will be made between mental health specialists and bot programmers. These feedback will end in bot reprograms that allow for a more fluid human-bot interaction. However, the mental health of the user will also be verified directly by the specialist, who in some moments will be behind the bot interacting live with the user.

During the whole process there will be at least a professional therapist and a bot programmer following the chat protocols in an integrated manner. This in order to have a more accurate cognitive blue-print of the user-patient. Nonetheless, the interaction with the bot should be always genuine and with no human influence during the process. The main reason is to respect the authenticity of the whole process and the expectations on the nature of the interaction generated by the user. Now, from the careful analysis of these written protocols the therapist will have more precise interpersonal elements for identifying more precisely the most suitable lines of conversation among which the patient will be more open and motivated to interact in a more fruitful manner.

Finally, the results described globally in the former sections showed the specific advantages that an hybrid methodology possesses for opening several cognitive components of people during (artificial) dialogues. Moreover, most of the disadvantages of a purely artificial interaction showed in former sections are essentially erased with the hybrid component of our proposal in the form of a continuous accompaniment of humans in both ways, invisible and visible, regarding the patient. In particular, this interbred method generates a strong sense of privacy and trust on the patient that stimulates naturally the level of openness and interest.

Acknowledgements Danny A. J. Gomez-Ramirez would like to thank the Institución Universitaria Pascual Bravo and to the Instituto Tecnológico Metropolitano (ITM) and to Visión Real Cognitiva S. A. S. for all the support. Special thanks to Gianny Rozo and to Diony González for all the support and kindness.

References

1. Abd-alrazaq, A., Alajlani, M., Alalwan, A.A., Bewick, B., Gardner, P., Househ, M.: An overview of the features of chatbots in mental health: a scoping review. Int. J. Med. Inf (2019)
2. Araujo, T.: Living up to the chatbot hype: the influence of anthropomorphic design cues and communicative agency framing on conversational agent and company perceptions. Comput. Human Behav. 183–189 (2018)
3. Ata, V., Griffith, C., Boatfield, C., Wang, X., Civitello, M., Bader, H., DeCero, E., Loggarakis, A.: User experiences of social support from companion chatbots in everyday contexts: thematic analysis. J. Med. Internet (2020)
4. Beaudry, J., Consigli, A., Clark, C., Robinson, K.J.: Getting ready for adult healthcare: designing a chatbot to coach adolescents with special health needs through the transitions of care. J. Pediatr. Nurs. 80–91 (2019)
5. Blogthinkbig.com. Una investigadora de stanford crea un chatbot para combatir la depresion (2018). https://blogthinkbig.com/esta-investigadora-de-stanford-ha-creado-un-chatbot-para-combatir-la-depresion

6. Ciechanowski, L., Przegalinska, A., Magnuski, M., Gloor, P.: In the shades of the uncanny valley: an experimental study of human-chatbot interaction. Future Generation Computer Systems (2018)
7. Cifuentes-Avellaneda, A., Rivera-Montero, D., Gil-Vera, C., Munrad-Rivera, R., Sanchez, S.M., Castaño, L.M., Royo, M., Rivillas-García, J.C.: Ansiedad, depresión y miedo: impulsores de la mala salud mental durante el distanciamiento fisico en colombia. Profamilia **1**(1), 1–3 (2020)
8. DANE. Geih mercado laboral-informacion julio 2020 (2020). https://www.dane.gov.co/index.php/estadisticas-por-tema/mercado-laboral/empleo-y-desempleo
9. de Gestión, G.: Integrada para la Salud Mental. Abece sobre la salud mental, sus trastornos y estigma. Ministerio de Salud y Proteccion Social, pp. 58–67 (2014)
10. Dokukinaa, I., Gumanova, J.: The rise of chatbots-new personal assistants in foreign language. Proc. Comput. Sci. 542–546 (2020)
11. Fangping, C., Dan, Z., Jing, L., Yi, G., Zhizhong, G., Didong, L.: Depression and anxiety among adolescents during covid-19: a cross-sectional study. Brain Behav. Immun. **88**, 36–38 (2020)
12. Gomez-Restrepo, C., Tamayo Martinez, N.: Trastornos depresivos y de ansiedad y factores asociados en la poblacion adulta colombiana, encuesta nacional de salud mental 2015. Revista Colombiana de Psiquiatria **45**(s1), 58–67 (2016)
13. Heraldo, E.: Ansiedad, uno de los trastornos que mas afectan a los colombianos (2019). https://www.elheraldo.co/entretenimiento/ansiedad-uno-de-los-trastornos-que-mas-afectan-los-colombianos-665526
14. Heung-yeung, S., Xiao-dong, H., Di, L.: From eliza to xiaoice: challenges and opportunities with social chatbots. Front. Inform. Technol. Electron. Eng. **19**(1), 10–26 (2018)
15. Hipertextual. De 'amigo' a psicologo 24 horas: los chatbots han sido los aliados inesperados en pandemia (2020). https://hipertextual.com/2020/06/chatbot-pandemia
16. Ho, A., Hancock, J., Miner, A.S.: Psychological, relational, and emotional effects of self-disclosure after conversations with a chatbot. J. Commun. 712–733 (2018)
17. Jooyoung, O., Sooah, J., Hyunji, K., Jae-Jin, K.: Efficacy of mobile app-based interactive cognitive behavioral therapy using t a chatbot for panic disorder. Int. J. Med. Inf. 1–8 (2020)
18. Kretzschmar, K., Tyroll, H., Pavarini, G., Manzini, A., Singh, I.: Can your phone be your therapist? young people's ethical perspectives on the use of fully automated conversational agents (chatbots) in mental health support. Biomed. Inf. Insights **11**, 1–9 (2019)
19. Liu, C., Stevens, C., Conrad, R., Hahm, H.: Evidence for elevated psychiatric distress, poor sleep, and quiality of lige concerns during the covid-19 pandemic among US young adults with suspected and reported psychiatric diagnoses. Psychiatry Res. 1–7 (2020)
20. Lòpez Gonzòlez, A.: El suicidio postpandemia, una epidemia anunciada. Notas de Politica **1**(1), 2–12 (2020)
21. Marroquín, B., Vine, V., Morgan, R.: Mental health during the covid-19 pandemic: effects of stay-at-home policies, social distancing behavior, and social resources. Psychiatry Res. 2–9 (2020)
22. Milenio. ¿deprimido? este programa de inteligencia artificial te da terapia psicologica (2020). https://www.milenio.com/tecnologia/yana-el-chatbot-que-brinda-apoyo-emocional
23. Min, P., Beirong, M., Yansong, L., Mingming, X., Xinran, S., Luyu, L., Yeqing, F., Tianyou, G., Jinying, Y., Zhijian, Y., Qiwen, D., Xiangyang, Z.: Prevalence, risk factors and clinical correlates of depression in quarantined t population during the covid-19 outbreak. J. Affect. Disord. 119–124 (2020)
24. Miner, A.S., Laranjo, L., Kocaballi, B.: Chatbots in the fight against the covid-19 pandemic. npj Digit. Med. (2020)
25. Minha, L., Sander, A., Nena, V.A., Hanwen, C., Enzo, L., Wijnand, I.: Caring for vincent: a chatbot for self-compassion. CHI 2019 (2019)
26. Organization (WHO): Trastornos mentales (2019). https://www.who.int/es/news-room/fact-sheets/detail/mental-disorders

27. Ozamiz-Etxebarria, N., Dosil-Santamaria, M., Picaza-Gorrochategui, M., Idoiaga-Mondragon, N.: Stress, anxiety, and depression levels in the initial stage of the covid-19 outbreak in a population sample in the northern spain. Cadernos de Saude Publica 1–10 (2020)
28. Picaza Gorrochategi, M., Eiguren Munitis, A., Dosil Santamaria, M., Ozamiz Etxebarria, N.: Brief report: stress, anxiety, and depression in people aged over 60 in the covid-19 outbreak in a sample collected in Northern Spain. Am. J. Geriatr. Psychiatry 993–998 (2020)
29. Shader, R.I.: Covid-19 and depression. Clin. Ther. **46**(6), 962–963 (2020)
30. Van der Velden, P.G., Contino Fonds Slachtofferhulp, C., Das, M., van Loon, P., van Loon, C., Bosmans, M.: Anxiety and depression symptoms, and lack of emotional support among the general population before and during the covid-19 pandemic. a prospective national study on prevalence and risk factors. J. Affect. Disord. 1–34 (2020)
31. Van Rheenen, T.E., Meyer, D., Neill, E., Phillipou, A., Tanb, E.J., Lin Toh, W., Rossell, S.L.: Mental health status of individuals with a mood-disorder during the covid-19 pandemic in Australia: Initial results from the collate project. J. Affect. Disord. **275**, 69–77 (2020)
32. Wanga, Z.-H., Yangb, H.-L., Yangb, Y.-Q., Liua, D., Lia, Z.-H., Zhanga, X.-R., Zhanga, Y.-J., Shena, D., Chena, P.-L., Songa, W.-Q., Wanga, X.-M., Wua, X.-B., Yangc, X.-F., Mao, C.: Prevalence of anxiety and depression symptom, and the demands for t psychological knowledge and interventions in college students during covid-19 epidemic: a large cross-sectional study. J. Affect. Disord. 188–193 (2020)
33. Zhong, B., Huang, Y., Liu, Q.: Mental health toll from the coronavirus: Social media usage reveals wuhan residents' depression and secondary trauma in the covid-19 outbreak. Comput. Human Behav. 2–9 (2020)

Semantic and Morpho-Syntactic Prevention's Guidelines for COVID-19 Based on Cognitively Inspired Artificial Intelligence and Data Mining. Case Study: Europe, North America, and South America

Yoe A. Herrera-Jaramillo, Danny A. J. Gómez-Ramírez, Johana C. Ortega-Giraldo, and Alex M. Ardila-Garcia

Abstract Based on a combination of cognitively inspired methods in artificial intelligence such as artificial mathematical intelligence and data mining, we study the correlation between the COVID-19 pandemic and the sentiment analysis (qualitative ontological nature) of tweets and their linguistic patterns from the presidents and the populations of five countries from Europe (Spain and the United Kingdom), North America (The United States of America), and South America (Chile and Colombia). The results show that tweets classified as negative are the most common in all presidential tweeter accounts, except in one country, Colombia. However, tweets classified as neutral are dominant in the population tweets in each country examined. Based on the results obtained and on some of the foundational cognitive techniques of artificial mathematical intelligence, we conclude by providing COVID-19 prevention guidelines at the linguistic and cognitive levels.

Y. A. Herrera-Jaramillo
Visión Real Cognitiva S. A. S. Itagü, Antioquia, Colombia

Institución Universitaria Tecnológico de Antioquia, Medellín, Colombia

D. A. J. Gómez-Ramírez (✉)
Parque Tech at the Institución Universitaria Pascual Bravo (Medellín, Colombia) Visión Real Cognitiva S. A. S. (Itagü, Antioquia, Colombia) and Instituto Tecnológico Metropolitano (ITM), Medellín, Colombia

J. C. Ortega-Giraldo
Visión Real Cognitiva S. A. S., Itagüí, Antioquia, Colombia
e-mail: jcog2583@outlook.com

A. M. Ardila-Garcia
Visión Real Cognitiva S. A. S., Medellín, Colombia

D. Oliva et al. (eds.), *Artificial Intelligence for COVID-19*, Studies in Systems, Decision and Control 358, https://doi.org/10.1007/978-3-030-69744-0_28

1 Introduction

The World Health Organization (WHO) declared the COVID-19 pandemic on 11 March 2020 after confirmation of more than 118,000 COVID-19 infections and 4,291 COVID-19 deaths in 114 countries [3]. COVID-19 is a highly contagious disease caused by a coronavirus (SARS-CoV-2) that is transmitted from person-to-person via saliva droplets or aerosols when coughing, sneezing, or speaking in close contact [1]. There is no known therapy or cure available for COVID-19 and a number of vaccines are being developed around the world [24]. The vast majority of people (around 80%) suffer non-severe symptoms [1] and can recover from COVID-19 at home, usually in one to two weeks. However, the remaining 20% require hospitalization, of which 20–30% must be treated in intensive care units (ICUs), of which approximately a third pass away [25]. The first COVID-19 outbreak was reported in China in December 2020 [29] and, in just ten months, there were over 30 million confirmed COVID-19 cases and nearly one million deaths around the world [2].

The worst COVID-19 death toll in the world is in the United States of America (USA) with over 200,000 (60.6/100,000 people) confirmed COVID-19 deaths [2]. The first confirmed case in the USA was in January 2020. There are nearly seven million confirmed COVID-19 cases in total in the USA [2] and daily confirmed cases range between 20,000 and 40,000, with daily peaks of nearly 80,000 cases in July 2020 (Fig. 1).

Two of the worst COVID-19 outbreaks in Latin America are in Chile and Colombia. Both countries confirmed their first COVID-19 case in the beginning of March 2020 and both countries have been affected similarly by COVID-19. Six months after the first case in Chile, there are over 450,000 confirmed COVID-19 cases and over 12,000 deaths (around 57.1 deaths/100,000 people) [2]. In Colombia, there are over 750,000 confirmed COVID-19 cases and over 25,000 deaths (around 50.0/100,000 people) over the same period [2]. In Chile, confirmed COVID-19 cases have never surpassed over 10,000 daily confirmed cases (Fig. 2), except for a single day in June 2020 when over 30,000 cases were reported. Daily confirmed COVID-19 cases in Colombia increased as testing capacity increased reaching over 10,000 confirmed daily cases in August 2020 (Fig. 3).

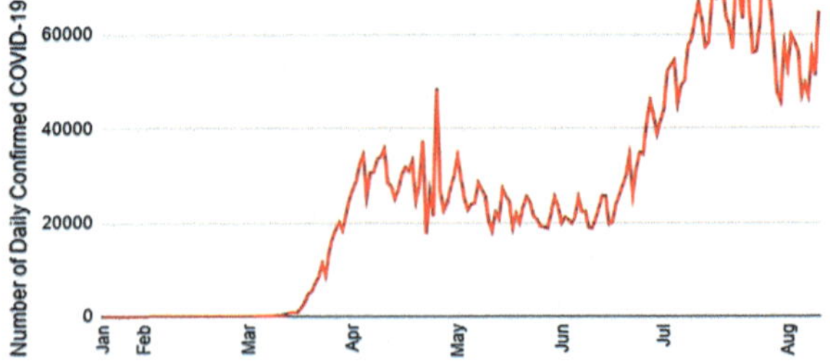

Fig. 1 Number of confirmed COVID-19 cases in the USA since its first confirmed case in January 2020 until 15 August 2020. *Data source* https://ourworldindata.org/coronavirus [23]

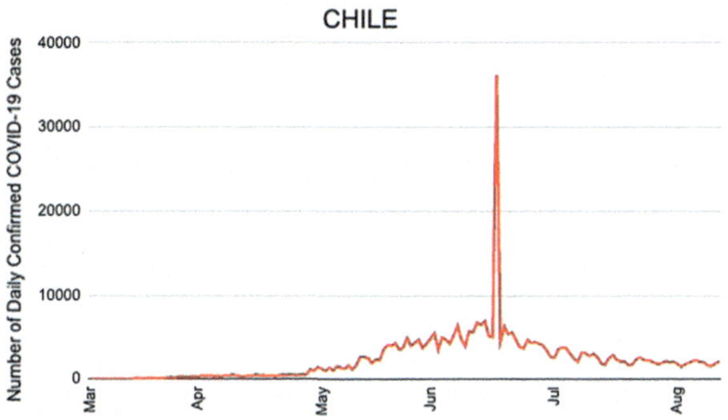

Fig. 2 Number of confirmed COVID-19 cases in Chile since its first confirmed case in March 2020 until 15 August 2020. *Data source* https://ourworldindata.org/coronavirus [23]

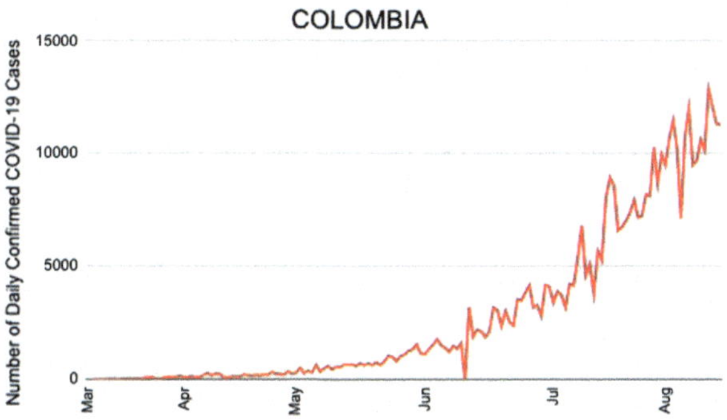

Fig. 3 Number of confirmed COVID-19 cases in Colombia since its first confirmed case in March 2020 until 15 August 2020. *Data source* https://ourworldindata.org/coronavirus [23]

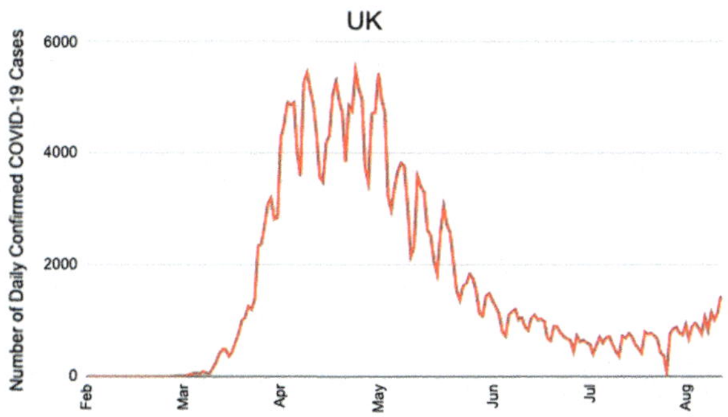

Fig. 4 Number of confirmed COVID-19 cases in the UK since its first confirmed case in February 2020 until 15 August 2020. *Data source* https://ourworldindata.org/coronavirus [23]

In Europe, the United Kingdom (UK) and Spain are two of the worst hit countries by COVID-19. There are over 400,000 confirmed cases in the UK and over 680,000 confirmed cases in Spain seven months after both countries reported their first cases in February 2020 [2]. Daily COVID-19 confirmed cases peaked in the UK between March and May 2020 with nearly 6,000 cases per day (Fig. 4) while Spain's daily confirmed cases peaked in March, April, and August with over 7,500 daily confirmed cases (Fig. 5). The COVID-19 death tolls in the UK and Spain are among the worst in Europe with over 40,000 (59.7/100,000 people) deaths in the UK and over 30,000 (63.8/100,000 people) deaths in Spain [2].

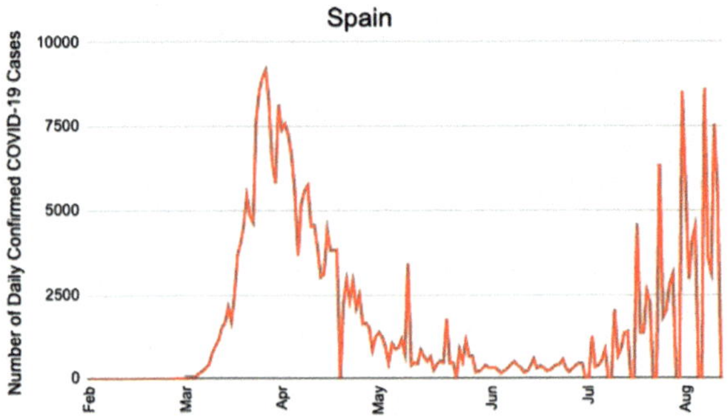

Fig. 5 Number of confirmed COVID-19 cases in Spain since its first confirmed case in February 2020 until 15 August 2020. *Data source* https://ourworldindata.org/coronavirus [23]

2 Preliminaries

2.1 Opinion Mining

In this section we describe the artificial intelligence techniques we used. The tools are part of the opinion mining and sentiment analysis theory. This field of study analyzes people's opinions, sentiments, evaluations, appraisals, attitudes, and emotions towards entities such as products, services, organizations, individuals, issues, events, topics, and their attributes (see [20]). Many different techniques are used to classify sentiments in texts, documents, tweets, and social app posts, and they range from Support Vector Machine, Logistic Regression, Deep Learning Neural Networks [30], Bayesian networks [27], among others.

The classification performed here is of the second level, that is, sentence-based classification [28] since we are analyzing tweets.

We perform the sentiment analysis of tweets from five different countries to assess the feelings of the inhabitants and contrast them with the tweets of the president or prime minister of their respective countries. The proposed technique is built, as illustrated in Fig. 6, in the following phases: data collection, pre-processing, feature extraction, sentiment analysis, and the classification algorithms.

2.1.1 Data Collection

Social media is a part of the daily life for most people nowadays. It is estimated that 51% of the world's population uses at least one social media app. One of the most popular social media apps is Twitter. It is estimated that around 330 million people have a Twitter account. People interact in Twitter by means of tweets. A tweet is a Twitter post and may include text, pictures, and emojis. The maximum length of text allowed in a tweet is 280 characters.

In this work, we retrieve and analyze tweets from users of five different countries, more precisely, ten tweet datasets from the following countries: The United States

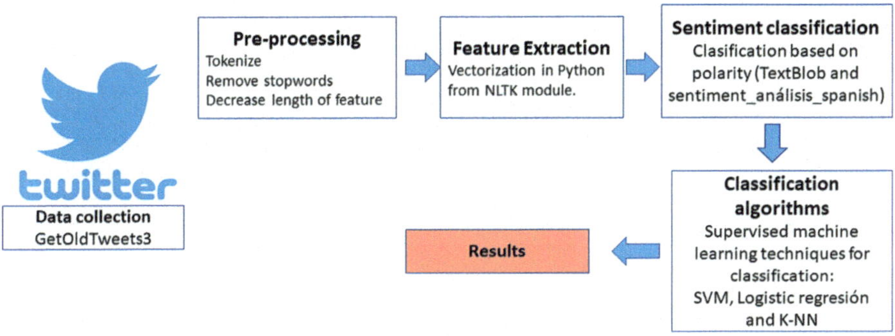

Fig. 6 Basic structure of the process of sentiment analysis

(USA), The United Kingdom (UK), Spain, Chile, and Colombia. There are two sets of tweets for each of the countries selected. One set for the president or prime minister and the other set for the population. The collection of tweets was obtained via Python with the help of the GetOldTweets3 module (https://pypi.org/project/GetOldTweets3/.) The day of the first confirmed COVID-19 case in each country was day 1 for each country. Then, we collected 20 tweets per day from day 1 until 15 August 2020 for each president or prime minister and for the population in each of the five selected countries. The search criteria used is shown below:

- For the tweets from the country's president or prime minister:
  - *setUsername* = president or prime minister Twitter username account.
  - *setTopTweets* = True.
  - *setSince* = day i.
  - *setUntil* = day i + 1.
  - *setMaxTweets*(20).
- For the tweets from the country's inhabitants:
  - *setNear* = city in the middle of the country.
  - *setWithin*("200mi").
  - *setTopTweets* = True.
  - *setSince* = day i.
  - *setUntil* = day i + 1.
  - *setMaxTweets*(20).

The total number of the collected tweets are shown in Table 1.

Table 1 Total number of collected tweets

Country	Number of tweets	Number of presidential tweets
Colombia	4,103	764
Chile	3,161	205
Spain	3,917	605
United Kingdom	4,120	446
United States of America	4,160	2,479

2.1.2 Pre-processing

A tweet may contain text, images, abbreviations, emojis, and other symbols. For this reason, the data collected have to be transformed or cleaned before use. The process of cleaning the data is known as pre-processing.

The first step in pre-processing is to separate the datasets by the country's language. That is, tweets from Colombia, Chile, and Spain make the group of Spanish speaking countries and the United Kingdom and the United States of America make the group of the English speaking countries. The following pre-processing steps were performed in Python using the frameworks of Natural Language Package ToolKit (NLPTK) and sklearn. We proceeded in the following order:

- Remove URLs, hashtags (#topic) and @username.
- Remove punctuation marks, symbols, numbers.
- Remove stopwords (Spanish and English).
- Make the tweets uniform by lowering the words.
- Delete repeated characters.

2.1.3 Feature Extraction

In this phase, we address the problem of attaining the most informative and compact set of features from the given data to improve the performance of machine learning models. We look for features that can characterize the opinions of Twitter users in the countries examined. The first step is tokenization of the text. Tokenization refers to the process of breaking the text in chunks, but with relevant meaning. These pieces are called tokens. Tokens can be words, phrases, or sentences. In this work we use words as tokens.

The method we use for this phase is the Bag of Words (BOW) method [26]. The compact quality refers to excluding irrelevant features from our model. There are several reasons to exclude irrelevant features, and in our study, we looked for compact feature sets to avoid overfitting problems. The tokenization of the tweets is performed by the module, resulting in a bag of words. Each tweet Tw can be turned into a vector in the vector space of dimension N, where N is the number of tokens and where $Tw[j]$ is the number of times that the token t_j is in the tweet Tw.

2.1.4 Sentiment Classification

For sentiment classification or analysis, it is extremely important to consider the language to be analyzed. Since we are dealing with Spanish speaking countries (Colombia, Chile, and Spain) and English-speaking countries (United States of America and the United Kingdom), care must be taken in the chosen method for the sentiment analysis. In this case, we use the module in Python called TextBlob to perform the sentiment analysis for the datasets of tweets from the United States of America and the United Kingdom. For Spanish-speaking countries we use sentiment_analysis_spanish module. The code was run in Google COLAB.

Both packages TextBlob and sentiment_analysis_spanish are of lexicographical type. These packages use a collection of words each with a value that represents the sentiment of the word. TextBlob values range from -1 to 1 and sentiment_analysis_spanish values range from 0 to 1. Then, a normalization is performed, where each value from 0 to 1 given by the sentiment_analysis_spanish API is transformed into its corresponding value from -1 to 1. Then, we consider that a word is positive if its sentiment is greater than 0, negative if its sentiment is less than 0, and neutral, otherwise. The sentiment of a tweet is then computed as the average of its constituting words.

The results obtained with these procedures are summarized in Fig. 7.

The results show that tweets classified as neutral (black color) are the dominant tweets in the population of each country examined. The countries that showed more positive tweets than negative tweets are Colombia, Chile, and Spain, which are Spanish-speaking countries. Only in Chile, we have a similar number of positive (blue color) and neutral tweets.

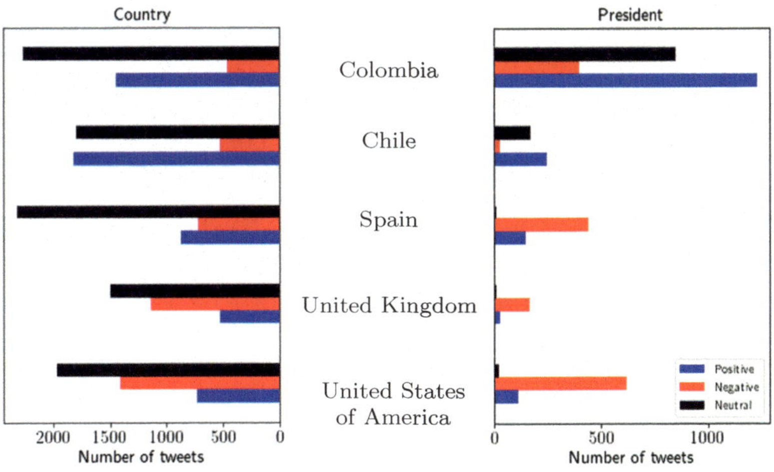

Fig. 7 Tweet sentiment analysis results

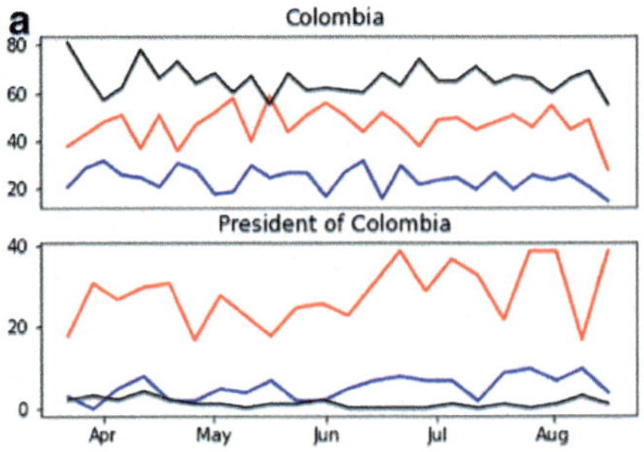

Fig. 8 **a** Colombia tweets polarity evolution through the COVID-19 pandemic. **b** Spain tweets polarity evolution through the COVID-19 pandemic

The datasets collected from the accounts of each of the presidents showed that tweets classified as negative (red color) are the most common in all but one country, Colombia. The tweets from Colombia's President Ivan Duque were positive most of the time (as measured by the package sentiment_analysis_spanish). In addition, the presidents from Spain and the United States of America were the two with the most negative tweets.

In addition, we examined the behavior of the polarity of the tweets from the Twitter users in these countries. We illustrate here the process made with two countries and the rest is left to the reader in Appendix 5. Figure 8 provides another way of appreciating how the polarity of the tweets changed during the time of the pandemic in Colombia. The mood of Colombian people (as suggested by the tweets analyzed) have been changing constantly during the Colombian COVID-19 lock-down, and the number of negative tweets is greater than the number of positive tweets.

On the other hand, Fig. 8b shows the evolution of Spain's tweets polarity. It is noticeable how the tweets of President Pedro Sánchez were negative, especially in March, precisely when the COVID-19 cases were peaking as shown above in Fig. 5.

Another country of particular interest is the United States of America. Figure 9 shows how the polarity of the tweets has changed during the six (6) months of the pandemic. It can be seen that June was the month when the population's tweets were positive.

2.1.5 Classification Algorithms

In this section we utilize the tools of Supervised Machine Learning for developing three classifiers. A classification algorithm learns from a labeled dataset (known as the training dataset) with known labels for each training input. When the algorithm is trained, that is, its parameters are tuned up, it is ready to predict the category or class for an input that may not be in the training dataset. These types of machines are then put to the test, with a testing set, that is, a set of inputs that have not passed through the machine and with known categories. Following the procedure in works like [19],

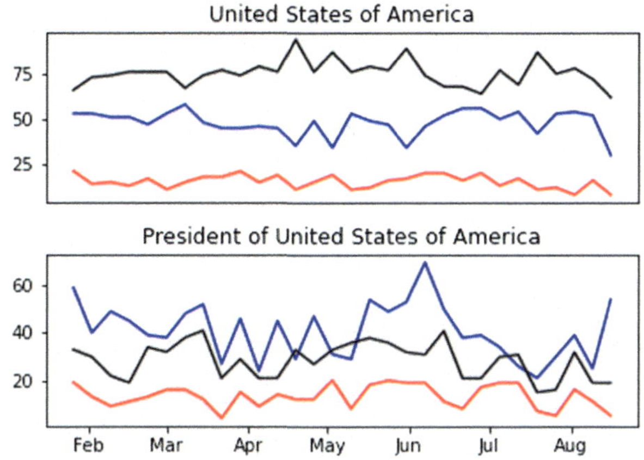

Fig. 9 United States of America tweets polarity evolution through the COVID-19 pandemic

we make a comparison between three sentiment classifiers of the supervised type with the dataset of classified tweets from the countries selected.

For the performance evaluation of a classifier, we use two metrics that are obtained by taking the weighted average of the accuracy ($Acurracy_i$) and precision ($Precision_i$) values for each class or category as given by Formulae (1) and (2), respectively.

$$Acurracy_i = \frac{TP_i + TN_i}{TP_i + TN_i + FP_i + FN_i} \tag{1}$$

$$Precision_i = \frac{TP_i}{TF_i + FP_i}. \tag{2}$$

where TP_i is the number of testing inputs correctly classified in its corresponding $i - th$ class; FP_i is the number of inputs which are wrongly classified in the category i; FN_i is the number of inputs from category i that are misclassified in another category and TN_i is the sum of the remaining entries of the diagonal of the confusion matrix, $C = [c_{ij}]$. The entries of this matrix c_{ij}, with $i \neq j$, are the number of testing items that are classified as belonging to class i, even though they are from class j. c_{ii} is the number of elements of class i correctly classified by the algorithm.

In respect to the weighted average for the evaluation of the technique, there are two options: (1) at the macro level consisting of assigning the same weight to every class and (2) at the micro level, assigning the same weight to each item, and in this case, larger classes will be heavier.

Support vector machine (SVM) [19]: This algorithm assigns a vector to each labeled training input. These vectors are mapped in a way that the members of the separate categories are divided by a gap as wide as possible. More specifically, the linear SVM separates categories with linear subspaces (hyperplanes, and the vectors which are orthogonal to these hyperplanes are the **support vectors**). During the testing phase, the vectors corresponding to testing inputs are mapped into the same

Table 2 Classifier performance evaluation

Classifier	Accuracy (%)	Precision micro (%)	Precision macro (%)
LR	**71.55**	**71.55**	**72.08**
k-NN	52.88	52.89	62.90
Linear SVM	70.00	70.00	69.54

space and they are predicted to belong to one of the categories. This is based on which side of the gap they fall in.

Logistic Regression (LR) [22]: Multinomial logistic regression is used to predict a nominal dependent variable given one or more independent variables. The formula of the model is given by Eq. 3.

$$P(Y = c) = \frac{1}{1 + e^{-\left(\beta_0 + \sum_{i=1}^{I} \beta_i x_i\right)}} \quad (3)$$

where the terms are: $C_1, C_2, \ldots, C_I$ are all possible categories of the dependent variable Y. $P(Y = c)$ is the probability that the dependent variable is equal to category "c." $\beta_i, i = 1, \ldots, I$ are the coefficients of the regression which, when transformed, express the importance of each variable in explaining the probability. $x_i, i = 1, \ldots, I$ are the independent variables.

***k*-Nearest neighborhood (*k*-NN)** [18]: This algorithm is part of the non-parametric classification technique. It is very effective in most of the cases and one of the most popular for text categorization and data mining. This method compares unknown inputs with known inputs, that is, the training inputs. This comparison is done by closeness as measured by Euclidean distance. Through the combination of a number of local distance functions based on individual attributes, a global distance function can be calculated. The distance is precisely the weighted of the point to the k nearest neighbors.

The best classifier: After some experimentation with the algorithm's possible configurations, the configurations with the best outcomes are selected. The results of the chosen configurations are given in Table 2. We split the collection of all the tweets from the seven datasets into a training part (75%) and a test part (the remaining 25%. For the k-NN method we use the linear algorithm $k = 3$ neighbors. As it can be appreciated, the Linear SVM algorithm outperformed the others soundly.

As can be seen in Table 2, the best classifier is the one given by the algorithm of Logistic Regression. The precision at the macro level is 72%. The linear SVM model also performed at a similar level. The k-NN precision is very low.

2.2 *Artificial Mathematical Intelligence*

The multidisciplinary research meta-project of artificial mathematical intelligence (AMI) is a multidisciplinary program for creating all the theoretical and computational foundations necessary for generating a universal mathematical artificial agent (UMAA) [4]. More specifically, AMI (or cognitive-computational metamathematics) involves the extension of a classic computational paradigm towards an extended multidisciplinary framework for *conceptual computation*, with all the (meta)mathematical preliminaries involved [10, 15]. Moreover, the first pillar of AMI encompasses the *New Cognitive Foundations' Program*, which involves the refinement of (meta)mathematical structures and frameworks like the physical numbers, Dathematics, and in a broader sense, the (cognitive) reality of mathematics and the mathematics of the (cognitive) reality, among others [7, 9, 14, 16].

The second fundamental pillar of AMI is the formalization of a sufficiently robust *taxonomy of seminal cognitive (metamathematical) mechanisms* used by the human mind during formal creation (for example see [5, 6, 8]) (for a more philosophical perspective about the conceptual substratum, please see [17], and in a more holistic context [21]). The quest for such a global taxonomy is not only important from a metamathematical and logic point of view, but also in an extended manner, from a mental and biological perspective. Effectively, one of the most ancient and important open questions in science is the intrinsic functioning of the mind. Such a query involves implicitly the identification of the grounding abilities used by the mind during abstract and concrete thinking [11].

The last pillar involves the specific generation of global pseudo-(pre)-code of conceptual computation, that is robust enough for implementing more holistic UMAA-s in initial mathematical sub-disciplines, and the potential and plausible extenstions of the AMI program to other related fields like physics and finances [12, 13].

In the context of the present work, we will focus on some of the most fundamental cognitive mechanisms used by our minds not only for creating mathematics, but also for structuring linguistic patterns, which includes semantic and morpho-syntactic constructs. In particular, for our subsequent analysis, we will fix our attention in the cognitive abilities of metaphorical thinking, analogical reasoning, and morpho-syntactic generalization and particularization [11].

3 Results and Discussion

3.1 *COVID-19 Daily Cases and Tweet Sentiment*

The number of new confirmed COVID-19 cases reported daily and the sentiment of presidential tweets varies considerably between the USA, the UK, Spain, Colombia, and Chile. The results show that the vast majority of tweets from the USA president are either positive or neutral (Fig. 9) during most of the outbreak (Fig. 1), even during the worst periods (June and July 2020) of the pandemic in the USA when daily new confirmed COVID-19 cases nearly quadrupled from 20,000 cases a day to 80,000 (Fig. 1). The USA's presidential tweet sentiment remained positive and neutral after June and July 2020 (Fig. 9) even though daily new COVID-19 cases remained high, between 40,000 and 70,000 (Fig. 1). Similarly, tweet sentiments obtained for the UK's prime minister during the UK's COVID-19 outbreak show that most of the UK's primer minister tweets are either positive or neutral (Fig. 14b), except during the worst period (April 2020) of the pandemic in the UK (Fig. 4). In April 2020, the UK reported over 40,000 new COVID-19 cases per day (Fig. 4), which coincides with the only period during which the UK's prime minister tweets are not positive or neutral, they are negative (Fig. 14b).

Tweet sentiments from the president of the USA (Fig. 9) and the UK's prime minister (Fig. 14b) showed a sharp contrast with the tweet sentiments obtained for the presidents of Spain (Fig. 8b), Chile (Fig. 14a), and Colombia (Fig. 8). Their tweets are mostly negative, not positive or neutral as obtained for the USA president (Fig. 9) and the UK's prime minister (Fig. 14b). Presidential tweet sentiment negativity dominated Spain's (Fig. 8b), Chile's (Fig. 14)a, and Colombia's (Fig. 8) presidential tweets during periods with the highest (over 10,000/day) and lowest incidence of new COVID-19 cases in each of these countries (Figs. 2, 3 and 5).

Presidential tweet sentiment during the COVID-19 pandemic does not seem to affect tweet sentiment of the general populations from the USA (Fig. 9), the UK (Fig. 14b), Spain (Fig. 8b), Chile (Fig. 14a), and Colombia (Fig. 8). This suggests that the population's sentiment does not to seem to be affected by presidential tweet sentiment, especially in Spain, Chile, and Colombia whose presidential tweets are negative and have remained negative during most of the COVID-19 pandemic. In addition, in each of the countries examined, the results show that tweet sentiment in the general population has been neutral or positive during most of the COVID-19 pandemic. The population's sentiment does not appear to change with increases nor reductions in daily new COVID-19 cases (Figs. 1, 2, 3, 4 and 5) in each of the countries examined.

3.2 Global Analysis from a Linguistic-Pragmatic Perspective

In this part, we will present a general inquiry of all the former health statistics regarding the development of COVID-19 in five representative countries and the corresponding sentiment analysis and word-clouds (see also the appendix). We focus specially on the relationship between the concrete spatio-temporal impact of COVID-19 per country and their corresponding linguistic patterns within a chosen temporal bound.

In the USA, one observes that the continuous growth in the number of infected people was accompanied by the predominance usage of words such as "thank," "great," "good," and "love", all with a positive component. In contrast, there were expressions that challenge the semantic veracity of the contextualized employment of words such as "fake news" and "never" in the corresponding tweets.

The United Kingdom has its worst development regarding the spread of the COVID-19 in the months of April and May. Then, the impact of this disease decreases significantly. At the same time, some of the most common words used in the analysed tweets are "great," "love," "day," "time," "amp," and "home." Most other words are neutral and a minority possess a negative connotation like "coronavirus."

In Spain, the worst sub-interval was at the beginning of April, with a reduction in the number of daily cases until the beginning of July, where a strong fluctuation per day was observed. This pattern was accompanied by an outstanding usage of words like "COVID-19," "España" (Spain), "Gobierno" (government), "Madrid," and "Love." There were almost no contrasting words.

In the Chilean context, the development of the COVID-19 pandemic was relatively severe showing the highest impact in the number of cases of infected people on a single day in the middle of June 2020. However, this spike was caused by an update on the official count of COVID-19 cases in Chile, where a large number of cases that were not included previously were added to the official report on a single day. After this spike in June, one observes a reduction in the number of cases per day. At the time, the main words used on the analysed tweets were "Chile," "Coronavirus," "Pandemia" (pandemic), "Persona" (person), "Salud" (health), "Gracia" (grace), and "Cuarentena" (quarantine). Surprisingly, in the Chilenian wordcloud one detects no word with a genuine negative connotation except for two ("coronavirus" and "pandemia") directly related with COVID-19.

In Colombia, there was an exponential spread in the number of infected people, beginning to be steeper in the middle of June 2020. In addition, the most used words in tweets during this time were "Pandemia" (pandemic), "país" (country), "Gobierno" (government), "Colombiano" (Colombian), "PrevencónYAcción" (PreventionAndAction), "Familia" (family), and "Gracia" (grace). Moreover, most of the additional words used can be classified as neutral e.g. "día" (day), "año" (year), "Bogotá," and "trabajo" (work).

4 General Conclusions and Semantic and Morpho-Syntactic Preventive Guidelines

Tweet sentiment analyses of presidential tweets and the general population from the USA, the UK, Spain, Chile, and Colombia show that presidential tweet sentiment does not appear to correlate with population tweet sentiment in each of the countries examined. In addition, presidential tweet sentiment and population tweet sentiment appeared not to change with spikes in new daily COVID-19 cases in each of the countries examined. On the other hand, by comparing the local impact that the coronavirus has in each of the five analysed countries with the corresponding linguistic development found on the word-clouds, we can suggest very fine semantic and morpho-syntactic preventive guidelines for overcoming COVID-19 along with all the preventive bio-security measures as follows. First, the usage of words with an essential positive an constructive inner meaning should be used very carefully, without over-using their semantic strength. Moreover, their original ontological impact should be highly protected specially by the country's leaders in order to guarantee that the credibility of the corresponding words will be mainly translated by most of the people. Second, an excessive focus of cognitive attention on the concept of COVID-19 (and all the primary synonyms) should be avoided. Instead of that, maintaining the highest medical accuracy on the description of the crucial factors should have a central focus on any kind of public communication. Otherwise, the common and particular subjective perception of this virus by the people would have a amplified negative impact on their unconscious mind, which could possible affect how people handle the pandemic in a less effective manner. Third, the usage of constructive, accurate and motivating words with notions related with COVID-19 could diminish negative mental effects. For instance, the usage of metaphors like "COVID-19 is a challenge that we will overcome united," are highly more desired than metaphors such as "COVID-19 is the worst pandemic ever."

Acknowledgements Danny A. J. Gomez-Ramirez would like to thank the Institución Universitaria Pascual Bravo, to the Institución Universitaria ITM (Instituto Tecnológico Metropolitano) and to Visión Real Cognitiva S. A. S. (Cognivisión) for all the support. He also wishes to thank Fabián Suarez, Ramiro Grisales, Ernesto Fajardo, William (Jake) Novoa, Sonya and Sandra Ramírez for all the empaphy and cooperation. Yoe Herrera thanks the Universidad Autónoma de Bucaramanga for their support.

5 Appendix

See (Figs. 10, 11, 12, 13, 14, 15, 16, 17, 18 and 19).

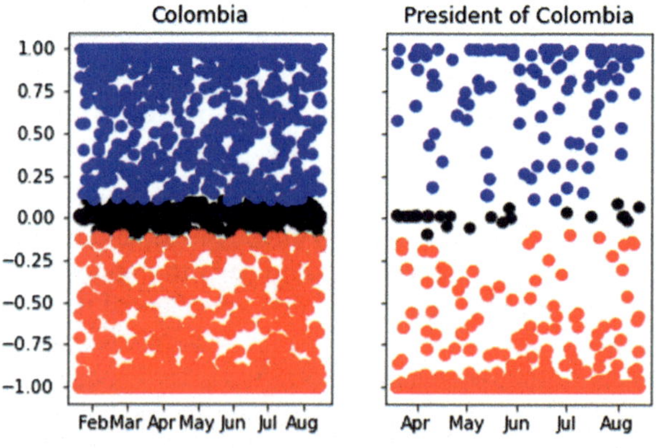

Fig. 10 Colombia tweets polarity

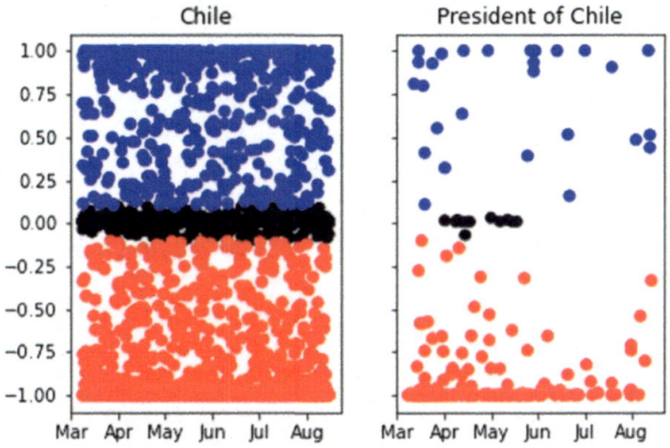

Fig. 11 Chile tweets polarity

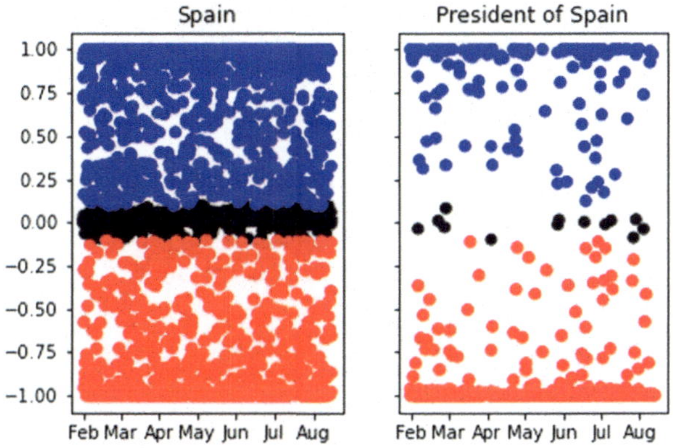

Fig. 12 Spain tweets polarity

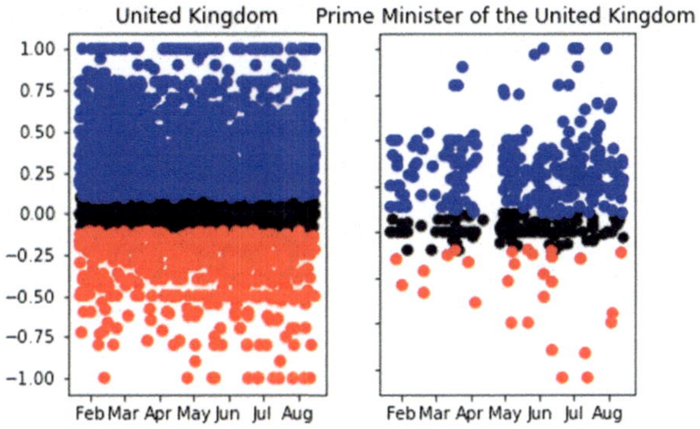

Fig. 13 United Kingdom tweets polarity

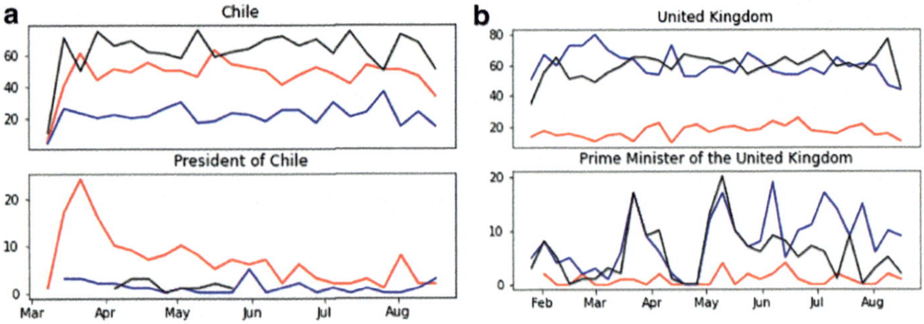

Fig. 14 **a** Chile tweets polarity evolution through the COVID-19 pandemic **b** United Kingdom tweets polarity evolution through the COVID-19 pandemic

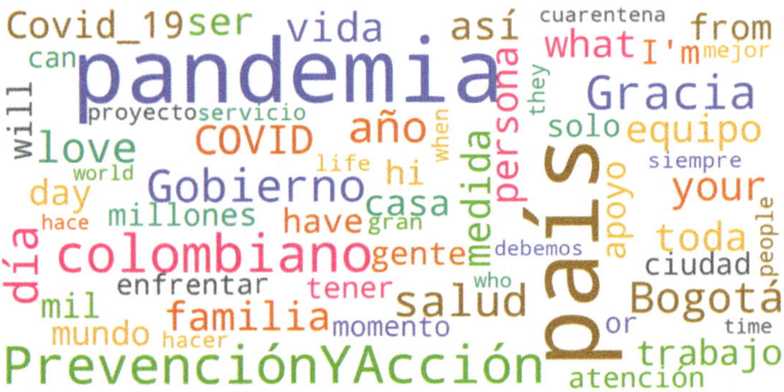

Fig. 15 Colombia tweets wordcloud

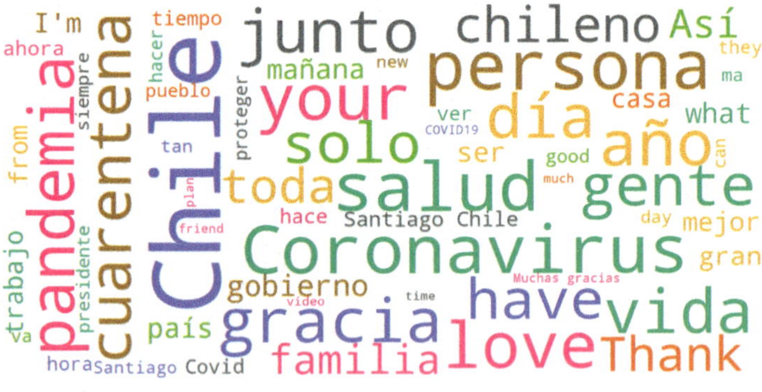

Fig. 16 Chile tweets wordcloud

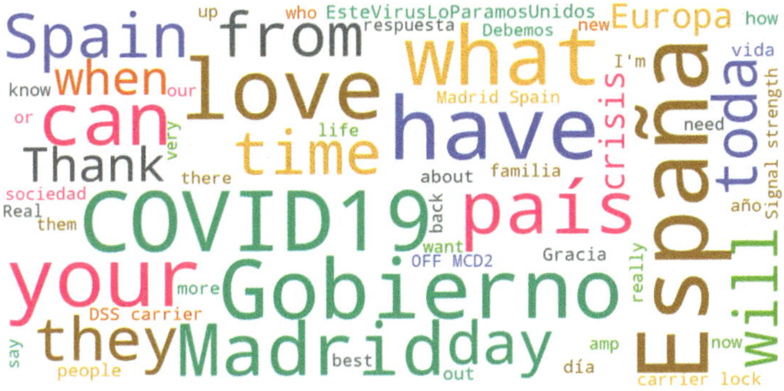

Fig. 17 Spain tweets wordcloud

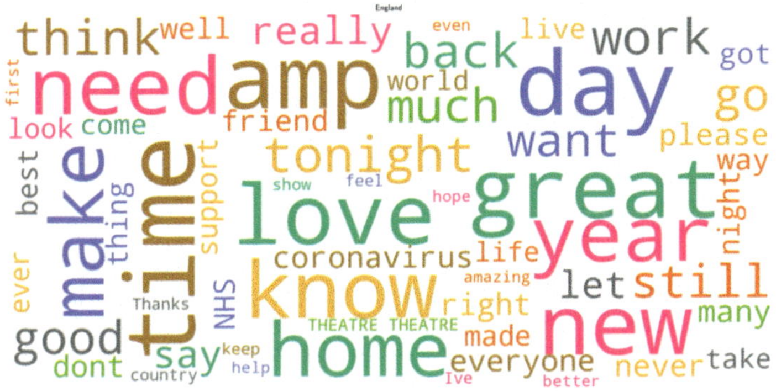

Fig. 18 United Kingdom tweets wordcloud

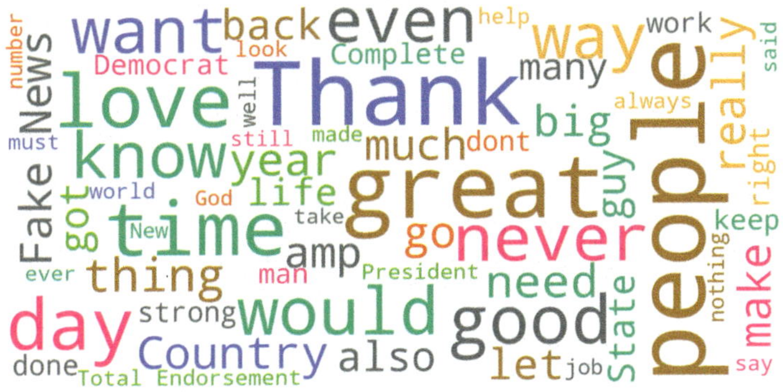

Fig. 19 United States of America tweets wordcloud

References

1. Abebe, E.C., Dejenie, T.A., Shiferaw, M.Y., Malik, T.: The newly emerged covid-19 disease: a systemic review. Virol. J. **17**(1), 1–8 (2020)
2. Dong, E., Du, H., Gardner, L.: An interactive web-based dashboard to track covid-19 in real time. Lancet Infect. Dis. (2020). https://doi.org/10.1016/S1473-3099(20)30120-1
3. General, W.D.: Who director-general's opening remarks at the media briefing on covid-19-11 March 2020. World Health Organization Website (2020). https://www.who.int/dg/speeches/detail/who-director-general-s-opening-remarks-at-the-media-briefing-on-covid-19. (11-Mar-2020)
4. Gomez-Ramirez, D.A.J.: Artificial Mathematical Intelligence: Cognitive, (Meta)mathemticial, Physical and Philosophical Foundations. Springer International Publishing (2020). ISBN 978-3-030-50272-0
5. Gómez-Ramírez, D.A.J.: Conceptual blending in mathematical creation/invention. In: Artificial Mathematical Intelligence, pp. 109–131. Springer, Cham (2020). https://doi.org/10.1007/978-3-030-50273-7_7
6. Gómez-Ramírez, D.A.J.: Conceptual substratum. In: Artificial Mathematical Intelligence, pp. 147–163. Springer, Cham (2020). https://doi.org/10.1007/978-3-030-50273-7_9
7. Gómez-Ramírez, D.A.J.: Dathematics: a meta-isomorphic version of "standard" mathematics based on proper classes. In: Artificial Mathematical Intelligence, pp. 91–105. Springer, Cham (2020). https://doi.org/10.1007/978-3-030-50273-7_6
8. Gómez-Ramírez, D.A.J.: Formal analogical reasoning in concrete mathematical research. In: Artificial Mathematical Intelligence, pp. 133–146. Springer, Cham (2020). https://doi.org/10.1007/978-3-030-50273-7_8
9. Gómez-Ramírez, D.A.J.: General considerations for the new cognitive foundations' program. In: Artificial Mathematical Intelligence, pp. 41–52. Springer, Cham (2020). https://doi.org/10.1007/978-3-030-50273-7_3
10. Gómez-Ramírez, D.A.J.: Global introduction to the artificial mathematical intelligence general program. In: Artificial Mathematical Intelligence, pp. 1–17. Springer, Cham (2020). https://doi.org/10.1007/978-3-030-50273-7_1
11. Gómez-Ramírez, D.A.J.: (Initial) global taxonomy of the most fundamental cognitive (meta-mathematical) mechanisms used in mathematical creation/invention. In: Artificial Mathematical Intelligence, pp. 165–198. Springer, Cham (2020). https://doi.org/10.1007/978-3-030-50273-7_10
12. Gómez-Ramírez, D.A.J.: Meta-modeling of classic and modern proofs and concepts. In: Artificial Mathematical Intelligence, pp. 201–249. Springer, Cham (2020). https://doi.org/10.1007/978-3-030-50273-7_11
13. Gómez-Ramírez, D.A.J.: The most outstanding (future) challenges towards global ami and its plausible extensions. In: Artificial Mathematical Intelligence, pp. 251–259. Springer, Cham (2020). https://doi.org/10.1007/978-3-030-50273-7_12
14. Gómez-Ramírez, D.A.J.: The physical numbers. In: Artificial Mathematical Intelligence, pp. 67–89. Springer, Cham (2020). https://doi.org/10.1007/978-3-030-50273-7_5
15. Gómez-Ramírez, D.A.J.: Some basic technical (meta)mathematical preliminaries for cognitive metamathematics. In: Artificial Mathematical Intelligence, pp. 19–38. Springer, Cham (2020). https://doi.org/10.1007/978-3-030-50273-7_2
16. Gómez-Ramírez, D.A.J.: Towards the (cognitive) reality of mathematics and the mathematics of the (cognitive) reality. In: Artificial Mathematical Intelligence, pp. 53–66. Springer, Cham (2020). https://doi.org/10.1007/978-3-030-50273-7_4
17. Gómez-Ramírez, D.A.J., Cardona, J.P.: Una aproximación multidisciplinaria a la formación del substrato ontológico-natural local de las estructuras matemáticas. In: Logos y Filosofía: Temas y Debates Contemporáneos, pp. 112–136. Editorial Bonaventuriana (2020)
18. Hota, S., Pathak, S.: Knn classifier based approach for multi-class sentiment analysis of twitter data. Int. J. Eng. Technol. **7**(3), 1372–1375 (2018). ISSN 2227-524X. 10.14419/ijet.v7i3.12656. https://www.sciencepubco.com/index.php/ijet/article/view/12656

19. Le, B., Nguyen, H.: Twitter sentiment analysis using machine learning techniques. In: Le Thi, H.A., Nguyen, N.T., Do, T.V. (eds.) Advanced Computational Methods for Knowledge Engineering, pp. 279–289. Springer International Publishing, Cham (2015). ISBN 978-3-319-17996-4
20. Liu, B.: Sentiment Analysis: Mining Opinions, Sentiments, and Emotions. Cambridge University Press (2015). https://doi.org/10.1017/CBO9781139084789
21. Lopez-Lopez, A.F. (ed.): Logos y Filosofía: Temas y Debates Contemporáneos. Editorial Bonaventuriana (2020). ISBN 978-958-8474-95-3
22. Maalouf, M.: Logistic regression in data analysis: an overview. Int. J. Data Anal. Tech. Strateg. **3**(3), 281 (2011). ISSN 1755-8050, 1755-8069. https://doi.org/10.1504/IJDATS.2011.041335. http://www.inderscience.com/link.php?id=41335
23. Roser, M., Ortiz-Ospina, E., Ritchie, H., Hasell, J.: Coronavirus pandemic (covid-19). In: Our World in Data (2020). https://ourworldindata.org/coronavirus
24. Moore, J.P., Klasse, P.: Covid-19 vaccines: "warp speed" needs mind melds, not warped minds. J. Virol. **94**(17) (2020)
25. Richardson, S., Hirsch, J.S., Narasimhan, M., Crawford, J.M., McGinn, T., Davidson, K.W., Barnaby, D.P., Becker, L.B., Chelico, J.D., Cohen, S.L., et al.: Presenting characteristics, comorbidities, and outcomes among 5700 patients hospitalized with covid-19 in the New York City area. Jama (2020)
26. Rudkowsky, E., Haselmayer, M., Wastian, M., Jenny, M., Emrich, Š., Sedlmair, M.: More than bags of words: Sentiment analysis with word embeddings. Commun. Methods Meas. **12**(2–3), 140–157 (2018). https://doi.org/10.1080/19312458.2018.1455817
27. Ruz, G.A., Henríquez, P.A., Mascareño, A.: Sentiment analysis of twitter data during critical events through bayesian networks classifiers. Future Generat. Comput. Syst. **106**, 92–104 (2020). ISSN 0167-739X. https://doi.org/10.1016/j.future.2020.01.005. http://www.sciencedirect.com/science/article/pii/S0167739X19303322
28. Saad, S., Saberi, B.: Sentiment analysis or opinion mining: a review. Int. J. Adv. Sci. Eng. Inf. Technol. **7**(5), 1660–1666 (2017.) ISSN 2088-5334. https://doi.org/10.18517/ijaseit.7.5.2137. http://ijaseit.insightsociety.org/index.php?option=com_content&view=article&id=9&Itemid=1&article_id=2137
29. Surveillances, V.: The epidemiological characteristics of an outbreak of 2019 novel coronavirus diseases (covid-19)–China, 2020. China CDC Weekly **2**(8), 113–122 (2020)
30. Wadawadagi, R., Pagi, V.: Sentiment analysis with deep neural networks: comparative study and performance assessment. Artif. Intell. Rev. **53**(8), 6155–6195 (2020). ISSN 1573-7462. https://doi.org/10.1007/s10462-020-09845-2

Applications of Artificial Intelligence and Molecular Immune Pathogenesis, Ongoing Diagnosis and Treatments for COVID-19

Balendra V. S. Chauhan, Akanksha Jaiswar, Ashish Bedi, Sneha Verma, Vivek Kumar Shrivastaw, and Ajitanshu Vedrtnam

Abstract The Coronavirus Disease (COVID-19) is an infectious disease caused by a newly discovered coronavirus. It is associated with infrequent epidemic derive by SARS-CoV-2 (Severe Acute Respiratory Syndrome Coronavirus 2) which started in Dec 2019 from Wuhan city, China and escalated throughout the world. The transmission of this SARS-CoV-2 has been reported as a third most pathogenic coronavirus for the human community after SARS-CoV (Severe Respiratory Syndrome Coronavirus) and MERS-CoV (Middle East Respiratory Syndrome Coronavirus) in 21st century. The aim of this chapter includes portraying the potential of artificial intelligence (AI) technology as a tool to analyse, evaluate, prevent and fight against the COVID-19. Additionally, there is an effort to summarize the molecular biology of this deadly virus, molecular immune pathogenesis, ongoing detection and therapeutic strategies of COVID-19 based on the present understanding of infection mechanism of MERS and SARS coronaviruses. On a broader aspect, this chapter also reports developments in vaccines and therapeutics to cure COVID-19 infection.

Keywords Covid-19 · MERS · SARS · Artificial intelligence · Pathogenesis · Diagnosis · Treatment

B. V. S. Chauhan
Department of Mechanical Engineering, Invertis University, Bareilly, U.P., India

A. Jaiswar
Mossakowski Medical Research Centre, Polish Academy of Sciences, Warsaw, Poland

A. Bedi
School of Life and Environmental Sciences, Deakin University, Geelong, Australia

S. Verma
School of Mathematics, Computer Science and Engineering, City University of London, London, UK

V. K. Shrivastaw
CSIR-Indian Institute of Petroleum, Dehradun, India

A. Vedrtnam (✉)
Departamento de Arquitectura, Escuela de Arquitectura-Universidad de Alcalá, Alcalá de Henares, Spain
e-mail: ajitanshu.m@invertis.org

D. Oliva et al. (eds.), *Artificial Intelligence for COVID-19*, Studies in Systems, Decision and Control 358, https://doi.org/10.1007/978-3-030-69744-0_29

Abbreviations

AI	Artificial Intelligence
CT	Computerized Tomography
VGG	Visual Geometry Group
SVM	Support Vector Machine
KNN	K-Nearest Neighbor
MLPNN	Multilayer Perceptron Neural Network
PCA	Principal Component Analysis
MRI	Magnetic Resonance Imaging
DBSCAN	Density Based Spatial Clustering of Applications with Noise
LSTM	Long Short-Term Memory
SEIR	Susceptible Exposed Infectious Recovered
BPNN	Backward Propagation Neural Network
GAN	Generative Adversarial Network
CNN	Convolutional Neural Network
NLP	Natural Language Processing (NLP)
NLG	Natural Language Generation (NLG)
NLU	Natural Language Understanding
ELMo	Embeddings from Language Models,
NLTK	Natural Language Toolkit (NLTK)
ULMFiT	Universal Language Model Fine Tuning
BERT	Bidirectional Encoder Representations from Transformers
ERNIE	Enhanced Representation through kNowledge IntEgration
GPT	Generative Pre-Training
BPT	Biopharma Trend Analytics
ANN	Artificial Neural Networks
SARS	Severe Acute Respiratory Syndrome
MERS	Middle East Respiratory Syndrome
COVID	Coronavirus Disease
RNA	Ribonucleic Acid
HCoV-HKU1	Human Coronavirus HKU1
ARDS	Acute Respiratory Distress Syndrome
ACE2	Angiotensin-Converting Enzyme 2
TMPRSS2	Transmembrane Serine Protease II
ERGIC	Endoplasmic Reticulum-Golgi Intermediate Compartment
ELISA	Enzyme-Linked Immunosorbent Assay
POCT	Point-of-care Testing
RdRp	RNA-Dependent RNA Polymerase Gene

1 Introduction

The deadly Coronavirus Disease (COVID-19) outbreak has already been declared as a pandemic, where the confirmed cases around the globe are above 22 million, the number of deaths has reached 787,686 on 20th August 2020 and these figures are still increasing alarmingly [1]. As a matter of fact, the mortality rate is increasing gradually, which is leading world into one of the drastic periods mankind has ever

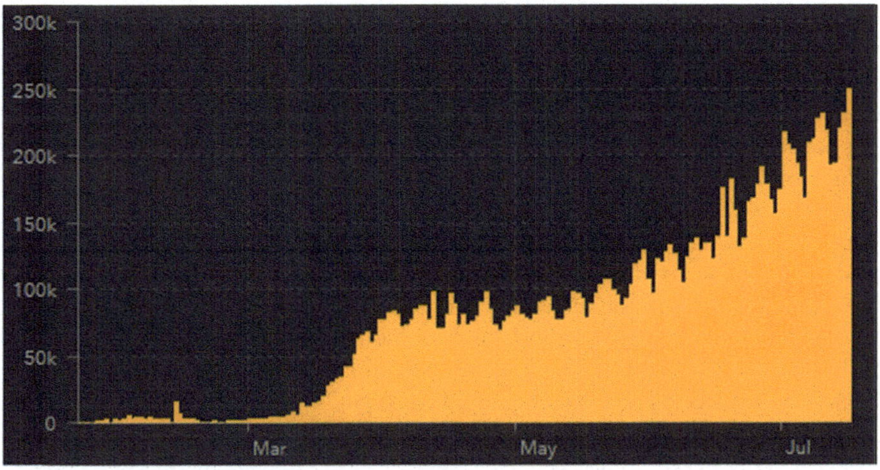

(a)

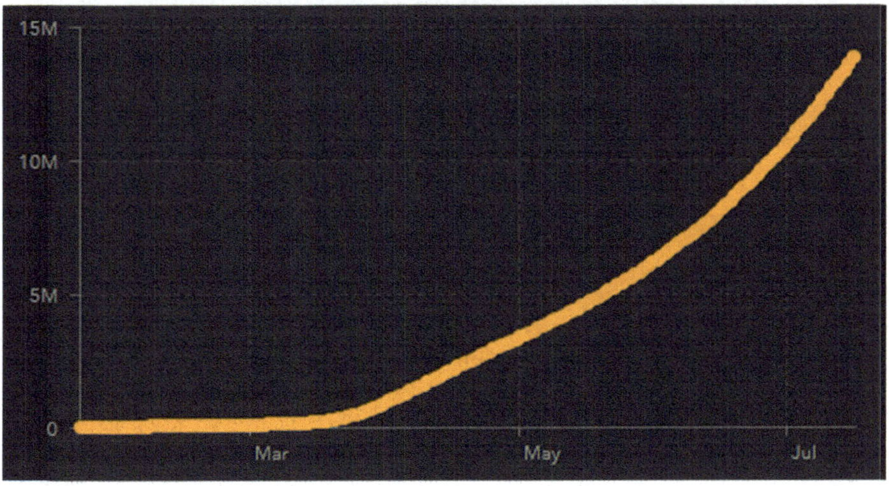

(b)

Fig. 1 (a) Worldwide number of cases found daily, (b) Worldwide Confirmed cases curve [1] seen. Figure 1 shows the pattern of number of cases that are being found globally till date (August 2020) [1].

To combat with the pandemic situation, countries are enforcing the social measures such as imposing lockdown in the country, sanitization, social distancing, abstain social meeting of people in large numbers, use of masks, restrictions in travelling etc. Humans are suffering with the situation, as wellbeing, economy and GDP is in jeopardy [2–17]. The world is striving for a technology, to control the situation, and AI has potential to tackle the situation [18].

Artificial Intelligence can assist in fighting COVID-19 by populace screening, clinical assistance, warning, and instructions about the disease control. AI is able to track the virus spread, spot the patients at high risk, assist in real-time governing of this disease, and by the investigation of patient's record; AI can prognosticate the mortality risk [19–23]. This chapter will discuss the overall strategy of AI based applications and conventional approach that could assist doctors in recognizing the symptoms of COVID-19. The flow chart (Fig. 2) reflects that the AI can assist in treatment with a high precision, while decreasing the unpredictability and treatment duration. The AI assist doctors by providing them a better control on symptoms recognition and analysis with paramount accuracy [24, 25]. The later part of the chapter deals with the molecular immune pathogenesis, ongoing diagnosis and treatment strategies. The diagnosis approaches such as molecular based approach, CT scans and other diagnostic methods, antiviral drugs, monoclonal antibody and plasma-based therapy and vaccine-based treatment are also briefly discussed.

2 Potential Application Areas for AI During Covid-19

This section briefly describes the application areas of AI at different stages of COVID-19 (Fig. 3).

2.1 Identification and Prognosis of the Infection

AI can quickly scan large number of people with high body temperature using thermal scanning in an automated manner. It can also monitor people maintaining social distance using facial recognition systems, computer vision camera systems and Infrared scans [26–28]. Models based on artificial neural networks such as GoogLeNet [29], Alexnet [30], VGG network [31], DenseNet [32], ZFNet [33], ResNet and ResNeXt [34] can be associated with AI for identification and prognosis of COVID-19. AI can rapidly examine the clinical symptoms, abnormal behaviour, laboratory tests, digital health records, heart & respiratory rate & other symptoms of COVID positive patient. The case history, treatment given and other clinical observations could be quickly analysed and thus, AI-based system can alert the patients and healthcare specialists well in time [35, 36]. AI enables risk evaluation, survival

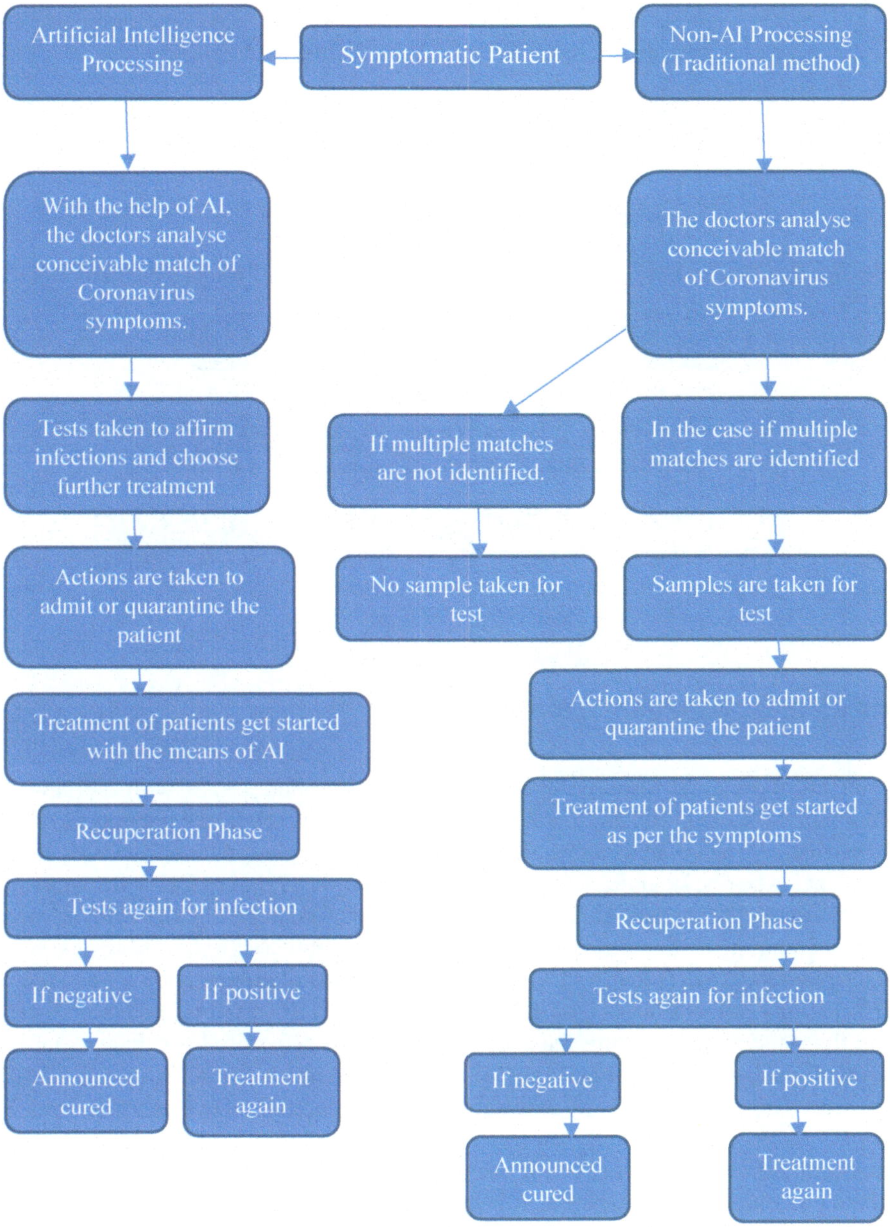

Fig. 2 Comparison of AI based and conventional approaches of treatment

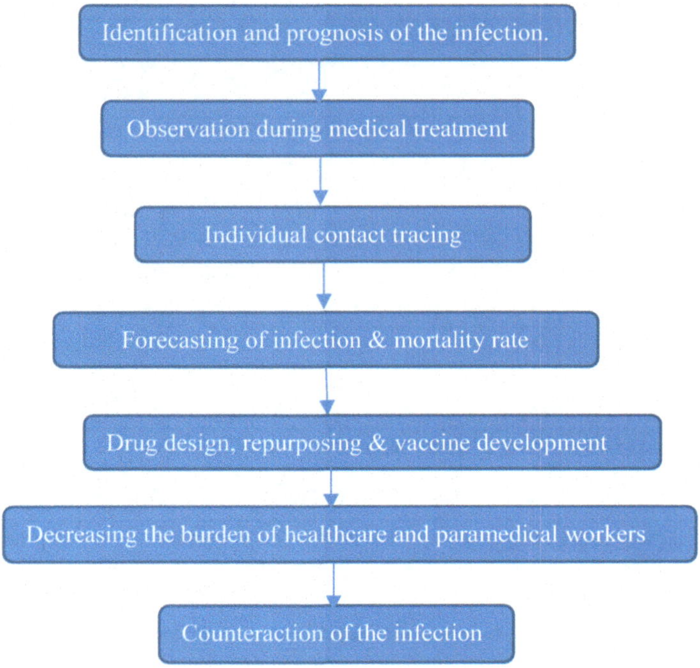

Fig. 3 Application areas of AI at different Stages of COVID-19

probability, medical resource planning at short time and assists with building up comprehensive analysis and managing system for the COVID 19 patients [37–43]. These data are calculated using automated complex calculations such as SVM, KNN, MLP, naive bayes, Logistic & Elasticnet regression [44], random forest, decision tree and nonparametric gaussian process methods [45]. AI can be clubbed with advance clinical imaging technologies like Computed tomography (CT) scan, Magnetic resonance imaging (MRI) scan and X-ray of different parts of human body for assistance in screening & identification of the positive cases [19, 46–63]. AI and Chest X-rays jointly assist in recognizing the unusual observations required for diagnosing the ground glass opacities in the lungs of affected persons suffering from COVID-19 disease. The degree of lungs damage could also be recognized using AI and X-rays. This is normally significant for critical patients. Despite of the challenges like inaccurate data predictions, continuous observation of physical behaviour, remedy given outcome, assurance of patient's privacy AI would surely assist in the effective administration of COVID-19 patients with minimal physical contact requirement.

2.2 Observation During Treatment

AI can fabricate a wise stage for programmed observation and forecast the spread of this infection. A neural framework can moreover be made to draw out the visual features of sickness and help progressively during examination and treatment of the Covid-19 patients [64–66]. These technologies have ability to provide regular updates of the patients and furthermore necessary precautions to be followed during complete treatment. Comprehensive analysis like sequence alignment via dynamic programming, heuristic & probabilistic approach and cluster analysis like hierarchical cluster, DBSCAN, k-means [67] & deep learning models uses viral genomes and protein data sequences to analyse physical & genetic changes to obtain phylogenetic tree which is useful in predicting secondary & tertiary structures of various protein. Although compilation of such a large database using deep learning models may take long training time but can be explainable once it is obtained [68–71].

2.3 Individual Contact Tracing

AI can assist in studying the level of contamination due to COVID-19 by distinguishing the'containment areas' and can effectively trace the contact of infected people and get them screened well in time. It can foresee the future course and likely return of infection. AI uses the anonymized mobile data, travel itinerary data, plant & animal disease networks, ecological data, temperature profiles, public announcements, news reports of foreign language, population distribution and scan database [72] for real time spread tracking, prior warnings & alerts for particular region. One such example is reported in literature as BlueDot [73] model of global Zika virus spread [74, 75]. It also uses forums, news outlets, social media interactions, and travel data in all dialects over the world to understand communities' responses to guidelines like social distancing during unlock phase, public aid understanding, detecting mental health problems [76–78].

2.4 Forecasting of Cases and Rate of Mortality

AI can trace and predict the behaviour of this deadly virus from available data, about the probability of contamination and its feasible spread. Moreover, it can also forecast the spread of infection and rate of mortality in infected area using case data of time series, populace of particular region and its demographic data [21, 79, 80]. These data are utilised by deep learning techniques like LSTM & recurrent networks and optimization methods [81] for highlighting the most infected areas in countries where strict measures would be needed. Different measurable, numerical and dynamic models have been utilized to effectively foresee the degree and spread of contagious illnesses through the populace [82–87]. Instead of conventional epidemiological models, informative driven models have the additional favourable position of versatile learning, recalibration based on pattern, adaptability and degree to enhance dependency on a more up to date comprehension of the sickness cycle like social distancing to control the spread of infection [88]. The Susceptible-Exposed-Infectious-Recovered (SEIR) demonstrating technique is most widely recognized method presently being utilized to foresee the zones and degree of COVID-19 spread [89, 90]. These strategies can likewise be utilized to decide different boundaries of the pandemic, for example, under-revealing of positive cases, precision of examination techniques and sufficiency of mediations [91, 92]. A model calculation attempted to propagate the constraints where Ebola was spread in a society located in China is already reported in literature [93]. Comparative models have additionally allowed to anticipate the development of Zika virus progressively in America and was resolved to about 85% exactness in assessments quantitatively [94]. It is reported that the backward propagation neural network (BPNN) exhibited most noteworthy prescient precision for demonstrating Zika infection transmission [95]. Researchers of Johns Hopkins University developed a Covid-19 gauge showing based on past published literature related to stochastic-metapopulation pandemic model [83].

However, a forecast model depends on accuracy of data and information available. In this worldwide pandemic, sharing of information across all networks is of central significance. It was one of the important obstructions in studying and demonstrating the Ebola infection pandemic during 2013 to 2016 [96]. World Health Organization (WHO) has suggested for an agreement on facilitated information sharing on COVID-19 pandemic to advance the network findings and investigation in AI area.

2.5 Drug Design, Repurposing and Vaccine Development

AI can assist in vaccine development by inspecting and analyzing the collected data on COVID-19. It uses data like protein sequence, viral genome, drug target interactions, various model of proteins, structures of protein, protein-protein interactions and database of transcriptome to discover vaccine and drug composition candidates to optimize clinical trials efficiently during the advancement of the vaccine [97–99]. Employed data are useful in drug analysis & its efficacy in a quick and reliable manner compare to conventional process. It can help in recognizing beneficial medications for the treatment of infected people. Innovative ways for the diagnosis of infected people and development of the vaccine simultaneously are reported in literature [100–102]. Advance calculations like Heuristic algorithm, combinatorics, theories based on graph & other robotic learning such as multitask CNN [98], auto-encoders [97] GAN [97, 103] and deep reinforcement learning [97, 104, 105] play a significant role in mining text to search possible candidates for evolution of vaccines and antiviral drugs using conclusive evidence from the treatment given, original research articles, libraries of drugs compounds & CORD-19 database. It also helps in understanding

Covid-19 transmission modes, risk factors, incubation period & genetics of virus including its origin and evolution [99, 106–112].

2.6 Decreasing the Burden of Healthcare and Paramedical Workers

Due to unexpected and huge increment in the number of Covid-19 patients, medical professionals are dealing with an exceptionally huge workload at their hand. AI can be utilized to lessen their burden by automating the decision-making process effectively without requirement physical contact of healthcare workers and patients [113–118]. The criticality of patient based on their medical history can be identified with the help of AI which enables better preparation strategies without requirement of specialists [119, 120]. Three major methods such as deep learning, transfer learning and NLP & NLG tools include techniques like recurrent networks and auto encoders, ELMo [121], NLTK [122], ULMFiT [123], Google's BERT [124], Transformer [125], Transformer-XL [126], ERNIE [127], XLNet [128], BPT [129], T5 [130] and OpenAI's GPT-2 [131] for different language related analysis are used for information extraction, relationship extraction, automatic summarization, sentiment analysis, semantic annotation, entity recognition, speech recognition & synthesis, segmentation of topic & modelling, machine translation and automated questions & answers. Thus, AI could contribute in decreasing the workload of the healthcare specialists by assisting them at different patient examination and treatment stages.

2.7 Counteraction of the Infection

Using real-time analysis of available data, AI can offer updated facts which help to counter this pandemic effectively. It would forecast the likely destinations of contamination, infection inflow, hospital beds requirement and medicinal services during an emergency. AI can also be useful for future infection and sickness counteraction using live update of COVID-19 related data and information. It recognizes behaviour, causes and explanations behind the virus spread. In coming days, AI will end up being a significant observation to battle against different pandemics. It can suggest a safety measure in the battle against numerous different diseases. AI can help medical experts in forming guidelines, posters, chatting robots, information to avoid spreading of any fake news regarding COVID-19 pandemic [132–140]. It uses simulation & demonstration data for training autonomous agencies through deep learning techniques, control & optimization, computer vision and transfer learning to make drones & robots for cleaning, disinfection, distance maintenance and easy delivery of medication as well [141–145]. In future, AI will assume an essential job in giving more attention and safety towards healthcare.

2.8 Preventive Strategies and Challenges Using Artificial Intelligence

Artificial Neural Networks (ANN) are already being utilized to predict antigen locations with a high thickness of covers called as antigen binding hotspots in the viral surface protein of SARS–CoV (Severe Acute Respiratory Syndrome Coronavirus) [146, 147]. Basically, it refers to the advancement of antibodies. Utilizing AI takes into consideration quick checking of the whole popular proteome, permitting quicker and less expensive antibody improvement. Turn around vaccinology and AI were effectively utilized to recognize potential antibodies target proteins in proteome of SARS-CoV-2 [148]. Similarly, AI was utilized earlier to foresee the problems of flu infection that are bound to source contamination in a populace and also for establishing the year's occasional flu immunization [149]. AI can be utilized to anticipate the hosts of newfound infections dependent on examination of nucleoprotein quality groupings and spike quality arrangements, with significant additional instrument for following back viral beginnings, particularly when the informational collection is huge and relative investigation is troublesome or tedious [149].

AI gives an energizing cluster of devices that are adaptable enough to permit their organization in any phase of the pandemic. With the enormous measure of information that is being created while contemplating an illness cycle, AI takes into account investigation and fast ID of examples that customary numerical and factual devices would set aside a long effort to determine. The adaptability, capacity to adjust dependent on another comprehension of the malady cycle, personal development as and when new information opens up, and the absence of human preference in the methodology of examination makes AI an exceptionally flexible novel device for overseeing novel contaminations. However, with such an upgraded capacity to get importance from a lot of information, there is a more prominent interest for better control during the assortment, stockpiling, and preparing of the information. Additionally, normalization of information structures across populace would permit these frameworks to adjust and gain from information over the globe, which was beyond the realm of imagination previously, and is considerably more significant in findings and dealing with a worldwide pandemic. Likewise, during another medical emergency, there will in general be significantly more "noise" in the information, and henceforth aimlessly taking care of this juvenile information, which is ridden with exceptions into an AI calculation ought to consistently be drawn nearer with alert.

3 The Virus: Virology

3.1 Molecular Structure

Role of AI in fighting the COVID-19 has been discussed so far in the chapter and now the aim is to explain the in-depth molecular structure of the virus and in the later sections the discussion will be made to use the knowledge of the molecular structure of the virus and move towards the artificial intelligence practices to predict and diagnose the disease caused by this virus.

Population genetics studies on SARS-CoV-2 viruses revealed that these viruses exist in two forms L and S with L form having higher transmission rate [150, 151]. SAR-CoV-2 is an enveloped, non-segmented, single stranded (positive sense) RNA non-segmented virus [152, 153]. This virus has a diameter of about 65-125 nm and length of 29.9 kb (Fig. 4, A) [154]. So far, four genera of coronavirus (alpha (α), beta (β), Delta (γ), Gamma (δ)) have been discovered. Human coronaviruses (HCoVs) have been pinpointed within α coronavirus (like HCoV-229E and NL63) and β coronavirus (MERS-CoV, SARS-CoV, HCoV-OC43 and HCoV-HKU1) genera [155–157]. Earlier, in December, 2019, samples were collected from individuals in Wuhan, China, showing the symptoms of mild illness to pneumonia (coughing, fever, and dyspnoea with Acute Respiratory Distress Syndrome (ARDS) led to the identification of a formerly unknown β-Coronavirus (β-CoV) strain which was present in all the patients [158]. The novel virus showed approx. ~ 88% sequence homology with mainly two SARS like coronaviruses (bat-derived: bat-SL-CoVZC45 and bat-SL-CoVZXC21) and ~ 50% similarity to the sequence of MERS (ORF1a/b). In another report SARS-CoV-2 genome showed approx. ~ 96.2% similarity to bat CoV-RaTG13, which suggests that bats can be the key reservoir of these viruses [159–161]. SARS-CoV-2 is a type of β-CoV and is named after these previously identified viruses.

Most of the viral RNAs (about two-third) are translated into two sub open reading frames (ORF1a and ORF1b) and produced two large polyproteins which are pp1a and pp1ab though rest of the ORFs (one-third of the genome) of SARS-CoV-2 encodes four structural proteins: spike (S) proteins, envelope (E) proteins, nucleocapsid (N) proteins and membrane (M) proteins. In addition, several accessory proteins are also encoded as well (Fig. 4, B) [162]. Sixteen non-structural proteins (nsp1-nsp16) are processed from the polyproteins (pp1a and pp1ab) and are involved in formation of the viral replicase transcriptase complex (Table 1, Fig. 4, A) [162–166].

The structural proteins (S, E, N, M proteins) forms the basic structure of SARS-CoV-2. The S protein, is a transmembrane glycoprotein that facilitates the attachment of virus envelop to targeted cells that serve as the host, by binding with the Angiotensin Converting Enzyme 2 (ACE2), which is expressed in the lower cells of the respiratory tract. S protein have a molecular weight of approx.150 kDa and it forms homotrimers that protrude from the surface of the virus. The furin-like protease of the host cell cleaves the S glycoprotein into 2 sub units viz. S1 subunit and S2 subunit, where S1 determines the range of host virus and facilitates cellular tropism

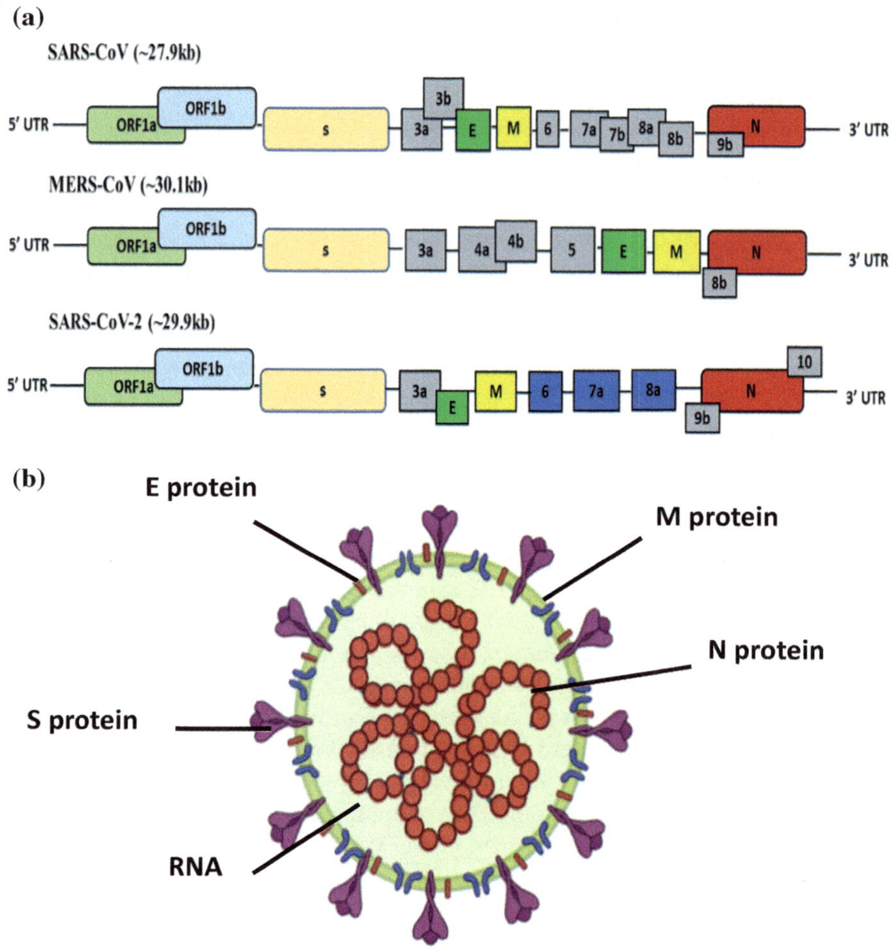

Fig. 4 Enveloped, non-segmented, single stranded positive sense RNA virus of approx. ~ 26-32 kb in size. Types- SARS-CoV, MERS-CoV and SARS-CoV-2, two-thirds of the genome ORF1a/b encodes for polyproteins (pp1a and pp1ab), forming the viral replicase transcriptase complex [154, 162]

with the receptor binding domain while S2 mediates entry of virus into the host cells by fusion of the viral and host membrane. [159, 162, 167].

Another structural protein, nucleocapsid (N) is basically localized in the Endoplasmic Reticulum-Golgi bodies (ER bodies) and is bound to viral RNA. This protein plays a role in replication of virus, and host cell response to viral infections [158, 168]. Moreover, N protein has been suggested to cause structural changes due to its ability to undergo high level of phosphorylation thereby enhancing the affinity of viral RNA [165].

Table 1 Role of structural and non-structural proteins of coronaviruses

S.No.	Structural protein (sp)	Protein length	Function
1.	Spike protein (S)	1,273 aa	Facilitates attachment of virus to target host cell by binding ACE2 receptors.
2.	Nucleocapsid protein (N)	419 aa	Bound to viral RNA and plays a role in viral imitation cycle and host cellular response to viral infections
3.	Membrane protein (M)	222 aa	Matrix protein determines the shape of the virus envelope and helps in viral assembly
4.	Envelope protein (E)	75 aa	Involved in the development and evolution of the virus
S.No.	**Non-structural Protein(nsp)**	**Protein length**	**Function**
1.	Nsp1	180 aa	suppressing type I IFN expression
2.	Nsp2	638 aa	Involved in mitochondrial biogenesis and binding to prohibition protein
3.	Nsp3	1945 aa	Promoting cellular degradation and blocked host innate immune response
4.	Nsp4	500 aa	To rearrange host cell membrane and interaction with all nsps
5.	Nsp5	306 aa	Involved in cytokine expression and role in cleavage of viral polyprotein
6.	Nsp6	290 aa	Contribution into structure of DMVs formation
7.	Nsp7	83 aa	complex Processivity clamp for RNA polymerase by arms hexadecameric complex and capable of both de novo initiation and primer extension
8.	Nsp8	198 aa	
9.	Nsp9	113 aa	Viral genomic RNA reproduction and RNA binding protein phosphatase
10.	Nsp10	139 aa	To evade immune Surveillance

(continued)

Table 1 (continued)

S.No.	Structural protein (sp)	Protein length	Function
11.	Nsp11	13 aa	unknown function
12.	Nsp12	932 aa	Replication enzyme (RNA-dependent RNA polymerase)
13.	Nsp13	601 aa	RNA helicase that unpacks viral genome material, 50 triphosphatase
14.	Nsp14	527 aa	Proofreading of viral genome
15.	Nsp15	346 aa	Role in viral endoribonuclease and chymotrypsin-like protease
16.	Nsp16	298 aa	Inhibit innate immunity regulation

The structure and shape of the corona virus envelope is determined by another important structural protein, called the M protein which have the ability to interact with all the other structural proteins. Binding of the M protein with the N proteins stabilizes the N protein-RNA complex within virion and it triggers the processes which are involved in viral assembly. The last and the smallest component in the SARS CoV structure is the E protein that plays a role in the construction and aging of this virus (Tables 1 and 2) [168].

Table 2 Accessories proteins of SARS-CoV2 [168]

No.	Accessories Proteins	Protein length	Function of Accessories Proteins
1.	ORF3a	275 aa	Required for virulence, infectivity, ion channel formation, and virus release
2.	ORF3b	22 aa	Essential for a potent IFN-1 antagonist
3.	ORF6	61 aa	karyopherin transportation
4.	ORF7a	121 aa	blocking the glycosylation of BST-2
5.	ORF7b	43 aa	structural component of the SARS-CoV virion
6.	ORF8	121 aa	enhances the downstream transcription of the N gene
7.	ORF9b	97 aa	activation of IRF-3
8.	ORF9c	XX aa	modulate IkB kinase and NF-kB signalling pathway
9.	ORF10	38 aa	stop codon

4 Molecular Immune Pathogenesis: Entry and Life Cycle of Coronavirus

The symptoms for SARS-CoV-2 appears after an average median incubation period of 5.1 days (approximately 95% CI. 4.5 to 5.8 days). In some cases, symptoms start in 11.5 days (CI. 8.2 to 15.6 days) of infection. Looking at the aforementioned data, it can be conservatively assumed that, 101 individual's data out of every 10,000 cases (99th percentile, 482) develop symptoms after 14 days of isolation, however, the 14 days of quarantine recommended for patients suspected with SARS-COV-2 infection remains virtually constant [169–171]. As mentioned in the first two sections, the Artificial Intelligence section is different from this approach and the chapter focuses on glorifying the AI approach.

This virus requires a median ACE2 as a receptor which are expressed in cells of the heart, kidneys, lungs (type II pneumocytes), and gastrointestinal tract to enter the human body. Sungnak et al. reported that, ACE2 receptor is highly expressed in the nasal epithelial cells, specifically goblet/secretory cells and ciliated cells throughout the respiratory tract [174]. The human and bat ACE2 receptors gets strongly attached to the binding domain of the S glycoprotein receptors, present at 331 to 524 residues [158]. Following binding, the host and the viral membrane fuse together [163] and the type II transmembrane serine protease (TMPRSS2) present on the surface of the host cell clears ACE2 and activates the S proteins which is attached to the receptor [172] leading to conformational changes thus allowing to the virus to enter the cells [173]. The viral RNA is the then released into the cytoplasm and is translated into protein in the nuclei (Fig. 5).

The SARS-COV-2 genome is accompanied by about 14 ORF and each one of them translates into several proteins (structural and non-structural) that are involved

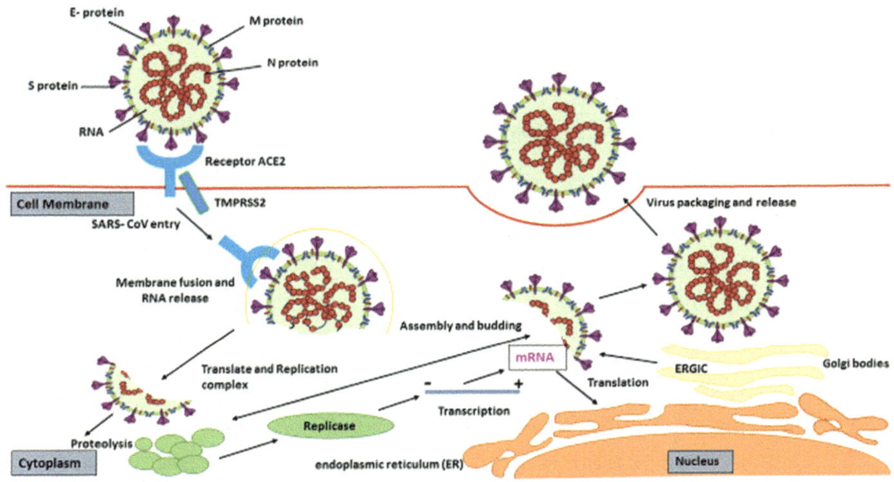

Fig. 5 Mechanism of entry and subsequent life cycle of SARS-COV

in the survival and virulence of this virus. During transformation, two overlapping large polypeptides (pp1a and pp1ab) are produced by ORF1a and ORF1b [162]. As mentioned earlier, the two polyproteins gets translated into sixteen non-structural proteins, some of which assemble with RdRp and helicase containing subunits, the nsp 12 canonical RdRp domain and AV nsp 9, together forming a unit known as replicase-transcriptase complex (RTC). This complex facilitates the transcription of endogenous viral genome to negative sense progeny genome and sub genomic RNA which are formed as an intermediate products and is followed by the RdRp mediated transcription to positive sense mRNAs [162, 164, 175]. The next step is the translation of the sub genomic proteins into structural glycoprotein (M, S, and E proteins) and also in accessory proteins that are then sequestered within the endoplasmic reticulum and carried to the endoplasmic reticulum-Golgi intermediate compartment (ERGIC). Meanwhile, the previously replicated genome program can directly join the N proteins to the nucleocapsid form and enter into the ERGIC. During this compartmentalisation, interaction between the nucleocapsids and other structural proteins takes place which results in synthesis of small wallet like vesicles that are directed out of the cells through exocytosis (Fig. 5).

5 Diagnosis of COVID-19

The patients with the SARS-CoV-2 infection usually present the typical respiratory symptoms such as cough, fever, shortness of breath and pneumonia. Due to overlapping symptoms of COVID-19 disease with symptoms of other respiratory diseases such pneumonia, it becomes difficult to diagnose SARS-CoV-2 in patients. Some important methods used for the diagnosis of COVID-19 includes nucleic acid detection, CT scan, immunological detection of viral antigen/antibody (like Point-of-care Testing (POCT) of IgM/IgG and also enzyme-linked immunosorbent assay (ELISA).

5.1 Molecular-Based Approach

The nucleic acid testing using real-time quantitative polymerase chain reaction (RT-qPCR) and the next generation sequencing is the main techniques for lab diagnosis of SARS-CoV-2 infection [176]. It has been shown that RT-qPCR is the most common and effective means for detecting pathogenic viral infections in respiratory secretions and blood [177]. This involves designing specific primers and probes from the viral genome targeting specific genes of SARSCoV- 2 [178]. Some of the key diagnostic targets for SARS-COV-2 detection are the ORF 1a and 1b, RNA-dependent RNA polymerase gene (RdRp), envelope (E), and nucleocapsid (N). During this time of crisis, the many countries are working together and have shared their protocols and provided specific sequences of target primers on the WHO public database [179].

However, one of the main drawbacks of RTqPCR technique is that sensitivity of 50%–79% has only been achieved for SARS-CoV detection. The efficiency, accuracy and sensitivity of this technique depends on the type of sample, the collected number of clinical specimens and on the protocol [180]. In addition to this, there are other shortcomings as well such as bio-safety hazards due to retention and operation of the patient samples, time taking nucleic acid detection procedure which increases the waiting time to get results back.

5.2 *CT Scans and Other Diagnostic Methods*

Many clinicians proposed the use of CT scans as a supporting diagnostic method due to high rate of false-negative results obtained by RTqPCR, It has been proposed that accurate detection of SARS-CoVID-19 in patients that were earlier screened negative for this viral infection can be done by combining RT-qPCR tests and chest CT scan. Analysis of the High-resolution CT (HRCT) scan images of individuals infected with SARS-CoV-2 have been helpful in early diagnosis and evaluation of disease severity in these patients [158, 181, 182]. However, this technique also has some limitations such as inability to distinguish SAR-COVID-2 infection from other viral pneumonia and false negative results.

Another promising and highly sensitive method is based on detection of target viral antigens or antibodies. Currently, immunological detection kits (POCT of IgM/IgG and ELISA) for detecting SARS-CoV-2 infection are being developed and tested by some companies. Previously, it has been reported that sensitivity of SARS-CoV N-based IgG ELISA (94.7%) was higher than the SARS-CoV S-based IgG ELISA (58.9%) [183], however, the sensitivity of SARS-CoV-2 IgG/IgM remains to be studied.

6 Current Approaches for Treatment of COVID-19

Medical researchers around the globe are continuously contributing in the development of specific treatment for SARS-CoV-2 but still lots of clinical trials have to be done. Currently, no clinically proven specific antiviral drug for treating SARS-CoV-2 infection is available in the market. However, other secondary treatment such as/generally oxygen therapy, conservation fluid management and the use of broad range antibiotics to treat secondary bacterial infections are being used for managing the viral infection. Deciphering the molecular structure and mechanism of SARS-CoV-2 has helped given us a fair idea of potential therapeutic targets and existing antiviral drugs can be repurposed or new drugs can be developed against this novel virus [167]. Based on the infection mechanisms of coronavirus [184] and the genome organization of SARS-CoV-2 [163], several potential targets for therapeutics have been identified and can be used to repurpose the currently available antiviral agents or design new strategies that are highly effective against this novel coronavirus.

6.1 Antiviral Drugs

Drugs that target viral RNA synthesis and replication process have shown promising results against SARS-CoV-2 infection. An adenosine analogue, remdesivir blocks viral RNA synthesis by inhibiting RdRp. This drug has been reported to be very effective against several RNA viruses including SARS and MERS-CoV in cultured cells [185], mice [186] and various non-human primate models [187, 188]. In a report, The Washington Department of Health stated that intravenous injection of remdesivir might be an effective treatment for SARS-CoV-2 infection [189]. In vitro testing of another drug named chloroquine demonstrated significant inhibition of the SARS-CoV-2 infection [190]. Several other nucleoside analogues, favipiravir, ribavirin and galidesivir, to name a few, are available and can be clinically tested against SARS-CoV-2 [191, 192]. Alternatively, effective treatment strategies can be developed by targeting some non-structural proteins such as chymotrypsin-like (3C-like protease, 3CLpro) and papain-like protease (PLP). These proteins are essential for viral replication process and inhibits the host innate immune responses [165]. Drugs such as cinanaserin and some flavonoids (3CL pro inhibitors) [193, 194], and diarylheptanoids (PLP inhibitors) can also be effectively used for SARS-CoV-2 treatment [195]. Another way to manage this viral infection involves blocking the ACE2 receptors that mediates entry of SARS-CoV-2 into the host cells [196].

6.2 Monoclonal Antibody and Plasma-Based Therapy

Plasma therapy have been shown to be an effective treatment for SARS-CoV [197] and MERS-CoV infections [198]. Similarly, plasma from patients recovering from SARA-infection is being used for preparing convalescent plasma and hyperimmune immunoglobulins. Moreover, SARS coronavirus-specific human monoclonal antibody such as SARS-CoV. CR3022, m396 and CR3014 can be used for neutralizing SARS-CoV-2 antigens in patients [199, 200]. These recombinant human monoclonal antibodies can be developed as potential treatment therapy against SARS-CoV-2.

6.3 Vaccine Based Treatment

SARS-CoV-2 is highly contagious and large number of people worldwide are still vulnerable to it. Prior activation of immune system by vaccines will lead to fast recovery by reducing disease severity and limit the spread of virus, thus controlling coronavirus outbreak. Several vaccination strategies against the SARS-CoV and MERS-CoV have been developed. These approaches involve in the use of live-attenuated or inactivated virus, viral vectors, subunit vaccines, recombinant DNA and protein-based vaccines have been tested in animals against SARS-CoV and MERS-CoV [199]. Vaccine development for SARS-CoV-2 is in progress and but following the standards vaccine should undergo multiple laboratory and clinical trials before it can be made publicly available.

7 Conclusion

The potential of artificial intelligence (AI) technology as a tool to analyse, evaluate, prevent and fight against the COVID-19 are fully described and they have proved to be the best technique to resolve the problem. Moreover, in conclusion, genomic analysis revealed that SARS-CoV-2 is a type of beta-coronavirus and is similar to previously reported coronavirus (SARS and MERS) in many respects. The interaction of virus with an individual's immune system is responsible for the disease and progression of COVID-19. An accurate and early diagnosis can limit the breakout of the disease. It is necessary to improve the sensitivity and accuracy of current techniques such as RTqPCR and CT scans. Moreover, there is an urgent need to develop rapid, fast, highly sensitive, cost effective and facile technologies for detecting COVID-19. Till date, there is no specific and effective therapeutics and vaccines available for treatment of COVID-19. Some medicines including hydroxychloroquine sulphate and chloroquine phosphate is provided as an Emergency Use Authorization (EUA) by USFDA for patients of COVID-19. However, more studies are needed to support the success of these drugs in the treatment. Plasma therapy has also emerged as an effective treatment against SARS-CoV-2 infection. Lots of research and clinical trials of vaccines and drugs are being conducted globally to develop a potential therapy or treatment for the disease. Several particulars included in this chapter may change as more research is carried out in this area.

References

1. https://www.arcgis.com/apps/opsdashboard/index.html#/bda7594740fd40299423467b48e9ecf6
2. Nicola, M., Alsafi, Z., Sohrabi, C., Kerwan, A., Al-Jabir, A., Iosifidis, C., Agha, M., Agha, R.: The socio-economic implications of the coronavirus and COVID-19 pandemic: a review. Int. J. Surg. (2020)
3. Maliszewska, M., Mattoo, A., Van Der Mensbrugghe, D.: The potential impact of COVID-19 on GDP and trade: a preliminary assessment (2020)
4. Fernandes, N.: Economic effects of coronavirus outbreak (COVID-19) on the world economy. Available at SSRN 3557504 (2020)

5. Makridis, C., Hartley, J.: The Cost of Covid-19: a Rough Estimate of the 2020 US GDP Impact. Special Edition Policy Brief (2020)
6. Wang, J., Tang, K., Feng, K., Lv, W.: High temperature and high humidity reduce the transmission of COVID-19. Available at SSRN 3551767 (2020)
7. McKibbin, W., Fernando, R.: The economic impact of COVID-19. Econ. Time of COVID-19 **19**, 45 (2020)
8. Iacus, S.M., Natale, F., Santamaria, C., Spyratos, S., Vespe, M.: Estimating and projecting air passenger traffic during the COVID-19 coronavirus outbreak and its socio-economic impact. Safety Science, p. 104791 (2020)
9. Boone, L., Haugh, D., Pain, N., Salins, V.: 2 Tackling the fallout from COVID-19. Economics in the Time of COVID-19, p. 37 (2020)
10. Baker, S.R., Bloom, N., Davis, S.J., Terry, S.J.: Covid-induced economic uncertainty (No. w26983). National Bureau of Economic Research (2020)
11. Sumner, A., Hoy, C., Ortiz-Juarez, E.: Estimates of the Impact of COVID-19 on Global Poverty. UNU-WIDER, April, pp. 800–809 (2020)
12. Dietrich, A., Keuster, K., Müller, G.J., Schoenle, R.: News and uncertainty about covid-19: Survey evidence and short-run economic impact (2020)
13. Maital, S., Barzani, E.: The Global Economic Impact of COVID-19: A Summary of Research. Samuel Neaman Institute for National Policy Research (2020)
14. Alvarez, F.E., Argente, D., Lippi, F.: A simple planning problem for covid-19 lockdown (No. w26981). National Bureau of Economic Research (2020)
15. Inoue, H., Todo, Y.: The propagation of the economic impact through supply chains: The case of a mega-city lockdown against the spread of COVID-19. Available at SSRN 3564898 (2020)
16. Gössling, S., Scott, D., Hall, C.M.: Pandemics, tourism and global change: a rapid assessment of COVID-19. J. Sustain. Tourism, 1–20 (2020)
17. Nicola, M., Alsafi, Z., Sohrabi, C., Kerwan, A., Al-Jabir, A., Iosifidis, C., Agha, M., Agha, R.: The socio-economic implications of the coronavirus pandemic (COVID-19): A review. Int. J. Surg. (London, England) **78**, 185 (2020)
18. Vaishya, R., Javaid, M., Khan, I.H., Haleem, A.: Artificial Intelligence (AI) applications for COVID-19 pandemic. Diabet. Metabolic Syndrome: Clin. Res. Rev. (2020)
19. Shi, F., Wang, J., Shi, J., Wu, Z., Wang, Q., Tang, Z., He, K., Shi, Y., Shen, D.: Review of artificial intelligence techniques in imaging data acquisition, segmentation and diagnosis for covid-19. IEEE Rev. Biomed. Eng. (2020)
20. Rao, A.S.S., Vazquez, J.A.: Identification of COVID-19 can be quicker through artificial intelligence framework using a mobile phone–based survey when cities and towns are under quarantine. Infect. Control Hosp. Epidemiol. **41**(7), 826–830 (2020)
21. Hu, Z., Ge, Q., Jin, L., Xiong, M.: Artificial intelligence forecasting of covid-19 in china. arXiv preprint arXiv:2002.07112
22. Alimadadi, A., Aryal, S., Manandhar, I., Munroe, P.B., Joe, B., Cheng, X.: Artificial intelligence and machine learning to fight COVID-19 (2020)
23. Mei, X., Lee, H.C., Diao, K.Y., Huang, M., Lin, B., Liu, C., Xie, Z., Ma, Y., Robson, P.M., Chung, M., Bernheim, A.: Artificial intelligence–enabled rapid diagnosis of patients with COVID-19. Nat. Med., 1–5 (2020)
24. McCall, B.: COVID-19 and artificial intelligence: protecting health-care workers and curbing the spread. The Lancet Digital Health **2**(4), e166–e167 (2020)
25. Naudé, W.: Artificial intelligence vs COVID-19: limitations, constraints and pitfalls. Ai & Society, p. 1
26. BBC News (2020). Coronavirus France: cameras to monitor masks and social distancing (2020). https://www.bbc.com/news/worldeurope-52529981
27. Singer, N., Sang-Hun, C.: As coronavirus surveillance escalates, personal privacy plummets. The New York Times (2020). https://www.nytimes.com/2020/03/23/technology/coronavirussurveillance-tracking-privacy.html

28. Reevell, P.: How Russia is using facial recognition to police its coronavirus lockdown. ABC News (2020). https://abcnews.go.com/International/russia-facial-recognition-policecoronavirus-lockdown/story?id=70299736
29. Szegedy, C., Liu, W., Jia, Y., Sermanet, P., Reed, S., Anguelov, D., Erhan, D., Vanhoucke, V., Rabinovich, A.: Going deeper with convolutions. In: Proceedings of the IEEE Conference on Computer Vision and Pattern Recognition, pp. 1–9 (2015)
30. Krizhevsky, A., Sutskever, I., Hinton, G.E.: Imagenet classification with deep convolutional neural networks. In: Advances in Neural Information Processing Systems, pp. 1097–1105 (2012)
31. Simonyan, K., Zisserman, A.: Very deep convolutional networks for large-scale image recognition. arXiv preprint (2014) arXiv:1409.1556
32. Huang, G., Liu, Z., Van Der Maaten, L., Weinberger, K.Q.: Densely connected convolutional networks. In Proceedings of the IEEE Conference on Computer Vision and Pattern Recognition, pp. 4700–4708 (2017)
33. Zeiler, M.D., Fergus, R.: Visualizing and understanding convolutional networks. In: European Conference on Computer Vision, pp. 818–833. Springer, Cham (2014)
34. He, K., Zhang, X., Ren, S., Sun, J.: Deep residual learning for image recognition. In: Proceedings of the IEEE Conference on Computer Vision and Pattern Recognition, pp. 770–778 (2016)
35. Xie, X., Zhong, Z., Zhao, W., Zheng, C., Wang, F., Liu, J.: Chest CT for typical 2019-nCoV pneumonia: relationship to negative RT-PCR testing. Radiology, p. 200343 (2020)
36. Luo, H., Tang, Q.L., Shang, Y.X., Liang, S.B., Yang, M., Robinson, N., Liu, J.P.: Can Chinese medicine be used for prevention of corona virus disease 2019 (COVID-19)? A review of historical classics, research evidence and current prevention programs. Chin. J. Integr. Med., 1–8 (2020)
37. Bala, P.C., Eisenreich, B.R., Yoo, S.B.M., Hayden, B.Y., Park, H.S., Zimmermann, J.: OpenMonkeyStudio: automated markerless pose estimation in freely moving macaques. bioRxiv (2020)
38. Pourhomayoun, M., Shakibi, M.: Predicting mortality risk in patients with COVID-19 using artificial intelligence to help medical decision-making. medRxiv (2020)
39. Feng, C., Huang, Z., Wang, L., Chen, X., Zhai, Y., Zhu, F., Chen, H., Wang, Y., Su, X., Huang, S., Tian, L.: A novel triage tool of artificial intelligence assisted diagnosis aid system for suspected COVID-19 pneumonia. In: Fever Clinics (2020)
40. Rahmatizadeh, S., Valizadeh-Haghi, S., Dabbagh, A.: The role of artificial intelligence in management of critical COVID-19 patients. J. Cell. Mol. Anesthesia **5**(1), 16–22 (2020)
41. Jiang, X., Coffee, M., Bari, A., Wang, J., Jiang, X., Huang, J., Shi, J., Dai, J., Cai, J., Zhang, T., Wu, Z.: Towards an artificial intelligence framework for data-driven prediction of coronavirus clinical severity. CMC: Comput. Mater. Continua **63**, 537–51 (2020)
42. Gutierrez, G.: Artificial intelligence in the intensive care unit. Crit. Care **24**, 1–9 (2020)
43. Yan, L., Zhang, H.T., Xiao, Y., Wang, M., Sun, C., Liang, J., Li, S., Zhang, M., Guo, Y., Xiao, Y., Tang, X.: Prediction of criticality in patients with severe Covid-19 infection using three clinical features: a machine learning-based prognostic model with clinical data in Wuhan. MedRxiv
44. Zou, H., Hastie, T.: Regularization and variable selection via the elastic net. J. R. Stat. Soc.: Series B (Stat. Methodol.) **67**(2), 301–320 (2005)
45. Williams, C.K., Rasmussen, C.E.: Gaussian Processes for Machine Learning, vol. 2. MIT Press Cambridge, MA, 493, p. 494 (2006)
46. Mei, X., Lee, H.C., Diao, K.Y., Huang, M., Lin, B., Liu, C., Xie, Z., Ma, Y., Robson, P.M., Chung, M., Bernheim, A.: Artificial intelligence–enabled rapid diagnosis of patients with COVID-19. Nature Medicine, pp. 1–5 (2020)
47. Zhang, K., Liu, X., Shen, J., Li, Z., Sang, Y., Wu, X., Zha, Y., Liang, W., Wang, C., Wang, K., Ye, L.: Clinically applicable AI system for accurate diagnosis, quantitative measurements, and prognosis of covid-19 pneumonia using computed tomography. Cell (2020)

48. Shi, H., Han, X., Jiang, N., Cao, Y., Alwalid, O., Gu, J., Fan, Y., Zheng, C.: Radiological findings from 81 patients with COVID-19 pneumonia in Wuhan, China: a descriptive study. Lancet Infect. Dis. (2020)
49. Lee, E.Y., Ng, M.Y., Khong, P.L.: COVID-19 pneumonia: what has CT taught us? Lancet. Infect. Dis **20**(4), 384–385 (2020)
50. Kang, H., Xia, L., Yan, F., Wan, Z., Shi, F., Yuan, H., Jiang, H., Wu, D., Sui, H., Zhang, C., Shen, D.: Diagnosis of coronavirus disease 2019 (covid-19) with structured latent multi-view representation learning. IEEE transactions on medical imaging (2020)
51. Ozturk, T., Talo, M., Yildirim, E.A., Baloglu, U.B., Yildirim, O., Acharya, U.R.: Automated detection of COVID-19 cases using deep neural networks with X-ray images. Comput. Biol. Med., 103792 (2020)
52. Khatami, A., Khosravi, A., Nguyen, T., Lim, C.P., Nahavandi, S.: Medical image analysis using wavelet transform and deep belief networks. Expert Syst. Appl. **86**, 190–198 (2017)
53. Khan, A.I., Shah, J.L., Bhat, M.M.: Coronet: A deep neural network for detection and diagnosis of COVID-19 from chest x-ray images. Comput. Methods Progr. Biomed., 105581 (2020)
54. Kooraki, S., Hosseiny, M., Myers, L., Gholamrezanezhad, A.: Coronavirus (COVID-19) outbreak: what the department of radiology should know. J. Am. Coll. Radiol. (2020)
55. Ardakani, A.A., Kanafi, A.R., Acharya, U.R., Khadem, N., Mohammadi, A.: Application of deep learning technique to manage COVID-19 in routine clinical practice using CT images: Results of 10 convolutional neural networks. Comput. Biol. Med., 103795 (2020)
56. Oh, Y., Park, S., Ye, J.C.: Deep learning covid-19 features on cxr using limited training data sets. IEEE Trans. Med. Imaging (2020)
57. Pereira, R.M., Bertolini, D., Teixeira, L.O., Silla Jr, C.N., Costa, Y.M.: COVID-19 identification in chest X-ray images on flat and hierarchical classification scenarios. Comput. Methods Progr. Biomed., 105532 (2020)
58. Fan, D.P., Zhou, T., Ji, G.P., Zhou, Y., Chen, G., Fu, H., Shen, J., Shao, L.: Inf-Net: Automatic COVID-19 Lung infection segmentation from CT Images. IEEE Trans. Med. Imaging (2020)
59. Brunese, L., Mercaldo, F., Reginelli, A., Santone, A.: Explainable deep learning for pulmonary disease and coronavirus COVID-19 detection from X-rays. Comput. Methods Programs Biomed. **196**, (2020)
60. Waheed, A., Goyal, M., Gupta, D., Khanna, A., Al-Turjman, F., Pinheiro, P.R.: Covidgan: Data augmentation using auxiliary classifier gan for improved covid-19 detection. IEEE Access **8**, 91916–91923 (2020)
61. Abdel-Basset, M., Mohamed, R., Elhoseny, M., Chakrabortty, R.K., Ryan, M.: A hybrid COVID-19 detection model using an improved marine predators algorithm and a ranking-based diversity reduction strategy. IEEE Access **8**, 79521–79540 (2020)
62. He, X., Yang, X., Zhang, S., Zhao, J., Zhang, Y., Xing, E., Xie, P.: Sample-efficient deep learning for COVID-19 diagnosis based on CT scans. medRxiv (2020)
63. Chen, J., Wu, L., Zhang, J., Zhang, L., Gong, D., Zhao, Y., Hu, S., Wang, Y., Hu, X., Zheng, B., Zhang, K.: Deep learning-based model for detecting 2019 novel coronavirus pneumonia on high-resolution computed tomography: a prospective study. MedRxiv (2020)
64. Haleem, A., Vaishya, R., Javaid, M., Khan, I.H.: Artificial Intelligence (AI) applications in orthopaedics: an innovative technology to embrace. J. Clin. Orthopaed. Trauma **11**, S80–S81 (2020)
65. Stebbing, J., Phelan, A., Griffin, I., Tucker, C., Oechsle, O., Smith, D., Richardson, P.: COVID-19: combining antiviral and anti-inflammatory treatments. Lancet. Infect. Dis. **20**(4), 400–402 (2020)
66. Biswas, K., Sen, P.: Space-time dependence of corona virus (COVID-19) outbreak. arXiv preprint arXiv:2003.03149
67. Ester, M., Kriegel, H. P., Sander, J., and Xu, X.: A density-based algorithm for discovering clusters in large spatial databases with noise. KDD **96**(34), 226–231 (1996)
68. Senior, A.W., Evans, R., Jumper, J., Kirkpatrick, J., Sifre, L., Green, T., Qin, C., Žídek, A., Nelson, A.W., Bridgland, A., Penedones, H.: Improved protein structure prediction using potentials from deep learning. Nature **577**(7792), 706–710 (2020)

69. Jumper, J., Tunyasuvunakool, K., Kohli, P., Hassabis, D., the AlphaFold Team: Computational predictions of protein structures associated with COVID-19, DeepMind website, 5 March 2020, https://deepmind.com/research/open-source/computationalpredictions-of-protein-structures-associated-with-COVID-19 (2020)
70. Nguyen, T.T., Abdelrazek, M., Nguyen, D.T., Aryal, S., Nguyen, D.T., Khatami, A.: Origin of Novel Coronavirus (COVID-19): a computational biology study using artificial intelligence. BioRxiv (2020)
71. Nguyen, T.T., Pathirana, P.N., Nguyen, T., Nguyen, H., Bhatti, A., Nguyen, D.C., Nguyen, D.T., Nguyen, N.D., Creighton, D., Abdelrazek, M.: Genomic mutations and changes in protein secondary structure and solvent accessibility of SARS-CoV-2 (COVID-19 virus). bioRxiv (2020)
72. Oak Ridge National Laboratory: LandScan Global Population Database. https://landscan.ornl.gov/ (2020)
73. Bogoch, I.I., Brady, O.J., Kraemer, M.U., German, M., Creatore, M.I., Kulkarni, M.A., Brownstein, J.S., Mekaru, S.R., Hay, S.I., Groot, E., Watts, A.: Anticipating the international spread of Zika virus from Brazil. The Lancet **387**(10016), 335–336 (2016)
74. Hou, X., Wang, B., Hu, W., Yin, L., Wu, H.: SolarNet: a deep learning framework to map solar power plants In China from satellite imagery. arXiv preprint arXiv:1912.03685
75. Perry, T.S.: Satellites and AI monitor Chinese economy's reaction to coronavirus. IEEE Spectrum 10
76. Abd-Alrazaq, A., Alhuwail, D., Househ, M., Hamdi, M., Shah, Z.: Top concerns of tweeters during the COVID-19 pandemic: infoveillance study. J. Med. Internet Res. **22**(4), (2020)
77. Li, S., Wang, Y., Xue, J., Zhao, N., Zhu, T.: The impact of COVID-19 epidemic declaration on psychological consequences: a study on active Weibo users. Int. J. Environ. Res. Public Health **17**(6), 2032 (2020)
78. Torales, J., O'Higgins, M., Castaldelli-Maia, J.M., Ventriglio, A.: The outbreak of COVID-19 coronavirus and its impact on global mental health. Int. J. Soc Psychiatry, 0020764020915212 (2020)
79. Yang, Z., Zeng, Z., Wang, K., Wong, S.S., Liang, W., Zanin, M., Liu, P., Cao, X., Gao, Z., Mai, Z., Liang, J.: Modified SEIR and AI prediction of the epidemics trend of COVID-19 in China under public health interventions. J. Thoracic Dis. **12**(3), 165 (2020)
80. Zheng, N., Du, S., Wang, J., Zhang, H., Cui, W., Kang, Z., Yang, T., Lou, B., Chi, Y., Long, H., Ma, M.: Predicting covid-19 in china using hybrid AI model. IEEE Trans. Cybern. (2020)
81. Hochreiter, S., Schmidhuber, J.: Long short-term memory. Neural Comput. **9**(8), 1735–1780 (1997)
82. Chae, S., Kwon, S., Lee, D.: Predicting infectious disease using deep learning and big data. Int. J. Environ. Res Public Health **15**(8), 1596 (2018)
83. Riad, M.H., Sekamatte, M., Ocom, F., Makumbi, I., Scoglio, C.M.: Risk assessment of Ebola virus disease spreading in Uganda using a two-layer temporal network. Sci. Rep. **9**(1), 1–17 (2019)
84. Venna, S.R., Tavanaei, A., Gottumukkala, R.N., Raghavan, V.V., Maida, A.S., Nichols, S.: A novel data-driven model for real-time influenza forecasting. IEEE Access **7**, 7691–7701 (2018)
85. Kucharski, A.J., Russell, T.W., Diamond, C., Liu, Y., Edmunds, J., Funk, S., Eggo, R.M., Sun, F., Jit, M., Munday, J.D., Davies, N.: Early dynamics of transmission and control of COVID-19: a mathematical modelling study. The Lancet Infect. Dis. (2020)
86. Gambhir, M., Bozio, C., O'Hagan, J.J., Uzicanin, A., Johnson, L.E., Biggerstaff, M., Swerdlow, D.L.: Infectious disease modeling methods as tools for informing response to novel influenza viruses of unknown pandemic potential. Clin. Infect. Dis. **60**(suppl_1), S11–S19 (2015)
87. Rasmussen, S.A., Redd, S.C., 2015. Using results from infectious disease modeling to improve the response to a potential H7N9 influenza pandemic. Clinical Infectious Diseases, 60(suppl_1), pp.S9-S10

88. Koo, J.R., Cook, A.R., Park, M., Sun, Y., Sun, H., Lim, J.T., Tam, C., Dickens, B.L.: Interventions to mitigate early spread of SARS-CoV-2 in Singapore: a modelling study. Lancet Infect. Dis. (2020)
89. Hamzah, F.B., Lau, C., Nazri, H., Ligot, D.V., Lee, G., Tan, C.L.: CoronaTracker: worldwide COVID-19 outbreak data analysis and prediction. Bull. World Health Organ. **1**, 32 (2020)
90. Wu, J.T., Leung, K., Leung, G.M.: Nowcasting and forecasting the potential domestic and international spread of the 2019-nCoV outbreak originating in Wuhan, China: a modelling study. The Lancet **395**(10225), 689–697 (2020)
91. Zhao, S., Musa, S.S., Lin, Q., Ran, J., Yang, G., Wang, W., Lou, Y., Yang, L., Gao, D., He, D., Wang, M.H.: Estimating the unreported number of novel coronavirus (2019-nCoV) cases in China in the first half of January 2020: a data-driven modelling analysis of the early outbreak. J. Clin. Med. **9**(2), 388 (2020)
92. Karako, K., Song, P., Chen, Y., Tang, W.: Analysis of COVID-19 infection spread in Japan based on stochastic transition model. Biosci. Trends (2020)
93. Zhang, P., Chen, B., Ma, L., Li, Z., Song, Z., Duan, W., Qiu, X.: The large scale machine learning in an artificial society: prediction of the Ebola outbreak in Beijing. Computational Intelligence and Neuroscience (2015)
94. Akhtar, M., Kraemer, M.U., Gardner, L.M.: A dynamic neural network model for predicting risk of Zika in real time. BMC Med. **17**(1), 171 (2019)
95. Jiang, D., Hao, M., Ding, F., Fu, J., Li, M.: Mapping the transmission risk of Zika virus using machine learning models. Acta Trop. **185**, 391–399 (2018)
96. Modjarrad, K., Moorthy, V.S., Millett, P., Gsell, P.S., Roth, C., Kieny, M.P.: Developing global norms for sharing data and results during public health emergencies. PLoS Med. **13**(1), (2016)
97. Zhavoronkov, A., Zagribelnyy, B., Zhebrak, A., Aladinskiy, V., Terentiev, V., Vanhaelen, Q., Bezrukov, D.S., Polykovskiy, D., Shayakhmetov, R., Filimonov, A., Bishop, M.: Potential non-covalent SARS-CoV-2 3C-like protease inhibitors designed using generative deep learning approaches and reviewed by human medicinal chemist in virtual reality (2020)
98. Nguyen, D., Gao, K., Chen, J., Wang, R., Wei, G.: Potentially highly potent drugs for 2019-nCoV. bioRxiv (2020)
99. Ge, Y., Tian, T., Huang, S., Wan, F., Li, J., Li, S., Yang, H., Hong, L., Wu, N., Yuan, E., Cheng, L.: A data-driven drug repositioning framework discovered a potential therapeutic agent targeting COVID-19. bioRxiv (2020)
100. Bobdey, S., Ray, S.: Going viral–Covid-19 impact assessment: a perspective beyond clinical practice. J. Marine Med. Soc. **22**(1), 9 (2020)
101. Sohrabi, C., Alsafi, Z., O'Neill, N., Khan, M., Kerwan, A., Al-Jabir, A., Iosifidis, C. and Agha, R.: World Health Organization declares global emergency: a review of the 2019 novel coronavirus (COVID-19). Int. J. Surg. (2020)
102. Chen, S., Yang, J., Yang, W., Wang, C., Bärnighausen, T.: COVID-19 control in China during mass population movements at New Year. The Lancet **395**(10226), 764–766 (2020)
103. Nguyen, D.D., Gao, K., Wang, M., Wei, G.W.: MathDL: mathematical deep learning for D3R Grand Challenge 4. J. Comput. Aided Mol. Des. **34**(2), 131–147 (2020)
104. Tang, B., He, F., Liu, D., Fang, M., Wu, Z., Xu, D.: AI-aided design of novel targeted covalent inhibitors against SARS-CoV-2. bioRxiv (2020)
105. Bung, N., Krishnan, S.R., Bulusu, G., Roy, A.: De novo design of new chemical entities (NCEs) for SARS-CoV-2 using artificial intelligence. ChemRxiv (2020)
106. Joshi, B.P., Bakrola, V.D., Shah, P., Krishnamurthy, R.: deepMINE-Natural language processing based automatic literature mining and research summarization for early stage comprehension in pandemic situations specifically for COVID-19. bioRxiv
107. Dong, M., Cao, X., Liang, M., Li, L., Liang, H., Liu, G.: Understand research hotspots surrounding COVID-19 and other coronavirus infections using topic modeling. medRxiv (2020)
108. Kuusisto, F., Page, D., Stewart, R.: Word embedding mining for SARS-CoV-2 and COVID-19 drug repurposing. F1000Research, 9(585), p. 585

109. Rao, A., Saipradeep, V.G., Joseph, T., Kotte, S., Sivadasan, N., Srinivasan, R.: Text and Network-Mining for COVID-19 Intervention Studies (2020)
110. Ahamed, S., Samad, M.: Information mining for covid-19 research from a large volume of scientific literature. arXiv preprint (2020). arXiv:2004.02085
111. Patel, J.C., Tulswani, R., Khurana, P., Sharma, Y.K., Ganju, L., Kumar, B., Sugadev, R.: Identification of pulmonary comorbid diseases network based repurposing effective drugs for COVID-19 (2020)
112. Duran-Frigola, M., Bertoni, M., Blanco, R., Martínez, V., Pauls, E., Alcalde, V., Turon, G., Villegas, N., Fernández-Torras, A., Pons, C., Mateo, L.: Bioactivity profile similarities to expand the repertoire of COVID-19 drugs. J. Chem. Inf. Model. (2020)
113. Smeulders, A.W., Van Ginneken, A.M.: An analysis of pathology knowledge and decision making for the development of artificial intelligence-based consulting systems. Anal. Quant. Cytol. Histol. **11**(3), 154–165 (1989)
114. Gozes, O., Frid-Adar, M., Greenspan, H., Browning, P.D., Zhang, H., Ji, W., Bernheim, A., Siegel, E.: Rapid ai development cycle for the coronavirus (covid-19) pandemic: Initial results for automated detection & patient monitoring using deep learning ct image analysis. arXiv preprint (2020). arXiv:2003.05037
115. Gugnani, P.: Coronavirus: It's Reactivation in Cured Patients and Role of Artificial Intelligence for Infected Patients. Available at SSRN 3589222 (2020)
116. Li, L., Qin, L., Xu, Z., Yin, Y., Wang, X., Kong, B., Bai, J., Lu, Y., Fang, Z., Song, Q., Cao, K.: Artificial intelligence distinguishes COVID-19 from community acquired pneumonia on chest CT. Radiology (2020)
117. Wan, K.H., Huang, S.S., Young, A.L., Lam, D.S.C.: Precautionary measures needed for ophthalmologists during pandemic of the coronavirus disease 2019 (COVID-19). Acta Ophthalmol. **98**(3), 221–222 (2020)
118. Pirouz, B., Shaffiee Haghshenas, S., Shaffiee Haghshenas, S., Piro, P.: Investigating a serious challenge in the sustainable development process: analysis of confirmed cases of COVID-19 (new type of coronavirus) through a binary classification using artificial intelligence and regression analysis. Sustainability **12**(6), 2427 (2020)
119. Gupta, R., Ghosh, A., Singh, A.K., Misra, A.: Clinical considerations for patients with diabetes in times of COVID-19 epidemic. Diabet Metabol Syndrome **14**(3), 211 (2020)
120. Gupta, R., Misra, A.: Contentious issues and evolving concepts in the clinical presentation and management of patients with COVID-19 infectionwith reference to use of therapeutic and other drugs used in Co-morbid diseases (Hypertension, diabetes etc). Diabetes Metabol. Syndrome: Clin. Res. Rev.
121. Peters, M.E., Neumann, M., Iyyer, M., Gardner, M., Clark, C., Lee, K., Zettlemoyer, L., 2018. Deep contextualized word representations. arXiv preprint (2020). arXiv:1802.05365
122. Bird, S., Klein, E., Loper, E., 2009. Natural Language Processing With Python: Analyzing Text With the Natural Language Toolkit. O'Reilly Media, Inc. (2020)
123. Howard, J., Ruder, S., 2018. Universal language model fine-tuning for text classification (2020). arXiv preprint arXiv:1801.06146
124. Devlin, J., Chang, M.W., Lee, K., Toutanova, K.: Bert: Pre-training of deep bidirectional transformers for language understanding (2018). arXiv preprint arXiv:1810.04805
125. Vaswani, A., Shazeer, N., Parmar, N., Uszkoreit, J., Jones, L., Gomez, A.N., Kaiser, Ł., Polosukhin, I.: Attention is all you need. In: Advances in Neural Information Processing Systems, pp. 5998–6008 (2017)
126. Dai, Z., Yang, Z., Yang, Y., Carbonell, J., Le, Q.V., Salakhutdinov, R.: Transformer-xl: Attentive language models beyond a fixed-length context (2019). arXiv preprint arXiv:1901.02860
127. Zhang, Z., Han, X., Liu, Z., Jiang, X., Sun, M., Liu, Q.: ERNIE: Enhanced language representation with informative entities (2019). arXiv preprint arXiv:1905.07129
128. Yang, Z., Dai, Z., Yang, Y., Carbonell, J., Salakhutdinov, R.R., Le, Q.V.: Xlnet: Generalized autoregressive pretraining for language understanding. In Advances in Neural Information Processing Systems, pp. 5753–5763 (2019)

129. Ye, Z., Guo, Q., Gan, Q., Qiu, X., Zhang, Z.: Bp-transformer: Modelling long-range context via binary partitioning (2019). arXiv preprint arXiv:1911.04070
130. Raffel, C., Shazeer, N., Roberts, A., Lee, K., Narang, S., Matena, M., Zhou, Y., Li, W., Liu, P.J.: Exploring the limits of transfer learning with a unified text-to-text transformer (2019). arXiv preprint arXiv:1910.10683
131. Radford, A., Wu, J., Child, R., Luan, D., Amodei, D., Sutskever, I.: Language models are unsupervised multitask learners. OpenAI Blog **1**(8), 9 (2019)
132. Martin, A., Nateqi, J., Gruarin, S., Munsch, N., Abdarahmane, I., Knapp, B.: An artificial intelligence-based first-line defence against COVID-19: digitally screening citizens for risks via a chatbot. bioRxiv (2020)
133. WHO and Facebook:. WHO Health Alert's Facebook Messenger Chatbot (2020). https://m.me/who
134. WHO and Rakuten Viber: WHO Viber Interactive Chatbot (2020). https://vb.me/82e535
135. WHO and WhatsApp: WHO's Health Alert on WhatsApp (2020). http://bit.ly/who-covid19-whatsapp
136. UNICEF's Europe and Central Asia Regional Office and the WHO Regional Office for Europe: HealthBuddy (2020). https://healthbuddy.info/
137. IBM: IBM Watson Assistant for Citizens (2020). https://www.ibm.com/au-en/watson/covid-response
138. Chatbot and Infermedica: COVID-19 Risk Assessment Chatbot (2020). https://www.chatbot.com/covid19-chatbot/
139. Barhead: Rona (COVID-19 Bot) (2020). https://barhead.com/technology/rona/
140. Health Service Executive Ireland: COVID 19 Chat Bot (2020). https://www.hse.ie/chatbot/covid/chatiframe.aspx
141. Yang, G.Z., Nelson, B.J., Murphy, R.R., Choset, H., Christensen, H., Collins, S.H., Dario, P., Goldberg, K., Ikuta, K., Jacobstein, N., Kragic, D.: Combating COVID-19—The role of robotics in managing public health and infectious diseases (2020)
142. Estrada, R., MA: The Uses of Drones in Case of Massive Epidemics Contagious Diseases Relief Humanitarian Aid: Wuhan-COVID-19 Crisis (2020)
143. Zeng, Z., Chen, P.J., Lew, A.A.: From high-touch to high-tech: COVID-19 drives robotics adoption. Tourism Geographies, pp. 1–11 (2020)
144. Tavakoli, M., Carriere, J., Torabi, A.: Robotics, smart wearable technologies, and autonomous intelligent systems for healthcare during the COVID-19 pandemic: An analysis of the state of the art and future vision. Adv. Intell. Syst., 2000071 (2020)
145. Nguyen, T.T., Nguyen, N.D., Nahavandi, S.: Deep reinforcement learning for multiagent systems: a review of challenges, solutions, and applications. IEEE Trans. Cybern. (2020)
146. Zhang, G.L., Khan, A.M., Srinivasan, K.N., August, J.T., Brusic, V.: Neural models for predicting viral vaccine targets. J. Bioinform. Comput. Biol. **3**(05), 1207–1225 (2005)
147. Soam, S.S., Bhasker, B., Mishra, B.N.: Improved prediction of MHC class I binders/non-binders peptides through artificial neural network using variable learning rate: SARS corona virus, a case study. In: Software Tools and Algorithms for Biological Systems, pp. 223–229. Springer, New York, NY (2011)
148. Ong, E., Wong, M.U., Huffman, A., He, Y.: COVID-19 coronavirus vaccine design using reverse vaccinology and machine learning. BioRxiv (2020)
149. Li, H., Sun, F.: Comparative studies of alignment, alignment-free and SVM based approaches for predicting the hosts of viruses based on viral sequences. Sci. Rep. **8**(1), 1–9 (2018)
150. Wrapp, D., et al.: Cryo-EM structure of the 2019-nCoV spike in the prefusion conformation. Science (2020). https://doi.org/10.1126/science.aax0902
151. Huang, C., et al.: 'Clinical features of patients infected with 2019 novel coronavirus in Wuhan. China', The Lancet. (2020). https://doi.org/10.1016/S0140-6736(20)30183-5
152. Tahir ul Qamar, M., et al.: Structural basis of SARS-CoV-2 3CLpro and anti-COVID-19 drug discovery from medicinal plants. J. Pharmaceut Anal. (2020). https://doi.org/10.1016/j.jpha.2020.03.009

153. Wu, F., et al.: A new coronavirus associated with human respiratory disease in China. Nature (2020). https://doi.org/10.1038/s41586-020-2008-3
154. Perlman, S., Netland, J.: Coronaviruses post-SARS: Update on replication and pathogenesis. Nat. Rev. Microbiol. (2009). https://doi.org/10.1038/nrmicro2147
155. Liu, D. X., Liang, J. Q., Fung, T.S.: Human Coronavirus-229E, -OC43, -NL63, and -HKU1. Reference Module in Life Sciences, B978–0-12-809633-8.21501-X (2020). https://doi.org/10.1016/B978-0-12-809633-8.21501-X
156. Ye, Z.W., Yuan, S., Yuen, K.S., Fung, S.Y., Chan, C.P., Jin, D.Y.: Zoonotic origins of human coronaviruses. Int. J. Biol. Sci. **16**(10), 1686–1697 (2020). https://doi.org/10.7150/ijbs.45472
157. T, W., et al.: Characterization of the receptor-binding domain (RBD) of 2019 novel coronavirus: implication for development of RBD protein as a viral attachment inhibitor and vaccine. Cell. Mol. Immunol. (2020). https://doi.org/10.1038/s41423-020-0400-4
158. Shereen, M.A., et al.: COVID-19 infection: Origin, transmission, and characteristics of human coronaviruses. J. Adv. Res. (2020). https://doi.org/10.1016/j.jare.2020.03.005
159. Guo, Y.R., et al.: The origin, transmission and clinical therapies on coronavirus disease 2019 (COVID-19) outbreak- A n update on the status. Military Med. Res. (2020). https://doi.org/10.1186/s40779-020-00240-0
160. Zheng, J.: SARS-coV-2: An emerging coronavirus that causes a global threat. Int. J. Biol. Sci. (2020). https://doi.org/10.7150/ijbs.45053
161. Fehr, A.R., Perlman, S.: Coronaviruses: An overview of their replication and pathogenesis. In: Coronaviruses: Methods and Protocols (2015). https://doi.org/10.1007/978-1-4939-2438-7_1
162. Masters, P.S.: The molecular biology of coronaviruses. Adv. Virus Res. (2006). https://doi.org/10.1016/S0065-3527(06)66005-3
163. Knoops, K., et al.: SARS-coronavirus replication is supported by a reticulovesicular network of modified endoplasmic reticulum. PLoS Biol. (2008). https://doi.org/10.1371/journal.pbio.0060226
164. Chen, Y., Liu, Q., Guo, D.: Emerging coronaviruses: genome structure, replication, and pathogenesis. J. Med. Virol. (2020). https://doi.org/10.1002/jmv.25681
165. Sun, L., et al.: Coronavirus papain-like proteases negatively regulate antiviral innate immune response through disruption of STING-mediated signaling. PLoS ONE (2012). https://doi.org/10.1371/journal.pone.0030802
166. Walls, A.C., et al.: Structure, function, and antigenicity of the SARS-CoV-2 spike glycoprotein. Cell (2020). https://doi.org/10.1016/j.cell.2020.02.058
167. Schoeman, D., Fielding, B.C.: Coronavirus envelope protein: Current knowledge. Virol. J. (2019). https://doi.org/10.1186/s12985-019-1182-0
168. Liu, D.X., Fung, T.S., Chong, K.K., Shukla, A., & Hilgenfeld, R.: Accessory proteins of SARS-CoV and other coronaviruses. Antiviral Res. **109**, 97–109. (2014). https://doi.org/10.1016/j.antiviral.2014.06.013
169. Linton, N.M., et al.: Incubation period and other epidemiological characteristics of 2019 novel coronavirus infections with right truncation: a statistical analysis of publicly available case data. J. Clin. Med. (2020). https://doi.org/10.3390/jcm9020538
170. Varia, M., et al.: Investigation of a nosocomial outbreak of severe acute respiratory syndrome (SARS) in Toronto, Canada. CMAJ (2003)
171. Rabi, F.A., et al.: Sars-cov-2 and coronavirus disease 2019: What we know so far. Pathogens (2020). https://doi.org/10.3390/pathogens9030231
172. Simmons, G., et al.: Proteolytic activation of the SARS-coronavirus spike protein: cutting enzymes at the cutting edge of antiviral research. Antiviral Res. (2013). https://doi.org/10.1016/j.antiviral.2013.09.028
173. Sungnak, W., et al.: SARS-CoV-2 Entry genes are most highly expressed in nasal goblet and ciliated cells within human airways. ArXiv (2020)
174. Posthuma, C.C., te Velthuis, A.J.W., Snijder, E.J.: Nidovirus RNA polymerases: Complex enzymes handling exceptional RNA genomes. Virus Res. (2017). https://doi.org/10.1016/j.virusres.2017.01.023

175. Zhou, P., et al.: A pneumonia outbreak associated with a new coronavirus of probable bat origin. Nature (2020). https://doi.org/10.1038/s41586-020-2012-7
176. Corman, V.M., et al.: Detection of 2019 novel coronavirus (2019-nCoV) by real-time RT-PCR. Eurosurveillance (2020). https://doi.org/10.2807/1560-7917.ES.2020.25.3.2000045
177. Williams, A.E., Chambers, R.C.: The mercurial nature of neutrophils: still an enigma in ARDS? Lung cellular and molecular physiology. Am. J. Physiol. **306**(3), L217–L230 (2014). https://doi.org/10.1152/ajplung.00311.2013
178. Channappanavar, R., Perlman, S.: Pathogenic human coronavirus infections: causes and consequences of cytokine storm and immunopathology. Seminars Immunopathol. (2017). https://doi.org/10.1007/s00281-017-0629-x
179. W., C.Y., et al.: Evaluation of reverse transcription-PCR assays for rapid diagnosis of severe acute respiratory syndrome associated with a novel coronavirus. J. Clin. Microbiol. (2003). https://doi.org/10.1128/JCM.41.10.4521
180. Pan, Y., Guan, H., Zhou, S., Wang, Y., Li, Q., Zhu, T., Hu, Q., Xia, L.: Initial CT findings and temporal changes in patients with the novel coronavirus pneumonia (2019-nCoV): a study of 63 patients in Wuhan. China. Eur. Radiol.s **30**(6), 3306–3309 (2020). https://doi.org/10.1007/s00330-020-06731-x
181. Chung, M., et al.: CT imaging features of 2019 novel coronavirus (2019-NCoV). Radiology (2020). https://doi.org/10.1148/radiol.2020200230
182. Woo, P.C.Y., et al.: Differential sensitivities of severe acute respiratory syndrome (SARS) coronavirus spike polypeptide enzyme-linked immunosorbent assay (ELISA) and SARS coronavirus nucleocapsid protein ELISA for serodiagnosis of SARS coronavirus pneumonia. J. Clin. Microbiol. (2005). https://doi.org/10.1128/JCM.43.7.3054-3058.2005
183. Groneberg, D.A., Hilgenfeld, R., Zabel, P.: Molecular mechanisms of severe acute respiratory syndrome (SARS). Respir. Res. (2005). https://doi.org/10.1186/1465-9921-6-8
184. Lo, M.K., et al.: 'GS-5734 and its parent nucleoside analog inhibit Filo-Pneumo-, and Paramyxoviruses. Sci. Rep. (2017). https://doi.org/10.1038/srep43395
185. Sheahan, T.P., et al.: Comparative therapeutic efficacy of remdesivir and combination lopinavir, ritonavir, and interferon beta against MERS-CoV. Nat. Commun. (2020). https://doi.org/10.1038/s41467-019-13940-6
186. de Wit, E., et al.: Prophylactic and therapeutic remdesivir (GS-5734) treatment in the rhesus macaque model of MERS-CoV infection. Proc. Natl. Acad. Sci. U.S.A. (2020). https://doi.org/10.1073/pnas.1922083117
187. Lo, M.K., et al.: Remdesivir (GS-5734) protects African green monkeys from Nipah virus challenge. Sci. Transl. Med. (2019). https://doi.org/10.1126/scitranslmed.aau9242
188. Holshue, M.L., et al.: First case of 2019 novel coronavirus in the United States. N. Engl. J. Med. (2020). https://doi.org/10.1056/NEJMoa2001191
189. Wang, M., et al.: Remdesivir and chloroquine effectively inhibit the recently emerged novel coronavirus (2019-nCoV) in vitro. Cell Res. (2020). https://doi.org/10.1038/s41422-020-0282-0
190. Zumla, A., et al.: Coronaviruses-drug discovery and therapeutic options. Nat. Rev. Drug Discovery (2016). https://doi.org/10.1038/nrd.2015.37
191. De Clercq, E.: New nucleoside analogues for the treatment of hemorrhagic fever virus infections. Chem. Asian J. (2019). https://doi.org/10.1002/asia.201900841
192. Chen, L., et al.: Cinanserin is an inhibitor of the 3C-Like proteinase of severe acute respiratory syndrome coronavirus and strongly reduces virus replication in vitro. J. Virol. (2005). https://doi.org/10.1128/jvi.79.11.7095-7103.2005
193. Jo, S., et al.: Inhibition of SARS-CoV 3CL protease by flavonoids. J. Enzyme Inhib. Med. Chem. (2020). https://doi.org/10.1080/14756366.2019.1690480
194. Park, J.Y., et al.: Diarylheptanoids from Alnus japonica inhibit papain-like protease of severe acute respiratory syndrome coronavirus. Biol. Pharmaceut. Bull. (2012). https://doi.org/10.1248/bpb.b12-00623
195. Li, W., et al.: Angiotensin-converting enzyme 2 is a functional receptor for the SARS coronavirus. Nature (2003). https://doi.org/10.1038/nature02145

196. Mair-Jenkins, J., et al.: The effectiveness of convalescent plasma and hyperimmune immunoglobulin for the treatment of severe acute respiratory infections of viral etiology: A systematic review and exploratory meta-analysis. J. Infect. Dis. (2015). https://doi.org/10.1093/infdis/jiu396
197. Koenig, K.L.: Identify-isolate-inform: A modified tool for initial detection and management of middle east respiratory syndrome patients in the emergency department. Western J. Emerg. Med. (2015). https://doi.org/10.5811/westjem.2015.7.27915
198. Zhang, L., Liu, Y.: Potential interventions for novel coronavirus in China: A systematic review. J. Med. Virol. (2020). https://doi.org/10.1002/jmv.25707
199. Graham, R.L., Donaldson, E.F., Baric, R.S.: A decade after SARS: Strategies for controlling emerging coronaviruses. Nat. Rev. Microbiol. (2013). https://doi.org/10.1038/nrmicro3143
200. Li, Q., et al.: Early transmission dynamics in Wuhan, China, of novel coronavirus-infected pneumonia. N. Engl. J. Med. (2020). https://doi.org/10.1056/NEJMoa2001316

Deep Learning for COVID-19

Suchandra Dutta, Avishake Adhikary, Dhrubasish Sarkar, Dipak K. Kole, and Premananda Jana

Abstract The devastating outbreak of the SARS-CoV-2 (Severe Acute Respiratory Syndrome-Coronavirus) also known as COVID-2019 has succeeded in introducing the danger to the worldwide living. Now COVID-19 is among the main potentially deadly issues in the world. Rapid and precise identification of COVID-19 infection is important to diagnose, make informed assumptions, and assure that patients receive care that aims to save people's health and life. The entire community is making enormous endeavors to tackle the spreading of such a horrible epidemic in forms of communications true, economy, information sources, safety equipment, existence-risk treatments, and many on this and many other tools. Coronavirus triggers a vast range of viral disease; however, it is a virus of the kind RNA which can affect all humans and animals. Coronavirus is now identified in this chapter uses a form of deep learning which is a sub-branch of artificial intelligence. This chapter suggests making use of the deep learning algorithms with such a view to recognizing its daily incremental behavior and predicting the potential accessibility of COVID-2019 throughout civilizations using real-time data knowledge. COVID-19 Quick diagnosis and It is necessary to identify high-risk patients with the worst diagnosis for early treatment and optimization of medical services. And the algorithm of deep learning helps to do that and helps to combat the COVID-19 and the deep learning algorithms are more time saving; less expensive; easy to operate. COVID-19 research

S. Dutta · A. Adhikary · D. Sarkar (✉)
Amity Institute of Information Technology, Amity University, Kolkata, India
e-mail: dsarkar@klk.amity.edu

S. Dutta
e-mail: duttasuchandra214@gmail.com

A. Adhikary
e-mail: avhishe.adhikary11@gmail.com

D. K. Kole
Department of CSE, Jalpaiguri Government Engineering College, Jalpaiguri, West Bengal, India
e-mail: dipak.kole@cse.jgec.ac.in

P. Jana
Netaji Subhas Open University, Kalyani, West Bengal, India
e-mail: prema_jana@yahoo.com

D. Oliva et al. (eds.), *Artificial Intelligence for COVID-19*, Studies in Systems, Decision and Control 358, https://doi.org/10.1007/978-3-030-69744-0_30

through deep learning involves the patient's x-rays of the lungs and the fundamental concept is to identify the ultrasound as impaired or usual COVID. In general, the issue is a collection of identification algorithms whereby we identify Standard normal v/s COVID-19 cases. There are several benefits and drawbacks to utilizing Deep Learning to solve these circumstances.

Keywords Covid-19 · Deep learning · Image recognition · Speech recognition · Machine learning

1 Introduction

The mystery novel coronavirus 2019 (COVID- 2019), which initially emerged during December 2019 in Wuhan city of China, circulated exponentially throughout the globe as well as has become a global epidemic. Presently COVID-19 is one of the many other life intimidating issues in the world. Rapid and precise recognition of COVID-19 infectious diseases is vital to identify, make better judgments, and ensure that patients receive medication that enables rescue people's lives. Coronavirus (COVID-2019) is a disease that is caused by a new virus that was previously unknown. The disease tends to cause lung infections with symptomatology such as cough, fever, and breathing difficulties in much more extreme cases. The COVID-19 family worldwide causes millions of deaths every day. Detecting the confirmed samples as soon as needed is important, to avoid the transmission of the disease and to prescribe medications harmed rapidly. Which also had a profound impact on both everyday life, global health as well as the world economies. Its requirement for indispensable testing equipment has risen because precise automatic tools and techniques are not accessible. A test, for major analysis the RT-PCR ("reverse transcription-polymerase chain reaction") is tested with oropharyngeal effusion followed by X-ray in the chest. If indeed the X-ray screenplay in the chest is normal, the patient may go home and take some rest. The patient must also be taken to the hospital if COVID-19 is confirmed. At the beginning phases, COVID-19 impacts almost all lungs with such an inherently external and subpleural allocation, especially in the lower labret and particularly the proximal sections. The lung CT scan is being used to identify COVID-19. The principal testing or diagnosing method used to recognize COVID-19 ought to be the CT scan as well as X-ray. The chest computed tomography (CT) and X-Ray is a quicker and easier procedure for managing COVID-19 in clinical practices by integrating the medical signs and symptoms.

Deep Learning is a machine learning model trained through neural networks and is used for the most complex and accurate results and is a subset of Machine Learning itself. These neural networks consist of neurons that either learn from the environment or can train themselves over and over. Deep Learning is being regularly used in the medical industry for a while now in areas like disease prediction, life rate prediction, predictions based on computer vision and so much more.

2 Overview of Deep Learning

Introduction to Deep Learning

To define deep learning, we need to define some other terms first:

(i) Artificial Intelligence
(ii) Machine Learning
(iii) Neurons
(iv) Neural Networks

Artificial Intelligence is the process of making any non-human thing in this world to make it think like humans. It is a far broader topic than machine learning and deep learning. Machine Learning is the process of creating a system for a machine that learns by itself using Artificial Intelligence and feeding itself data. It is a subset of Artificial Intelligence and is the superset of Deep Learning. Neurons in computer science terms are defined as a mathematical function that takes some input and gives some output. Neural Networks are chains of neurons as defined earlier and user input of one function and feeds the output of the function to another function in a sort of chained mechanism. A single function is also capable of feeding output produced by it to itself.

Now to define 'Deep Learning' we say that it is the subset of Machine Learning that uses neural networks to perform tasks exactly like the way a human might try to perform, using Artificial Intelligence.

There are a thousand number of deep learning models that are performed to execute real-life tasks. Some of the most popular models are:

(i) Deep Belief Net
(ii) CNN's
(iii) RNNs
(iv) Reinforcement Learning etc.

The deep learning model that we applied to our application as discussed later is called CNN or Convolutional Neural Networks.

CNN's are generally used in performing real-life tasks related to computer vision. The CNNs model later in the application also learns by itself to produce more accurate outputs based on the data it already produces. And the CNN model used here uses zero performance drops on the application itself and rather utilizes the server that generates the outcome.

3 COVID-19 Recognition and Dismember from X-Ray Image with the Help of the Deep-Learning Algorithm

Coronavirus was identified in the deep learning system that is a sub-branch of artificial intelligence. Despite hundreds number of deaths reported the amount of verified COVID-19 deaths has reached millions of people. The WHO ("World Health

Organization") also declared COVID-2019 to be a worldwide pandemic. In essence, COVID-19 lung data was correlated to pneumonia and normal lung data because pneumonia is one of the signs of COVID-19. mention in [1] beware of the similarities among the structured image and initial image of a stack.If configured the photo in a specific context along with size state or color pixel level), the performance obtained in this analysis would have not been obtained.

For Renovation of images:

- ***Method of fuzzy color***

The Fuzzy theory is recognized based on its level of precision and it is the next stage is unstable. Fuzzy Color [mention at Fig. 1] implementations play an essential role. In the study mention in [1] of images as well as the conclusions drawn depend on the similarity as well as various features used to distinguish colors. Each one of the input images as in Fuzzy color methodology comprises triple input variations (red, green, and blue → RGB). A specific output parameter is transferred because of the method. The amounts of input and output are calculated by the testing results.

The rationale everything behind the methodology of Fuzzy Color is to break the input data through blurred frames. The pixels within the image do have a membership degree from each window, and affiliation levels are determined proportion to the gap between the window and the pixel. Image variation is acquired with a membership degree.

The procedure for Fuzzy Color is to establish the Output-Input End. The measurements of the photos are in this phase every blurry window is illustrated, and the overall output picture is generated. Thus, each pixel's width value is represented as an affiliation level mention in [2–4]. They reconstructed the entire dataset using the Fuzzy Color methodology of the Python codes mention in [1].

- ***Stacking method***

Stacking of images is a method [mentioned at Fig. 2] in virtual image processing, incorporating numerous pictures are captured or restored at various focal lengths. It is a method often used to enhance image consistency within the dataset. By merging

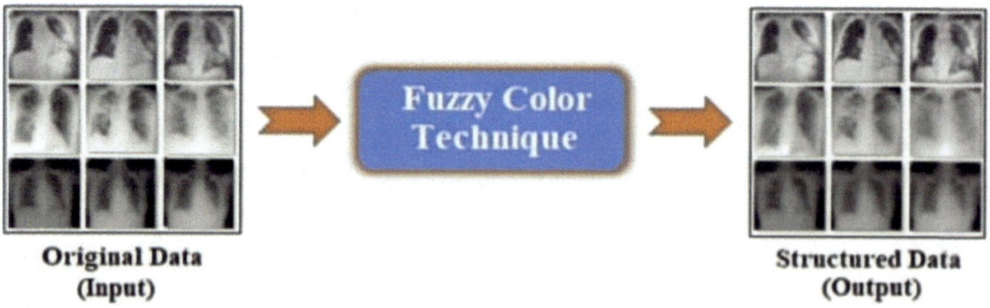

Fig. 1 Fuzzy color technique [1]

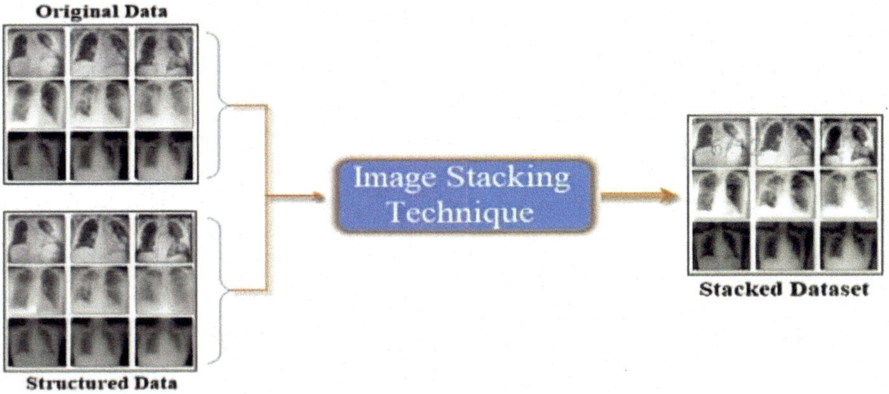

Fig. 2 Image stacking technique [1]

at least two images in such a row and splitting the image into two sections, such a method helps to remove the noises from the main image.

Those are all context and shadow pieces. Although the first pictures are analyzed in the backdrop, the second one is superimposed on a backdrop image. Parameters like transparency, comparison, visibility, and a combined ratio of the two images are essential here. Mention in [5], the more precise those ratios, the smaller the amount of noise in the pictures, and the greater the ratio of performance.

The Stacking method mention in [6] was used with the Python and Pillow libraries.

The positive outcome of the Fuzzy methodology would continue to make the stacking methodology a success.

Advantages (benefit) for using this approach:

1. When analyzing the X-ray images of COVID-19 victims, it has a 100 percent rate of effectiveness in identifying the COVID-19 virus.
2. The deep-learning frameworks used throughout the suggested method (MobileNetV2 & Squeeze Net) include lower complexity relative to several other deep learning algorithms. It will enable build momentum and efficiency over time.
3. It also helps to reduce the interruption in each image in the data and offers stacking methodology with effective functionality.

Difficulties that are facing during to use of these methods-

1. Unless the sample image sizes in the database are small, a full output cannot be obtained. Regardless of the re-compress criterion, treating often quite low-resolution images still is a hurdle for the methods.
2. The pixel density components of the actual pictures and the formalized images must be the equivalent in the Stacking methodology.

CONVOLUTION NEURAL NETWORK (CNN):

As all know that the condition of the Coronavirus, which is horrible, to overcome that situation, all people need to do manual testing.

Manual testing has been one of the key things which requires being undertaken and already has begun in most parts of the world, while the real-life scenario can also be recognized, and correct decisions should be made. However, the limitations of this testing process involve a limited supply of testing kits, expensive and unreliable blood testing; usually, that test took approximately 5–6 h for a blood test to produce the response.

Therefore, the aim is to use the Deep Learning method can solve such conditions through good as well as a more effective diagnosis. So, because the infection is extremely infectious as soon as researchers produce the outcomes the lesser scenarios in the country and that's why people should use Convolution Neural Network (CNN) to even getting our job completed.

Although the two X-rays that means normal. People's chest X -rays and COVID-19 affected people's chest X-rays have not been numbered, CNN may tend to differentiate among the two X-rays.

4 COVID-19 Recognition and Dismember from Computed Tomography (CT) Scan with the Help of the Deep-Learning Algorithm

Radio-graphic studies have shown tremendous predictive and therapeutic significance against COVID-19 in computed tomography (CT). In COVID-19 diagnosis, e.g., CT displayed a far better capacity by far than RT-PCR for sick people from COVID-19, mention in [8] CT scans often revealed simultaneous lung defects comprising of ground-glass opacities (GGO).

Mention in [9] anomalies as well as alterations have been noticed in habitual CT, except in symptom-less patients.As just a prevalent clinical instrument, the CT scan can be easily as well as quickly acquired without introducing considerable costs. Developing a responsive screening tool with a CT scan image must speed up the treatment decisions and enhance the RT-PCR ("real-time reverse transcription-polymerase chain reaction") approach. But on the other side, forecasting individualized diagnosis and treatment by using CT scan images can define potentially more serious conditions patients who may be more probable to be intense or need immediate healthcare assistant.

Deep learning (DL) as a technique of artificial intelligence clearly shows impressive outcomes in helping the evaluation of lung disease utilizing CT scan images Profiting from of the high learning capability of characteristics, DL could even instantaneously extract functionalities which are associated with health outcomes of CT scan images.

Properties acquired from DL prototypes that represent high-dimensional conceptual modifier keys that are challenging for most people to understand however closely linked to patient results. Mention in [10] that contrast to established DL models, we intend to get a completely automated DL framework for predictive and therapeutic evaluation of COVID-19.

Completely automated deep learning framework for therapeutic COVID-19 also Forecast analyzes → The conceptual DL framework consisted of 3 components: automated differentiation of the lungs, Repression of the non-lung region, and predictive and therapeutic examination of COVID 19. Two DL mechanisms became interested throughout this DL system: DenseNet121-FPN to chest CT image lung optimization, including adaptive threshold COVID-19Net for COVID- 19 predictive and therapeutic research mention in [7].

Such an innovative DL framework is efficient and accurate in medical application, despite needing any living human-assisted transcription. The DL mechanism discovers lung functions could even represent correlation among operational anomalies in the micro-level lung as well as CT scan images in the chest.

Used for controlled pulmonary optimization of covid-19 patients:

Consistently utilized CT scan of the chest contains several – anti-lung regions like musculature, back, as well as outer organ open area. Fully automated DL design, as well as model (DenseNet121-FPN), used to fragment lung regions in the chest CT scan to concentrate on the analysis of lung region.

Delusive lung region (pulmonary) found through the DL method

Mention in [11] researchers can envision a lung through DL simulation algorithms. A region that makes the DL framework the much more focus. Such DL's considered questionable Lung regions typically showed irregular features associated with radiologists' Performance. Besides, several problematic lung regions identified by DL displayed a strong correlation to Immune regions potentially.

As DL is also an end-to-end design of forecasting which studies explicit interfaces the inference method of the DL framework is beneficial to illustrate explicitly seen among lung CT picture and COVID-19. Convolution layers filtration is a very significant element of the DL framework.

5 Speech-Recognition Method Using Deep Learning Algorithm for the Fight Against the Coronavirus

Deep learning is widely recognized because of its effectiveness in image recognition, however yet other primary use of the technique is speech recognition for example Alexa from Amazon or as well as voice recognition typing or can say texting. Deep learning improves speech recognition through call centers throughout the COVID-19 recession.

Speech recognition technology is a system that is equipped to interpret, decode, and translate the data of people's speech to textual content. Speech recognition at even the very core point transforms sounds waves into different characters, as well as eventually phrases. The said program extracts phrases, decodes it, and evaluates the composite tones. To decode everything that is said, the visual image of those sounds, as well as tones, develops computational study.

The benefit of deep learning for recognition of speech derives from the versatility and predictive ability of deep neural networks which are becoming increasingly available currently.

Methods for speaking recognition are highly effective in improving operating performance and lowering excessive expenses. That is precisely whatever the healthcare industry requires throughout a period when the COVID-19 epidemic impacts humans.

Working procedure

Technology for voice recognition as well as speech recognition utilizes by NLP ("Natural Language Processing") and deep learning as well as the neural networks to decompose speech to pieces it might understand. It turns such modules into a digital form and evaluates information parts.

The system focuses on a database of documented speaking terms and phrases, and creates assumptions about the different sounds, creating a theory over what the consumer says.

A crucial challenge in reliably translating the right phrases is the audio variation produced for much the similar words provided sounds, or intonation (i.e. same words but different sound as well as pronunciation). Here in this technique, the understanding of tone is not sufficient. A huge issue mostly with methodology is the failure of the deep neural network to classify character, which appears to render pronunciation and semantic failures. The remedy is just to combine the acoustic model (described earlier) with such a word framework that can recognize meaning.

To be effective, speech recognition technology wants to be willing to recognize, for example, the difference among original names as well as common terms (for instance, "Cook" in "James Cook" is a title), or distinguish among homophones (terms with the same sound albeit with different meaning).

Advanced speech recognition, provided an understandable text, starts with the processing of seismic waves by using fast & furious transform (FFT) and the concatenation of blocks from adjacent frames to create a 'spectrogram' [mentioned in Fig. 3]. The aim is to reduce the complexity of the multivariate regression sound information in a manner that allows for the prediction of characters.

Analysis among spectrogram frameworks as well as the projected real characters is best accomplished with deep neural networks. Different methods are historically used following sound quality, pronunciation, and language; rather, deep neural networks produce increasingly reliable translations by enabling more versatility in interpreting words with differing noises.

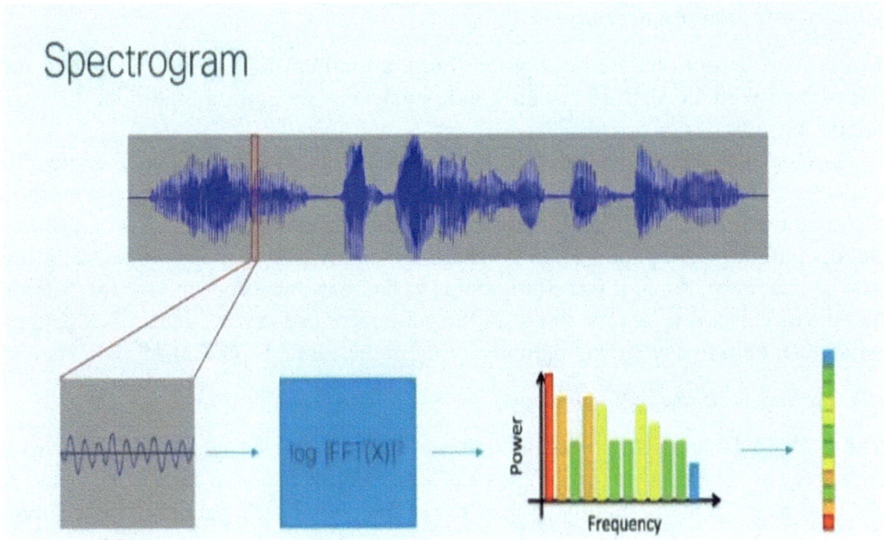

Fig. 3 Spectrogram [12]

Thus, a speech recognition obstacle is to create an intellectual mechanism not just to 'hear' voice yet often to interact and argue with outlets of information and centralized relations that make up concepts throughout the actual world.

Speech to script methods is the necessity of the period that we are passing throughout that period of the COVID-19 epidemic. Transferring technology from speech to script helps boost operational efficiency for healthcare sector organizations.

Speech recognition has many applications for EMR (Electronic Medical Records). Such applications can vary from aggregating information from clinical records to assisting with medical studies or diagnosing and treating clients. Precise is incredibly important in any direction.

The digital healthcare technology is the way to go until the patient safety is the necessity of a few time. Through healthcare technology serving even an important role in the battle opposed to the COVID-19 outbreak, that's where speech to texting technology and text processing technologies come into the equation and the benefits of telehealth, as well as health care technology, are accentuated. Telemedicine or remote healthcare is particularly effective in cases where clients are distant in proportion to the distances or are moving frequently. The ongoing COVID-19 issue, nonetheless, allows digital-care solutions such as telemedicine services essential worldwide. The deep-leaning use as well as help for some several reasons, the reasons are given below.

(i) Errors in turning decreased:

Errors like disruptions are not a good thing, a moment as well when the hospitals are packed with COVID-19 patients and physicians are getting treatment through a telephone call.

As speech to script conversion technologies has been in position, all data which is collected from the telephone conversation is recorded by the technology and modified throughout the client's EMR (Electronic Medical Records). It guarantees that perhaps the document of the patients can be shared instantly, – this means processing time now is near zero. Also, it incredibly helps to decrease waiting time for the patients, and the time is a very crucial thing for the patients or can say for the serious patients, which can help to save many patients living in the case of COVID-19 patients also.

(ii) Dealing with the call workload:

The COVID-19 had also compelled the health sector to be a sector with all arms on the roof. The workload of calls in the healthcare sectors is one of the crucial issues for the healthcare centers, mainly in the time of the COVID-19 pandemic. For solving this problem many healthcare sectors can take the help of deep-learning technology as well as speech recognition methodology.

The doctors, nurses, and medical staffs in healthcare centers are so preoccupied with treating patients who have acquired the disease that so few of them are accessible to manage to the phone calls. To fewer physicians managing the telephone and a stream of phone conversations streaming in. Telehealth technology is what many turns to as nobody tries to make the drive to a health care center.

(iii)Going to ensure accurateness and reducing inaccuracy:

Another crucial problem is the handwritten prescription of doctors, which doctors can give to their patients for prescriptive medicine. But the main problem is, a prescription from a physician is still one which leaves everyone puzzled. A doctor's prescription can mislead both patients and pharmacy. Most doctors do use handwritten prescriptions even though the adequacy rating is substantially lower.

All information about prescriptions, departure notes, etc. are registered and translated through text and in case of electronic health records. This technique can help to remove the hassle of calling the physician to make clear what has been mentioned. In this way, deep learning can help to solve the above problem.

6 Equivocal Lung Area Detection with the Help of Deep Learning

The COVID-19 enhanced information qualified detector offers better output measurements and is reliable for diagnosing X-ray (The use of X-Ray images of the lung area as well the chest is suggested for COVID-19 diagnosis since X-rays are easily achieved close-by hospitals or clinics or healthcare centers are reasonably fast as well

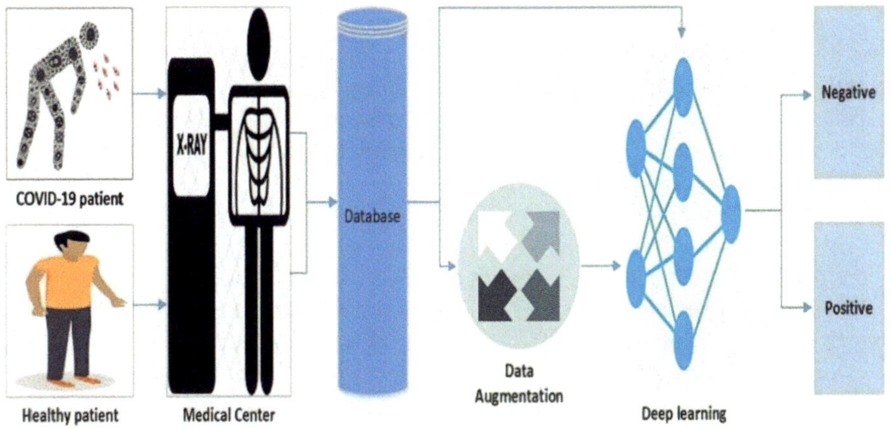

Fig. 4 Working procedure of deep-learning in the time of COVID-19 [16]

as at low cost.) and CT scan of the lung area of the COVID-19 patients. Detection of the lung area of the patients helps to detect that who is affected by the COVID-19 and who is not affected by the COVID-19.

Mention in [13]. The implementation of modern artificial intelligence (AI) technologies, as well as deep-learning combined by chest as well as lung area of the COVID-19 patients' radiography (for example CT-scan and X-Ray), can help to diagnose such epidemic accurately and also can enable to resolve the issue of the absence of qualified doctors in rural village areas. The latest results taken from radiology Imaging technology as well as laser scanners indicate that all these photographs provide prominent COVID-19 virus details.

Mention in [14, 15] that an RT-PCR ("Real-Time Reverse transcription-polymerase Chain Reaction") is perhaps among the most favored testing methodology widely used during the treatment of COVID-19. Radiographic scans of the chest to detect the lung area of the COVID-19 patients including CT (computed tomography) as well as X-ray serve important functions inaccurate detection and medication of such an epidemic. Because of the lower susceptibility of 60–70% to RT-PCR, however, though unfavorable outcomes are produced, signs can indeed be identified by analyzing individual radiological scans. The technique for detecting COVID-19 pneumonia, which may be considering an RT-PRC scanning device.

As discussed in the 3rd and 4th points, by CT-scan and X-ray using deep-learning doctors can easily detect the C0VID-19 affected people (Fig. 4).

7 Future Supposition by Deep Learning Algorithm

DL is often used as a collection of dynamic artificial neural network platforms, aimed at understanding the conceptual projection of an ideal treatment diagnosis among data sets. The conceptual elements in the DL framework are described as textures and thus are incorporated to replicate the brain inference method.

DL in the future might give us the possibility to use unsupervised learning in a better way to mimic the behavior of a human, that might also help in creating better neural networks and perform more complex tasks that are performed in the medical field, such as more accurate mortality rate and disease predictions, more accurate pandemic and big data predictions, more accurate NLPs that might help in contributing to communication with doctors around the world and newer deep learning model architectures that might help in creating and executing more memory efficient tasks, execute tasks faster and create more accurate predicted results, and which thus can create more efficient neural network model architectures.

Deep learning might also help in creating more complex graphical system design architectures based on the 3D CNNs that might help in identifying images on a different level. The 3D CNNs might also help in predicting the rate and calculating the possibility of impossible operational tasks that are performed by the doctors and might also help in simulating the human and other research domain architectures.

8 Proposed Method

8.1 Concept of Using Deep Learning in Our Application

Our concept was to combine mobile computer vision and deep learning. We created an application for a medicine shop and the primary idea was to implement an online pharmacy consisting of two sides—the user and the shopkeeper. The user's side (patient side) consists of a camera to send the existing document of prescription and the provider's side consists of a list of containers where the shop owner can see whenever the patient has made any request. Whenever the patient makes a request the deep learning model paired with computer vision checks for signs of how the document might be incorrect or fraud. If the document is incorrect then the user is prompted to retake the image of the document and send it to the shopkeeper or provider.

The application also consists of a server that handles multiple user requests and makes it easy to access the database from anywhere in the world. The shopkeeper then receives the request from the server and then confirms the order of the patient asking for medicine as a request. This concept and the application were made from scratch using the latest technologies and the memory-efficient practices to reduce memory and file size usage, which led to an application of 5 Mb (even after installation).

This lightweight application can also be installed in a minimum android version of 7.0+ which satisfies more than 90% of the current and higher version of the android users in the world and ensures the maximum level of security without hampering the maximum number of users.

Accuracy of the model:

We took sample images of 1024*768 resolution from a 5mp primary camera sensor in good to moderate lighting conditions and we were able to produce output like this:

Top Images	Recognition Accuracy (%)	Matching Matrices (Out of 786432)
Top One	95	747110.40
Top Three	97.25	764805.20
Top Five	97.75	768737.28
Top Ten	98.25	772669.44
Denial	**1.75**	**137625.60**

Thus the model is extremely successful in producing accurate results even in moderate lighting conditions.

DIAGRAMMATIC REPRESENTATION: (Fig. 5)

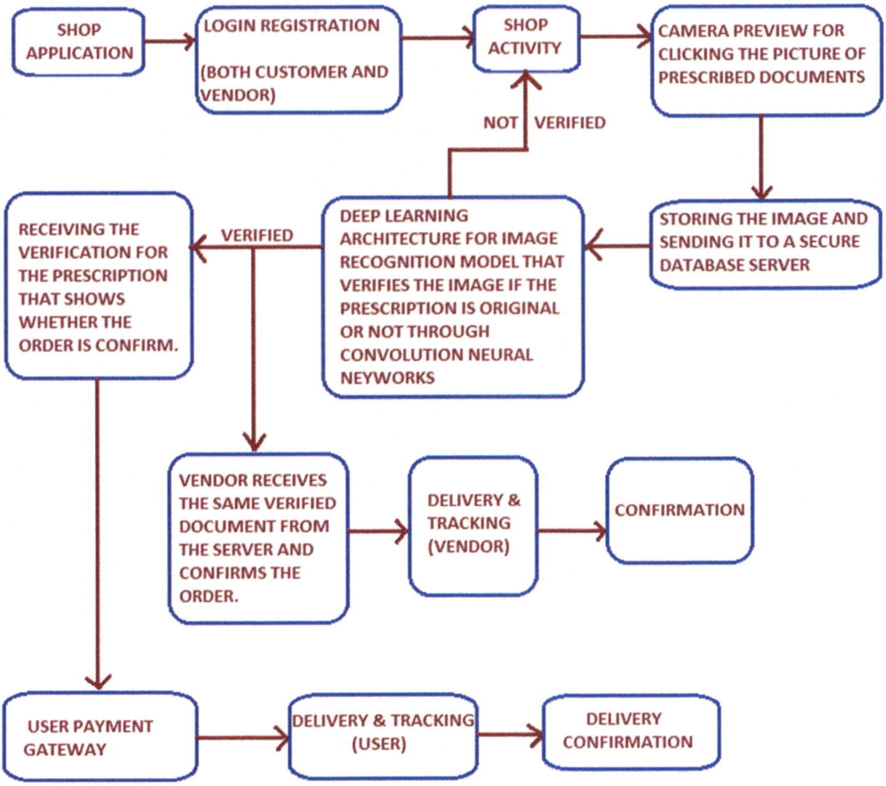

Fig. 5 Diagrammatic representation of the proposed model

9 Conclusion

People afflicted by COVID-19 are expected to experience irreversible lung problems as well as breathing problems which can cause death earlier on. COVID-19 identification was achieved utilizing deep learning methods. Even though it is crucial to monitor the increasingly and internationally spreading COVID-19, AI technologies are being used to conduct it efficiently and consistently.

Applicational predictions based on Deep Learning are getting more commonly used in the healthcare sector and more and more complex tasks in healthcare are being executed with the help of neural networks and complex deep learning models.

The more data that is generated by the millions on devices every day is helping the models create more accurate predictions and helping researchers the ability to create newer models based on training data and testing data.

Future models will also be satisfying more complex and greater tasks that will be executed with the help of deep learning architectures. The health care sector will also tend to benefit from these models which are going to predict more accurate results and are surely going to help mankind.

References

1. Togaçar, M, Ergen B., Comert, Z.: COVID-19 detection using deep learning models to exploit Social Mimic Optimization and structured chest X-ray images using fuzzy color and stacking approaches, Computers in Biology and Medicine 121103805, Contents lists available at ScienceDirect Computers in Biology and Medicine, (5–8) journal homepage: http://www.elsevier.com/locate/compbiomed (2020). article
2. Bardak, T., Bardak, S.: Prediction of wood density by using red-green-blue (RGB) color and fuzzy logic techniques. J. Polytech. **20**, 979–984 (2017). https://doi.org/10.2339/politeknik.369132. 2017. https://doi.org/10.2339/politeknik.369132
3. Arnal J., Súcar L.: Hybrid filter based on fuzzy techniques for mixed noise reduction in color images. Appl. Sci. **10** (2020). https://doi.org/10.3390/
4. Soto-Hidalgo, J.M., Sanchez, D., Chamorro-Martínez, J., Martínez-Jim enez, P.M.: Color comparison in fuzzy color spaces (2019), https://doi.org/10.1016/j.fss.2019.09.013
5. Elleboudy, N.A., Ezz Eldin, H.M., Azab, S.M.S.: Focus stacking technique in identification of forensically important Chrysomya species (Diptera: Calliphoridae), 5–10 Egypt, J. (2016). https://doi.org/10.1016/j.ejfs.2016.06.001
6. Gingold, Y.: Image stack: simple code to load and process image stacks. https://github.com/yig/imagestack, 2019 March 11, 2020
7. Wang, S., Zha, Y., Li, W., et al.: A fully automatic deep learning system for COVID-19 diagnostic and prognostic analysis. Eur. Respir. J., 13–20 (2020). https://doi.org/10.1183/13993003.00775-2020
8. Ai, T., Yang, Z., Hou, H., Zhan, C., Chen, C., Lv, W., Tao, Q., Sun, Z., Xia, L.: Correlation of Chest CT and RT-PCR testing in coronavirus disease 2019 (COVID-19) in China: A Report of 1014 Cases
9. Wang, S., Shi, J., Ye, Z., Dong, D., Yu, D., Zhou, M., Liu, Y., Gevaert, O., Wang, K., Zhu, Y., Zhou, H., Liu, Z., Tian, J.: Predicting EGFR mutation status in lung adenocarcinoma on computed tomography image using deep learning. Eur. Respir. J. (2019)

10. Wang, S.,, Kang, B., Ma, J., Zeng, X., Xiao, M., Guo, J., Cai, M., Yang, J., Li, Y., Meng, X., Xu, B.: A deep learning algorithm using CT images to screen for Corona Virus Disease (COVID-19) (2020)
11. Selvaraju, R.R., Cogswell, M., Das, A., Vedantam, R., Parikh, D., Batra, D.: Grad-cam: Visual explanations from deep networks via gradient-based localization (2017)
12. https://medium.com/@ODSC/deep-learning-for-speech-recognition-cbbebab15f0d
13. Ozturk, T., Talo, M., Yildirim, E.A., Baloglu, U.B., Yildirim, O., Acharya, U.R.: Automated detection of COVID-19 cases using deep neural networks with X-ray images (2020). http://www.elsevier.com/locate/compbiomed, (2–10)computers in biology and medicine 121 (2020) 103792 (2020)
14. Kanne, J.P., Little, B.P., Chung, J.H., Elicker, B.M., Ketai, L.H.: Essentials for radiologists on COVID-19: an update—radiology scientific expert panel. Radiology, 4–9 (2020), https://doi.org/10.1148/radiol.2020200527
15. Lee, E.Y., Ng, M.Y., Khong, P.L.: COVID-19 pneumonia: what has CT taught us? Lancet Infect
16. Alazab, M., Awajan, J., Mesleh, A., Abraham, A., Jatana, V., Alhyari, S.: COVID-19 Prediction and Detection Using Deep Learning, pp. 3–4, 29 May 2020. https://www.researchgate.net/publication/341980921

Factors Affecting Medical Mask Purchase Decision in Covid19 Pandemic

Bui Huy Khoi, Nguyen Thi Ngan, and Luu Quang Vinh

Abstract This paper aims to analyze the influence of Product (PRO), Service quality elements (SER), Psychological factor (PSY), Brand (BRA) on the purchasing decision of medical masks in the covid19 pandemic in Vietnam. Data was collected Vietnam consumers who are living in Ho Chi Minh City habitually usually use the medical mask. We used R 4.0.2 for analyzing statistics. The results of this study indicate that the Psychological factor (PSY) and Brand (BRA) had an important and positive influence on purchasing decisions the products from the medical mask is 37.77%. Product (PRO) and Service quality elements (SER) are not related to the purchasing decision. Applications of this study give implications to enhance to buy the medical mask in product market development. Previous studies revealed that using linear regression. This study uses the optimal choice by the AIC method.

Keywords Covid19 pandemic · Medical mask · Akaike's information criteria · Medical mask purchase decision

1 Introduction

As COVID-19 has had a major effect worldwide, 2020 has taken a track distinct from the years before. As for humans, it has brought deep changes to our lives and the nature of our lives [5]. As today's world finds itself embroiled in one of the biggest health and humanitarian crises that were seen in the last century, the global implications of Covid-19 remain difficult to gauge [17]. The collateral effects of the war against the virus include the paralysis of productive activity, with significant global economic and social consequences [2]. One of the industries most vulnerable

Authors Contribution Three authors contribute to the paper. Bui Huy Khoi contributed to the study of data and the gathering of research-related references. Nguyen Thi Ngan contributed to the compilation of data and the manuscript was revised. Luu Quang Vinh conducted a data survey.

B. H. Khoi (✉) · N. T. Ngan · L. Q. Vinh
Industrial University of Ho Chi Minh City, Ho Chi Minh City, Vietnam
e-mail: buihuykhoi@iuh.edu.vn

D. Oliva et al. (eds.), *Artificial Intelligence for COVID-19*, Studies in Systems, Decision and Control 358, https://doi.org/10.1007/978-3-030-69744-0_31

to health and safety challenges, political transitions, economic crises, natural catastrophes [4]. The COVID-19 pandemic is an infectious pandemic with the agent of the virus SARS-CoV-2, happening on a global scale. From the beginning of December 2019 to the beginning of September 2020, the COVID pandemic has spread in 210 countries/regions, with nearly 33.5 million cases and more than 1 million deaths [16]. Up to now, the pandemic is still spreading in many countries, complicatedly happening in Europe, countries in Asia and America, negatively affecting all socio-economic activities in the world, including Vietnam. In which, almost all economic sectors and fields are affected negatively. Due to the increasingly complicated situation of COVID-19 in Vietnam, the demand for medical equipment such as gloves, disinfectant water … especially the price of masks has increased sharply. The market has witnessed a scarcity of these products, which has pushed the selling price 3–4 times higher than the normal price. The medical mask market suddenly increases in demand. Meanwhile, the supply of masks is still limited. Many factories export the page's lack of raw materials, difficult to import … These reasons make prices soar.

The pandemic of the COVID-19 coronavirus is affecting a global health crisis. According to the World Health Organization (WHO), one of the most important methods of security is wearing a face mask in public areas. Owing to the COVID-19 coronavirus outbreak all over the world, the tendency of bringing medical masks in public is growing. People used to wear masks before Covid-19 to safeguard their health from air pollution [13]. An individual normally wears a mask to protect himself, but at the same time, preventing others from breathing in their respiratory drops has a significant impact on public health. This is also an effective way to transmit the SARS-CoV-2 virus since it has spread because there are no signs of an infected person. Mass masking is also underpinned by the fundamentals of public health. First, wearing a mask is that controlling the hazard at the source is at least as important as the method of minimizing the hazard (washing hands). The benefits of mass masking can also be seen as interventions that provide moderate individual benefits but large population benefits. Wearing a mass mask to control the source of infection is a useful complement to social distance and hand hygiene during the COVID-19 pandemic. In the global response to the pandemic, mass masking has changed the emphasis from self-defense to altruism and is a sign of social solidarity.

Consumer choice results from the quality expectations before and quality experience after the purchase [15]. Many studies have shown that when buying, consumers usually choose a product with a brand (BRA) that assurances a certain quality. These consumer's psychological behavior (PSY) is crucial for marketers seeking to increase buying decisions and is a significant factor affecting consumer intention [18]. The research of Baedowy et al. [1] shows that product variables (PRO) and service quality (SER) have a significant influence on purchasing decisions. In this paper, we have designed an empirical study in the context of purchasing decision the medical mask in Vietnam to examine its factors to protect consumer's health in Covid19 Pandemic:

$$\mathrm{PQ} = \beta_0 + \beta_1 \mathrm{PRO} + \beta_2 \mathrm{SER} + \beta_3 \mathrm{PSY} + \beta_4 \mathrm{BRA}$$

Code: Product (PRO), Service quality elements (SER), Psychological factor (PSY), Brand (BRA), and β is the regression estimate coefficient of the dependent variable.

PQ: The decision to purchase the face mask in the Covid19 Pandemic.

2 Methodology

2.1 Research Approach

In this study, collecting information for our quantitative analysis, questionnaires were used. The respondents' survey responses were the primary method for gathering information. The research was conducted in the year 2020. The research included questions about the status of the determinants that affected the decision to buy. According to Hair et al. [10] to use factor analysis, the minimum sample size should be 50, preferably 100, and the item/measurement ratio is 5: 1. With 4 independent variables, 1 dependent variable, and 21 items on the official scale, based on the sample size calculation stated, the author needs a sample size of at least 105. Respondents were selected using conventional methods, and a total of 134 consumers living in How Chi Minh City, Vietnam. Our study population consisted of 50 (37.3%) men and 84 (62.7%) women. Their income and jobs are shown in Table 1.

Our study is composed of four Jobs. The student accounts for the highest proportion. We use the 5-point Likert scale to evaluate the level of consent for the related factors. Therefore, this paper also uses the 5-point Likert scale to evaluate the level of consent for all observed variables, with 1: Disagree… and 5: Agree in Table 2.

Blinding

For the duration of the study, all study staff and respondents were blinded. No one from the outside world had any contact with the study participants.

Table 1 Job and income

Job	Number	Percentages (%)	Income	Number	Percentage (%)
Student	108	80.6	Lower 5 mill VND	108	80.6
Worker	11	8.2			
Officer	11	8.2	From 5 to10 mill VND	16	11.9
Teacher	4	3.0	Higher 10 to 20 mill VND	10	7.5
Total	134	100.0	Total	134	100.0

Table 2 Factor and item

Unit	Factor and item	Mean
PRO	Product	3.77
PRO1	Wearing a medical mask will help prevent COVID-19 infection	4.24
PRO2	The prices of medical masks during the COVID-19 pandemic environment are just right for your purchase	2.66
PRO3	Quality is the top concern when buying medical masks	4.41
SER	Service quality elements	3.08
SER1	When buying, you will be assisted in choosing the appropriate medical mask	3.48
SER2	When you buy a medical mask, you will be delivered to your doorstep	3.01
SER3	When purchasing a medical mask, you will be rewarded with medical-related items	2.74
PSY	Psychological factor	3.35
PSY1	You use a medical mask during the COVID pandemic environment to protect your health	4.55
PSY2	Because you see around you many people poured out to buy medical masks	2.69
PSY3	Masks have antibacterial effects and prevent infection	3.87
PSY4	If the COVID-19 pandemic environment does not break out, you will not purchase medical masks	2.28
BRA	Brand	4.07
BRA1	When buying a medical mask, you will buy one that has a well-known brand name	3.75
BRA2	Branded medical masks will give you peace of mind to use	4.28
BRA3	The brand will bring positive emotions to consumers when buying	4.18
PQ	Purchase decision	3.92
PQ1	The quality of the medical mask will affect your buying decision	4.30
PQ2	The characteristics of the medical mask will influence your purchasing decision	4.19
PQ3	The service that when you buy the mask attached also influences your buying decision.	3.57
PQ4	Psychological factors that influence your decision to buy a medical mask	3.55
PQ5	The brand of the medical mask you buy will influence your buying decision	3.99

3 Results

3.1 Akaike Information Criterion Selection

AIC (Akaike's Information Criteria) was utilized to choose the best model by R software. AIC has been used in the theoretical context for model selection. And when multicollinearity occurs, the AIC approach can handle multiple independent variables. As a regression model, AIC can be applied, estimating one or more dependent

Table 3 Akaike information criterion selection

Model	AIC
PQ = f (PRO, SER, PSY, BRA)	−174.75
PQ = f (PSY, BRA)	−175.66

Table 4 The second coefficients

PQ	Estimate	Std. error	t-value	P-value	Decision
Cons	1.27174	0.29822	4.264	0.000003	Supported
PSY	0.28651	0.06919	4.141	0.000004	Supported
BRA	0.41458	0.05986	6.926	0.000000	Supported

variables from one or more independent variables. An essential and useful measurement for deciding a complete and straightforward model is the AIC. Based on the AIC information standard, a model with a lower AIC is selected. The best model will stop when the minimum AIC value in Table 3 [3].

In the above results, R reports show every step of searching the optimal model. The first step is to start with all 04 independent variables with AIC = −174.75. The second step is to find a model, R stops with a model of 02 independent variables (PSY, BRA) in Table 3 with AIC = −175.66.

All variables have a P-value greater than 0.05 [12], so they are correlated with PQ, which are in Table 4. Psychological factor (PSY) and Brand (BRA) affected the decision to purchase the face mask in the Covid19 Pandemic (PQ) with the estimates of PSY and BRA being 0.28651 and 0.41458.

Variance Inflation Factor

The multicollinearity phenomenon occurs when there is a high degree of correlation between the independent variables in the regression models. Gujarati and Porter [9] showed some signs of multicollinearity in the model when the VIF coefficient is greater than 10.

According to Table 5, VIF for the independent variables is smaller than 10 [14], so there is no collinearity between the independent variables.

Heteroskesdaticity

One of the fundamental assumptions of the classical linear regression model is that the random error must have a constant (Homoskedasticity). Obviously, in practice, this assumption is unlikely to exist. On the contrary, if the variance of the random error for each observation is different, we meet heteroscedasticity.

Table 5 Variance inflation factor (VIF)

INDICATOR	PSY	BRA
VIF	1.056087	1.056087

Table 6 Heteroskesdaticity

Source	chi2	df	p
Goldfeld-Quandt test	1.812	64	0.009349

Table 7 Autocorrelation Test

Durbin-Watson		Test for autocorrelation
1.9196	p-value = 0.3185	

Table 8 Model Test

Indicator	Value
Adjusted R-squared	0.3777
F-statistic	41.37
p-value	0.00000

Goldfeld-Quandt test shows that P-value = 0.009349 and lower than 0.05 [7], so it can be concluded that there is no heteroskedasticity in Table 6.

Autocorrelation

Durbin-Watson Test shows that there is no autocorrelation from the model in Table 7 because p-value = 0.3185 is greater than 0.05 [6].

Model Test

According to the results from Table 8, the Brand (BRA) and the Psychological factor (PSY) are related to the purchasing decision (PQ) of the products from the medical mask is 37.77% in Table 8. The above analysis shows the regression equation below is statistically significant [8].

$$PQ = 1.27174 + 0.28651\ PSY + 0.41458\ BRA$$

4 Discussion

PSY: Positive sign (+): positive relationship: When the Psychological factor (PSY) increases by 1 point, the purchasing decision (Y) of the medical mask will increase by 0.28651 points.

BRA: Positive sign (+): positive relationship: When the Brand (BRA) increases by 1 point, the purchasing decision (Y) of the medical mask will increase by 0.41458 points.

5 Conclusion

This article aims to concentrate on the quantitative model and the results of the application for the purchasing decision (PQ) to create the consumption market from the medical mask in the Covid19 Pandemic Environment. Through the tests, it can be affirmed: The factors influencing purchasing decision (PQ) in the order of importance are the Brand (BRA) and the Psychological factor (PSY) will increase purchasing decision (PQ).

6 Implications

In the world, the pandemic is still happening complicatedly and unpredictable. Being subjective, losing vigilance, and ignoring epidemic prevention measures will lead to unpredictable consequences. Currently, the risk of outbreaks again is very high. Sources from outside can attack the water at any time. In the context, regional countries and the world are in turmoil with the new COVID-19 pandemic wave, the risk will increase for Vietnam as the number of entries increases. In Vietnam, there has been a requirement to force people to wear masks when participating in events in public places, on public transport. Vietnam requires all passengers (including Vietnamese and foreigners) to wear a mask properly during their time onboard, during check-in, while at the airport or airport. Passengers and escorts are required to wear masks within airports and airports. So, Vietnamese firms produce medical masks that should do implications as follows [11].

First, Vietnamese businesses need to plan activities to improve the Brand (BRA) of products and the Psychological factor (PSY) of customers in the Covid19 Pandemic Environment. Enterprises need to focus on regular advertising and especially take advantage of advertising right on their products. This is a factor for customers to get to know the business and improve its brands such as a well-known brand name (3.75), positive emotions to consumers (4.18), and peace of mind to use (4.28).

The second, Vietnamese businesses create good psychology for their customers such as purchase medical masks in the COVID-19 pandemic (2.28), buy medical masks when people poured out to bargain (2.69), antibacterial effects and prevent infection (3.87), and use a medical mask during the in Covid19 Pandemic Environment to protect customer's health (4.55).

Acknowledgements This research is funded by the Industrial University of Ho Chi Minh City, Vietnam.

References

1. Baedowy, M., Sumarwan, U., Setiawan, I.: Factors influencing consumer intention and decision to purchase plastic waste recycle machine. Indonesian J. Bus. Entrepreneur. (IJBE) **6**, 163–163 (2020)
2. Bapuji, H., Patel, C., Ertug, G., Allen, D.G.: Corona crisis and inequality: why management research needs a societal turn. J. Manage. **46**, 1205–1222 (2020)
3. Burnham, K.P., Anderson, D.R.: Multimodel inference: understanding AIC and BIC in model selection. Sociol. Methods Res. **33**, 261–304 (2004)
4. Çakar, K.: Tourophobia: fear of travel resulting from man-made or natural disasters. Tourism Rev., 22 (2020)
5. Chen, C., Zhang, Y., Xu, A., Chen, X., Lin, J.: Reconstruction of meaning in life: meaning made during the pandemic of COVID-19. Int. J. Mental Health Promot. 2020
6. Durbin, J., Watson, G.S.: Testing for serial correlation in least squares regression. III. Biometrika **58**, 1–19 (1971)
7. Godfrey, L.G.: Testing for multiplicative heteroskedasticity. J Econometr. **8**, 227–236 (1978)
8. Greene, W.H.: Econometric Analysis. Pearson Education India (2003)
9. Gujarati, D.N., Porter, D.: Basic Econometrics. Mc Graw-Hill International Edition (2009)
10. Hair, J.F., Black, W.C., Babin, B.J., Anderson, R.E., Tatham, R.L.: Multivariate Data Analysis, vol. 6. Pearson Prentice Hall, Upper Saddle River, NJ (2006)
11. HaiYen: Newsletter COVID-19 in 24 h: Raise vigilance, strictly follow the practice of wearing masks to prevent pandemics (Vietnamese) [Online] (2020). https://suckhoedoisong.vn/ban-tin-dich-covid-19-trong-24h–n182287.html
12. Hill, R.C., Griffiths, W.E., Lim, G.C.: Principles of Econometrics. Wiley, New York (2018)
13. Loey, M., Manogaran, G., Taha, M.H.N., Khalifa, N.E.M.: A hybrid deep transfer learning model with machine learning methods for face mask detection in the era of the COVID-19 pandemic. Measurement **167**, (2020)
14. Miles, J.: Tolerance and variance inflation factor. Statistics Reference Online, Wiley StatsRef (2014)
15. Mondelaers, K., Verbeke, W., Huylenbroeck, G.V.: Importance of health and environment as quality traits in the buying decision of organic products. Br. Food J. **111**, 1120–1139 (2009)
16. News. 2020. https://news.google.com/covid19/map?hl=vi&gl=VN&ceid=VN%3Avi [Online]
17. Sánchez-Cañizares, S. M., Cabeza-Ramírez, L. J., Muñoz-Fernández, G., Fuentes-García, F.J.: Impact of the perceived risk from Covid-19 on intention to travel. Current Issues in Tourism, 1–15 (2020)
18. Shiau, W.-L., Luo, M.M.: Factors affecting online group buying intention and satisfaction: A social exchange theory perspective. Comput. Hum. Behav. **28**, 2431–2444 (2012)

Classification Approach for COVID-19 Gene Based on Harris Hawks Optimization

Essam H. Houssein, Muhammad Ahmad, Mosa E. Hosney, and Manuel Mazzara

Abstract A number of COVID-19 outbreak classification and prediction methods have been proposed and are being applied around the globe to make the right decision and to enforce proper control measures. Among these methods, simple statistical and epidemiological methods have received much attention whereas, for the long term prediction, the standard methods do not perform well due to the lack of essential data and high-level of uncertainty. Thus, the essential robustness and generalization abilities of these methods need to be improved. Therefore, this work proposed a new hybrid Harris Hawks Optimization (HHO) combined with the Support Vector Machine (SVM) method called HHO-SVM. The HHO-SVM is applied on a big Gene Expression Cancer (RNA-Seq) dataset which comprises more than 20531 features to identify the critical Gene that causes the COVID-19. The experimental results revealed that HHO-SVM outperformed than Grey Wolf Optimizer (GWO), Particle Swarm Optimization (PSO), Moth Flame Optimization (MFO), Slap Swarm Algorithm (SSA) and Genetic Algorithms (GA's). We further investigate that the most critical Gene is Tmprss2 which causes Prostate Cancer is the same Gene that causes COVID-19 through the ACE2 receptor.

Keywords COVID-19 · Harris Hawks Optimization · Support Vector Machine · Emerging infectious disease · Mathematical modelling · Wuhan

---

E. H. Houssein (✉)
Faculty of Computers and Information, Minia University, Minia, Egypt
e-mail: essam.halim@mu.edu.eg

M. Ahmad
Department of Computer Science, National University of Computer and Emerging Sciences, Islamabad, Pakistan

M. E. Hosney
Faculty of Computers and Information, Luxor University, Luxor, Egypt

M. Mazzara
Institute of Software Development and Engineering, Innopolis University, Innopolis 420500, Russia

D. Oliva et al. (eds.), *Artificial Intelligence for COVID-19*, Studies in Systems, Decision and Control 358, https://doi.org/10.1007/978-3-030-69744-0_32

1 Introduction

The World Health Organization (WHO) termed the infectious disease as COVID-19 that belongs to a large family of well-known Coronavirus diseases such as Severe Acute Respiratory Syndrome Coronavirus-2 (SARS-CoV-2) [1]. SARS-CoV-2 is an enveloped virus having a large, trimeric spike glycoproteins (S) essential for identification and recognition of host receptors for several types of Coronaviruses along with host cell membranes and fusion of viral entry into cells [2, 3]. SARS-CoV-2 is a severe pathogen for human beings that strongly infects hepatic, respiratory, neurologic, and gastrointestinal diseases [4, 5].

The outbreaks of two well-known coronaviruses namely MERS-CoV 2012 and SARS-CoV 2003 have shown and revealed that the transmission is done from animal-to-animal and from human-to-human subject to the conditions [6]. Back in 2016, different countries suffered due to the spread of $2019 - nCoV$ which also belongs to the coronaviruses family. The practitioner concluded that Coronavirus originated in later bats and pangolins because it has more resemblance to two bat-derived new Coronavirus strains [7]. However, based on the previous and current research, one can conclude that the source of COVID-19 is not yet confirmed, thus, more investigations are required.

SARS-CoV-2 is considered as a part of big Coronavirus family recognized as the "crown-like appearance of spikes on this new Coronavirus surface". There are many other family members of this infectious virus, include SARS-CoV-2, the Syndrome Coronavirus (SARS-CoV), and the Middle East Respiratory Syndrome Coronavirus (MERS-CoV) is beta Coronaviruses and are likely to be associated with an animal reservoir. In recent years, MERS-CoV [8] and the likelihood of zoonotic[1] transmission of above-discussed Coronavirus families transferred from animals-to-human subjects. However, there is no clear evidence which confirms the source for COVID-19 (or other Coronaviruses) whereas, many early identified cases were certainly linked to the seafood and live animal market. Based on the previous knowledge regarding the other Coronaviruses mentioned above, experts assume that COVID-19 also spread from individual to individual through close physical contact [9]. M.A. Shereen et al., have summarized the pathogenicity and emergence of COVID-19 infection as well as the previous coronaviruses such as MERS-CoV and SARS-CoV [10].

The number of identified cases and confirmed deaths is increasing with every passing day and almost approaches to $37,601,848$ and $1,077,799$ respectively reported in 235 countries till 13 Oct 2020 [2] [11]. The rapid spread of this infectious disease as shown in Fig. 1 (https://covid19.who.int/) is quite dangerous, alarming, and requires more strict actions, plans, and policies. Therefore, it is very crucial to build accurate forecasting approaches to identify cases in the coming days to enact the essential security, safety plans, and precautionary measures. WHO labeled this infectious disease as a new Coronavirus disease (COVID-19) which has not been seen before in

[1] https://www.medicinenet.com/script/main/art.asp?articlekey=12958.

[2] https://www.who.int/emergencies/diseases/novel-Coronavirus-2019.

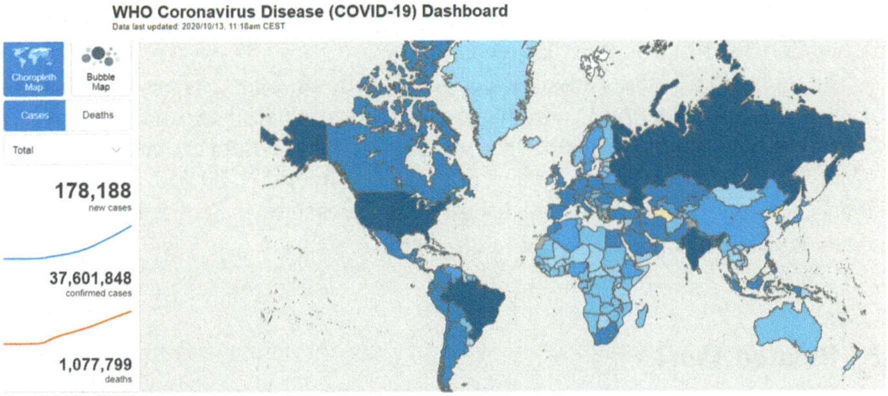

Fig. 1 Current (COVID-19) outbreak situation around the Globe

humans and declared "Public Health Emergency of International Concern (PHEIC)". Based on the aforementioned facts which could be considered as a foundation for the future as well as current works of this field to adapt not only the existing techniques for these new classes of problems but to invent or explore the latest optimization methods [12].

Recently, many meta-heuristic algorithms [13] have been used to overcome the high processing time and accuracy problems. However, several meta-heuristic algorithms have been proposed in the recent years such as; Archimedes optimization algorithm [14], Lévy flight distribution [15] and Henry gas solubility optimization [16]. Since many fields of science need optimization, meta-heuristic algorithms have been applied successfully to solve many optimization problems in different domains, such as drug design [17, 18], Maximizing lifetime of wireless sensor networks [19, 20], Bioinformatics [21], Chemical compound activities [22], Renewable energy [23], Optimization problems [24, 25] and Feature selection [26–29].

In the same context regarding to the COVID-19 disease classification and prediction, for instance, the marine predators' algorithm (MPA) [30] and Salp swarm algorithm (SSA) [31]. In general speaking, several prediction and classification methods have been proposed to make the right decision for the COVID-19 outbreak. The epidemiological and statistical methods lack when it comes to the long term prediction due to the high-level of uncertainty. Thus, the essential robustness and generalization abilities of these methods need to be improved. Consequently, this paper proposed a new classification method that combined the Harris Hawks optimization (HHO) with the Support Vector Machine (SVM) classifier. The proposed HHO-SVM approach is evaluated on a big Gene Expression Cancer (RNA-Seq) dataset which comprises more than 20531 features to identify the critical Gene that causes the COVID-19. The experimental results revealed that the proposed HHO-SVM outperformed the well-know meta-heuristic algorithms such as the Grey Wolf Optimizer (GWO), Particle Swarm Optimization (PSO), Moth Flame Optimization (MFO), Slap Swarm Algorithm (SSA), and Genetic Algorithms (GA's). We further investigate that the most critical Gene is Tmprss2 which causes Prostate Cancer is the same Gene that causes COVID-19 through ACE2 receptors.

The remainder of the study is structured as follows: Sect. 2 presents a summary of related works. Section 3, introduces the various material and methods used in this paper such as Harris Hawks Optimization (HHO) and Support Vector Machines (SVMs). Meanwhile, Sect. 4 explains the proposed hybrid HHO with the SVM classifier. The experimental result and discussion are presented in Sect. 5. Finally, Sect. 6 concludes the paper with possible future research stems.

2 Related Works

Chavez et al. [9], presented an emergency physician with an indication of the most recent understanding of COVID-19 and advice on the evaluation and management of patients with doubted COVID-19. Also, Li et al. [32], concentrated on recent advancement concerning the formation of $SARS - CoV2$ and features of COVID-19, such as etiology, epidemiological, and pathogenesis characteristics. Al-qaness, et al. [31], presented a new forecasting model just to identify the number of confirmed COVID-19 cases in China in the upcoming days based upon prior knowledge or confirmed cases.

Zhao et al. [33], Tang et al. [34] and Nishiura et al. [35] presented the studies to estimate and deal with the transmission riks and infection rate of new COVID-19, respectively. Bansal [36] applied Google and PubMed search engines to present a chronicle review on several patients with acute cardiac injury or having cardiovascular disease during illness. The authors further explained that the optimum management of such patients is based on an adequate understanding of the interplay among CV disease and COVID-19. Bai et al. [37] developed a diagnose model called "COVID-19 Intelligent Diagnosis and Treatment Assistant Program (nCapp). The nCapp model is based on the Internet of Things (IoT) to early diagnose and further to improve the treatment of COVID-19 patients using medical technologies. nCapp model classifies the COVID-19 patients into mild, moderate, severe, or critical pneumonia.

In the same context, Ozturk et al. [38] proposed a deep neural network model for automatic COVID-19 detection using raw chest X-ray images. The automatic COVID-19 detection is obtained the following accuracy 87.02% and 98.08% for both multi-class and binary classification respectively. M. Abdel-Basset et al. hybridized the marine predators' algorithm (MPA) with ranking diversity reduction (RDR) using X-Ray image segmentation for COVID-19 detection [30]. In [39], with some of the COVID-19 patients, the variations witnessed in computed tomography that can lead to the detection of nucleic acid tests are identified. Whereas, Liu et al. [40] conduct a study on 73 COVID-19 patients based on initial Computed Tomography features and follow-up with disease severity using Computed Tomography manifestations.

Long et al. [41], a real-time reverse for COVID-19 pneumonia named transcriptase-polymerase chain reaction using the diagnostic values of Computed tomography is proposed. The authors proved that the real-time reverse transcriptase-polymerase chain reaction may produce false-negative results than the patients with typical Computed Tomography with negative real-time reverse transcriptase-polymerase chain reaction results. Besides, Sohrabi et al. [42] reviewed the current state of encompassing awareness of this global outbreak COVID-19. Eventually, in [43], the chest Computed Tomography scans over twenty-one COVID-19 symptomatic patients is reported.

The most effective approach to control this outbreak is to test either the existing antiviral drugs are good enough to treat related viral infections or not. There are many antiviral drugs such as interferon, ribavirin, corticosteroids, and lopinavir-ritonavir for the possible treatment of MERS and SARS patients whereas the effectiveness of some of these antiviral drugs remains controversial [44]. Therefore any forecast is reliable due to the high uncertainty and complex societal political factors involved with the limited knowledge of this outbreak influence the widespread of COVID-19. Another important factor involved is the limited availability of reliable data for experimental evaluation. The data samples and their descriptions are often scarce whenever an epidemic started. Thus, while having a limited number of training examples, finding the forecasting model that offers a forecast at the best efforts is a big hurdle not only the practitioners but the machine learning community as well.

The work [45] proposed three data mining approaches to handle the small sample size problems for COVID-19 prediction. A bioinspired metaheuristic "Coronavirus Optimization Algorithm (COVA)" was proposed in [46] to predict the spreads of COVID-19 and how it infects healthy individuals. An infectious virus dynamics Susceptible, Exposed, Infectious, and Removed (SEIR) model was proposed in [47]. The authors only consider estimating the outbreak trends in Wuhan, China.

To overcome the limitations of previous works, this paper proposed a simple yet effective HHO-SVM classification method. A big dataset of COVID-19 patients is used to evaluate the performance of the HHO-SVM method compared to the 6 well-reputed metaheuristic method. The comparative methods include; Moth-Flame Optimization (MFO) [48], Whale Optimization Algorithm (WOA) [49], Salp Swarm Algorithm (SSA) [50], Grey Wolf Optimizer (GWO) [51], Genetic Algorithms (GAs) [52], and Particle Swarm Optimization (PSO) [53]. In a nutshell, the following specific contributions are made in this work:

- A new classification approach called HHO-SVM is proposed.
- HHO is used to attain the optimum number of informative features and for SVM parameter optimization.
- The efficiency of the proposed HHO-SVM is assessed over a big Gene Expression Cancer (RNA-Seq) dataset to detect the caused gene of COVID-19.
- HHO-SVM can discover the confirmed gene for the COVID-19 by accuracy equal to 95.68%.

3 Materials and Methods

This section presents the ground for Harris Hawks Optimization (HHO) and the Support Vector Machines (SVM).

3.1 *Overview of Harris Hawks Optimization*

A new population-based nature-inspired Harris Hawks Optimization (HHO) method was first proposed by Heidari et al. [54]. The HHO is inspired by the chasing style of Harris Hawks in nature and its cooperative behavior called surprise pounce. The following subsection illustrates the process of HHO.

3.1.1 Exploration Stage

The exploration stage of HHO includes the Harris Hawks perch arbitrarily on some positions and hold to detect a prey depending upon the following strategies.

$$X(t+1) = \begin{cases} -r_1(|X_{rand}(t) - 2r_2X(t)|) + \\ X_{rand}(t) & q \geq 0.5 \\ -r_3(LB + r_4(UB - LB)) + \\ X_{rabbit}(t) - X_m(t) & q < 0.5 \end{cases} \tag{1}$$

where $X(t)$ and $X(t+1)$ are the position vector of Hawks at current and $(t+1)th$ iteration, respectively. $X_{rabbit}(t)$ be the rabbit position, q and r_1, r_2, r_3, r_4 are random numbers between the closed interval of [0, 1] which are updated with respect the number of iterations. UB and LB are lower and upper bounds for the said variables. $X_{rand}(t)$ and X_m are randomly selected and the average position of Hawk from its current population, respectively. The X_m of Hawks can be computed using Eq. 2:

$$X_m(t) = \frac{1}{N}\sum_{i=1}^{N} X_i(t) \tag{2}$$

where N be the total number of Hawks and $X_i(t)$ denote the location of Hawk at tth iteration.

3.1.2 HHO Shift: Exploration to Exploitation

In the HHO transition phase i.e., exploration to exploitation, the energy of a rabbit can be model as:

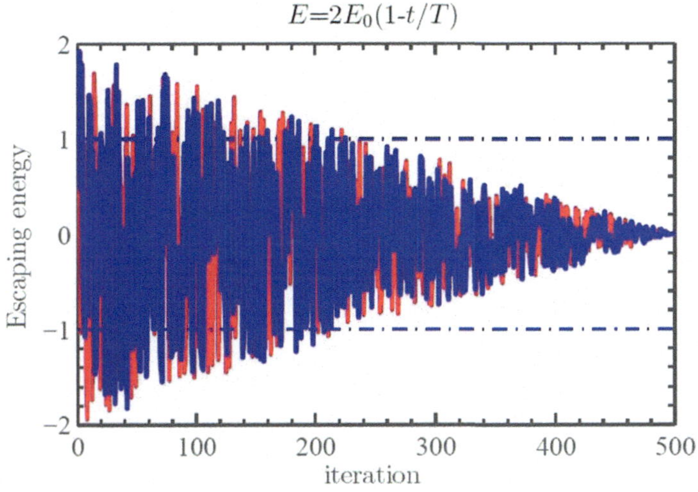

Fig. 2 Behavior of E in 2 different runs with 500 iterations

$$E = 2E_0 - 2E_0\frac{t}{T} \tag{3}$$

where T be the maximum number of iterations, E_0 and E are the initial state of energy and escaping energy of the prey, respectively. Furthermore, the time dependency of E is shown in Fig. 2.

3.1.3 Exploitation Phase

Soft Besiege: Soft Besiege's behavior can be modeled as:

$$X(t+1) = \Delta X(t) - E|J\Delta X(t)| \tag{4}$$

with

$$\Delta X(t) = X_{rabbit}(t) - X(t) \tag{5}$$

where $\Delta X(t)$ be the difference among the current location and the position vector of the rabbit at tth iteration. r_5 be the random number chosen from the closed interval $[0, 1]$, and $J = 2 - 2r_5$ is known as a random jump strength of the rabbit throughout the escaping procedure and its values changes randomly with respect to the iterations to simulate the nature of rabbit motions.

Hard Besiege: The Hard Basieges update the current positions using Eq. 6:

$$X(t+1) = X_{rabbit}(t) - E|\Delta X(t)| \tag{6}$$

Soft Besiege with progressive rapid dives: To perform or update the Soft Basieges one can assume that the Hawks can be evaluated based on their future moves as defined in Eq. 7:

$$Y = X_{rabbit}(t) - E|J\Delta X(t)| \tag{7}$$

One can assume that future move dive based on the LF-based patterns using the expression given below:

$$Z = Y + S \times LF(D) \tag{8}$$

where S be the random vector of size $1 \times D$, D be the dimension of the given problem and LF be the levy flight function that can be computed using Eq. 9:

$$LF(x) = 0.01 \times \frac{u \times \sigma}{|v|^{\frac{1}{\beta}}} \tag{9}$$

where

$$\sigma = \left(\frac{\Gamma(1+\beta) \times sin(\frac{\pi\beta}{2})}{\Gamma(\frac{1+\beta}{2}) \times \beta \times 2^{(\frac{\beta-1}{2})}} \right)^{\frac{1}{\beta}} \tag{10}$$

where u and v inside (0, 1), default β is equal to 1.5. Hence, Eq. (15) is performed in the soft besiege phase to update the Hawk's positions as follows:

$$X(t+1) = \begin{cases} Y & if \ F(Y) < F(X(t)) \\ Z & if \ F(Z) < F(X(t)) \end{cases} \tag{11}$$

where Y and Z can easily be computed using Eqs. 7 and 8, respectively.

Hard besiege with progressive rapid dives: The similar rule is employed to perform the Hard Besiege conditions:

$$X(t+1) = \begin{cases} Y & if \ F(Y) < F(X(t)) \\ Z & if \ F(Z) < F(X(t)) \end{cases} \tag{12}$$

where Y and Z can easily be computed using the expressions defined in Eqs. 13 and 14, respectively.

$$Y = X_{rabbit}(t) - E|JX_{rabbit}(t) - X_m(t)| \tag{13}$$

$$Z = Y + S \times LF(D) \tag{14}$$

where $X_m(t)$ can be computed using the expression shown in Eq. 2.

3.2 *Support Vector Machines*

Among the most popular methods for regression and classification problems, Support Vector Machine (SVM) is regarding the most common classifier and initially introduced in [55]. SVM has been deployed for several real-world applications for instance bioinformatics, biometrics, cheminformatics, and remote sensing [56]. The SVM hierarchy works in two phases as the training examples are used to build the model for classification later the trained model is used to classify an unknown example. The tuning parameters of SVM are considered as key to success for any classification problems. These parameters include kernel and penalty parameters [57]. The penalty is important to maintain a trade-off between maximizing the decision margin while minimizing the training error [58]. Whereas, the kernel parameters are used to map the low dimensional input feature space to a higher dimensional feature space. These two parameters are labeled as a backbone to control the performance of SVM for any classification problem. SVM works while separating several known classes using the concept of hyperplanes and achieved remarkable results in linearly separable data examples [59] as shown in Fig. 3.

4 The Proposed HHO-SVM Method

The proposed HHO-SVM method is hybridized with HHO and SVM for classification as well as for feature optimization i.e., not only to select the optimum number of quality features but to optimize the SVM parameters. In HHO, X_{rabbit} as the location

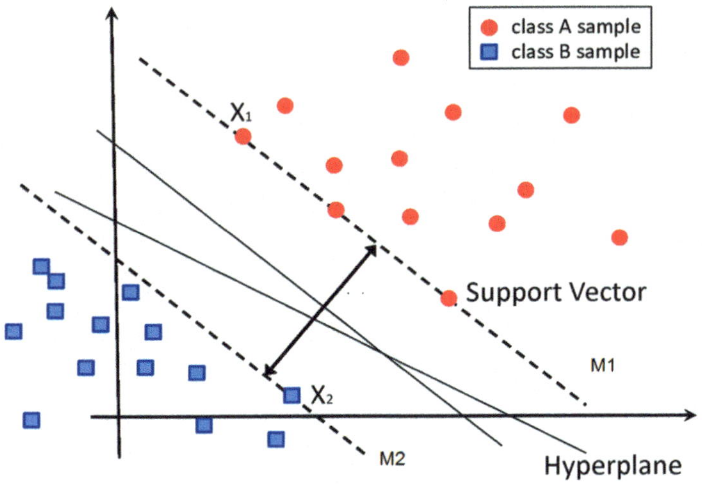

Fig. 3 Structure of SVM used for a classification task

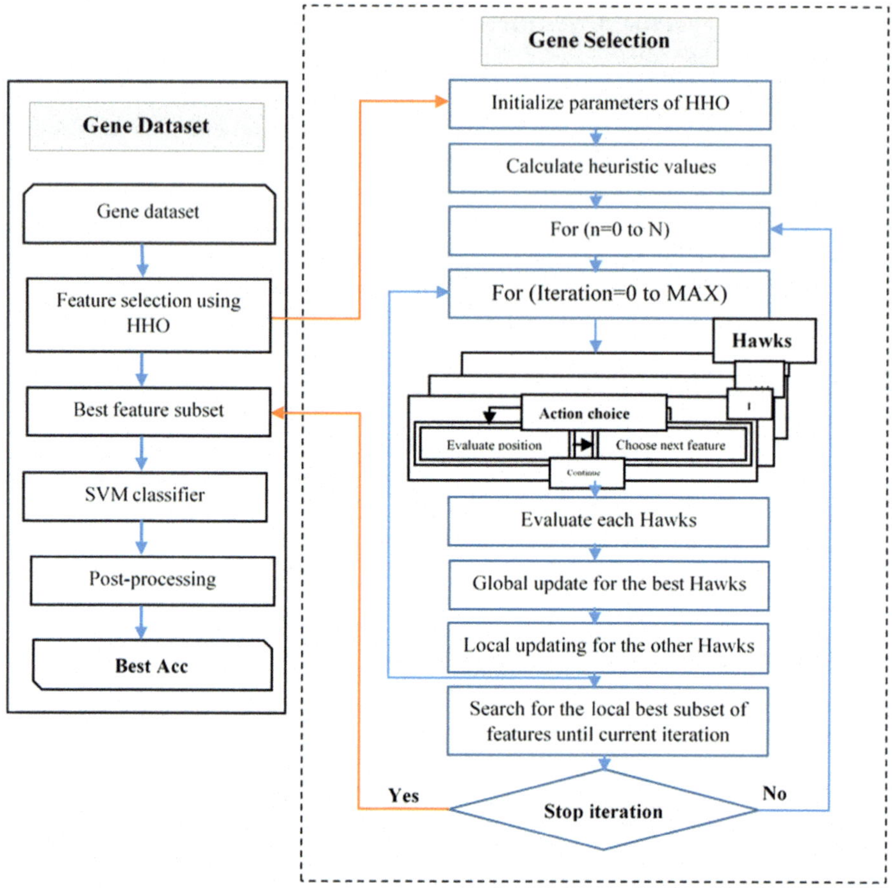

Fig. 4 Flowchart of The proposed HHO-SVM model

of the rabbit i.e., the best location of the rabbit can be considered as SVM parameters, and the optimum selected feature vectors. Whereas the X_{rabbit} fitness is deliberated as the overall classification accuracy for all cross-validation folds applied to evaluate preys location. For each location fitness evaluation, SVM is trained using 3 training folds and validated against 5 validation folds. The validation strategy has been further discussed in the following sections. The flowchart of the proposed HHO-SVM approach is presented in Fig. 4 shows both the phases of the proposed HHO-SVM approach, i.e., optimum feature selection and parameter optimization as well as the classification and validation. Furthermore, the Algorithm 1 presents the flow of our proposed HHO-SVM classification approach. Algorithm 1, provides the algorithmic framework of HHO-SVM classification approach.

Algorithm 1 Pseudocode of HHO-SVM classification approach.

Input: Training sets (Folds) $(T1, T2 \ldots Tn)$
Input: Validation sets (Folds) $(V1, V2 \ldots Vn)$
Output: Classification accuracy
Initialization: The population size N, maximum number of iterations T,data set D ,group classifier G,feature X and new fitness function HHO-SVM $(fobj)$, the random population $X_i (i = 1, 2, \ldots, N)$
while (stopping condition is not met) **do**
  Calculate the new fitness values of hawks
  Set X_{rabbit} as the location of rabbit (best location)
  for (each hawk (X_i)) **do**
    Update the initial energy E_0 and jump strength J ▷ `E0=2rand()-1, J=2(1-rand())`
    Update the E using Eq. (3)
    if ($|E| \geq 1$) **then** ▷ `Exploration phase`
      Update the location vector using Eq. (1)
    end if
    if ($|E| < 1$) **then** ▷ `Exploitation phase`
      if ($r \geq 0.5$ and $|E| \geq 0.5$) **then** ▷ Soft besiege
        Update the location vector using Eq. (4)
      else if ($r \geq 0.5$ and $|E| < 0.5$) **then** ▷ Hard besiege
        Update the location vector using Eq. (6)
      else if ($r < 0.5$ and $|E| \geq 0.5$) **then** ▷ Soft besiege with progressive rapid dives
        Update the location vector using Eq. (15):
        Call the feature selection method.
        Call the SVM classifier.

$$X(t+1) = \begin{cases} Y \; if LF(fobj(D, G, Y)) < LF(fobj(D, G, X((t)) * X((t) \\ Z \; if LF(fobj(D, G, Z)) < LF(fobj(D, G, X((t)) * X((t) \end{cases} \tag{15}$$

      else if ($r < 0.5$ and $|E| < 0.5$) **then** ▷ Hard besiege with progressive rapid dives
        Update the location vector using Eq. (15).
        Call the feature selection method.
        Call the SVM classifier.
      end if
    end if
  end for
end while
Return *The best accuracy*

4.1 Validation Strategy

For each patient, all data is partitioned into a 30% cut off set for Testing and a 70% set for training and validation. During the optimization process, the testing set is partitioned into 5 folds (5 training and 5 validation sets) for cross-validation at each fitness evaluation step where model accuracy is the average of 5 accuracy values from 5 folds of training and validation as mentioned earlier in this section (Fitness Function). When the model is optimized with the highest accuracy, it is tested against the 30% cut off data set in 5 folds of cross-validation.

4.2 *Fitness Function*

In this work, the classification accuracy is selected as a solution qualifier through the search process. Classification accuracy lies in the range [0, 1], and each search agent is assigned 5 accuracy values. Each candidate solution is used to evaluate along with the number of iterative processes to verify the performance of HHO. Meanwhile, in classification, the dataset should be divided into training and test subsets; then, the fitness function of the proposed HHO method is defined in Eq. 16 as follows:

$$Fitness\ function\ (fobj) = \alpha + \beta \frac{|R|}{|C|} - G \tag{16}$$

$$\beta = \alpha \tag{17}$$

where R be the classification error and C represents the total number of features for a given dataset D. β refer to the subset length and α represents the classification performance defined in the range [0, 1]. T is a necessary condition and G is a group column for the specific classifier. Each step in algorithm compared with T as well as the obtained fitness value must be greater than it, to maximize the solution.

5 Experimental Results and Discussion

In order to perform the experiments and comparisons, it is necessary to configure the parameters of the problem. In this way, the number of search agents is 200, the problem dimensions 20531 for data set. Meanwhile, the number of iterations 1000, number experiments (runs) 30, α is the fitness function 0.99, β in the fitness function 0.01, lower bound 0 and upper bound 4. For comparative purposes, they have used the standard version the Harris Hawks optimization (HHO) that of them provides better results. The selected metaheuristics and the proposal have the same elements in the population and all of them are randomly initialized. The internal parameters for all the algorithms are provided in Table 1.

5.1 *Results Discussion and Analysis*

All the listed experiments are performed over 1000 iterations and 30 independent runs. The experimental setup, including the description of the datasets, and statistics results will be illustrated in the following subsections.

Table 1 The parameters setting of competitor algorithms used in the comparison and evaluation

Methods	Parameters
PSO	$Agents\ number = 50$
	$Velocity = 65$
MFO	$Agents\ number = 50$
	$B = 1$
GWO	$Agents\ number = 50$
	$Number\ domination = 100$
SSA	$Agents\ number = 50$
	$L = 2$ and $C = rand$
HHO	$Agents\ number = 50$
	E_0 variable change from $-1\ to\ 1$ (Default)
	$Beta = 1.5$
GA	selector is a Binary Tournament selection
	$Crossover\ is\ single\ point = 0.7$
	$Mutation\ is\ multi - Point = 0.05$
WOA	$b = 1$

5.1.1 Dataset Description

The performance of the competitors' algorithms are assessed on $RNA - Seq$ cancer benchmark dataset obtained from the UCI Machine Learning Repository.[3] $RNA - Seq$ having 20531 dimensions and 801 instances as one of the effects of COVID19 that is related to the cancer gene as prostate cancer [60] that indicates the $SARS - CoV - 2$ and $SARS - CoV$ uses the receptor $ACE2$ as a point entry and the serine protease $TMPRSS2$ for S protein priming.

5.1.2 Statistical Results

In this subsection, the SVM is used for the classification task. Following the previous methodology, in the first experiment, iterations are set to 1000 for each of the 30 runs. The experimental results are reported in Table 2. In this experiment, the HHO based on SVM obtains the best mean and standard deviation (std), and the fourth in CPU time.

[3] Available at http://archive.ics.uci.edu/ml/datasets/gene+expression+cancer+RNA-Seq.

Table 2 The statistical measurements values obtained by the competitor algorithms using the SVM classifier with 1000 iterations

Methods	Mean	Std	Best	Worst	CPU time
Cancer RNA-Seq UCI dataset					
PSO	8.55E+01	2.49E-02	85.492	85.192	1.181
MFO	8.87E+01	2.48E-02	88.716	87.481	1.971
GWO	9.05E+01	2.47E-01	90.503	89.399	1.920
SSA	9.48E+01	2.37E-02	93.773	92.673	1.571
GA	8.20E+01	2.60E-02	81.955	80.555	1.360
HHO	9.79E+01	2.31E-02	95.881	94.081	1.968
WOA	9.29E+01	2.45E-02	91.871	90.430	1.971

5.1.3 Classification Results

Since SVM is one of the most promising methods of classification, its performance needs to be analyzed. In the first experiment, iterations are set to 1000, the experimental results are reported in Table 3. In this experiment, the HHO based on SVM obtains the best mean and standard deviation (Std), also for maximizing the classification accuracy solution, specificity, precision, and F-measure.

5.1.4 The Graphical Representation

This section aims to investigate the convergence of the HHO-SVM approach presented in this paper along the iterative process. The convergence curves plotted in Fig. 5 provides evidence that the HHO-SVM obtained over, the best results compared with the original HHO along with stopping criteria (1000 iterations). Also, the Box-plot is demonstrated in Fig. 6 indicates that the proposed HHO-SVM approach

Table 3 The classification measurements values obtained by the competitor algorithms using the SVM classifier with 1000 iterations

Methods	Accuracy	Specificity	Precision	F-measure
PSO	85.492	53.102	63.981	46.667
MFO	87.985	33.150	47.450	33.150
GWO	90.238	57.082	65.091	49.147
SSA	93.573	59.922	68.971	51.197
HHO	**95.681**	61.522	69.690	51.846
GA	81.550	50.902	59.951	42.167
WOA	91.576	58.132	67.181	50.037

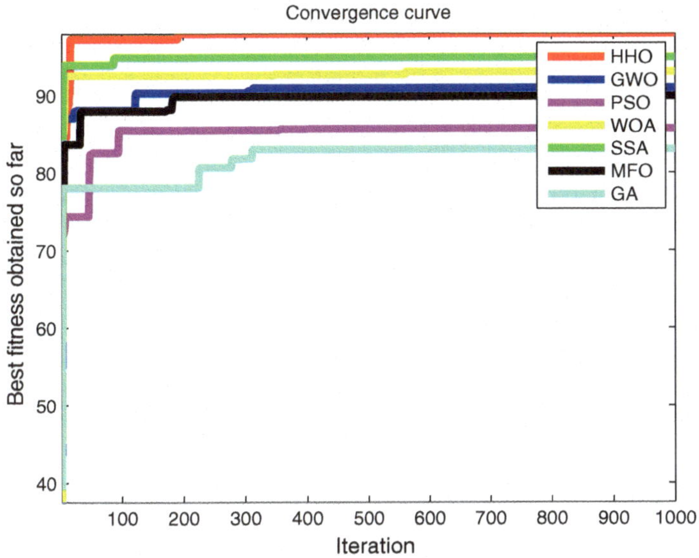

Fig. 5 The convergence curve of the HHO-SVM approach and the competitor algorithms

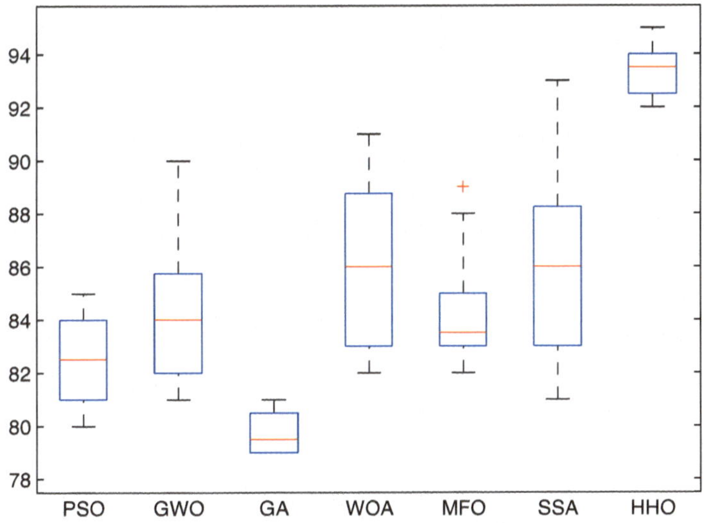

Fig. 6 The Box-plot of the HHO-SVM approach and the competitor algorithms

was achieved the best results compared with the 6 common competitor algorithms along stop criteria (1000 iterations).

5.1.5 Discussion

To sum up the aforementioned observations,

- The $ACE2$ enzyme [61] excited the outer surface such as cell membranes of i.e. cells arteries, lungs, kidneys, heart, and intestines and spur the different cleavage of angiotensin so it is responsible for lowers blood pressure. Consequently, $ACE2$ is used as an entry point into cells for some diseases such as COVID-19.
- The transmembrane protease serine ($TMPRSS2$) enzyme is lived in the human body and is encoded by the $TMPRSS2$ $Gene$ [62]. $TMPRSS2$ $Gene$ is considered a part of the serine protease family and used to encodes a protein. Serine proteases are also known to be involved in a lot of pathological and physiological processes. The protease domain of this protein is thought to be secreted and cleaved into cell media after auto cleavage. $TMPRSS2$ was used to be down-regulated in androgen-independent prostate cancer tissue and up-regulated by androgenic hormones in prostate cancer cells.
- The recent emergence of pathogenic $SARS - CoV - 2$ and its hurried international and national spread poses a global health emergency because the cellular entry of this new COVID-19 depends on the binding of several viral proteins (S) to cells S receptors and protein priming by host cell proteases [60]. The disclosure that cellular factors can be used by $SARS - CoV - 2$ for entry could provide insight into revealed therapeutic targets and viral transmission. $SARS - CoV - 2$ is depending on the receptor $ACE2$ and the serine protease $TMPRSS2$ for the priming of the protein S. A $TMPRSS2$ inhibitor approved for clinical use blocked entry and may be a treatment option.
- In the same context, Hoffmann et al. [60], investigate that $SARS - 2 - S$ and $SARS - S$ negotiated the entry into the same cell also, contains the amino acid residues required for interaction with the $SARS - S$ entry the receptor $ACE2$. Analysis of part of the receptor-binding domain (RBD), several receptor binding motifs (RBM) that come into contact with $ACE2$ revealed that most of the amino acid residues essential for the binding of $ACE2$ per $SARS - S$ were kept in $SARS - 2 - S$ so on the other hand, most of these residues which were absent from the S proteins of $SARSrCoV$ were previously found not to use $ACE2$ for entry.
- Based on the obtained results for RNA-Seq cancer data sets, the HHO-SVM approach maximizes the accuracy and reduces the number of features selected. In addition, the obtained Std of the HHO-based SVM classifier has been increased directly with increases in the number of iterations. Notably, the obtained accuracy $= 95.68\%$ is evidence that can be observed to reveal the following; (1) $ACE2$ also serves as an entry point into cells for COVID-19, (2) $TMPRSS2$ is an enzyme that exists in humans and is coded by the $TMPRSS2$ and is used to code a protein considered belongs to the family of serine proteases.

6 Conclusion

The generalized outbreak prediction models are essential for delivering intuitions into the spread and consequences of this spreadable disease. However, the standard epidemiological and statistical models do not perform well for long term prediction of COVID-19 due to the lack of data and high uncertainty. Therefore, this work proposed a hybrid approach consisting of Harris Hawks Optimization (HHO) combined with Support Vector Machine (SVM) termed (HHO-SVM). Therefore, the main objective of this work is to overcome the aforementioned difficulties to identify the critical Gene which causes COVID-19. The experimental results on Gene expression Cancer (RNA-Seq - consist of more than 20531 features) reveal that the HHO-SVM enhances the optimization process compared to the 6 well-known optimization algorithms. One can conclude that the HHO-SVM can determine the most critical Gene, i.e., "$tmprss2\ Gene$" causes COVID-19 from $ACE2$ which is also known to cause prostate cancer. The HHO-SVM results reported in this work have a high ability of generalization for long-term prediction.

Our recommendations to reduce disease outbreaks: to control this new COVID-19 virus in numerous regions, it is required to appropriately manage the suspected patients of having COVID-19, furthermore, immediately identify the patients, and isolate the source of COVID-19 infection, cut off the transmission route between the source city and prevent viral transmission from these potential patients or virus carriers. In the future, the proposed HHO'SVM approach can be used as a feature selection paradigm for high-dimensional problems containing many instances to increase the classification rate and decrease the selection ratio of the attributes.

Conflict of interest The authors declare that there is no conflict of interest.

References

1. Hui, D.S., Azhar, E.I., Madani, T.A., Ntoumi, F., Kock, R., Dar, O., Ippolito, G., Mchugh, T.D., Memish, Z.A., Drosten, C., et al.: The continuing 2019-ncov epidemic threat of novel coronaviruses to global health'the latest 2019 novel coronavirus outbreak in wuhan, china. Int. J. Infect. Dis. **91**, 264–266 (2020)
2. Kirchdoerfer, R.N., Wang, N., Pallesen, J., Wrapp, D., Turner, H.L., Cottrell, C.A., Corbett, K.S., Graham, B.S., McLellan, J.S., Ward, A.B.: Stabilized coronavirus spikes are resistant to conformational changes induced by receptor recognition or proteolysis. Sci. Rep. **8**(1), 1–11 (2018)
3. Belouzard, S., Millet, J.K., Licitra, B.N., Whittaker, G.R.: Mechanisms of coronavirus cell entry mediated by the viral spike protein. Viruses **4**(6), 1011–1033 (2012)
4. Zhao, S., Lin, Q., Ran, J., Musa, S.S., Yang, G., Wang, W., Lou, Y., Gao, D., Yang, L., He, D., et al.: Preliminary estimation of the basic reproduction number of novel coronavirus (2019-ncov) in china, from 2019 to 2020: A data-driven analysis in the early phase of the outbreak. Int. J. Infect. Dis. **92**, 214–217 (2020)
5. Chen, Y., Liu, Q., Guo, D.: Emerging coronaviruses: genome structure, replication, and pathogenesis. J. Med. Virol. **92**(4), 418–423 (2020)

6. Wang, L.-F., Shi, Z., Zhang, S., Field, H., Daszak, P., Eaton, B.T.: Review of bats and sars. Emerg. Infect. Dis. **12**(12), 1834 (2006)
7. Lu, R., Zhao, X., Li, J., Niu, P., Yang, B., Wu, H., Wang, W., Song, H., Huang, B., Zhu, N., et al.: Genomic characterisation and epidemiology of 2019 novel coronavirus: implications for virus origins and receptor binding. The Lancet **395**(10224), 565–574 (2020)
8. de Wit, E., van Doremalen, N., Falzarano, D., Munster, V.J.: Sars and mers: recent insights into emerging coronaviruses. Nat. Rev. Microbiol. **14**(8), 523 (2016)
9. Chavez, S., Long, B., Koyfman, A., Liang, S.Y.: Coronavirus disease (covid-19): a primer for emergency physicians. Am. J. Emerg, Med (2020)
10. Shereen, M.A., Khan, S., Kazmi, A., Bashir, N., Siddique, R.: Covid-19 infection: origin, transmission, and characteristics of human coronaviruses. J. Adv. Res. (2020)
11. W.H.O. (WHO): Confirmed covid 19 cases. World Health Organization (2020). https://www.who.int/emergencies/diseases/novel-coronavirus-2019
12. Organization, W.H., et al.: Coronavirus disease 2019 (covid-19): situation report, 67. World Health Organization (2020)
13. Houssein, E.H., Mina, Y., Aboul, E.: Nature-inspired algorithms: a comprehensive review. In: Hybrid Computational Intelligence: Research and Applications. CRC Press, p. 1 (2019)
14. Hashim, F.A., Hussain, K., Houssein, E.H., Mabrouk, M.S., Al-Atabany, W.: Archimedes optimization algorithm: a new metaheuristic algorithm for solving optimization problems. In: Applied Intelligence, pp. 1–21 (2020)
15. Houssein, E.H., Saad, M.R., Hashim, F.A., Shaban, H., Hassaballah, M.: Lévy flight distribution: a new metaheuristic algorithm for solving engineering optimization problems. Eng. Appl. Artif. Intell. **94**, 103731 (2020)
16. Hashim, F.A., Houssein, E.H., Mabrouk, M.S., Al-Atabany, W., Mirjalili, S.: Henry gas solubility optimization: a novel physics-based algorithm. Futur. Gener. Comput. Syst. **101**, 646–667 (2019)
17. Houssein, E.H., Hosney, M.E., Elhoseny, M., Oliva, D., Mohamed, W.M., Hassaballah, M.: Hybrid harris hawks optimization with cuckoo search for drug design and discovery in chemoinformatics. Sci. Rep. **10**(1), 1–22 (2020)
18. Houssein, E.H., Hosney, M.E., Oliva, D., Mohamed, W.M., Hassaballah, M.: A novel hybrid Harris hawks optimization and support vector machines for drug design and discovery. Comput. Chem. Eng. **133**, 106656 (2020)
19. Houssein, E.H., Saad, M.R., Hussain, K, Zhu, W., Shaban, H., Hassaballah, M.: Optimal sink node placement in large scale wireless sensor networks based on harris' hawk optimization algorithm. In: IEEE Access, vol. 8, pp. 19 381–19 397 (2020)
20. Ahmed, M.M., Houssein, E.H., Hassanien, A.E., Taha, A., Hassanien, E.: Maximizing lifetime of large-scale wireless sensor networks using multi-objective whale optimization algorithm. Telecommun. Syst. **72**(2), 243–259 (2019)
21. Hashim, F.A., Houssein, E.H., Hussain, K., Mabrouk, M.S., Al-Atabany, W.: A modified henry gas solubility optimization for solving motif discovery problem. Neural Comput. Appl. **32**(14), 10 759–10 771 (2020)
22. Hussien, A.G., Hassanien, A.E., Houssein, E.H.: Swarming behaviour of salps algorithm for predicting chemical compound activities. In: 2017 Eighth International Conference on Intelligent Computing and Information Systems (ICICIS), IEEE, pp. 315–320 (2017)
23. Houssein, E.H.: Machine learning and meta-heuristic algorithms for renewable energy: a systematic review. In: Advanced Control and Optimization Paradigms for Wind Energy Systems. Springer, pp. 165–187 (2019)
24. Ewees, A.A., Abd Elaziz, M., Houssein, E.H.: Improved grasshopper optimization algorithm using opposition-based learning. Expert Syst. Appl. **112**, 156–172 (2018)
25. Tharwat, A., Houssein, E.H., Ahmed, M.M., Hassanien, A.E., Gabel, T.: Mogoa algorithm for constrained and unconstrained multi-objective optimization problems. Appl. Intell. **48**(8), 2268–2283 (2018)
26. Hussien, A.G., Houssein, E.H., Hassanien, A.E.: A binary whale optimization algorithm with hyperbolic tangent fitness function for feature selection. In: 2017 Eighth International Conference on Intelligent Computing and Information Systems (ICICIS), pp. 166–172. IEEE (2017)

27. Hussien, A.G., Hassanien, A.E., Houssein, E.H., Bhattacharyya, S., Amin, M.: S-shaped binary whale optimization algorithm for feature selection. In: Recent Trends in Signal and Image Processing, pp. 79–87. Springer (2019)
28. Neggaz, N., Houssein, E.H., Hussain, K.: An efficient henry gas solubility optimization for feature selection. Expert Syst. Appl. 113364 (2020)
29. Hussien, A.G., Hassanien, A.E., Houssein, E.H., Amin, M., Azar, A.T.: New binary whale optimization algorithm for discrete optimization problems. Eng. Optim. **52**(6), 945–959 (2020)
30. Abdel-Basset, M., Mohamed, R., Elhoseny, M., Chakrabortty, R.K., Ryan, M.: A hybrid covid-19 detection model using an improved marine predators algorithm and a ranking-based diversity reduction strategy. IEEE Access (2020)
31. Al-qaness, M.A., Ewees, A.A., Fan, H., Abd El Aziz, M.: Optimization method for forecasting confirmed cases of covid-19 in china. J. Clin. Med. **9**(3), 674 (2020)
32. Li, H., Liu, S.-M., Yu, X.-H., Tang, S.-L., Tang, C.-K.: Coronavirus disease 2019 (covid-19): current status and future perspective. Int. J. Antimicrob. Agents 105951 (2020)
33. Zhao, S., Musa, S.S., Lin, Q., Ran, J., Yang, G., Wang, W., Lou, Y., Yang, L., Gao, D., He, D., et al.: Estimating the unreported number of novel coronavirus (2019-ncov) cases in china in the first half of january 2020: a data-driven modelling analysis of the early outbreak. J. Clin. Med. **9**(2), 388 (2020)
34. Tang, B., Wang, X., Li, Q., Bragazzi, N.L., Tang, S., Xiao, Y., Wu, J.: Estimation of the transmission risk of the 2019-ncov and its implication for public health interventions. J. Clin. Med. **9**(2), 462 (2020)
35. Nishiura, H., Kobayashi, T., Yang, Y., Hayashi, K., Miyama, T., Kinoshita, R., Linton, N.M., Jung, S.-M., Yuan, B., Suzuki, A., et al.: The rate of underascertainment of novel coronavirus (2019-ncov) infection: estimation using japanese passengers data on evacuation flights (2020)
36. Bansal, M.: Cardiovascular disease and covid-19. Diabetes Metab. Syndr. Clin. Res, Rev (2020)
37. Bai, L., Yang, D., Wang, X., Tong, L., Zhu, X., Bai, C., Powell, C.A.: Chinese experts' consensus on the internet of things-aided diagnosis and treatment of coronavirus disease 2019. Clin. eHealth (2020)
38. Ozturk, T., Talo, M., Yildirim, E.A., Baloglu, U.B., Yildirim, O., Acharya, U.R.: Automated detection of covid-19 cases using deep neural networks with x-ray images. Comput. Biol. Med. 103792 (2020)
39. Bernheim, A., Mei, X., Huang, M., Yang, Y., Fayad, Z.A., Zhang, N., Diao, K., Lin, B., Zhu, X., Li, K., et al.: Chest ct findings in coronavirus disease-19 (covid-19): relationship to duration of infection. Radiology 200463 (2020)
40. Liu, K.-C., Xu, P., Lv, W.-F., Qiu, X.-H., Yao, J.-L., Jin-Feng, G., et al.: Ct manifestations of coronavirus disease-2019: retrospective analysis of 73 cases by disease severity. Eur. J. Radiol. 108941 (2020)
41. Long, C., Xu, H., Shen, Q., Zhang, X., Fan, B., Wang, C., Zeng, B., Li, Z., Li, X., Li, H.: Diagnosis of the coronavirus disease (covid-19): rrt-pcr or ct? Eur. J. Radiol. 108961 (2020)
42. Sohrabi, C., Alsafi, Z., O'Neill, N., Khan, M., Kerwan, A., Al-Jabir, A., Iosifidis, C., Agha, R.: World health organization declares global emergency: a review of the 2019 novel coronavirus (covid-19). Int. J, Surg (2020)
43. Chung, M., Bernheim, A., Mei, X., Zhang, N., Huang, M., Zeng, X., Cui, J., Xu, W., Yang, Y., Fayad, Z.A., et al.: Ct imaging features of 2019 novel coronavirus (2019-ncov). Radiology 200230 (2020)
44. Wang, M., Cao, R., Zhang, L., Yang, X., Liu, J., Xu, M., Shi, Z., Hu, Z., Zhong, W., Xiao, G.: Remdesivir and chloroquine effectively inhibit the recently emerged novel coronavirus (2019-ncov) in vitro. Cell Res. **30**(3), 269–271 (2020)
45. Fong, S.J., Li, G., Dey, N., Crespo, R.G., Herrera-Viedma, E.: Finding an accurate early forecasting model from small dataset: a case of 2019-ncov novel coronavirus outbreak (2020). arXiv:2003.10776
46. Martínez-Álvarez, F., Asencio-Cortés, G., Torres, J., Gutiérrez-Avilés, D., Melgar-García, L., Pérez-Chacón, R., Rubio-Escudero, C., Riquelme, J., Troncoso, A.: Coronavirus optimization algorithm: a bioinspired metaheuristic based on the covid-19 propagation model (2020). arXiv:2003.13633

47. Wang, H., Wang, Z., Dong, Y., Chang, R., Xu, C., Yu, X., Zhang, S., Tsamlag, L., Shang, M., Huang, J., et al.: Phase-adjusted estimation of the number of coronavirus disease 2019 cases in wuhan, china. Cell Discov. **6**(1), 1–8 (2020)
48. Mirjalili, S.: Moth-flame optimization algorithm: A novel nature-inspired heuristic paradigm. Knowl. Based Syst. **89**, 228–249 (2015)
49. Mirjalili, S., Lewis, A.: The whale optimization algorithm. Adv. Eng. Softw. **95**, 51–67 (2016)
50. Mirjalili, S., Gandomi, A.H., Mirjalili, S.Z., Saremi, S., Faris, H., Mirjalili, S.M.: Salp swarm algorithm: a bio-inspired optimizer for engineering design problems. Adv. Eng. Softw. **114**, 163–191 (2017)
51. Mirjalili, S., Mirjalili, S.M., Lewis, A.: Grey wolf optimizer. Adv. Eng. Softw. **69**, 46–61 (2014)
52. Holland, J.H.: Genetic algorithms. Sci. Am. **267**(1), 66–73 (1992)
53. Eberhart, R., Kennedy, J.: A new optimizer using particle swarm theory. In: Proceedings of the Sixth International Symposium on Micro Machine and Human Science, 1995. MHS'95, pp. 39–43. IEEE (1995)
54. Heidari, A.A., Mirjalili, S., Faris, H., Aljarah, I., Mafarja, M., Chen, H.: Harris hawks optimization: algorithm and applications. Futur. Gener. Comput. Syst. **97**, 849–872 (2019)
55. Cortes, C., Vapnik, V.: Support-vector networks. Mach. Learn. **20**(3), 273–297 (1995)
56. Ahmad, M., Khan, A., Khan, A., Mazzara, M., Distefano, S., Sohaib, A., Nibouche, O.: Spatial prior fuzziness pool-based interactive classification of hyperspectral images. Remote Sens. **11**(5) (2019)
57. Ahmad, M., Khan, A.M., Hussain, R.: Graph-based spatial spectral feature learning for hyperspectral image classification. IET Image Proc. **11**(12), 1310–1316 (2017)
58. Ahmad, M., Protasov, S., Khan, A.M., Hussain, R., Khattak, A.M., Khan, W.A.: Fuzziness-based active learning framework to enhance hyperspectral image classification performance for discriminative and generative classifiers. PLoS ONE **13**(1), e0188996 (2018)
59. Tharwat, A., Hassanien, A.E., Elnaghi, B.E.: A ba-based algorithm for parameter optimization of support vector machine. Pattern Recogn. Lett. **93**, 13–22 (2017)
60. Hoffmann, M., Kleine-Weber, H., Schroeder, S., Krüger, N., Herrler, T., Erichsen, S., Schiergens, T.S., Herrler, G., Wu, N.-H., Nitsche, A., et al.: Sars-cov-2 cell entry depends on ace2 and tmprss2 and is blocked by a clinically proven protease inhibitor. Cell (2020)
61. Rodrigues Prestes, T.R., Rocha, N.P., Miranda, A.S., Teixeira, A.L., Simoes-e Silva, A.C.: The anti-inflammatory potential of ace2/angiotensin-(1–7)/mas receptor axis: evidence from basic and clinical research. Current Drug Targets **18**(11), 1301–1313 (2017)
62. Li, X., Baek, G., Ramanand, S.G., Sharp, A., Gao, Y., Yuan, W., Welti, J., Rodrigues, D.N., Dolling, D., Figueiredo, I., et al.: Brd4 promotes dna repair and mediates the formation of tmprss2-erg gene rearrangements in prostate cancer. Cell Rep. **22**(3), 796–808 (2018)

Printed by Printforce, the Netherlands